NONDESTRUCTIVE TESTING HANDBOOK

Third Edition

Volume 7

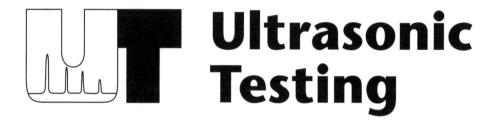 **Ultrasonic Testing**

Technical Editors
Gary L. Workman
Doron Kishoni

Editor
Patrick O. Moore

 American Society for Nondestructive Testing

Errata
You can check for errata for this and other ASNT publications at asnt.org

ISBN: 978-1-57117-105-4 (print)
ISBN: 978-1-57117-283-9 (ebook)

first printing 5/07
second printing 11/10, with new impositions for pages vii, 39, 100, 102, 103, 105, 106
third printing 8/13
fourth printing 6/19
ebook 7/13 (ebooks contain all corrections and updates, including the latest errata)

Printed in the United States of America

Published by:
The American Society for Nondestructive Testing Inc.
1711 Arlingate Lane
Columbus, OH 43228-0518
asnt.org

ASNT Mission Statement:
ASNT exists to create a safer world by advancing scientific, engineering, and technical knowledge in the field of nondestructive testing.

ASNT Code of Ethics:
The ASNT *Code of Ethics* was developed to provide members of the Society with broad ethical statements to guide their professional lives. In spirit and in word, each ASNT member is responsible for knowing and adhering to the values and standards set forth in the Society's Code. More information, as well as the complete version of the *Code of Ethics*, can be found on ASNT's website, asnt.org.

President's Foreword

The mission of the American Society for Nondestructive Testing (ASNT) is to create a safer world through the promotion of the nondestructive testing (NDT) profession and the application of its technologies. Our society has a strong volunteer tradition and a talented staff. Together, they provide opportunities for NDT professionals to improve their skills and apply their talents through the exchange of information and experiences relating to NDT. Because of the nature of our work, our customers expect NDT professionals to perform at the highest possible level with little room for error. ASNT aids their initial and continued professional development through published materials and numerous activities — international, national and local. The *NDT Handbook* series continues to be one of the finest examples of what society volunteers and staff can accomplish when focused on a goal and working together to accomplish it.

ASNT's future depends on the creation, improvement and sharing of information so that safety and reliability stay at the forefront of product development and inservice evaluation of existing components. This volume of the *NDT Handbook* represents the efforts of many dedicated professionals who have embraced change and given freely of their time with the mission of making a difference in their profession. There were scores of individual contributors and reviewers, both volunteers and staff, in an essential ongoing partnership.

A special thanks is due to Handbook Coordinator Harb Hayre and to Technical Editors Gary Workman and Doron Kishoni for their commitment to this project. Their editing required an in-depth understanding of the technology. The job is long and tedious and must be driven first from the heart and then from the mind.

I also thank *NDT Handbook* Editor Patrick Moore and other ASNT staff for their guidance and continued pursuit of excellence. They have made sacrifices necessary to ensure quality and value to our members.

To our volunteers: you are our greatest asset. You do not appear on the financial balance sheet, but you make this society great. I would like to challenge each NDT professional to get involved in making our professional organization better, especially if you feel that important information is missing from any society publication. Each of you has unique knowledge and experiences. The volunteers who worked on this *NDT Handbook* were willing to share their expertise. When you study this volume, you will learn from their knowledge and experiences.

Please consider an active role in succeeding volumes of the *NDT Handbook*. Your participation will allow future readers to gain from your wisdom and experiences.

Again thanks to all who contributed.

Marvin W. Trimm
ASNT President, 2006-2007

Foreword

Aims of a Handbook

The volume you are holding in your hand is the seventh in the third edition of the *Nondestructive Testing Handbook*. In the beginning of each volume, it has been useful to state the purposes and nature of the *NDT Handbook* series.

Handbooks exist in many disciplines of science and technology, and certain features set them apart from other reference works. A handbook should ideally give the basic knowledge necessary for an understanding of the technology, including both scientific principles and means of application.

The typical reader may be assumed to have completed three years of college toward a degree in mechanical engineering or materials science and hence has the background of an elementary physics or mechanics course. Additionally, this volume provides a positive reinforcement for the use of computer based media that enhances its educational value and enlightens all levels of education and training.

Standards, specifications, recommended practices and inspection procedures may be discussed in a handbook for instructional purposes, but at a level of generalization that is illustrative rather than comprehensive. Standards writing bodies take great pains to ensure that their documents are definitive in wording and technical accuracy. People writing contracts or procedures should consult the actual standards when appropriate.

Those who design qualifying examinations or study for them draw on handbooks as a quick and convenient way of approximating the body of knowledge. Committees and individuals who write or anticipate questions are selective in what they draw from any source. The parts of a handbook that give scientific background, for instance, may have little bearing on a practical examination except to provide the physical foundation to assist handling of more challenging tasks. Other parts of a handbook are specific to a certain industry. This handbook provides a collection of perspectives on its subject to broaden its value and convenience to the nondestructive testing community.

The present volume is a worthy addition to the third edition. The editors, technical editors, ASNT staff, many contributors and reviewers worked together to bring the project to completion. For their scholarship and dedication, I thank them all.

Gary L. Workman
Handbook Development Director

Preface

The *Nondestrucive Testing Handbook: Ultrasonic Testing* continues to include a broad range of techniques and applications as shown in this handbook. This third edition volume builds upon the very extensive and in-depth information contained in the second edition and brings additional robust and up-to-date information on this rapidly changing field. Ultrasonic techniques are used for discontinuity detection, material property characterization and physical measurements such as thickness gaging. Many ultrasonic concepts that were primarily research topics for the second edition have now matured into well defined applications in the third edition. This volume offers more extensive contributions of techniques such as phased arrays, guided waves, laser ultrasonics and newer signal processing techniques; as well as a broader range of applications in the aerospace industry. We continue to profit from international contributions, promoting a larger knowledge base for nondestructive testing worldwide.

The third edition of *Ultrasonic Testing* includes many changes in the way ultrasonic inspections are performed because of advances in computer technology. New equipment and techniques enable improved data collection and analysis, both in the laboratory and in the field. These advances in technology also provide improved imaging capability and better understanding of ultrasonic measurements with theory.

This volume represents the work of many in the field who were able to contribute their time and effort to provide latest state-of-the-art information. In addition, many volunteers were able to review and return comments in short order. We are indebted to both groups for bringing this volume to publication in less than two years. We are also indebted to the Ultrasonic Testing Committee in ASNT's Technical and Education Council and to Harb Hayre, who provided support as the handbook coordinator. We also wish to express our gratitude to Patrick Moore and his staff for their thoroughness and diligence in preparing the volume for publication in a timely manner.

Gary L. Workman
Doron Kishoni
Technical Editors

Editor's Preface

It was a different world when ASNT was founded in 1941. The United States was not yet an ally in World War II. Acoustic tests using inaudibly high frequencies were called *supersonic* in the 1940s because that term had not yet been co-opted by aircraft traveling faster than sound. The first edition of the *Nondestructive Testing Handbook* was published in 1959. Ten years earlier, its editor, Robert McMaster, had published an extensive survey of nondestructive testing patents. At that time, in 1949, ultrasonic tests were called *mechanical vibration tests* and were lumped together with various modulus measurements and sonic techniques. In the 1950s, ultrasonic testing became well established as a method for discontinuity detection.

ASNT published the ultrasonic volume of the second edition in 1991, in time for ASNT's 50th anniversary. The text files for that volume were keyed entirely by ASNT staff working on a Wang™ word processor. Images in illustrations were all shot, imposed and archived as hard copy images and did not exist digitally, not anywhere. The text files for that book were archived and survived as ASCII files until 2003, when they were converted to word processing files formatted for use in desktop publishing.

The second edition *Ultrasonic Testing* remains the single largest book that ASNT has ever published. The technical editors for that volume were Robert Green and Albert Birks; the staff editor was Paul McIntire. The good effects of their work on the second edition have survived into the third. Half of the 1991 volume has been updated and survives as more than half of this 2007 edition.

Planning by ASNT's Ultrasonic Committee for the third edition became earnest at a meeting in Austin in Spring 2004. The book became more streamlined in concept as the committee agreed to eliminate redundancies in its coverage from one chapter to the next and to focus on providing information useful to Level II and Level III inspectors. The outline omitted reference tables available elsewhere and theoretical analyses of interest to a few. The committee affirmed the vision of the series as instructional. The result is the concise treatment of the subject in the book you are holding.

A fourth of ASNT's membership and half of its certification holders are overseas. Gradually and irrevocably, the United States is changing to international units of measurement. This volume's technical review is especially indebted to close attention by volunteers from the United States Metric Association. The accuracy and omnipresence of international units in the third edition of the *NDT Handbook* help to ensure that the series will be of value both to the world that ASNT serves and to posterity.

Likewise, alloys throughout are identified according to the Unified Numbering System.

I would personally like to thank members of ASNT staff who helped to make this book better. Hollis Humphries and Joy Grimm produced many excellent graphics. Grimm also laid out the chapters, and Humphries proofed the book and produced its CD-ROM version.

People listed as contributors in the acknowledgments below were also reviewers but are listed once, as contributors.

Patrick O. Moore
NDT Handbook Editor

Acknowledgments

For the chapter on electric power applications, the contributor and editors would like to thank Jay L. Fisher and Southwest Research Institute; Grady Lapleder and IHI Southwest Technologies; and Michael Moles and Olympus NDT.

For information on piezoelectric materials, the first part of Chapter 3 is indebted to the Vernitron Division of Morgan Matroc.

The first three parts of Chapter 14 are indebted to volunteers of Boeing Aerospace. Some information on airframes is from second edition contributions from Douglas Aircraft Company, now part of Boeing Aerospace.

Handbook Development Committee

Gary L. Workman, University of Alabama, Huntsville
Michael W. Allgaier, Mistras
David R. Bajula, Acuren Inspection
Albert S. Birks, Naval Surface Warfare Center
Richard H. Bossi, Boeing Aerospace
Lisa Brasche, Iowa State University
James E. Cox, Zetec, Incorporated
David L. Culbertson, El Paso Corporation
James L. Doyle, Jr., NorthWest Research Associates
Nat Y. Faransso, KBR
Robert E. Green, Jr., Johns Hopkins University
Gerard K. Hacker, Teledyne Brown Engineering
Harb S. Hayre, Ceie Specs
Eric v.K. Hill
Frank A. Iddings
Charles N. Jackson, Jr.
Morteza K. Jafari, Fugro South
Timothy E. Jones, American Society for Nondestructive Testing
John K. Keve, DynCorp Tri-Cities Services
Doron Kishoni, Business Solutions USA
Xavier P.V. Maldague, University Laval
George A. Matzkanin, Texas Research Institute
Ronnie K. Miller
Scott D. Miller, Saudi Aramco
Mani Mina, Technology Resource Group
David G. Moore, Sandia National Laboratories
Patrick O. Moore, American Society for Nondestructive Testing
Stanislav I. Rokhlin, Ohio State University
Frank J. Sattler

Fred Seppi, Williams International
Kermit A. Skeie
Roderic K. Stanley, NDE Information Consultants
Stuart A. Tison, Millipore Corporation
Noel A. Tracy, Universal Technology Corporation
Satish S. Udpa, Michigan State University
Mark F.A. Warchol, Alcoa
Glenn A. Washer, University of Missouri — Columbia
George C. Wheeler

Contributors

Laszlo Adler
George A. Alers
Theodore L. Allen
David R. Bajula, Acuren Inspection
Yoseph Bar-Cohen, Jet Propulsion Laboratory
Anmol S. Birring, NDE Associates
Richard H. Bossi, Boeing Aerospace
Byron B. Brenden
Frederick Anthony Bruton, Southwest Research Institute
Francis H. Chang
Dale E. Chimenti, Iowa State University
Brozia H. Clark, Jr.
Laura M. Harmon Cosgriff, Cleveland State University and NASA Glenn Research Center
John C. Duke, Jr., Virginia Polytechnic Institute
David S. Forsyth, Advanced Materials, Manufacturing, and Testing Information and Analysis Center
Hormoz Ghaziary, Advanced NDE Associates
Lawrence O. Goldberg, Seatest Services
Matthew J. Golis, Advanced Quality Concepts
Karl F. Graff, Edison Welding Institute
Robert E. Green, Jr., Johns Hopkins University
Andrew L. Gyekenyesi, Ohio Aerospace Institute and NASA Glenn Research Center
Donald J. Hagemaier
Stephen D. Hart
Howard Hartzog, The Timken Company
Edmund G. Henneke, II, Virginia Polytechnic Institute and State University
Amos E. Holt, Southwest Research Institute
Gregory A. Hudkins, ExxonMobil
Alain Jungman, Université Paris
Lawrence W. Kessler, Sonoscan

Butrus Pierre T. Khuri-Yakub, Stanford University
Doron Kishoni, Business Solutions USA
Francesco Lanza di Scalea, University of California, San Diego
Eric I. Madaras, NASA Langley Research Center
D.K. Mak
Ajit K. Mal, University of California at Los Angeles
Richard E. Martin, Cleveland State University and NASA Glenn Research Center
John Mittleman, United States Navy, Naples, Italy
Michael Moles, Olympus NDT Canada
Jean-Pierre Monchalin, Industrial Materials Research Institute, National Research Council Canada
Peter B. Nagy, University of Cincinnati
John S. Popovics, University of Illinois
William H. Prosser, National Aeronautics and Space Administration
Joseph L. Rose, Pennsylvania State University
Donald J. Roth, National Aeronautics and Space Administration
G.P. Singh, Karta Technology
Roderic K. Stanley, NDE Information Consultants
Marvin W. Trimm, Savannah River National Laboratory
Alex Vary
Roger D. Wallace
Gary L. Workman, University of Alabama, Huntsville

Reviewers

Ronald Alers, Sonic Sensors of EMAT Ultrasonics
Gary E. Alvey, Naval Aviation Depot, Cherry Point
Sony Baby, Regional Engineering College, India
Mohamad Behravesh, Electric Power Research Institute
Bruce Berger, Signet Testing Laboratories
Albert S. Birks
Kaydell C. Bowles, Sandvik Special Metals
Lisa Brasche, Iowa State University
Donald E. Bray
John A. Brunk
Robert H. Bushnell
James R. Cahill, GE Inspection Technologies
Thomas N. Claytor, Los Alamos National Laboratory
David R. Culbertson, El Paso Corporation
B. Boro Djordjevic, Materials and Sensors Technologies
James B. Elder, Savannah River National Laboratory
Dale Ensminger
Ying Fan, General Electric Research
Nat Y. Faransso, KBR
James R. Frysinger, College of Charleston
David P. Harvey, Wah Chang

Donald E. Harvey, Tennessee Valley Authority
Harb S. Hayre, CEIE Specs
Gary E. Heath, All Tech Inspection
Dietmar Henning, Sector-Cert
James W. Houf, American Society for Nondestructive Testing
G. Huebschen, Fraunhofer Institut für Zerstörungsfreie Prüfverfahren
Nelson N. Hsu, National Institute of Standards and Technology
D.R. Johnson, Oak Ridge National Laboratory
Don M. Jordan, University of South Carolina
Sang Kim, Southwest Research Institute
David S. Kupperman, Argonne National Laboratory
Lloyd P. Lemle, Jr.
George A. Matzkanin, Texas Research Institute
Bruce W. Maxfield, Industrial Sensors
Eugene A. Mechtly
Scott D. Miller, Saudi Arabian Oil Company, Dhahran
Ricky L. Morgan, Smith Emery Company
Robert Murner, Jentek Sensors
Emmanuel P. Papadakis
Ramesh J. Rao Pardikar, Bharat Heavy Electricals, India
Jean Perdijon, France
Robert F. Plumstead, Municipal Testing Laboratory
William C. Plumstead, Sr., PQT Services
Randy Plis
Jason Riggs, All Trans Tek
Scott D. Ritzheimer, Integritesting
Piervincenzo Rizzo, University of Pittsburgh
Stanislav I. Rokhlin, Ohio State University
H.J. Salzburger, Fraunhofer Institut für Zerstörungsfreie Prüfverfahren
Frank J. Sattler
Robert L. Saunders, Ellwood City Forge
Simon D. Senibi, Boeing Aerospace
William A. Simpson, Oak Ridge National Laboratory
R. Lowell Smith
R.W. Smith, Xactex Corporation
Graham H. Thomas, Lawrence Livermore National Labs
R. Bruce Thompson, Iowa State University
Nancy J. Verdick, Alcoa
James W. Wagner, Emory University
Mark F.A. Warchol, Alcoa
Glenn A. Washer, University of Missouri, Columbia
Brad S. Whiteleather, Pechiney Rolled Products
Andrew James Woodrow, Jr., US Steel
Gary J. Zimak, Northrop Grumman

CONTENTS

Introduction to Ultrasonic Testing

Marvin W. Trimm, Savannah River National Laboratory, Aiken, South Carolina (Parts 1 and 2)

Karl F. Graff, Edison Welding Institute, Columbus, Ohio (Part 3)

Part 1. Nondestructive Testing

Definition

Nondestructive testing (NDT) has been defined as comprising those methods used to test a part or material or system without impairing its future usefulness.[1] The term is generally applied to nonmedical investigations of material integrity.

Nondestructive testing is used to investigate specifically the material integrity or properties of the test object. A number of other technologies — for instance, radio astronomy, voltage and amperage measurement and rheometry (flow measurement) — are nondestructive but are not used specifically to evaluate material properties. Radar and sonar are classified as nondestructive testing when used to inspect dams, for instance, but not when they are used to chart a river bottom.

Nondestructive testing asks "Is there something wrong with this material?" In contrast, performance and proof tests ask "Does this component work?" It is not considered nondestructive testing when an inspector checks a circuit by running electric current through it. Hydrostatic pressure testing is a form of proof testing that sometimes destroys the test object.

A gray area in the definition of *nondestructive testing* is the phrase *future usefulness*. Some material investigations involve taking a sample of the test object for a test that is inherently destructive. A noncritical part of a pressure vessel may be scraped or shaved to get a sample for electron microscopy, for example. Although future usefulness of the vessel is not impaired by the loss of material, the procedure is inherently destructive and the shaving itself — in one sense the true test object — has been removed from service permanently.

The idea of future usefulness is relevant to the quality control practice of sampling. Sampling (that is, less than 100 percent testing to draw inferences about the unsampled lots) *is* nondestructive testing if the tested sample is returned to service. If steel bolts are tested to verify their alloy and are then returned to service, then the test is nondestructive. In contrast, even if spectroscopy used in the chemical testing of many fluids is inherently nondestructive, the testing is destructive if the samples are poured down the drain after testing.

Nondestructive testing is not confined to crack detection. Other anomalies include porosity, wall thinning from corrosion and many sorts of disbonds. Nondestructive material characterization is a field concerned with properties including material identification and microstructural characteristics — such as resin curing, case hardening and stress — that have a direct influence on the service life of the test object.

Methods and Techniques

Nondestructive testing has also been defined by listing or classifying the various techniques.[1-3] This approach to *nondestructive testing* is practical in that it typically highlights methods in use by industry.

In the *Nondestructive Testing Handbook*, the word *method* is used for a group of test techniques that share a form of probing energy. The ultrasonic test method, for example, uses acoustic waves at a higher frequency than audible sound. Infrared and thermal testing and radiographic testing are two test methods that use electromagnetic radiation, each in a defined wavelength range. The word *technique*, in contrast, denotes a way of adapting the method to the application. Through-transmission immersion testing is a technique of the ultrasonic method, for example.

Purposes of Nondestructive Testing

Since the 1920s, the art of testing without destroying the test object has developed from a laboratory curiosity to an indispensable tool of fabrication, construction, manufacturing and maintenance processes. No longer is visual testing of materials, parts and complete products the principal means of determining adequate quality. Nondestructive tests in great variety are in worldwide use to detect variations in structure, minute changes in surface finish, the presence of cracks or other physical discontinuities, to measure the thickness of materials and coatings and to determine other characteristics of industrial products.

How is nondestructive testing useful? Why do thousands of industrial concerns buy the test equipment, pay the subsequent operating costs of the testing and even reshape manufacturing processes to fit the needs and findings of nondestructive testing? Modern nondestructive tests are used by manufacturers (1) to ensure product integrity and in turn reliability, (2) to avoid failures, prevent accidents and save human life (see Figs. 1 and 2), (3) to make a profit for the user, (4) to ensure customer satisfaction and maintain the manufacturer's reputation, (5) to aid in better product design, (6) to control manufacturing processes, (7) to lower manufacturing costs, (8) to maintain uniform quality levels and (9) to ensure operational readiness.

These reasons for widespread and profitable nondestructive testing are sufficient in themselves but parallel developments have contributed to the technology's growth and acceptance.

Increased Demand on Machines

In the interest of greater performance and reduced cost for materials, the design engineer is often under pressure to reduce weight. Weight can sometimes be reduced by substituting aluminum alloys, magnesium alloys or composite materials for steel or iron but such light parts may not be the same size or design as those they replace. The tendency is also to reduce the size. These pressures on the designer have subjected parts of all sorts to increased stress levels. Even such commonplace objects as sewing machines, sauce pans and luggage are also lighter and more heavily loaded than ever before. The stress to be supported is

seldom static. It often fluctuates and reverses at low or high frequencies. Frequency of stress reversals increases with the speeds of modern machines, so components tend to fatigue and fail more rapidly.

Another cause of increased stress on modern products is a reduction in the safety factor. An engineer designs with certain known loads in mind. On the supposition that materials and workmanship are never perfect, a safety factor of 2, 3, 5 or 10 is applied. However, a lower factor is often used that depends on considerations such as cost or weight.

New demands on machinery have also stimulated the development and use of new materials whose operating characteristics and performance are not completely known. These new materials could create greater and potentially dangerous problems. For example, an aircraft part was built from an alloy whose work hardening, notch resistance and fatigue life were not well known. After relatively short periods of service, some of the aircraft using these parts suffered disastrous failures. Sufficient and proper nondestructive tests could have saved many lives.

As technology improves and as service requirements increase, machines are subjected to greater variations and to wider extremes of all kinds of stress, creating an increasing demand for stronger or more damage tolerant materials.

Engineering Demands for Sounder Materials

Another justification for nondestructive tests is the designer's demand for sounder

FIGURE 1. Fatigue cracks contributed to damage to aircraft fuselage in flight (April 1988).

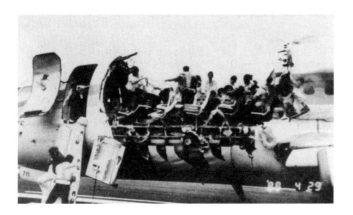

FIGURE 2. Boilers operate with high internal steam pressure. Material discontinuities can lead to sudden, violent failure with possible injury to people and property.

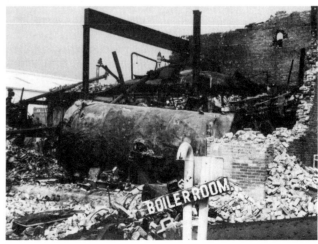

materials. As size and weight decrease and the factor of safety is lowered, more emphasis is placed on better raw material control and higher quality of materials, manufacturing processes and workmanship.

An interesting fact is that a producer of raw material or of a finished product sometimes does not improve quality or performance until that improvement is demanded by the customer. The pressure of the customer is transferred to implementation of improved design or manufacturing. Nondestructive testing is frequently called on to deliver this new quality level.

Public Demands for Greater Safety

The demands and expectations of the public for greater safety are apparent everywhere. Review the record of the courts in granting high awards to injured persons. Consider the outcry for greater automobile safety as evidenced by the required automotive safety belts and the demand for air bags, blowout proof tires and antilock braking systems. The publicly supported activities of the National Safety Council, Underwriters Laboratories, the Occupational Safety and Health Administration, the Federal Aviation Administration and other agencies around the world are only a few of the ways in which this demand for safety is expressed. It has been expressed directly by passengers who cancel reservations following a serious aircraft accident. This demand for personal safety has been another strong force in the development of nondestructive tests.

Rising Costs of Failure

Aside from awards to the injured or to estates of the deceased and aside from costs to the public (because of evacuation occasioned by chemical leaks, for example), there are other factors in the rising costs of mechanical failure.

These costs are increasing for many reasons. Some important ones are (1) greater costs of materials and labor, (2) greater costs of complex parts, (3) greater costs because of the complexity of assemblies, (4) a greater probability that failure of one part will cause failure of others because of overloads, (5) the probability that the failure of one part will damage other parts of high value and (6) part failure in an integrated automatic production machine, shutting down an entire high speed production line. When production was carried out on many separate machines, the broken one could be bypassed until repaired. Today, one machine is often tied into the production of several others. Loss of such production is one of the greatest losses resulting from part failure.

Applications of Nondestructive Testing

Nondestructive testing is a branch of materials science that is concerned with all aspects of the uniformity, quality and serviceability of materials and structures. The science of nondestructive testing incorporates all the technology for process monitoring and detection and measurement of significant properties, including discontinuities, in items ranging from research test objects to finished hardware and products in service. By definition, nondestructive test methods provide a means for examining materials and structures without disruption or impairment of serviceability. Nondestructive testing makes it possible for internal properties or hidden discontinuities to be revealed or inferred.

Nondestructive testing is becoming increasingly vital in the effective conduct of research, development, design and manufacturing programs. Only with appropriate nondestructive testing methods can the benefits of advanced materials science be fully realized.

Classification of Methods

In 1984, the National Materials Advisory Board (NMAB) Ad Hoc Committee on Nondestructive Evaluation adopted a system that classified techniques into six major method categories: visual, penetrating radiation, magnetic-electrical, mechanical vibration, thermal and chemical/electrochemical.[3] A modified version is presented in Table 1.[1]

Each method can be completely characterized in terms of five principal factors: (1) energy source or medium used to probe the object (such as X-rays, ultrasonic waves or thermal radiation); (2) nature of the signals, image or signature resulting from interaction with the object (attenuation of X-rays or reflection of ultrasound, for example); (3) means of detecting or sensing resultant signals (photoemulsion, piezoelectric crystal or inductance coil); (4) means of indicating or recording signals (meter deflection, oscilloscope trace or radiograph); and (5) basis for interpreting the results (direct or indirect indication, qualitative or quantitative and pertinent dependencies).

The objective of each method is to provide information about one or more of the following material parameters: (1) discontinuities and separations (cracks, voids, inclusions, delaminations and others); (2) structure or malstructure (crystalline structure, grain size, segregation, misalignment and others); (3) dimensions and metrology (thickness, diameter, gap size, discontinuity size and others); (4) physical and mechanical properties (reflectivity, conductivity, elastic modulus, sonic velocity and others); (5) composition and chemical analysis (alloy identification, impurities, elemental distributions and others); (6) stress and dynamic response (residual stress, crack growth, wear, vibration and others); (7) signature analysis (image content, frequency spectrum, field configuration and others); and (8) abnormal sources of heat.

Material characteristics in Table 1 are further defined in Table 2 with respect to specific objectives and specific attributes to be measured, detected and defined.

The limitations of a method include conditions to be met for method application (access, physical contact, preparation and others) and requirements to adapt the probe or probe medium to the object examined. Other factors limit the detection or characterization of discontinuities, properties and other attributes and limit interpretation of signals or images generated.

Classification Relative to Test Object

Nondestructive test techniques may be classified according to how they detect indications relative to the surface of a test object. Surface methods include liquid penetrant testing, visual testing, grid testing and moiré testing. Surface/near-surface methods include tap, holographic, shearographic, magnetic particle and electromagnetic testing. When surface or near-surface methods are applied during intermediate manufacturing processes, they provide preliminary assurance that volumetric methods performed on the completed object or component will reveal few rejectable discontinuities. Volumetric methods include radiography, ultrasonic testing, acoustic emission testing and less widely used methods such as acoustoultrasonic testing and magnetic resonance imaging. Through-boundary techniques include leak testing, some infrared thermographic techniques, airborne ultrasonic testing and certain techniques of acoustic emission testing. Other less easily classified methods are material identification, vibration analysis and strain gaging.

No one nondestructive test method is all revealing. In some cases, one method

TABLE 1. Nondestructive test method categories.

Categories	Detection Objectives
Basic Categories	
Mechanical and optical	color, cracks, dimensions, film thickness, gaging, reflectivity, strain distribution and magnitude, surface finish, surface flaws, through-cracks
Penetrating radiation	cracks; density and chemistry variations; elemental distribution; foreign objects; inclusions; microporosity; misalignment; missing parts; segregation; service degradation; shrinkage; thickness; voids
Electromagnetic and electronic	alloy content; anisotropy; cavities; cold work; local strain, hardness; composition; contamination; corrosion; cracks; crack depth; crystal structure; electrical conductivities; flakes; heat treatment; hot tears; inclusions; ion concentrations; laps; lattice strain; layer thickness; moisture content; polarization; seams; segregation; shrinkage; state of cure; tensile strength; thickness; disbonds; voids
Sonic and ultrasonic	crack initiation and propagation; cracks, voids; damping factor; degree of cure; degree of impregnation; degree of sintering; delaminations; density; dimensions; elastic moduli; grain size; inclusions; mechanical degradation; misalignment; porosity; radiation degradation; structure of composites; surface stress; tensile, shear and compressive strength; disbonds; wear
Infrared and thermal	anisotropy, bonding; composition; emissivity; heat contours; plating thickness; porosity; reflectivity; stress; thermal conductivity; thickness; voids; cracks; delaminations; heat treatment; state of cure; moisture; corrosion
Chemical and analytical	alloy identification; composition; cracks; elemental analysis and distribution; grain size; inclusions; macrostructure; porosity; segregation; surface anomalies
Auxiliary Categories	
Image generation	dimensional variations; dynamic performance; anomaly characterization and definition; anomaly distribution; anomaly propagation; magnetic field configurations
Signal image analysis	data selection, processing and display; anomaly mapping, correlation and identification; image enhancement; separation of multiple variables; signature analysis

or technique may be adequate for testing a specific object or component. However, in most cases, it takes a series of test methods to do a complete nondestructive test of an object or component. For example, if surface cracks must be detected and eliminated and if the object or component is made of ferromagnetic material, then magnetic particle testing would be the appropriate choice. If the material is aluminum or titanium, then the choice would be liquid penetrant or electromagnetic testing. However, if internal discontinuities are to be detected, then ultrasonic testing or radiography would be chosen. The exact technique in each case would depend on the thickness

TABLE 2. Objectives of nondestructive test methods.

Objectives	Attributes Measured or Detected
Discontinuities and Separations	
Surface anomalies	roughness, scratches, gouges, crazing, pitting, imbedded foreign material
Surface connected anomalies	cracks, porosity, pinholes, laps, seams, folds, inclusions
Internal anomalies	cracks, separations, hot tears, cold shuts, shrinkage, voids, lack of fusion, pores, cavities, delaminations, disbonds, poor bonds, inclusions, segregations
Structure	
Microstructure	molecular structure; crystalline structure and/or strain; lattice structure; strain; dislocation; vacancy; deformation
Matrix structure	grain structure, size, orientation and phase; sinter and porosity; impregnation; filler and/or reinforcement distribution; anisotropy; heterogeneity; segregation
Small structural anomalies	leaks (lack of seal or through-holes), poor fit, poor contact, loose parts, loose particles, foreign objects
Gross structural anomalies	assembly errors; misalignment; poor spacing or ordering; deformation; malformation; missing parts
Dimensions and Metrology	
Displacement; position	linear measurement; separation; gap size; discontinuity size, depth, location and orientation
Dimensional variations	unevenness; nonuniformity; eccentricity; shape and contour; size and mass variations
Thickness; density	film, coating, layer, plating, wall and sheet thickness; density or thickness variations
Physical and Mechanical Properties	
Electrical properties	resistivity; conductivity; dielectric constant and dissipation factor
Magnetic properties	polarization; permeability; ferromagnetism; cohesive force, susceptibility
Thermal properties	conductivity; thermal time constant and thermoelectric potential; diffusivity; effusivity; specific heat
Mechanical properties	compressive, shear and tensile strength (and moduli); Poisson's ratio; sonic speed; hardness; temper and embrittlement
Surface properties	color, reflectivity, refraction index, emissivity
Chemical Composition and Analysis	
Elemental analysis	detection, identification, distribution and/or profile
Impurity concentrations	contamination, depletion, doping and diffusants
Metallurgical content	variation; alloy identification, verification and sorting
Physiochemical state	moisture content; degree of cure; ion concentrations and corrosion; reaction products
Stress and Dynamic Response	
Stress, strain, fatigue	heat treatment, annealing and cold work effects; stress and strain; fatigue damage and residual life
Mechanical damage	wear, spalling, erosion, friction effects
Chemical damage	corrosion, stress corrosion, phase transformation
Other damage	radiation damage and high frequency voltage breakdown
Dynamic performance	crack initiation, crack propagation, plastic deformation, creep, excessive motion, vibration, damping, timing of events, any anomalous behavior
Signature Analysis	
Electromagnetic field	potential; intensity; field distribution and pattern
Thermal field	isotherms, heat contours, temperatures, heat flow, temperature distribution, heat leaks, hot spots, contrast
Acoustic signature	noise, vibration characteristics, frequency amplitude, harmonic spectrum, harmonic analysis, sonic emissions, ultrasonic emissions
Radioactive signature	distribution and diffusion of isotopes and tracers
Signal or image analysis	image enhancement and quantization; pattern recognition; densitometry; signal classification, separation and correlation; discontinuity identification, definition (size and shape) and distribution analysis; discontinuity mapping and display

and nature of the material and the types of discontinuities that must be detected.

Value of Nondestructive Testing

The contribution of nondestructive testing to profits has been acknowledged in the medical field and in the computer and aerospace industries. However, in industries such as heavy metals, nondestructive testing may be accepted reluctantly because its contribution to profits may not be obvious to management. Nondestructive testing is sometimes thought of only as a cost item and can be curtailed by industry downsizing. When a company cuts costs, two vulnerable areas are quality and safety. When bidding contract work, companies add profit margin to all cost items, including nondestructive testing, so a profit should be made on the nondestructive testing. The attitude toward nondestructive testing is positive when management understands its value.

Nondestructive testing should be used as a control mechanism to ensure that manufacturing processes are within design performance requirements. When used properly, nondestructive testing saves money for the manufacturer. Rather than costing the manufacturer money, nondestructive testing should add profits to the manufacturing process.

Other Nondestructive Test Methods

To optimize nondestructive testing, it is necessary first to understand the principles and applications of all the methods. This volume features ultrasonic testing (Fig. 3) — one of many nondestructive test methods. The following section briefly describes several other methods and the applications associated with them.

Visual Testing

Principles. Visual testing (Fig. 4) is the observation of a test object, either directly with the eyes or indirectly using optical instruments, by an inspector to evaluate the presence of surface anomalies and the object's conformance to specification. Visual testing should be the first

FIGURE 3. Classic setups for ultrasonic testing: (a) longitudinal wave technique; (b) shear wave technique.

(a)

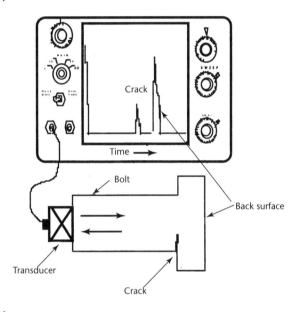

(b)

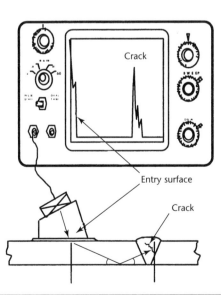

FIGURE 4. Visual test using a borescope to view the interior of a cylinder.

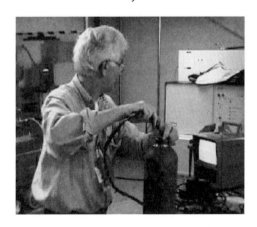

nondestructive test method applied to an item. The test procedure is to clean the surface, provide adequate illumination and observe. A prerequisite necessary for competent visual testing of an object is knowledge of the manufacturing processes by which it was made, of its service history and of its potential failure modes, as well as related industry experience.

Applications. Visual testing provides a means of examining a variety of surfaces. It is the most widely used method for detecting surface discontinuities associated with various structural failure mechanisms. Even when other nondestructive tests are performed, visual tests often provide a useful supplement. When the eddy current testing of process tubing is performed, for example, visual testing is often performed to verify and more closely examine the surface condition. The following discontinuities may be detected by a simple visual test: surface discontinuities, cracks, misalignment, warping, corrosion, wear and physical damage.

Liquid Penetrant Testing

Principles. Liquid penetrant testing (Fig. 5) reveals discontinuities open to the surfaces of solid and nonporous materials. Indications of a wide variety of discontinuity sizes can be found regardless of the configuration of the test object and regardless of discontinuity orientations. Liquid penetrants seep into various types of minute surface openings by capillary action. The cavities of interest can be very small, often invisible to the unaided eye. The ability of a given liquid to flow over a surface and enter surface cavities depends principally on the following: cleanliness of the surface, surface tension of the liquid, configuration of the cavity, contact angle of the liquid, ability of the liquid to wet the surface, cleanliness of the cavity and size of the surface opening of the cavity.

Applications. The principal industrial uses of liquid penetrant testing include postfabrication testing, receiving testing, in-process testing and quality control, testing for maintenance and overhaul in the transportation industries, in-plant and machinery maintenance testing and testing of large components. The following are some of the typically detected discontinuities: surface discontinuities, seams, cracks, laps, porosity and leak paths.

Magnetic Particle Testing

Principles. Magnetic particle testing (Fig. 6) is a method of locating surface and near-surface discontinuities in ferromagnetic materials. It depends on the fact that when the test object is magnetized, discontinuities that lie in a direction generally transverse to the direction of the magnetic field will cause a magnetic flux leakage field to be formed at and above the surface of the test object. This leakage field and therefore the discontinuity are detected with fine ferromagnetic particles applied over the surface, some of the particles being gathered and held to indicate the discontinuity's location, size, shape and orientation. Magnetic particles are applied over a surface as dry particles or as wet particles in a liquid carrier such as water or oil.

Applications. The principal industrial uses of magnetic particle testing include final, receiving and in-process testing; testing for quality control; testing for maintenance and overhaul in the transportation industries; testing for plant and machinery maintenance; and testing of large components. Some of the typically detected discontinuities are surface discontinuities, seams, cracks and laps.

FIGURE 6. In magnetic particle testing, particles gather where lines of magnetic flux leak from a discontinuity.

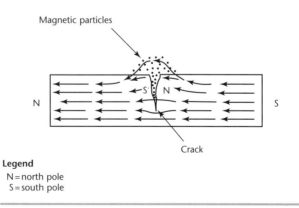

Legend
N = north pole
S = south pole

FIGURE 5. Liquid penetrant indication of cracking.

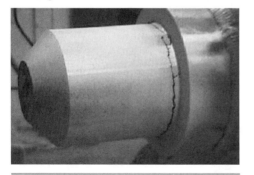

Eddy Current Testing

Principles. Based on electromagnetic induction, eddy current testing (Fig. 7) is perhaps the best known of the techniques in the electromagnetic test method. Eddy current testing is used to identify or differentiate among a wide variety of physical, structural and metallurgical conditions in electrically conductive ferromagnetic and nonferromagnetic metals and metal test objects. The method is based on indirect measurement and on correlation between the instrument reading and the structural characteristics and serviceability of the test objects.

FIGURE 7. Electromagnetic testing: (a) representative setup for eddy current test; (b) in-service detection of discontinuities.

(a)

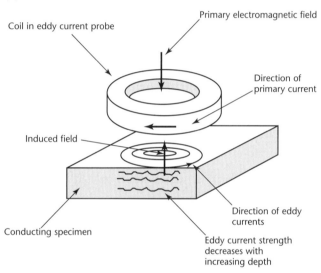

(b)

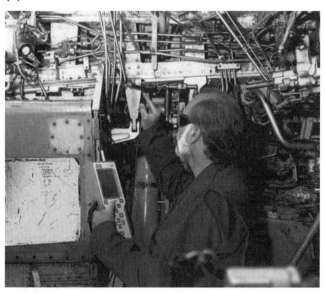

With a basic system, the test object is placed within or next to an electric coil in which high frequency alternating current is flowing. This excitation current establishes an electromagnetic field around the coil. This primary field causes eddy current to flow in the test object because of electromagnetic induction. Inversely, the eddy currents affected by all characteristics (conductivity, permeability, thickness, discontinuities and geometry) of the test object create a secondary magnetic field that opposes the primary field. This interaction affects the coil voltage and can be displayed in various ways.

Eddy currents flow in closed loops in the test object. Their two most important characteristics, amplitude and phase, are influenced by the arrangement and characteristics of the instrumentation and test object. For example, during the test of a tube, the eddy currents flow symmetrically in the tube when discontinuities are not present. However, when a crack is present, then the eddy current flow is impeded and changed in direction, causing significant changes in the associated electromagnetic field.

Applications. An important industrial use of eddy current testing is on tubing. For example, eddy current testing is often specified for quality control in tube mills, thin wall tubing in pressurized water reactors, steam generators, turbine condensers and air conditioning heat exchangers. Eddy current testing is also used in aircraft maintenance. The following are some of the typical material characteristics that can be evaluated by eddy current testing: cracks, inclusions, dents and holes; grain size and hardness; coating and material thickness; dimensions and geometry; composition, conductivity or permeability; and alloy composition.

Radiographic Testing

Principles. Radiographic testing (Fig. 8) is based on the test object's differential absorption of penetrating radiation — either electromagnetic radiation of very short wavelength or particulate radiation (X-rays, gamma rays and neutrons). Different portions of an object absorb different amounts of penetrating radiation because of variations in density, thickness or absorption characteristics caused by composition variations. These variations in the absorption of the penetrating radiation can be monitored by detecting the unabsorbed radiation that passes through the object.

This monitoring may be in different forms. The traditional form is through radiation sensitive film. Radioscopic sensors provide digital images. X-ray computed tomography is another radiographic technique.

Applications. The principal industrial uses of radiographic testing involve testing of castings and weldments, particularly where there is a critical need to ensure freedom from internal discontinuities. Radiographic testing is often specified for thick wall castings and for weldments in steam power equipment (boiler and turbine components and assemblies). The method can also be used on forgings and mechanical assemblies, although with mechanical assemblies radiographic testing is usually limited to testing for conditions and proper placement of components. Radiographic testing is used to detect inclusions, lack of fusion, cracks, corrosion, porosity, leak paths, missing or incomplete components and debris.

Acoustic Emission Testing

Principles. Acoustic emissions are stress waves produced by sudden movement in stressed materials. The classic source of acoustic emission is discontinuity related deformation processes such as crack growth and plastic deformation. Sudden movement at the source produces a stress wave that radiates into the structure and excites a sensitive piezoelectric transducer. As the stress in the material is raised, emissions are generated. The signals from one or more transducers are amplified and measured to produce data for display and interpretation.

The source of acoustic emission energy is the elastic stress field in the material. Without stress, there is no emission. Therefore, an acoustic emission test is

usually carried out during a controlled loading of the structure. This can be a proof load before service; a controlled variation of load while the structure is in service; a fatigue, pressure or creep test; or a complex loading program. Often, a structure is going to be loaded hydrostatically anyway during service and acoustic emission testing is used because it gives valuable additional information about the expected performance of the structure under load. Other times, acoustic emission testing is selected for reasons of economy or safety and a special loading procedure is arranged to meet the needs of the acoustic emission test.

Applications. Acoustic emission is a natural phenomenon occurring in the widest range of materials, structures and processes. The largest scale events observed with acoustic emission testing are seismic and the smallest are small dislocations in stressed metals.

The equipment used is highly sensitive to any kind of movement in its operating frequency (typically 20 to 1200 kHz). The equipment can detect not only crack growth and material deformation but also such processes as solidification, friction, impact, flow and phase transformations. Therefore, acoustic emission testing is also used for in-process weld monitoring, for detecting tool touch and tool wear during automatic machining, for detecting wear and loss of lubrication in rotating equipment, for detecting loose parts and loose particles, for structural monitoring in service (Fig. 9), for preservice proof testing and for detecting and monitoring leaks, cavitation and flow.

Leak Testing

Principles. Leak testing is concerned with the flow of liquids or gases from

FIGURE 8. Representative setup for radiographic testing.

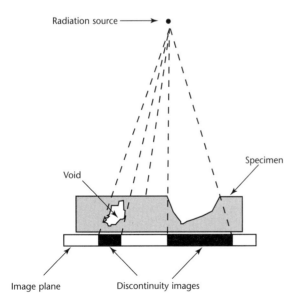

FIGURE 9. Acoustic emission monitoring of floor beam on a suspension bridge.

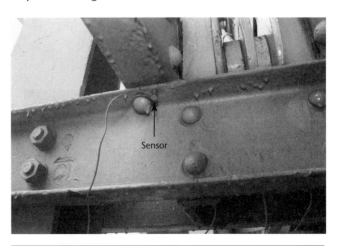

pressurized components or into evacuated components. The principles of leak testing involve the physics of fluid (liquids or gases) flowing through a barrier where a pressure differential or capillary action exists.

Leak testing encompasses procedures that fall into these basic functions: leak location, leakage measurement and leakage monitoring. There are several subsidiary methods of leak testing, entailing tracer gas detection (Fig. 10), pressure change measurement, observation of bubble formation, acoustic emission leak testing and other principles.

Applications. Like other forms of nondestructive testing, leak testing has an impact on the safety and performance of a product. Reliable leak testing decreases costs by reducing the number of reworked products, warranty repairs and liability claims. The most common reasons for performing a leak test are to prevent the loss of costly materials or energy; to prevent contamination of the environment; to ensure component or system reliability; and to prevent an explosion or fire.

Infrared and Thermal Testing

Principles. Conduction, convection and radiation are the primary mechanisms of heat transfer in an object or system. Electromagnetic radiation is emitted from all bodies to a degree that depends on their energy state.

Thermal testing involves the measurement or mapping of surface temperatures when heat flows from, to or through a test object. Temperature differentials on a surface, or changes in surface temperature with time, are related to heat flow patterns and can be used to detect discontinuities or to determine the heat transfer characteristics of an object. For example, during the operation of an electrical breaker, a hot spot detected at an electrical termination may be caused by a loose or corroded connection (Fig. 11). The resistance to electrical flow through the connection produces an increase in surface temperature of the connection.

Applications. There are two basic categories of infrared and thermal test applications: electrical and mechanical. The specific applications within these two categories are numerous.

Electrical applications include transmission and distribution lines, transformers, disconnects, switches, fuses, relays, breakers, motor windings, capacitor banks, cable trays, bus taps and other components and subsystems.

Mechanical applications include insulation (in boilers, furnaces, kilns, piping, ducts, vessels, refrigerated trucks and systems, tank cars and elsewhere), friction in rotating equipment (bearings,

FIGURE 10. Leakage measurement dynamic leak testing using vacuum pumping: (a) pressurized system mode for leak testing of smaller components; (b) pressurized envelope mode for leak testing of larger volume systems.

(a)

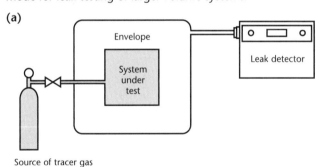

Source of tracer gas

(b)

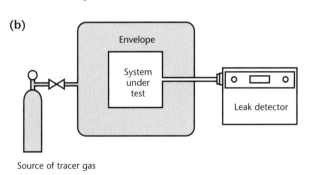

Source of tracer gas

FIGURE 11. Infrared thermography of automatic transfer switches for an emergency diesel generator. Hot spots appear bright in thermogram (inset).

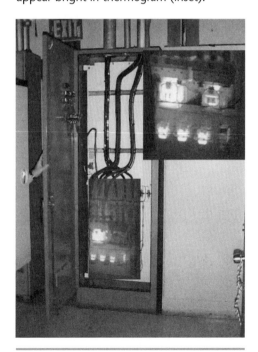

couplings, gears, gearboxes, conveyor belts, pumps, compressors and other components) and fluid flow (steam lines; heat exchangers; tank fluid levels; exothermic reactions; heating, ventilation and air conditioning systems; leaks above and below ground; cooling and heating; tube blockages; environmental assessment of thermal discharge; boiler or furnace air leakage; condenser or turbine system leakage; pumps; compressors; and other system applications).

Other Methods

There are many other methods of nondestructive testing, including optical methods such as holography, shearography and moiré imaging; material identification methods such as chemical spot testing, spark testing and spectroscopy; strain gaging; and acoustic methods such as vibration analysis and tapping.

PART 2. Management of Ultrasonic Testing

Selection of Ultrasonic Testing[4]

Ultrasonic testing is an important method within the broad field of nondestructive testing. Ultrasonic techniques usually fall into one of the following categories: internal discontinuity detection, cross section evaluation (thickness testing) or bond characterization. Some techniques can be subdivided even further. Cross section evaluation (thickness testing, corrosion mapping and others) is the most widely used application as applied to new and inservice components used in various industries. Thicknesses of structural materials can be measured from a micrometer to a meter with accuracies of better than one percent. The method can also be used to determine physical properties, structure, grain size and elastic constants.

Ultrasonic instrumentation is designed to detect structural characteristics of a component. These characteristics range from simple cross sectional thickness to complex geometries for various fabrication or inservice discontinuities.

As a result, specific applications have been developed using ultrasonic testing. Some examples are: detecting discontinuities in fabricated structures such as airframes, piping and pressure vessels, ships, bridges, motor vehicles, machinery; detecting the impending failure in high stressed components that are exposed to the various modes of fatigue; and quantifying liquid level or presence of liquids in single-wall components.

Advantages of Ultrasonic Testing

Modern ultrasonic test techniques offer an economical means for high speed, large or small scale testing of materials and structures such as those found in nearly every industry. Many of the materials used in industry today can be evaluated by one or more of the ultrasonic techniques using various equipment types (digital thickness gage, manual discontinuity detectors, remote automated scanning systems and others).

When proper techniques are coupled with appropriate equipment, ultrasonic tests are highly sensitive (permitting detection of minute discontinuities), penetrate very thick or long sections of materials, provide required information to accurately measure the location and size of discontinuities, provide rapid evaluation of materials (by manual or automated means) and require access from only one side of the test object.

Limitations of Ultrasonic Testing

Ultrasonic testing may be limited by component geometry (size, contour, surface roughness, complexity and discontinuity orientation) and undesirable internal structure characteristics (grain size, grain orientation, acoustic impedance differences of joined material and others). Because most ultrasonic techniques require some type of couplant to eliminate air between the transducer and the test surface, component compatibility with the couplant and test object temperature can become a factor. Ultrasonic equipment compatibility with the test environment (temperature, radiation levels, electrical interference and others) may also affect the effectiveness of testing The final potential limitation is the skill of the inspector as it relates to the ultrasonic technique and knowledge of the component characteristics.

Management of Ultrasonic Testing Programs

Management of an ultrasonic testing program requires consideration of many items before it can produce the desired results. Six basic questions must be answered before a true direction can be charted. They are as follows.

1. Are regulatory requirements in place that mandate program characteristics?
2. What is the magnitude of the program that will provide desired results?
3. What provisions must be made for personnel safety and for compliance with environmental regulations?
4. What is the performance date for a program to be fully implemented?
5. Is there a cost benefit of ultrasonic testing?
6. What are the available resources in personnel and money?

Once these questions are answered, then a recommendation can be made to determine the type of inspection agency. Three primary types of agencies responsible for inspection are (1) service companies, (2) consultants and (3) in-house programs.

Although these are the main agency types, some programs may, routinely or as needed, require support personnel from a combination of two or more of these sources. Before a final decision is made, advantages and disadvantages of each agency type must be considered.

Service Companies

1. Who will identify the components within the facility to be examined?
2. Will the contract be for time and materials or have a specific scope of work?
3. If a time and materials contract is awarded, who will monitor the time and materials charged?
4. If a scope of work is required, who is technically qualified to develop and approve it?
5. What products or documents (test reports, trending, recommendations, root cause analysis and others) will be provided once the tests are completed?
6. Who will evaluate and accept the product (test reports, trending, recommendations, root cause analysis and others) within the service company?
7. Do the service company workers possess qualifications and certifications required by contract and by applicable regulations?
8. Do the service company workers require site specific training (confined space entry, electrical safety, hazardous materials and others) or clearance to enter and work in the facility?
9. Does the service company retain any liability for test results?

Consultants

1. Will the contract be for time and materials or have a specific scope of work?
2. If a scope of work is required, who is technically qualified to develop and approve it?
3. Who will identify the required qualifications of the consultant?
4. Is the purpose of the consultant to develop or update a program or is it to oversee and evaluate the performance of an existing program?
5. Will the consultant have oversight responsibility for tests performed?

6. What products (trending, recommendations, root cause analysis and others) are provided once the tests are completed?
7. Who will evaluate the consultant's performance (test reports, trending, recommendations, root cause analysis and other functions) within the sponsoring company?
8. Does the consultant possess qualifications and certifications required by contract and by applicable regulations?
9. Does the consultant require site specific training (confined space entry, electrical safety, hazardous materials and others) or clearance to enter and work in the facility?
10. Does the consultant retain any liability for test results?

In-House Programs

1. Who will determine the scope of the program, such as which techniques will be used?
2. What are the regulatory requirements (codes and standards) associated with program development and implementation?
3. Who will develop a cost benefit analysis for the program?
4. How much time and what resources are available to establish the program?
5. What are the qualification requirements (education, training, experience and others) for personnel?
6. Do program personnel require additional training (safety, confined space entry or others) or qualifications?
7. Are subject matter experts required to provide technical guidance during personnel development?
8. Are procedures required to perform work in the facility?
9. If procedures are required, who will develop, review and approve them?
10. Who will determine the technical specifications for test equipment?

Test Procedures for Ultrasonic Testing

The conduct of test operations (in-house or contracted) should be performed in accordance with specific instructions from an expert. Specific instructions are typically written as a technical procedure. In many cases, codes and specifications will require that a technical procedure be developed for each individual test. In other cases, the same procedure is used repeatedly.

The procedure can take many forms. A procedure may comprise general instructions that address only major aspects of test techniques. Or a procedure may be written as a step-by-step process requiring a supervisor's or a qualified/certified worker's signature after each step. The following is a typical format for an industrial procedure.

1. The *purpose* identifies the intent of the procedure.
2. The *scope* establishes the latitude of items, tests and techniques covered and not covered by the procedure.
3. *References* are specific documents from which criteria are extracted or are documents satisfied by implementation of the procedure.
4. *Definitions* are needed for terms and abbreviations that are not common knowledge to people who will read the procedure.
5. Statements about *personnel requirements* address specific requirements to perform tasks in accordance with the procedure — issues such as personnel qualification, certification and access clearance.
6. *Equipment* characteristics, calibration requirements and model numbers of qualified equipment must be specified.
7. The test *procedure* provides a sequential process to be used to conduct test activities.
8. *Acceptance criteria* establish component characteristics that will identify the items suitable for service (initial use or continued service).
9. *Reports* (records) provide the means to document specific test techniques, equipment used, personnel, activity, date performed and test results.
10. *Attachments* may include (if required) items such as report forms, instrument calibration forms, qualified equipment matrix, schedules and others.

Once the procedure is written, an expert in the subject evaluates it. If the procedure meets identified requirements, the expert will approve it for use. Some codes and standards also require the procedure to be qualified — that is, demonstrated to the satisfaction of a representative of a regulatory body or jurisdictional authority.

Test Specifications for Ultrasonic Testing[4]

An ultrasonic test specification must anticipate a number of issues that arise during testing.

Means of Generating and Detecting Ultrasonic Signals

The generation and detection of ultrasonic waves for testing are accomplished by interaction between transducer element(s) and an ultrasonic instrument. The transducer element is in a device referred to as a *search unit* or as a *probe*. Transducers containing piezoelectric elements (the most commonly used transducer material) are used to transmit and detect ultrasonic signals. The ultrasonic instrument has an electronic pulse circuit that provides a controlled electrical pulse to activate a piezoelectric element within the search unit. Once activated, the probe transmits an ultrasonic wave into the test object. Another required element for sound transmission is the couplant between the search unit and component. The couplant provides a compatible medium for the ultrasonic sound to travel from the probe to the test object. Sound travels through a homogeneous material at a constant speed. Depending on the ultrasonic technique (through transmission or pulse echo), the ultrasonic sound will be received by reentering the same or another search unit. The search unit will convert the mechanical sound energy into an electrical pulse that the instrument processes and displays as a signal or digital value. The display represents a time of flight or distance (thickness) traveled within the component. This information can be used to evaluate the condition or to measure the section thickness of the test object.

Ultrasonic Test Frequencies

A single ultrasonic test system can be used for many different measurements through the selection of test frequencies. These frequencies are usually those that correspond to bandwidths that match the resonant frequency of the ultrasonic transducer designed for a specific application. Frequency is measured in hertz (Hz). The range of audible frequencies for most adult humans is about 0.02 to 20 kHz. Most industrial ultrasonic tests are made in the frequency range between 1 and 15 MHz.

Most ultrasonic test equipment provides several fixed frequency steps. Thus, appropriate frequencies can be readily selected by the inspector to meet requirements of the test and to match the search unit selected. Lower frequencies are typically used in applications where it is desirable to minimize sound attenuation as a result of material grain size or for long distances. Higher test frequencies are used for applications where increased sensitivity is required and sound attenuation is not a problem.

Interpretation

Interpretation may be complex, especially before a procedure has been established. The interpreter must have a knowledge of the following: (1) the underlying physical process, including wave propagation in the test item, (2) techniques and equipment used for data acquisition and display, (3) details about the item being examined (configuration, material properties, fabrication process, potential discontinuities and intended service conditions) and (4) possible sources of noise that might be mistaken for meaningful ultrasound.

After interpretation, acceptance criteria are applied in a phase called *evaluation.*

Reliability of Test Results

When a test is performed, there are four possible outcomes: (1) a rejectable discontinuity can be found when one is present, (2) a rejectable discontinuity can be missed even when one is present, (3) a rejectable discontinuity can be indicated when none is present and (4) no rejectable discontinuity is found when none is present. A reliable testing process and a qualified inspector should find all discontinuities of concern with no discontinuities missed (no errors as in case 2 above) and no false calls (case 3 above).

To approach this goal, the probability of finding a rejectable discontinuity must be high and the inspector must be both proficient in the testing process and motivated to perform with maximum efficiency. An ineffective inspector may accept test objects that contain discontinuities, with the result of possible inservice part failure. The same inspector may reject parts that do not contain rejectable discontinuities, with the result of unnecessary scrap and repair. Neither scenario is desirable.

Ultrasonic Test Standards

Traditionally, the purpose of specifications and standards has been to define the requirements that goods or services must meet. As such, they are intended to be incorporated into contracts so that both the buyer and provider have a well defined description of what one will receive and the other will provide.

Standards have undergone a process of peer review in industry and can be invoked with the force of law by contract or by government regulation. In contrast, a specification represents an employer's instructions to employees and is specific to a contract or workplace. Many a specification originates as a detailed description either as part of a purchaser's

requirements or as part of a vendor's offer. Specifications may be incorporated into standards through the normal review process. Standards and specifications exist in three basic areas: equipment, processes and personnel.

1. Standards for ultrasonic equipment include criteria that address transducers and other parts of a system.
2. ASTM International and other organizations publish standards for test techniques. Some other standards are for quality assurance procedures and are not specific to a test method or even to testing in general. Tables 3 to 6 list some standards used in ultrasonic testing. The United States Department of Defense has replaced most military specifications and standards with industry consensus specifications and standards. A source for nondestructive test standards is the *Annual Book of ASTM Standards.*[5]
3. Qualification and certification of testing personnel are discussed below with specific reference to recommendations of *ASNT Recommended Practice No. SNT-TC-1A.*[6]

Personnel Qualification and Certification

One of the most critical aspects of the test process is the qualification of testing personnel. Nondestructive testing is sometimes referred to as a *special process.* The term simply means that it is very difficult to determine the adequacy of a test by merely observing the process or the documentation generated at its conclusion. The quality of the test is largely dependent on the skills and knowledge of the inspector.

The American Society for Nondestructive Testing (ASNT) has been a world leader in the qualification and certification of nondestructive testing personnel since the 1960s. (Qualification demonstrates that an individual has the required training, experience, knowledge and abilities. Certification provides written testimony that an individual is qualified.) By the twenty-first century, the American Society for Nondestructive Testing had instituted three major programs for the qualification and certification of nondestructive testing personnel.

TABLE 3. Some standards for ultrasonic testing.

American Bureau of Shipping

ABS 30   *Ultrasonic Examination of Carbon Steel Forgings for Tall Shafts*

American Petroleum Institute

API RP 5UE   *Recommended Practice for Ultrasonic Evaluation of Pipe Imperfections*

API RP 2X   *Recommended Practice for Ultrasonic Examination of Offshore Structural Fabrication and Guidelines for Qualification of Ultrasonic Technicians*

API SPEC 5L   *Specification for Line Pipe*

API SPEC 6A   *Specification for Wellhead and Christmas Tree Equipment*

American Welding Society

AWS G1.2   *Specification for Standardized Ultrasonic Welding Test Specimen for Thermoplastics*

AWS C3.8   *Specification for the Ultrasonic Examination of Brazed Joints*

ASME International

ASME BPVC   *Boiler and Pressure Vessel Code*

Deutsches Institut für Normung [German Institute for Standardization]

DIN 25435 P1   *Inservice Inspections for Primary Circuit Components of Light Water Reactors; Remote-Controlled Ultrasonic Inspection*

DIN 54123   *Non-Destructive Test; Ultrasonic Method of Testing Claddings, Produced by Welding, Rolling and Explosion*

DIN 65455   *Aerospace — Seamless Tubes in Steel, Nickel and Titanium Alloys — Ultrasonic Inspection*

Manufacturers Standardization Society of the Valve and Fittings Industry

MSS SP-94   *Quality Standard for Ferritic and Martensitic Steel Castings for Valves, Flanges, and Fittings and Other Piping Components — Ultrasonic Examination Method*

Pipe Fabrication Institute

PFI ES-20   *Wall Thickness Measurement by Ultrasonic Examination*

PFI ES-30   *Random Ultrasonic Examination of Butt Welds*

SAE International

SAE AMS 2154   *Inspection, Ultrasonic, Wrought Metals, Process for*

SAE AMS 2628   *Ultrasonic Immersion Inspection Titanium and Titanium Alloy Billet Premium Grade*

SAE AMS 2630B   *Inspection, Ultrasonic Product over 0.5 inch (12.7 mm) Thick*

SAE AMS 2631B   *Ultrasonic Inspection, Titanium and Titanium Alloy Bar and Billet*

SAE AMS 2632A   *Inspection, Ultrasonic, of Thin Materials 0.50 inch (12.7 mm) and under in Cross-Sectional Thickness*

SAE AMS 2633B   *Ultrasonic Inspection, Centrifugally-Cast, Corrosion-Resistant Steel Tubular Cylinders*

SAE AMS 2634B   *Ultrasonic Inspection, Thin Wall Metal Tubing*

SAE AS 7114/3   *NADCAP Requirements for Nondestructive Testing Facility Ultrasonic Survey*

SAE J 428   *Ultrasonic Inspection*

1. *Recommended Practice No. SNT-TC-1A* provides guidelines to employers for personnel qualification and certification in nondestructive testing. This recommended practice identifies the attributes that should be considered when qualifying nondestructive testing personnel. It requires the employer to develop and implement a written practice, a procedure that details the specific process and any limitation in the qualification and certification of nondestructive testing personnel.[6]

2. ANSI/ASNT CP-189, *Standard for Qualification and Certification of Nondestructive Testing Personnel* resembles *SNT-TC-1A* but establishes specific requirements for the qualification and certification of Level I and II nondestructive testing personnel. For Level III, CP-189 references an examination administered by the American Society for Nondestructive Testing. However, CP-189 is a consensus standard as defined by the American National Standards Institute (ANSI). It is recognized as the American standard for nondestructive testing. It is not considered a recommended practice; it is a national standard.[7]

TABLE 4. Ultrasonic testing standards published by ASTM International.

ASTM A 388   *Standard Practice for Ultrasonic Examination of Heavy Steel Forgings*
ASTM A 418   *Standard Test Method for Ultrasonic Examination of Turbine and Generator Steel Rotor Forgings*
ASTM A 435   *Standard Specification for Straight-Beam Ultrasonic Examination of Steel Plates*
ASTM A 503   *Standard Specification for Ultrasonic Examination of Forged Crankshafts*
ASTM A 531M   *Standard Practice for Ultrasonic Examination of Turbine-Generator Steel Retaining Rings*
ASTM A 577M   *Standard Specification for Ultrasonic Angle-Beam Examination of Steel Plates*
ASTM A 578M   *Standard Specification for Straight-Beam Ultrasonic Examination of Plain and Clad Steel Plates for Special Applications*
ASTM A 609M   *Standard Practice for Castings, Carbon, Low-Alloy, and Martensitic Stainless Steel, Ultrasonic Examination Thereof*
ASTM A 745M   *Standard Practice for Ultrasonic Examination of Austenitic Steel Forgings*
ASTM A 898M   *Standard Specification for Straight Beam Ultrasonic Examination of Rolled Steel Structural Shapes*
ASTM A 939   *Standard Test Method for Ultrasonic Examination from Bored Surfaces of Cylindrical Forgings*
ASTM B 548   *Standard Test Method for Ultrasonic Inspection of Aluminum-Alloy Plate for Pressure Vessels*
ASTM B 594   *Standard Practice for Ultrasonic Inspection of Aluminum-Alloy Wrought Products for Aerospace Applications*
ASTM B 773   *Standard Guide for Ultrasonic C-Scan Bond Evaluation of Brazed or Welded Electrical Contact Assemblies*
ASTM C 133   *Standard Test Method for Measuring Ultrasonic Velocity in Advanced Ceramics with Broadband Pulse-Echo Cross-Correlation Method*
ASTM C 1332   *Standard Test Method for Measurement of Ultrasonic Attenuation Coefficients of Advanced Ceramics by Pulse-Echo Contact Technique*
ASTM D 4883   *Standard Test Method for Density of Polyethylene by the Ultrasound Technique*
ASTM D 6132   *Standard Test Method for Nondestructive Measurement of Dry Film Thickness of Applied Organic Coatings Using an Ultrasonic Gage*
ASTM E 114   *Standard Practice for Ultrasonic Pulse-Echo Straight-Beam Examination by the Contact Method*
ASTM E 127   *Standard Practice for Fabricating and Checking Aluminum Alloy Ultrasonic Standard Reference Blocks*
ASTM E 164   *Standard Practice for Ultrasonic Contact Examination of Weldments*
ASTM E 213   *Standard Practice for Ultrasonic Examination of Metal Pipe and Tubing*
ASTM E 214   *Standard Practice for Immersed Ultrasonic Examination by the Reflection Method Using Pulsed Longitudinal Waves*
ASTM E 273   *Standard Practice for Ultrasonic Examination of the Weld Zone of Welded Pipe and Tubing*
ASTM E 317   *Standard Practice for Evaluating Performance Characteristics of Ultrasonic Pulse- Echo Examination Instruments and Systems without the Use of Electronic Measurement Instruments*
ASTM E 428   *Standard Practice for Fabrication and Control of Steel Reference Blocks Used in Ultrasonic Examination*
ASTM E 494   *Standard Practice for Measuring Ultrasonic Velocity in Materials*
ASTM E 587   *Standard Practice for Ultrasonic Angle-Beam Examination by the Contact Method*
ASTM E 588   *Standard Practice for Detection of Large Inclusions in Bearing Quality Steel by the Ultrasonic Method*
ASTM E 664   *Standard Practice for the Measurement of the Apparent Attenuation of Longitudinal Ultrasonic Waves by Immersion Method*
ASTM E 797   *Standard Practice for Measuring Thickness by Manual Ultrasonic Pulse-Echo Contact Method*
ASTM E 1001   *Standard Practice for Detection and Evaluation of Discontinuities by the Immersed Pulse-Echo Ultrasonic Method Using Longitudinal Waves*
ASTM E 1065   *Standard Guide for Evaluating Characteristics of Ultrasonic Search Units*
ASTM E 1158   *Standard Guide for Material Selection and Fabrication of Reference Blocks for the Pulsed Longitudinal Wave Ultrasonic Examination of Metal and Metal Alloy Production Material*
ASTM E 1315   *Standard Practice for Ultrasonic Examination of Steel with Convex Cylindrically Curved Entry Surfaces*
ASTM E 1324   *Standard Guide for Measuring Some Electronic Characteristics of Ultrasonic Examination Instruments*
ASTM E 1454   *Standard Guide for Data Fields for Computerized Transfer of Digital Ultrasonic Testing Data*
ASTM E 1495   *Standard Guide for Acousto-Ultrasonic Assessment of Composites, Laminates, and Bonded Joints*
ASTM E 1774   *Standard Guide for Electromagnetic Acoustic Transducers (EMATs)*
ASTM E 1816   *Standard Practice for Ultrasonic Examinations Using Electromagnetic Acoustic Transducer (EMAT) Techniques*
ASTM E 1901   *Standard Guide for Detection and Evaluation of Discontinuities by Contact Pulse-Echo Straight-Beam Ultrasonic Methods*
ASTM E 1961   *Standard Practice for Mechanized Ultrasonic Examination of Girth Welds Using Zonal Discrimination with Focused Search Units*
ASTM E 1962   *Standard Test Method for Ultrasonic Surface Examinations Using Electromagnetic Acoustic Transducer (EMAT) Techniques*
ASTM E 2001   *Standard Guide for Resonant Ultrasound Spectroscopy for Defect Detection in Both Metallic and Non-Metallic Parts*
ASTM E 2192   *Standard Guide for Planar Flaw Height Sizing by Ultrasonics*
ASTM E 2223   *Standard Practice for Examination of Seamless, Gas-Filled, Steel Pressure Vessels Using Angle Beam Ultrasonics*
ASTM E 2373   *Standard Practice for Use of the Ultrasonic Time of Flight Diffraction (TOFD) Technique*
ASTM E 2375   *Standard Practice for Ultrasonic Examination of Wrought Products*
ASTM F 1512   *Standard Practice for Ultrasonic C-Scan Bond Evaluation of Sputtering Target-Backing Plate Assemblies*

TABLE 5 Ultrasonic testing standards published by international organizations for Europe and the world.

European Committee for Standardization

EN 583	*Non-Destructive Testing — Ultrasonic Examination*
EN 1330-4	*Non Destructive Testing — Terminology — Part 4: Terms Used in Ultrasonic Testing*
EN 1712	*Non-Destructive Testing of Welds — Ultrasonic Testing of Welded Joints Acceptance Levels*
EN 1713	*Non-Destructive Testing of Welds — Ultrasonic Testing Characterization of Indications in Welds*
EN 1714	*Non-Destructive Testing of Welds — Ultrasonic Testing of Welded Joints*
EN 10160	*Ultrasonic Testing of Steel Flat Product of Thickness Equal or Greater than 6 mm (Reflection Method)*
EN 10228	*Non-Destructive Testing of Steel Forgings*
EN 10246	*Non-Destructive Testing of Steel Tubes*
EN 10306	*Iron and Steel — Ultrasonic Testing of H Beams with Parallel Flanges and IPE Beams*
EN 10307	*Non-Destructive Testing — Ultrasonic Testing of Austenitic and Austenitic-Ferritic Stainless Steel Flat Products of Thickness Equal to or Greater than 6 mm (Reflection Method)*
EN 10308	*Non-Destructive Testing — Ultrasonic Testing of Steel Bars*
EN 12223	*Non-Destructive Testing — Ultrasonic Examination — Specification for Calibration Block No. 1*
EN 12504	*Testing Concrete — Part 4: Determination of Ultrasonic Pulse Velocity*
EN 12668	*Non-Destructive Testing — Characterization and Verification of Ultrasonic Examination Equipment*
EN 12680	*Founding — Ultrasonic Examination*
EN 13100-3	*Non Destructive Testing of Welded Joints in Thermoplastics Semifinished Products — Part 3: Ultrasonic Testing*
EN 14127	*Non-Destructive Testing — Ultrasonic Thickness Measurement*
EN 27963	*Welds in Steel — Calibration Block No. 2 for Ultrasonic Examination of Welds*
ENV 583-6	*Non-Destructive Testing — Ultrasonic Examination — Part 6: Time-Of-Flight Diffraction Technique As a Method for Detection and Sizing of Discontinuities*
ENV 14186	*Advanced Technical Ceramics — Ceramic Composites — Mechanical Properties at Room Temperature, Determination of Elastic Properties by an Ultrasonic Technique*
PREN 2003-8	*Aerospace Series Acceptance Criteria for Ultrasonic Inspection of Billets, Bars, Plates and Forgings in Steel, Titanium, Titanium Alloys, Aluminum Alloys and Heat Resisting Alloys*

International Organization for Standardization

ISO 2400	*Welds in Steel — Reference Block for the Calibration of Equipment for Ultrasonic Examination*
ISO 4386-1	*Plain Bearings — Metallic Multilayer Plain Bearings — Part 1: Non-Destructive Ultrasonic Testing of Bond*
ISO 5577	*Non-Destructive Testing — Ultrasonic Inspection — Vocabulary*
ISO 5948	*Railway Rolling Stock Material — Ultrasonic Acceptance Testing*
ISO 7963	*Welds in Steel — Calibration Block No. 2 for Ultrasonic Examination of Welds*
ISO 9303	*Seamless and Welded (except Submerged Arc-Welded) Steel Tubes for Pressure Purposes — Full Peripheral Ultrasonic Testing for the Detection of Longitudinal Imperfections*
ISO 9305	*Seamless Steel Tubes for Pressure Purposes — Full Peripheral Ultrasonic Testing for the Detection of Transverse Imperfections*
ISO 9764	*Electric Resistance and Induction Welded Steel Tubes for Pressure Purposes — Ultrasonic Testing of the Weld Seam for the Detection of Longitudinal Imperfections*
ISO 9765	*Submerged Arc-Welded Steel Tubes for Pressure Purposes — Ultrasonic Testing of the Weld Seam for the Detection of Longitudinal and/or Transverse Imperfections*
ISO 10124	*Seamless and Welded (except Submerged Arc-Welded) Steel Tubes for Pressure Purposes — Ultrasonic Testing for the Detection of Laminar Imperfections*
ISO 10332	*Seamless and Welded (except Submerged Arc-Welded) Steel Tubes for Pressure Purposes — Ultrasonic Testing for the Verification of Hydraulic Leak-Tightness*
ISO 10375	*Non-Destructive Testing — Ultrasonic Inspection — Characterization of Search Unit and Sound Field*
ISO 10423	*Petroleum and Natural Gas Industries — Drilling and Production Equipment — Wellhead and Christmas Tree Equipment*
ISO 10543	*Seamless and Hot-Stretch-Reduced Welded Steel Tubes for Pressure Purposes — Full Peripheral Ultrasonic Thickness Testing*
ISO 11496	*Seamless and Welded Steel Tubes for Pressure Purposes — Ultrasonic Testing of Tube Ends for the Detection of Laminar Imperfections*
ISO 12094	*Welded Steel Tubes for Pressure Purposes — Ultrasonic Testing for the Detection of Laminar Imperfections in Strips/Plates Used in the Manufacture of Welded Tubes*
ISO 12710	*Non-Destructive Testing — Ultrasonic Inspection — Evaluating Electronic Characteristics of Ultrasonic Test Instruments*
ISO 12715	*Ultrasonic Non-Destructive Testing — Reference Blocks and Test Procedures for the Characterization of Contact Search Unit Beam Profiles*
ISO 13663	*Welded Steel Tubes for Pressure Purposes — Ultrasonic Testing of the Area Adjacent to the Weld Seam for the Detection of Laminar Imperfections*
ISO 17640	*Non-Destructive Testing of Welds — Ultrasonic Testing of Welded Joints*
ISO 18175	*Non-Destructive Testing — Evaluating Performance Characteristics of Ultrasonic Pulse-Echo Testing Systems without the Use of Electronic Measurement Instruments*
ISO 22825	*Non-Destructive Testing of Welds — Ultrasonic Method — Testing of Welds in Austenitic Steels and Nickel Based Alloys*

TABLE 6. Ultrasonic testing standards published by three Pacific Rim organizations.

Japanese Standards Association

JSA G 0582   *Ultrasonic Examination for Steel Pipes and Tubes*
JSA G 0584   *Ultrasonic Examination for Arc Welded Steel Pipes*
JSA G 0587   *Methods of Ultrasonic Examination for Carbon and Low Alloy Steel Forgings*
JSA G 0801   *Ultrasonic Examination of Steel Plates for Pressure Vessels*
JSA G 0802   *Ultrasonic Examination of Stainless Steel Plates*
JSA G 0901   *Classification of Structural Rolled Steel Plate and Wide Flat for Building by Ultrasonic Test*
JSA H 0516   *Ultrasonic Inspection of Titanium Pipes and Tubes*
JSA K 7090   *Testing Method for Ultrasonic Pulse Echo Technique of Carbon Fibre Reinforced Plastic Panels*
JSA Z 2344   *General Rule of Ultrasonic Testing of Metals by Pulse Echo Technique*
JSA Z 2345   *Standard Test Blocks for Ultrasonic Testing*
JSA Z 2350   *Method for Measurement of Performance Characteristics of Ultrasonic Probes*
JSA Z 2351   *Method for Assessing the Electrical Characteristics of Ultrasonic Testing Instrument Using Pulse Echo Technique*
JSA Z 2352   *Method for Assessing the Overall Performance Characteristics of Ultrasonic Pulse Echo Testing Instrument*
JSA Z 2354   *Method for Measurement of Ultrasonic Attenuation Coefficient of Solid by Pulse Echo Technique*
JSA Z 2355   *Methods for Measurement of Thickness by Ultrasonic Pulse Echo Technique*
JSA Z 3060   *Method for Ultrasonic Examination for Welds of Ferritic Steel*
JSA Z 3062   *Methods and Acceptance Criteria of Ultrasonic Examination for Gas Pressure Welds of Reinforcing Deformed Bars*
JSA Z 3070   *Methods for Automatic Ultrasonic Testing for Welds of Ferritic Steel*
JSA Z 3080   *Methods of Ultrasonic Angle Beam Examination for Butt Welds of Aluminium Plates*
JSA Z 3081   *Methods of Ultrasonic Angle Beam Examination for Welds of Aluminium Pipes and Tubes*
JSA Z 3082   *Methods of Ultrasonic Examination for T Type Welds of Aluminium Plates*
JSA Z 3871   *Standard Qualification Procedure for Ultrasonic Testing Technique of Aluminium and Aluminium Alloy Welds*

Korean Standards Association

KSA B 0521   *Methods of Ultrasonic Angle Beam Testing and Classification of Test Results for Welds of Aluminium Pipes and Tubes*
KSA B 0522   *Method of Ultrasonic Testing and Classification of Test Results for T Type Welds in Aluminium Plates*
KSA B 0532   *Method for Measurement of Ultrasonic Attenuation Coefficient of Solid by Pulse Echo Technique*
KSA B 0533   *Methods for Measurement on Ultrasonic Velocity of Solid by Pulse Technique Using Reference Test Pieces*
KSA B 0534   *Method for Assessing the Overall Performance Characteristics of Ultrasonic Pulse Echo Testing Instrument*
KSA B 0535   *Method for Measurement of Performance Characteristics of Ultrasonic Probes*
KSA B 0536   *Methods for Measurement of Thickness by Ultrasonic Pulse Echo Technique*
KSA B 0537   *Methods for Assessing the Electrical Characteristics of Ultrasonic Testing Instrument Using Pulse Echo Technique*
KSA B 0817   *General Rule of Ultrasonic Testing of Metals by the Pulse Echo Technique*
KSA B 0831   *Standard Test Blocks for Ultrasonic Testing*
KSA B 0896   *Methods of Ultrasonic Manual Testing and Classification of Test Results for Steel Welds*
KSA B 0897   *Method of Ultrasonic Angle Beam Testing and Classification of Test Results for Butt Welds in Aluminium Plates*
KSA D 0040   *Classification of Structural Rolled Steel Plate for Building by Ultrasonic Test*
KSA D 0075   *Ultrasonic Inspection of Titanium Pipes and Tubes*
KSA D 0233   *Ultrasonic Examination of Steel Plates for Pressure Vessels*
KSA D 0250   *Ultrasonic Examination of Steel Pipes and Tubes*
KSA D 0252   *Ultrasonic Examination for Arc Welded Steel Pipes*
KSA D 0273   *Methods of Ultrasonic Examination for Gas Pressure Welds of Reinforcing Deformed Bars*

Standards Australia International

SAI AS 1065   *Non-Destructive Testing — Ultrasonic Testing of Carbon and Low Alloy Steel Forgings*
SAI AS 1710   *Non-Destructive Testing — Ultrasonic Testing of Carbon and Low Alloy Steel Plate — Test Methods and Quality Classification*
SAI AS 2083   *Calibration Blocks and Their Methods of Use in Ultrasonic Testing*
SAI AS 2207   *Non-Destructive Testing — Ultrasonic Testing of Fusion Welded Joints in Carbon and Low Alloy Steel*
SAI AS 2452.3   *Non-Destructive Testing — Determination of Thickness — Use of Ultrasonic Testing*
SAI AS 2824   *Non-Destructive Testing — Ultrasonic Methods — Evaluation and Quality Classification of Metal Bearing Bonds*
SAI AS/NZS 2574   *Non-Destructive Testing — Ultrasonic Testing of Ferritic Steel Castings*

3. The *ASNT Central Certification Program (ACCP)*, unlike *SNT-TC-1A* and CP-189, is a third party certification process that identifies qualification and certification attributes for Level II and Level III nondestructive testing personnel. The American Society for Nondestructive Testing certifies that the individual has the skills and knowledge for many nondestructive test method applications. It does not remove the responsibility for the final determination of personnel qualification from the employer. The employer evaluates an individual's skills and knowledge for application of company procedures using designated techniques and equipment identified for specific tests.[8]

Excerpts from Recommended Practice No. SNT-TC-1A

To give a general idea of the contents of these documents, the following items are excerpted from *Recommended Practice No. SNT-TC-1A*.[6] The original text is arranged in outline format and includes recommendations that are not specific to ultrasonic testing.

Scope ... This Recommended Practice has been prepared to establish guidelines for the qualification and certification of [nondestructive testing] personnel whose specific jobs require appropriate knowledge of the technical principles underlying the nondestructive tests they perform, witness, monitor, or evaluate. ... This document provides guidelines for the establishment of a qualification and certification program....

Written Practice ... The employer shall establish a written practice for the control and administration of [nondestructive testing] personnel training, examination and certification. ... The employer's written practice should describe the responsibility of each level of certification for determining the acceptability of materials or components in accordance with the applicable codes, standards, specifications and procedures. ...

Education, Training and Experience Requirements for Initial Qualification ... Candidates for certification in [nondestructive testing] should have sufficient education, training and experience to ensure qualification in those [nondestructive testing] methods in which they are being considered for certification. ... Table 6.3.1A [see Table 5 in this *Nondestructive Testing Handbook* chapter, for ultrasonic testing] lists the recommended training and experience factors to be considered by the employer in establishing written practices for initial qualification of Level I and II individuals ...

Training Programs ... Personnel being considered for initial certification should complete sufficient organized training to become thoroughly familiar with the principles and practices of the specified [nondestructive testing] method related to the level of certification desired and applicable to the processes to be used and the products to be tested. ...

Examinations ... For Level I and II personnel, a composite grade should be determined by simple averaging of the results of the general, specific and practical examinations described below. ... Examinations administered for qualification should result in a passing composite grade of at least 80 percent, with no individual examination having a passing grade less than 70 percent. ...

Practical [Examination for NDT Level I and II] ... The candidate should demonstrate ... ability to operate the necessary [nondestructive testing] equipment [and to] record and analyze the resultant information to the degree required. ... At least one ... specimen should be tested and the results of the [nondestructive testing] analyzed by the candidate. ...

Certification ... Certification of all levels of [nondestructive testing] personnel is the responsibility of the employer. ... Certification of [nondestructive testing] personnel shall be based on demonstration of satisfactory qualification in accordance with [sections on education, training, experience and examinations] as described in the employer's written practice. ... Personnel certification records shall be [retained] by the employer. ...

Recertification ... All levels of [nondestructive testing] personnel shall be recertified periodically in accordance with [one of the following:] continuing satisfactory technical performance [or reexamination in] those portions of the examinations ... deemed necessary by the employer's [NDT] Level III. ... Recommended maximum recertification intervals are [five years for Level I and II and five years for Level III]. ...

These recommendations from the 2006 edition of *Recommended Practice No. SNT-TC-1A* are cited only to provide an idea of items that must be considered in the development of an in-house nondestructive testing program. Because the text above is excerpted, those developing a personnel qualification program should consult the complete text of *SNT-TC-1A* and other applicable procedures and practices. If an outside agency is contracted for ultrasonic test services, then the contractor must have a qualification and certification program to satisfy most codes and standards.

The minimum number of questions that should be administered in the written examination for ultrasonic test personnel is as follows: 40 questions in the general examination and 20 questions in the specific examination. The number of questions is the same for Level I and

Level II personnel. Table 7 shows required hours of experience for Levels I and II.

Central Certification

Another standard that may be a source for compliance is published by the International Organization for Standardization (ISO). The work of preparing international standards is normally carried out through technical committees of this worldwide federation of national standards bodies. Each ISO member body interested in a subject for which a technical committee has been established has the right to be represented on that committee. International organizations, governmental and nongovernmental, in liaison with the International Organization for Standardization, also take part in the work.

Technical Committee ISO/TC 135, Non-Destructive Testing Subcommittee SC 7, Personnel Qualification, prepared international standard ISO 9712, *Non-Destructive Testing — Qualification and Certification of Personnel.*[9] In its statement of scope, ISO 9712 states that it "specifies the qualification and certification of personnel involved in non-destructive testing . . . in one or more of the following methods: acoustic emission testing; eddy current testing; infrared thermographic testing; leak testing (hydraulic pressure tests excluded); magnetic particle testing; penetrant testing; radiographic testing; strain testing; ultrasonic testing; visual testing (direct unaided visual tests and visual tests carried out during the application of another NDT method are excluded)."

TABLE 7. Recommended training and experience for ultrasonic testing personnel according to *Recommended Practice No. SNT-TC-1A.*[6]

	Level I	Level II
High school graduate[a]	40 h	40 h
Two years of college[b]	30 h	40 h
Work experience[c]	210 h	630 h

a. Or equivalent.

b. Completion with a passing grade of at least two years of engineering or science study in a university, college or technical school.

c. Minimum work experience per level. Note: For Level II certification, the experience shall consist of time as Level I or equivalent. If a person is being qualified directly to Level II with no time at Level I, the required experience shall consist of the sum of the times required for Level I and Level II and the required training shall consist of the sum of the hours required for Level I and Level II.

Safety in Ultrasonic Testing

To manage an ultrasonic testing program, as with any testing program, the first obligation is to ensure safe working conditions. The following are components of a safety program that may be required or at least deserve serious consideration.

1. Before work is to begin, identify the safety and operational rules and codes applicable to the areas, equipment and systems to be tested.
2. Provide proper safety equipment (protective barriers, hard hats, safety harnesses, steel toed shoes, hearing protection and others).
3. Before the test, perform a thorough visual survey to determine all the hazards and to identify necessary safeguards to protect personnel and equipment.
4. Notify operative personnel to identify the location and specific material, equipment or systems to be tested. In addition, state, federal and company lockout/tagout procedures should be followed. Be aware of equipment that may be operated remotely or may be started by time delay.
5. Be aware of any potentially explosive atmospheres. Determine whether it is safe to take test equipment into the area.
6. Do not enter any roped off or no entry areas without permission and approval.
7. When working on or around moving or electrical equipment, the inspector should remove pens, watches, rings or objects in pockets that may touch (or fall into) energized equipment.
8. Know interplant communication and evacuation systems.
9. Never let unqualified personnel operate equipment independently from qualified supervision.
10. Keep a safe distance between the inspector and any energized equipment. In the United States, these distances can be found in documents from the Occupational Safety and Health Administration, the National Fire Prevention Association (*National Electric Code*),[10] the Institute of Electrical and Electronics Engineers (*National Electrical Safety Code*)[11] and other organizations.
11. Be aware of the personnel responsibilities before entering a confined space. All such areas must be tested satisfactorily for gas and oxygen levels before entry and periodically thereafter. If odors are noticed or if unusual sensations such as ear aches, dizziness or difficulty in breathing are experienced, leave the area immediately.

Most facilities in the United States are required by law to follow the requirements in the applicable standard. Two occupational safety and health standards in the United States that should be reviewed are *Occupational Safety and Health Standards* for general industry[12] and the *Occupational Safety and Health Standards for the Construction Industry*.[13] Personnel safety is always the first consideration for every job.

Part 3. History of Ultrasonic Testing[14]

Early Developments in High Frequency Acoustics

Ultrasonics is a branch of acoustics dealing with frequencies above the audible range. While developments in the field of acoustics can be traced far back into antiquity, the study of ultrasonics originated in the nineteenth century. The use of ultrasonic waves for nondestructive testing is even more recent, beginning in the late 1920s. Developments since the 1930s have made ultrasonic testing a widely used nondestructive test method.

From the period of development in the 1800s through the 1930s, the term *ultrasonics* was not associated with high frequency acoustic studies but despite its recent origin the term is used for convenience when discussing earlier developments.[15]

Studies of High Frequency Acoustic Events[16]

It is not known when humans became aware of sounds that could not be heard. Investigations on the pitch limits of the human ear led to studies by the French physicist Felix Savart (1830) in which a large toothed wheel was used to generate frequencies up to 24 kHz. For similar research, Francis Galton (1883) invented a whistle capable of generating 80 kHz. Thorough studies on the pitch limits of audibility were carried out by R. Koenig (1899) using tuning forks.

Before the age of electroacoustics, detection of high frequency acoustic waves was difficult but many ingenious detection devices were reported. John Tyndall observed the effects of sound waves on gas flames and thus developed the *sensitive flame* as a detection technique. August Kundt discovered that dust figures in tubes permitted an accurate means of measuring acoustic wavelength.

The famous acoustician John William Strutt (Lord Rayleigh) (Fig. 12) made many early contributions to the field of ultrasonics, including the development of the rayleigh disk used to measure acoustic pressure. The well known rayleigh surface wave, which plays a prominent role in ultrasonic testing and surface acoustic wave devices, was actually predicted by Rayleigh from efforts to analyze seismic phenomena.[17]

Discoveries in Acoustics

Accurate measurements of sound speed in iron pipes were made as early as 1808. In 1826, underwater sound velocity was measured by Charles Colladon and Daniel Sturm in Lake Geneva, Switzerland. George Stokes included the effects of viscosity in deriving theoretical expressions for sound speed. The Russian physicist Petr Lebedev succeeded in explaining the absorption mechanism in acoustic waves that had puzzled many leading researchers before the turn of the century. Lebedev was notable for developing the first true ultrasonic system, comprising a high frequency sound generator and an acoustic grating detector.

Among Rayleigh's many contributions was the analysis of the wave pattern of a high frequency piston generator, a critical factor in understanding the radiation fields of modern ultrasonic transducers.

FIGURE 12. John William Strutt (1842-1919).

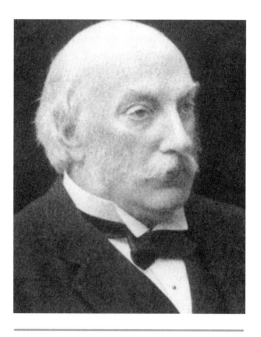

Transduction Mechanisms

Two electrical-to-mechanical transduction mechanisms that would dominate twentieth century ultrasonics, magnetostriction and piezoelectricity, were discovered in the 1800s. James Prescott Joule, most famous for his studies in thermodynamics, was responsible for identifying and systematically studying the magnetostrictive effect in the 1840s.

The piezoelectric effect, the most widely used phenomenon for ultrasonic wave generation and detection, was the last of the electroacoustic transduction mechanisms to be discovered. Although there were many earlier observations, in 1880 the brothers Jacques-Paul and Pierre Curie were credited with the discovery of the direct piezoelectric effect (the generation of an electric field by mechanical pressure). The inverse effect was observed less than a year later.[18]

Developments in Electroacoustics

The golden age of electroacoustics was opened by James Clerk Maxwell's classic *Treatise on Electricity* and closed by the Curie brothers' discovery of piezoelectricity. During this period, the principia of acoustics were published in Lord Rayleigh's *Theory of Sound*. At the time, the book was said by many to be so definitive as to close the field of acoustics to further scientific inquiry.

An important event in electroacoustics was the invention of the telephone by Alexander Graham Bell in 1876. The device greatly stimulated interest and study in the field and had a dramatic influence on the development of acoustics and ultrasonics. It was said that, because of Bell's invention, "we know much more than might ever have been reasonably expected from mere human curiosity about the way that the human being hears and speaks."[19]

Origins of Practical Ultrasonics

The seminal event that initiated the chain of developments toward modern ultrasonics was the sinking of the Titanic after collision with an iceberg in 1912. This famous disaster brought forth many schemes for avoiding icebergs and other underwater obstacles. Some of these techniques now seem curious or amusing, such as the proposal by Hiram Maxim that ships be fitted with low frequency generators and sensitive *ears* so they might navigate after the fashion of bats.

However, Lewis Fry Richardson in England did set forth well founded schemes for obstacle avoidance. He patented two techniques for echo ranging that involved generating narrow beams of sound and discriminating between transmitted and reflected signals but no practical implementation was recorded.

In the United States, R.A. Fessenden, working for the Submarine Signal Company, developed low frequency (540 to 1100 Hz) piston oscillators that could successfully detect icebergs and also found use as depth detectors.

Ultrasonic Detection of Submarines

With the outbreak of World War I, attention was turned to the need for detecting a different sort of underwater obstacle, the submarine. It may be said that modern ultrasonics and ultrasonic testing were born in the sea because their antecedents are directly traceable to efforts at submarine detection in World War I.

Key developments leading to modern ultrasonics started in France in 1915. A young Russian electrical engineer, M. Constantin Chilowsky proposed a plan for submarine detection that revived the original echo ranging ideas of Lewis Richardson. For evaluation, Chilowsky's proposals were forwarded to Paul Langevin, a physicist acclaimed for work on magnetics, ionization and relativity theory.[20]

Langevin recommended that work proceed on evaluating the echo ranging ideas and was asked to head the effort, working in cooperation with Chilowsky. A program was started in Langevin's laboratory with tests first being done in a 6 x 3 x 1.5 m (20 x 10 x 5 ft) tank. Langevin initially considered using the piezoelectric effect but discarded that approach in favor of *singing condensers* and carbon button microphones. Poulsen arc generators were used to drive the transducers.

Tests in the Seine River and later at a naval base at Toulon showed the ability to transmit signals up to 1850 m (6000 ft) and to receive echoes from target plates at distances of about 150 m (500 ft). Chilowsky and Langevin were coinventors on patents for this early ultrasonic application but soon severed their working relationship.

Piezoelectric Experiments

Langevin continued the studies on submarine detection and began to reexamine the use of the piezoelectric effect. The recent availability of French designed high frequency vacuum tube amplifiers and quartz crystals of significant size provided more favorable circumstances for new tests. Using quartz as a receiver, signals were detected at distances up to 6 km (3.7 mi).

The use of quartz crystal generators led to spectacular results. At a fundamental frequency of 150 kHz, the output power was estimated at 1 kW. Langevin reported that "fish placed in the beam in the neighborhood of the source ... were killed immediately and certain observers experienced a painful sensation on plunging the hand in this region."[21]

Sandwich Transducers

There then followed a critical invention in ultrasonics. Although the quartz transducers were encouraging, very high voltages were required to drive the systems. Furthermore, there was a limited supply of large quartz crystals. These considerations led Langevin to conceive of the steel quartz steel sandwich, where the overall resonance of the transducer was determined by the thickness of the composite assembly and not just by the quartz thickness.

The design evolved to one comprising several pieces of quartz cemented between steel plates (Fig. 13). The overall assembly had a large ratio of diameter to wavelength and could radiate a narrow beam of sound. These developments led to signals' being returned from a submarine at distances up to 1.5 km (0.9 mi).

FIGURE 13. Langevin's sandwich transducer.

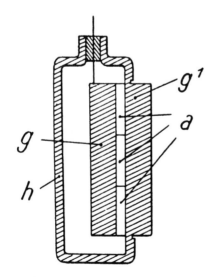

Legend
  a. Quartz.
  g. Steel plate.
  g¹. Steel plate.
  h. Housing.

Despite its tremendous potential, the development of ultrasonic detection came too late in World War I to combat the submarine. However, the science of ultrasonics had advanced greatly. Furthermore, the new discoveries were widely disseminated in the United Kingdom and the United States, so the stage was set for progress after the war.

Early Ultrasonic Nondestructive Testing

Discontinuity Detection

The practical application of ultrasonic technologies developed rapidly in the 1920s. While progress was made in underwater detection systems, whole new areas of use also emerged: piezoelectric resonators for frequency control appeared and the ultrasonic interferometer was invented. In the 1920s, intense ultrasonic waves were used for cavitation, heating, emulsifying and levitation and acoustooptic phenomena were reported.

In about 1929, the use of ultrasonics for material testing was reported. Two researchers, S.Y. Sokolov of the Soviet Union and O. Mühlhauser of Germany, share credit for first applying ultrasound to the nondestructive testing of materials.

Sokolov proposed an ultrasonic through-transmission technique to find hidden discontinuities in metals. Sokolov had started working with the piezoelectric properties of quartz soon after beginning his teaching career at the Leningrad Electro-Technical Institute. By 1929, he headed an acoustics laboratory at the Institute and was investigating a wide range of uses for ultrasonics. Many of Sokolov's concepts in ultrasonics, which were to include microscopy and imaging systems, were far in advance of electronics and optical technology of the 1930s and achieved fruition only after many years had passed.

Mühlhauser (1931) had the first patent in the area of ultrasonic nondestructive testing. Both his and Sokolov's techniques were based on continuous ultrasonic waves and the concept that discontinuities in a material would screen some of the energy from a receiving transducer. Others who contributed in this area of ultrasonics in the 1930s included D.S. Shraiber, F. Kruse, A. Giacomini and A.B. Giacomini.[22,23]

Acoustooptics and Imaging Tubes

Sokolov went on to devise an innovative system for discontinuity detection that used acoustooptic effects. This system transmitted waves through the test object into an illuminated liquid medium. A diffraction pattern was formed, with differences in the pattern being used to distinguish test objects with and without discontinuities. In a further simplification, Sokolov eliminated the diffraction approach and used a light beam reflected from the surface of a liquid insonified by waves transmitted through the test object. This was the original concept of the liquid surface levitation converter and may actually have been proposed by Sokolov as early as 1929.

In yet another pioneering contribution, Sokolov devised an ultrasonic image tube based on the piezoelectric effect. He found that piezoelectric crystals damped on one side do not resonate as a whole when excited at the fundamental frequency. Instead, the crystals resonate point by point in accord with the incident sound energy. Sokolov's patent for this type of testing (Fig. 14) was granted in the United States in 1937.[22]

At about the same time, he also conducted very extensive investigations into the properties of the langevin sandwich transducer. This included

FIGURE 14. United States Patent 2164125 by Sokolov (1937).[22]

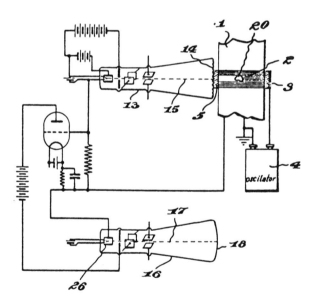

Legend
1. Test block.
2. Acoustic rays.
3. First piezo quartz plate.
4. Generator.
5. Second piezo quartz plate.
13. Cathode ray tube.
14. Small metal electrodes.
15. Electron ray.
16. Second cathode ray tube.
17. Oscillating ray tube.
18. Screen.
20. Gap (artificial discontinuity).
26. Sleeve of second cathode ray tube.

(1) determining the natural frequencies of various configurations from 10 kHz to 130 MHz and (2) the use of a piezoelectric pickup for mapping the distribution of vibration amplitude on the surface of the transducer.

Development of Modern Ultrasonic Testing

Wartime Developments

The decade of the 1940s opened with World War II in progress and saw major developments in the field of ultrasonic nondestructive testing. Many of the new testing techniques were used or refined in wartime production environments.

For example, R. Pohlman developed an image cell using a suspension of aluminum dust in xylene to detect acoustic waves. The small platelets of aluminum oriented themselves with the intensity of acoustic pressure over the face of the cell, thus acting as minute rayleigh disks and presenting an image (Fig. 15). This was incorporated into ultrasonic test systems and used by German industry during World War II. Inspection of shell casings was a particular application.

Continuous Ultrasonic Waves

A distinguishing characteristic of these nondestructive tests was the use of continuous ultrasonic waves. Discontinuity detection was based on a decrease in transmitted acoustic intensity, in much the same way as radiographic testing. This approach had limitations, including the generation of standing waves, lack of acoustic transparency of certain materials and the need to access both material surfaces. There were also sensitivity problems — discontinuities might intercept only a small portion of the transmitted energy and thus cause only a slight change in the received energy.

FIGURE 15. Pohlman's image cell.

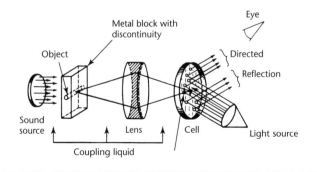

Because ultrasonic pulse echo concepts had been developed in the 1930s for submarine detection (known in the United States as *sonar*), there is little doubt that pulse echo techniques were also considered for nondestructive testing. However, scaling down the sonar concept to measure small time intervals was beyond the capabilities of electronics in the early 1930s.

Work on radar started in 1935, achieved practical use by 1938 and provided opportunities for ultrasonic applications. The electronic developments for pulse echo radar were directly applicable to ultrasonic technology.

Firestone's Discontinuity Detector

In 1940, Floyd Firestone, an associate professor of physics at the University of Michigan, filed application for a patent on a discontinuity detection device and measuring instrument (Fig. 16) that used ultrasonic pulse reflection.[24-26] Firestone had received his early training from acoustic authorities Dayton Miller at Case Western Reserve University and Paul Sabine at the Riverbanks Laboratory of Acoustics and had been working in acoustics for many years at Michigan.

During the 1930s, Firestone was pioneering the mobility technique of analyzing vibrating systems. His pulse echo instrument for ultrasonic testing, called the *Reflectoscope*, eliminated most of the difficulties inherent in a continuous wave system. For example, the sensitivity problem was completely transformed because a discontinuity was shown by the *presence* of a signal rather than by a slight change in a continuous signal level.

Other Discontinuity Detectors

Independently, work was being done in the United Kingdom at the same time, directed by D.O. Sproule of Hughes and Sons, London. In 1940, a subcommittee of the Alloy Steels Research Committee asked the company to examine ultrasonic techniques of discontinuity detection. Continuous wave techniques using a pohlman cell were tried and discarded. By 1942, Sproule devised the pulse echo technique, using separate sending and receiving transducers. For a number of years, dual transducers distinguished the British approach from the American technique where a single transducer was used.[27]

Postwar investigations by the British revealed that Sproule and Firestone were not alone in their developments. F. Kruse in Germany, who at the time of his doctoral thesis in 1938 was discouraged over the prospects of ultrasonic nondestructive testing, had also developed a discontinuity detector similar to the Firestone and Sproule instruments. In 1941, Sokolov also devised a nondestructive test technique involving ultrasonic pulses and pulse frequency modulation concepts. This was based on earlier concepts of E. Heidemann in Berlin and was ultimately used in thickness gaging.

FIGURE 16. United States Patent 2280226 by Firestone for pulse echo ultrasonic testing (1942).[25]

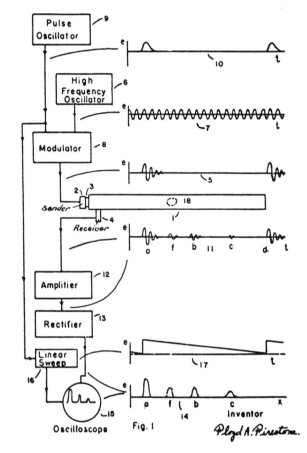

Legend
1. Metal bar (test object).
2. Transmitting piezo crystal.
3. Thin film of oil.
4. Receiving piezo crystal.
5. Graph.
6. High frequency oscillator.
7. Graph.
8. Modulator.
9. Pulse oscillator.
10. Graph.
11. Graph.
12. Linear amplifier.
13. Rectifier.
14. Graph showing indications.
15. Cathode ray oscilloscope.
16. Linear sweep oscillator.
17. Output voltage.
18. Artificial discontinuity.
a. Initial transmitted pulse.
b. First reflected pulse.
c. Second voltage train, from reflected signal.
d. Voltage generated by waves as they pass receiving crystal.
e. Signal (vertical) potential or voltage.
f. Reflection from discontinuity.
t. Time (horizontal).

Pulse Echo Development

Commercial pulse echo ultrasonic test instruments appeared in 1943, with Sperry Products producing the Firestone instrument and Kelvin and Hughes Limited, London, producing the Sproule instrument. Many further contributions were made by Firestone and his coworkers, including (1) transverse wave testing of welds, (2) techniques for damping transducers and (3) in 1946 the use of surface waves in nondestructive testing.

The Krautkrämer brothers developed pulse echo instruments in Germany.[28]

Immersion testing techniques were introduced in 1948 by Donald Erdman. He also pioneered the use of B-scan ultrasonic testing. With Erdman as president, Electrocircuits Company was formed in 1951 to market ultrasonic immersion testing units.[29]

In 1959, there was litigation between Sperry Products and Electrocircuits over numerous claims of the Firestone patents, some as they related to immersion testing. Defense of the Firestone claims involved comparisons with early Langevin developments in depth sounding and Sokolov ultrasonic test techniques of the 1930s.

The techniques of ultrasonic nondestructive testing were soon applied to diverse nonindustrial uses ranging from medical imaging to the measurement of backfat on hogs. By 1955, the pulse echo technique was the dominant ultrasonic test technique.[30]

Other Techniques

Not all ultrasonic testing during the 1940s was with pulse echo techniques. Based on United States Patent 2 431 233 by W.S. Erwin and G.M. Rassweiler, General Motors company in 1947 built an instrument (called the *Sonigage*) which measured resonance in order to gage thickness. Branson Instruments, founded by Norman Branson in 1946, introduced the *Audigage* (under the Erwin patent) and the *Vidigage*, both resonance thickness testers. The Magnaflux Corporation marketed a similar instrument known as the *Sonizon*. Beginning early in the 1950s, these instruments found wide use in applications such as testing of rails, pipe and plate.[31,32]

In another related development, the phenomenon of acoustic emission from metal test objects was documented with observations by W.P. Mason in 1948 and J. Kaiser in 1950. Acoustic emission techniques were broadly developed and soon became important nondestructive test techniques with their own unique applications.[33] Although the field of acoustic holography was years away as a formal discipline, precursors of acoustic holograms were first made in 1950.

Conclusion

Developments in ultrasonics in the years following 1955 have been rapid and extensive. Ultrasonic imaging techniques have greatly progressed and the need to extract exact data from ultrasonics has led to the development of more quantitative test techniques.

Techniques for generation and detection of ultrasound have evolved around lasers and electromagnetic acoustic transducers. The promise of ultrasonics, conceived in the nineteenth century, remains strong as the method continues to develop in the twenty-first century.

PART 4. Measurement Units for Ultrasonic Testing

Origin and Use of International System

In 1960, the General Conference on Weights and Measures established the International System of Units. *Le Systéme International d'Unités* (SI) was designed so that a single set of measurement units could be used by all branches of science, engineering and the general public. Without SI, the *Nondestructive Testing Handbook* series would contain a confusing mix of obsolete centimeter-gram-second (CGS) units, imperial units and the units preferred by certain localities or scientific specialties.

SI is the modern version of the metric system and ends the division between metric units used by scientists and metric units used by engineers and the public. Scientists have given up their units based on centimeter and gram and engineers have abandoned the kilogram-force in favor of the newton. Electrical engineers have retained the ampere, volt and ohm but changed all units related to magnetism.

Table 8 lists the seven SI base units. Table 9 lists derived units with special names. Table 10 gives examples of conversions to SI units. In SI, the unit of time is the second (s) but hour (h) is recognized for use with SI.

For more information, the reader is referred to the information available through national standards organizations and specialized information compiled by technical organizations.[34-37]

TABLE 8. SI base units.

Quantity	Unit	Symbol
Length	meter	m
Mass	kilogram	kg
Time	second	s
Electric current	ampere	A
Temperature	kelvin	K
Amount of substance	mole	mol
Luminous intensity	candela	cd

Multipliers

In science and engineering, very large or very small numbers with units are expressed by using the SI multipliers, prefixes of 10^3 intervals (Table 11). The multiplier becomes a property of the SI unit. For example, a millimeter (mm) is 0.001 meter (m). The preferred volume unit is cubic meter (m^3). The volume unit cubic centimeter (cm^3) is $(0.01\ m)^3$ or $10^{-6}\ m^3$. Unit submultiples such as the centimeter, decimeter, dekameter and hectometer are avoided in scientific and technical uses of SI because of their variance from the convenient 10^3 or 10^{-3} intervals that make equations easy to manipulate.

TABLE 9. SI derived units with special names.[a]

Quantity	Units	Symbol	Relation to Other SI Units[b]
Capacitance	farad	F	$C{\cdot}V^{-1}$
Catalytic activity	katal	kat	$s^{-1}{\cdot}mol$
Conductance	siemens	S	$A{\cdot}V^{-1}$
Energy	joule	J	$N{\cdot}m$
Frequency (periodic)	hertz	Hz	$1{\cdot}s^{-1}$
Force	newton	N	$kg{\cdot}m{\cdot}s^{-2}$
Inductance	henry	H	$Wb{\cdot}A^{-1}$
Illuminance	lux	lx	$lm{\cdot}m^{-2}$
Luminous flux	lumen	lm	$cd{\cdot}sr$
Electric charge	coulomb	C	$A{\cdot}s$
Electric potential[c]	volt	V	$W{\cdot}A^{-1}$
Electric resistance	ohm	Ω	$V{\cdot}A^{-1}$
Magnetic flux	weber	Wb	$V{\cdot}s$
Magnetic flux density	tesla	T	$Wb{\cdot}m^{-2}$
Plane angle	radian	rad	1
Power	watt	W	$J{\cdot}s^{-1}$
Pressure (stress)	pascal	Pa	$N{\cdot}m^{-2}$
Radiation absorbed dose	gray	Gy	$J{\cdot}kg^{-1}$
Radiation dose equivalent	sievert	Sv	$J{\cdot}kg^{-1}$
Radioactivity	becquerel	Bq	$1{\cdot}s^{-1}$
Solid angle	steradian	sr	1
Temperature, celsius	degree celsius	°C	K
Time[a]	hour	h	3600 s
Volume[a]	liter	L	dm^3

a. Hour and liter are not SI units but are accepted for use with the SI.
b. Number one (1) expresses a dimensionless relationship.
c. Electromotive force.

TABLE 10. Examples of conversions to SI units.

Quantity	Measurement in Non-SI Unit	Multiply by	To Get Measurement in SI Unit
Angle	minute (min)	$2.908\,882 \times 10^{-4}$	radian (rad)
	degree (deg)	$1.745\,329 \times 10^{-2}$	radian (rad)
Area	square inch (in.^{2})	645	square millimeter (mm^2)
Distance	angstrom (Å)	0.1	nanometer (nm)
	inch (in.)	25.4	millimeter (mm)
Energy	British thermal unit (BTU)	1.055	kilojoule (kJ)
	calorie (cal), thermochemical	4.184	joule (J)
Power	British thermal unit per hour (BTU·h^{-1})	0.293	watt (W)
Specific heat	British thermal unit per pound degree fahrenheit (BTU·lb$_m^{-1}$·°F^{-1})	4.19	kilojoule per kilogram per kelvin (kJ·kg^{-1}·K^{-1})
Force	pound force	4.448	newton (N)
Torque (couple)	foot-pound (ft-lb$_f$)	1.36	newton meter (N·m)
Pressure	pound force per square inch (lb$_f$·in.$^{-2}$)	6.89	kilopascal (kPa)
Frequency (cycle)	cycle per minute	60^{-1}	hertz (Hz)
Illuminance	footcandle (ftc)	10.76	lux (lx)
	phot (ph)	10 000	lux (lx)
Luminance	candela per square foot (cd·ft^{-2})	10.76	candela per square meter (cd·m^{-2})
	candela per square inch (cd·in.$^{-2}$)	1 550	candela per square meter (cd·m^{-2})
	footlambert (ftl)	3.426	candela per square meter (cd·m^{-2})
	lambert	$3\,183\ (=10\,000 \div \pi)$	candela per square meter (cd·m^{-2})
	nit (nt)	1	candela per square meter (cd·m^{-2})
	stilb (sb)	10 000	candela per square meter (cd·m^{-2})
Radioactivity	curie (Ci)	37	gigabecquerel (GBq)
Ionizing radiation exposure	roentgen (R)	0.258	millicoulomb per kilogram (mC·kg^{-1})
Mass	pound (lb$_m$)	0.454	kilogram (kg)
Temperature (increment)	degree fahrenheit (°F)	0.556	kelvin (K) or degree celsius (°C)
Temperature (scale)	degree fahrenheit (°F)	(°F − 32) ÷ 1.8	degree celsius (°C)
Temperature (scale)	degree fahrenheit (°F)	(°F − 32) ÷ 1.8 + 273.15	kelvin (K)

TABLE 11. SI prefixes and multipliers.

Prefix	Symbol	Multiplier
yotta	Y	10^{24}
zetta	Z	10^{21}
exa	E	10^{18}
peta	P	10^{15}
tera	T	10^{12}
giga	G	10^{9}
mega	M	10^{6}
kilo	k	10^{3}
hecto[a]	h	10^{2}
deka[a]	da	10
deci[a]	d	10^{-1}
centi[a]	c	10^{-2}
milli	m	10^{-3}
micro	μ	10^{-6}
nano	n	10^{-9}
pico	p	10^{-12}
femto	f	10^{-15}
atto	a	10^{-18}
zepto	z	10^{-21}
yocto	y	10^{-24}

a. Avoid these prefixes (except in dm^3 and cm^3) for science and engineering.

In SI, the distinction between upper and lower case letters is meaningful and should be observed. For example, the meanings of the prefix m (milli) and the prefix M (mega) differ by nine orders of magnitude.

Units for Acoustics

Pressure, Displacement and Related Quantities

Acoustic emission is a shock wave inside a stressed material, where a displacement ripples through the material and moves its surface. A transducer on that surface undergoes this displacement as a pressure. The pressure is measured as force per unit area in pascal (Pa), equivalent to newton per square meter (N·m^{-2}). The signal from the transducer is sometimes related to speed (m·s^{-1}), displacement (m) or acceleration (m·s^{-2}).

Properties of piezoelectric transducers are related to electric charge: a pressure on the element creates a charge (measured in coulomb) on the electrodes. A rapidly changing pressure alters the charge fast enough to allow the use of either voltage or charge amplifiers. After this, signal processing may analyze and store data in terms of distance in meter (m), speed in meter per second ($m \cdot s^{-1}$), acceleration in meter per second per second ($m \cdot s^{-2}$), signal strength in volt second ($V \cdot s$), energy in joule (J), signal in volt (V) or power in watt (W).

Radian

The radian (rad) is the international unit for measurement of plane angle and is equal to the angle subtended by an arc from the center of a circle and equal to its radius. The radian is used in theoretical physics. Physical measurements are in degrees. The degree (deg) is approved for use with the International System of Units.

Hertz

Frequencies usually correspond to bandwidths for specific applications. Frequency is measured in hertz (Hz), where 1 Hz equals one cycle per second.

Decibel

The term *loudness* refers to amplitude in audible frequencies. Some acoustic waves are audible; others have frequencies above or below audible frequencies (ultrasonic or subsonic, respectively). A signal at an inaudible frequency has measurable amplitude but is not called *loud* or *soft*.

A customary unit for measuring the amplitude of an acoustic signal is the decibel (dB), one tenth of a bel (B). The decibel is extensively used in acoustics and electronics. The decibel is not a fixed measurement unit but rather expresses a logarithmic ratio between two conditions of the same dimension (such as voltage or energy). In auditory acoustics, an arbitrary sound pressure such as 20 µPa can be used for the reference level of 0 dB. In acoustics, the reference level 0 dB_{AE} is defined as a signal of 1 µV at the transducer before any amplification.

The fundamental decibel is:

$$(1) \quad N_{dB} \;=\; 10 \log_{10} \frac{P}{P_0}$$

where P is the measured power and P_0 is the reference power in watts. The power is a square function of voltage:

$$(2) \quad N_{dB} \;=\; 10 \log_{10} \left(\frac{V}{V_0} \right)^2$$
$$\phantom{(2) \quad N_{dB} } \;=\; 20 \log_{10} \frac{V}{V_0}$$

where V is the measured potential and V_0 is the reference potential in volts.

Bel and decibel are not units in the International System of Units but are accepted for use with that system. There are often two definitions given for the decibel, so voltage decibel is sometimes written *dB(V)*.

References

1. *Nondestructive Testing Handbook,* second edition: Vol. 10, *Nondestructive Testing Overview.* Columbus, OH: American Society for Nondestructive Testing (1996).
2. Wenk, S.A. and R.C. McMaster. *Choosing NDT: Applications, Costs and Benefits of Nondestructive Testing in Your Quality Assurance Program.* Columbus, OH: American Society for Nondestructive Testing (1987).
3. *Nondestructive Testing Methods.* TO33B-1-1 (NAVAIR 01-1A-16) TM1-1500-335-23. Washington, DC: Department of Defense (January 2005).
4. *Nondestructive Testing Handbook,* second edition: Vol. 7, *Ultrasonic Testing.* Columbus, OH: American Society for Nondestructive Testing (1991).
5. *Annual Book of ASTM Standards:* Section 3, *Metals Test Methods and Analytical Procedures.* Vol. 03.03, *Nondestructive Testing.* West Conshohocken, PA: ASTM International (2005).
6. *Recommended Practice No. SNT-TC-1A.* Columbus, OH: American Society for Nondestructive Testing (2001).
7. ANSI/ASNT CP-189, *Standard for Qualification and Certification of Nondestructive Testing Personnel.* Columbus, OH: American Society for Nondestructive Testing (2001).
8. *ASNT Central Certification Program (ACCP),* Revision 4 (March 2005). Columbus, OH: American Society for Nondestructive Testing (2005).
9. ISO 9712, *Non-Destructive Testing — Qualification and Certification of Personnel,* third edition. Geneva, Switzerland: International Organization for Standardization (2005).
10. NFPA 70, *National Electric Code,* 2005 edition. Quincy, MA: National Fire Prevention Association (2005).
11. *National Electrical Safety Code,* 2002 edition. New York, NY: Institute of Electrical and Electronics Engineers (2002).
12. 29 CFR 1910, *Occupational Safety and Health Standards* [*Code of Federal Regulations:* Title 29, *Labor*]. Washington, DC: United States Department of Labor, Occupational Safety and Health Administration; United States Government Printing Office.
13. 29 CFR 1926, *Occupational Safety and Health Standards for the Construction Industry* [*Code of Federal Regulations:* Title 29, *Labor*]. Washington, DC: United States Department of Labor, Occupational Safety and Health Administration; United States Government Printing Office.
14. Graff, K. "Historical Overview of Ultrasonic Test Development." *Nondestructive Testing Handbook,* second edition: Vol. 7, *Ultrasonic Testing.* Columbus, OH: American Society for Nondestructive Testing (1991): p 23-32.
15. Heuter, T. and R. Bolt. *Sonics.* New York, NY: Wiley (1955): p 353.
16. Graff, K. "A History of Ultrasonics." *Physical Acoustics.* Vol. 15. New York, NY: Academic Press (1981): p 1-97.
17. Schuster, A. "Obituary Notice of John William Strutt, Baron Rayleigh, 1842-1919." *Proceedings of the Royal Society, London.* Series A 98 (1920): p i.
18. Cady, W.G. *Piezoelectricity.* New York, NY: McGraw-Hill (1946). New York, NY: Dover (1964).
19. Hunt, F.V. *Electroacoustics.* Cambridge, MA: Harvard University Press (1954).
20. "Oeuvres Scientific de Paul Langevin." Paris, France: Centre National de la Recherche Scientific (1950).
21. Lindsay, R.B. "The Story of Acoustics." *Journal of the Acoustical Society of America.* Vol. 39. New York, NY: Acoustical Society of America (1966): p 630.
22. Sokolov, S. United States Patent 2 164 125, *Means for Indicating Flaws in Materials* (1937).
23. McMaster, R.C. and S.A. Wenk. "A Basic Guide for Management's Choice of Non-Destructive Tests." *Symposium on the Role of Non-Destructive Testing in the Economics of Production.* Special Technical Publication 112. West Conshohocken, PA: ASTM International (1951).

24. Firestone, F. "The Supersonic Reflectoscope, an Instrument for Inspecting the Interior of Solid Parts by Means of Sound Waves." *Journal of the Acoustical Society of America*. Vol. 17, No. 3. New York, NY: Acoustical Society of America (1946): p 287.

25. Firestone, F. United States Patent 2 280 226, *Flaw Detecting Device and Measuring Instrument* (1942).

26. Straw, R. "Do You Hear What I Hear? The Early Days of Pulse-Echo Ultrasonics." *Materials Evaluation*. Vol. 42, No. 1, Columbus, OH: American Society for Nondestructive Testing (January 1984): p 24-28. Erratum, Vol. 42, No. 4 (April 1984): p 382.

27. Desch, C., D. Sproule and W. Dawson. "The Detection of Cracks in Steel by Means of Supersonic Waves." *Welding Journal Research Supplement*. Vol. 26. Miami, FL: American Welding Society (1946): p 6.

28. Krautkrämer, H. "The Founding of a German Ultrasonic Firm." *Materials Evaluation*. Vol. 42, No. 13. Columbus, OH: American Society for Nondestructive Testing (December 1984): p 1554-1559.

29. Moore, P.O. "The Water's Fine: The Origin of Immersion Ultrasonic Testing, 1945-57." *Materials Evaluation*. Vol. 43, No. 1. Columbus, OH: American Society for Nondestructive Testing (January 1985): p 60-66.

30. "Cary E. Hohl and Ultrasonic Testing." *Materials Evaluation*. Vol. 47, No. 5. Columbus, OH: American Society for Nondestructive Testing (May 1989): p 493-495.

31. Erwin, W.S. United States Patent 2 431 233, *Supersonic Measuring Means* (1947).

32. Moore, P.O. "Good Vibrations: The Development of Ultrasonic Resonance Testing, 1944-55." *Materials Evaluation*. Vol. 42, No. 12. Columbus, OH: American Society for Nondestructive Testing (November 1984): p 1450-1454, 1456.

33. Drouillard, T.F. "History of Acoustic Emission Testing." *Nondestructive Testing Handbook*, third edition: Vol. 6, *Acoustic Emission Testing*. Columbus, OH: American Society for Nondestructive Testing (2005): p 21-24.

34. IEEE/ASTM SI 10, *American National Standard for Use of the International System of Units (SI): The Modernized Metric System*. New York, NY: International Institute of Electrical and Electronics Engineers. West Conshohocken, PA: ASTM International (2002).

35. Taylor, B.N. *Guide for the Use of the International System of Units (SI)*. National Institute of Standards and Technology Special Publication 811, 1995 edition. Washington, DC: United States Government Printing Office (1995).

36. Taylor, B.N., ed. *Interpretation of the SI for the United States and Federal Government and Metric Conversion Policy*. NIST Special Publication 814, 1998 edition. Washington, DC: United States Government Printing Office (1998).

37. Taylor, B.N., ed. *The International System of Units (SI)*, 2001 edition. NIST Special Publication 330. Washington DC: United States Government Printing Office (2001).

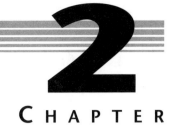

Ultrasonic Wave Propagation[1]

Edmund Henneke, II, Virginia Polytechnic Institute and State University, Blacksburg, Virginia

Dale E. Chimenti, Iowa State University, Ames, Iowa (Part 3)

Part 1. Introduction to Wave Propagation

This chapter describes fundamental concepts necessary to mathematically and physically describe the phenomena of wave propagation. These phenomena are basic to the propagation of ultrasonic waves used for nondestructive testing of materials.

Definition of Wave and Wave Properties

A wave is a disturbance that conveys energy through space in a manner that depends on both position and time. The disturbance can be thought of physically as the amount of displacement of a material point away from its equilibrium position or, when measured using ultrasonic techniques, as the value of the measured signal in volts. The most common example of a wave propagating in one dimension may be represented graphically by Fig. 1 and mathematically by the simple expression:

$$(1) \quad D(x,t) = A \sin(\omega t - kx)$$

where A is the amplitude (volt) of the disturbance, that is, the magnitude of particle displacement signal; $D(x,t)$ is the value of a disturbance in space at some position x and time t; k is the wave

number; and ω is the angular frequency (radians per second).

This simplest wave is often referred to as a *sine wave*. The quantity $(\omega t - kx)$ is called the *phase angle* as its value in radians at a specific location x and time t represents the phase of the sine function.

This elementary mathematical form for a sine wave can be used to define several important properties of a wave: frequency (or period), wavelength (or wave number) and velocity. In the following discussion, *velocity* merely means *speed* and is not a vector. Frequency and wavelength are physical characteristics of the wave represented in Eq. 1 in terms of angular frequency and wave number for mathematical convenience. The frequency is the number of times the wave progresses through one complete oscillation in a unit time, usually taken to be a second. The reciprocal of frequency, or period τ, is often used to describe this wave property. Period is the length of time in seconds that it takes a wave to complete one cycle. The frequency is commonly expressed in cycles per second, called *hertz* (Hz). In Fig. 2a, if each tic mark along the horizontal axis represents

FIGURE 1. Directions of particle vibration: (a) longitudinal wave, also call *pressure wave*, (b) transverse wave, also called *shear wave*.

(a)

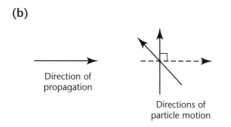

Direction of propagation   Directions of particle motion

(b)

Direction of propagation

Directions of particle motion

FIGURE 2. Harmonic plane wave showing definitions of wavelength, period and velocity: (a) wave 1; (b) wave 2.

(a)

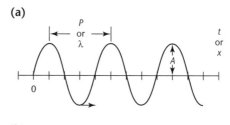

(b)

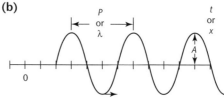

Legend
A = amplitude of sine wave
P = period, used with time axis t
t = time
x = distance axis
λ = wavelength, used with distance axis x

0.1 s, the frequency of the wave shown is 1 cycle per 0.4 s = 2.5 Hz. As shown in Eq. 1, the angular frequency ω is often used instead of frequency, where angular frequency ω is related to wave frequency f:

(2) $\omega = 2\pi f$

The wavelength λ is the distance in space between two successive maxima (or minima, crossings of the X axis with positive slope) of the sine wave. Again referring to Fig. 1, the wave shown has a wavelength, λ = 4 units of distance (in the metric system, the unit of distance is normally meter or a fraction of meter such as millimeter, micrometer or nanometer). Again, as shown in Eq. 1, rather than using wavelength, the concept of wave number is often used. The wave number k is the number of wavelengths λ contained in unit distance scaled by the factor 2π:

(3) $k = \dfrac{2\pi}{\lambda}$

When an ultrasonic wave propagates through a material, you can imagine sitting at a material point inside the medium and feeling a vibratory motion as the wave passes by. To follow this motion through one cycle of the wave, initially you are at a static equilibrium position (ignoring thermal motion). As the wave begins to pass by, you will begin to be displaced or moved away from equilibrium in a positive direction. Then, 0.1 s later, you will have been displaced a maximum amplitude A away from equilibrium. As time progresses, you move back toward the equilibrium position until, 0.2 s after time zero, you have returned to the starting point. As time continues, you continue to move beyond in the negative direction. Then, 0.1 s later (0.3 s after time zero) you have reached a maximum displacement in the negative direction, –A. The next 0.1 s finds you once again returning to equilibrium until, 0.4 s after time zero, you have returned to the starting point once again and are ready to begin the cycle all over again. For the wave shown in Fig. 2, 2.5 of these cycles will be completed in 1 s because the frequency for this wave is 2.5. (Or in terms of period, it will take you 0.4 s to complete one cycle, so τ = 0.40 s.)

The wavelength and the frequency are directly related to another important wave property — *phase velocity*. The phase velocity of a wave is the speed at which a specific point or phase on the wave (for simplicity, think about the maximum positive amplitude) propagates through the material. In simple terms, returning to imagining that you are sitting at a material point and your colleague is sitting at another material point a distance x away in the positive x direction — the phase velocity would be the speed with which the maximum displacement A propagates from you to your colleague. If t is the time it takes the maximum displacement to reach your colleague after passing by you, then the phase speed v is:

(4) $v = \dfrac{x}{t} = \dfrac{\lambda}{\tau} = f\lambda = \dfrac{\omega}{k}$

That is, the phase velocity is simply the distance x traveled in time t by a phase point (such as the maximum displacement) and this speed can also be found by dividing the wavelength (the distance between two successive maxima) by the period of the wave (the time it takes for the wave to complete one cycle of motion). The other expressions for phase velocity follow immediately from the respective definitions for frequency, angular frequency and wave number.

Waves having a form more complex than a simple sine function, including those typically used in nondestructive testing, may be represented within certain limits as finite or infinite sums of sine waves differing by finite phase angles (such sums are required mathematically to represent periodic waves) or as an infinite sum (that is, an integral mathematical form) of sine waves differing by infinitesimal phase angles (the mathematical form necessary to represent nonperiodic waves). Examples are shown in Fig. 3.

Because any wave can be represented mathematically as a sum or integral of sine waves, it suffices for this discussion

FIGURE 3. General forms of waves: (a) finite sum of sine waves (periodic wave); (b) infinite number of sine waves varying by infinitesimally close frequencies (wave pulse).

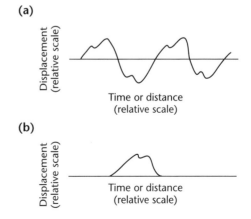

(a)

Displacement (relative scale)

Time or distance (relative scale)

(b)

Displacement (relative scale)

Time or distance (relative scale)

to consider the propagation of a sine wave in the form of Eq. 1 (or a completely equivalent form in three-dimensional space). In the following text, only forms equivalent to Eq. 1 are considered.

Other important concepts of wave propagation need to be introduced. Returning to Fig. 3, two types of waves are shown: a periodic wave and a nonperiodic wave. A periodic wave is one that reproduces itself repetitively after a certain time period τ. As already noted, a periodic wave can be represented by a finite or infinite sum of sine waves differing from each other by a finite difference in their phase angle $(\omega t - kx)$. Each phase angle can be represented by $n(\omega_n t - k_n x)$ where n is an integer. Each wave will have a different angular frequency ω_n and a different wave number k_n. As already noted, the phase velocity of each sine wave is equal to $(\omega_n \cdot k_n^{-1})$.

A nonperiodic wave might be continuous in time and space (something in appearance like Fig. 3a except that there will be no successive repetition of the form of the wave) or a pulse which has a finite length as in Fig. 3b. Most ultrasonic testing is performed using a pulse form. The pulse itself will travel through space at a wave speed known as the *group velocity*, so called simply because the pulse is composed of a sum (or group) of individual sine waves. Each of these sine waves propagates through the material and continue to sum together to form the pulse. The wave pulse form can be thought of as the sum of each of these individual sine waves at any specific time. The group velocity can be shown mathematically to be equivalent to $d\omega \cdot (dk)^{-1}$, that is, the derivative of the angular frequency with respect to the wave number.

Theoretically, a material that is strictly linear elastic (that is, the relationship between stress and strain is linear and elastic) can be shown to have a linear relationship between the angular frequency and the wave number, such that $\omega = c \cdot k$, where c is a constant. Hence, $\omega \cdot k^{-1} = d\omega \cdot (dk)^{-1} = c$ for linear elastic materials; the phase velocity and the group velocity are identical for linear elastic materials.

Although many materials of engineering interest can be approximated as linear elastic, none of these materials is *exactly* linear elastic. All real materials possess the property of having a nonlinear relationship between angular frequency and wave number and the phase speed and group speeds are *not* equal although the values may be close in value (differing perhaps only in the first or second decimal place). That is, $\omega_n \cdot k_n^{-1}$ for a given sine wave numbered n will have a different phase speed from the $(n + 1)$st

sine wave, or the $(n + 2)$nd sine wave, and so on.

For pulse waveforms, then, each sine wave combined to form the shape of the pulse at a specific instant of time t_0 will at a later instant of time t have traveled to a different point in space because each sine wave composing the pulse has a different phase speed. Thus, at time t, the sine waves will add together to form a new, different shape of the pulse. If the speed at which each individual sine wave propagates is known, this new envelope shape of the pulse can be calculated. If the shape of a pulse changes in form as the wave propagates, the material is called *dispersive*. Mathematically, a material is said to be dispersive if the angular frequency depends nonlinearly on the wave number or, equivalently, if the phase velocity and group velocity are unequal.

Other phenomena involving the interaction of waves in various media are of interest to nondestructive testing. When a wave interacts with a material boundary such as an internal surface bounding on a discontinuity or an external surface, part of the wave will scatter or reflect, depending on the size of the boundary relative to the wavelength of the incident wave. If the boundary is large in comparison with the wavelength of the incident wave, the wave will be reflected from the boundary. The angle of reflection is equal to the angle of incidence, just as with the reflection of light. If the boundary is much smaller than the wavelength, the wave is *scattered*, that is, some portion of the wave energy is reflected in all directions. A major portion of the wave will pass through the small object, the relative amount depending on the relative size of the wavelength and boundary of the object and on the relative difference of the acoustic properties (fundamentally related to the relative wave speeds) of the material and the object. For nondestructive testing, often the scattered or reflected wave can be detected and its energy content or its time of arrival relative to that of the incident wave can be used to interpret the size and location of the reflecting or scattering surface. This information is obviously critical to the detection of internal discontinuities.

When the boundary between two different materials is large compared to the wavelength of the incident wave, some portion of energy of the wave will be reflected at the boundary and some portion of energy will be *refracted*, that is, transmitted with a change in propagation direction into the second material. The refraction angle, or change in propagation direction, is related to the incident angle and the ratio of the phase velocities of the two materials.

As a wave propagates in any material, a variety of inelastic mechanisms remove energy from the wave and the wave is said to *attenuate*. Eventually the attenuation of the wave will decrease its energy to a level that cannot be detected. The attenuation of a wave is often measured by the attenuation coefficient α such that the amplitude as a function of time can be written $A(t) = A_0 e^{-\alpha t}$ where A_0 is the displacement of the wave at time $t = 0$.

Types of Waves

Plane Waves

In three dimensions, it is necessary to consider a wave propagating in a direction described by the direction of propagation relative to the chosen three-dimensional axes: X, Y and Z. In this case, Eq. 1 is written in the more general form:

$$(5) \quad u(x,y,z,t) = \left(A_x \boldsymbol{i} + A_y \boldsymbol{j} + A_z \boldsymbol{k}\right) \\ \times \cos\left(k_x x + k_y y + k_z z - \omega t\right)$$

where $A_x \boldsymbol{i}$, $A_y \boldsymbol{j}$ and $A_z \boldsymbol{k}$ are the amplitudes of the components of the disturbance in the X, Y and Z directions, respectively; k_x, k_y and k_z are the components of a wave vector in three dimensions; and $\boldsymbol{u}$ is the disturbance at point (x,y,z) and time t.

The wave vector $\boldsymbol{k}$ is the three-dimensional analog of the wave number k. The wave vector has a magnitude k (which is the wave number of the wave and equal to the reciprocal of the wavelength λ times 2π) pointing in a direction in space in which the wave is propagating. All other quantities have the same definitions given above for the one-dimensional wave. Waves of the form given by Eq. 5 are called *plane waves*. In three-dimensions, a plane wave is a disturbance that has the same phase describing a plane in space. The phase of a wave is a particular value of the angle argument of the sine function. Mathematically, this means that a constant value of phase is the equation of a plane:

$$(6) \quad k_x x + k_y y + k_z z - \omega t = \phi$$

where ϕ is a constant value of an angle.

Two types, or modes, of plane waves will propagate in isotropic, elastic solids — longitudinal or transverse waves. Longitudinal waves propagate such that the particle disturbance in the solid material vibrates parallel to the direction of wave propagation (Fig. 4). Longitudinal modes are also called *dilational* or *irrotational*. Longitudinal waves are

identical to sound waves that travel through the atmosphere or any gas — as they propagate, local volume changes caused by compression and rarefaction of small material volumes occur (hence the term *dilational*). Transverse waves propagate such that the particle disturbance in the solid material vibrates in a direction perpendicular to the direction of wave propagation (Fig. 4). Transverse waves are also called *shear* or *equivoluminal*. Transverse waves are identical to the vibration motion of a plucked string (such as on a violin or guitar.) For plucked strings, the wave travels along the string, causing vibration of the string particles in a direction perpendicular to the string. Transverse modes do not cause local changes in volume as they propagate.

Spherical Waves

Distinguished from plane waves, spherical waves are described by a disturbance that has a particular value of phase on a spherical surface in three-dimensional space. If the wave is spherically symmetric, it may be mathematically represented as:

$$(7) \quad u(r,t) = \frac{A}{r} \cos\left(k_r r - \omega t\right)$$

where k_r is the wave vector in the radial direction and r is the radial distance (meter) from the origin.

Surface Waves

Surface waves are constrained to propagate along the surface of a solid or liquid surface. Their energy is concentrated in a relatively small region about one wavelength or so deep near the

FIGURE 4. Path of a point on the surface displaced by the passage of rayleigh surface wave.

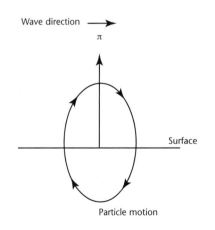

surface. The disturbance of a surface wave can be represented mathematically by multiplying the amplitude of the wave by a factor that causes the amplitude to decay, or attenuate, in a direction perpendicular to the surface (see the discussion of rayleigh waves elsewhere in this volume).

Propagation in Anisotropic Materials

All metals and alloys are crystalline materials, that is, their atoms or molecules occupy a symmetric, defined position in space under thermodynamic equilibrium conditions. Most such materials used in engineering structures are elastically isotropic because they are composed of a very large number of randomly oriented, small crystals. Elastically isotropic means that their elastic properties are the same in all directions. Some modern day engineering structural materials, such as advanced composites or specially prepared single-crystal alloys, are especially designed and used in engineering structures to take advantage of their elastic anisotropic properties. For example, an advanced composite material composed of unidirectional single fibers is much stiffer elastically in the direction parallel to the fibers than it is perpendicular to the fiber direction. The stiffness parallel to the fiber direction can be five to fifteen times greater than that perpendicular to the fiber direction. The difference in mechanical properties as a function of direction has a dramatic effect on wave propagation. In anisotropic materials, three distinct wave modes can propagate. These modes are distinct in that each of the three propagates with a different phase speed. Each of these waves also has a distinct direction of particle vibration motion. Normally, one of these waves will have a vibration disturbance that is nearly parallel to the direction of propagation (and therefore called the *quasilongitudinal* mode) whereas the other two modes have particle vibration directions that are nearly perpendicular to the direction of propagation (and are called the *quasi transverse* modes). The three directions of particle displacements are always mutually perpendicular to each other, just as the three coordinate axes of a three-dimensional coordinate system are mutually perpendicular. The quasilongitudinal mode travels with a phase speed that is almost always the fastest of the three modes.

Another interesting effect of anisotropy on wave propagation is that the group velocity of the wave will travel in a direction different than the direction of propagation. This can lead to reflection from a surface that one might think is parallel to the direction of wave propagation, for example when an ultrasonic test is performed on a cylindrical test object. When an ultrasonic transducer is placed on the end of the test object, the wave is usually expected to propagate along the axis of the test object (as always happens for isotropic materials) and to have little or no interaction with the side wall of the test object. For an anisotropic material, the deviation of the group velocity from the direction of propagation, which will still be down the axis of the material, can cause reflection from the side wall.

Mathematical study of wave propagation in anisotropic materials leads to many interesting observations but is beyond the scope of this chapter.

PART 2. Wave Propagation in Isotropic Materials

Plane Body Waves

An infinite medium containing a linear, elastic, homogeneous isotropic material has a constitutive equation (a relation between stresses and strains in the material):

$$(8) \quad \sigma_{xx} = (\lambda + 2\mu)\epsilon_{xx} + \lambda\left(\epsilon_{yy} + \epsilon_{zz}\right)$$

$$(9) \quad \sigma_{yy} = (\lambda + 2\mu)\epsilon_{yy} + \lambda\left(\epsilon_{xx} + \epsilon_{zz}\right)$$

$$(10) \quad \sigma_{zz} = (\lambda + 2\mu)\epsilon_{zz} + \lambda\left(\epsilon_{xx} + \epsilon_{yy}\right)$$

$$(11) \quad \sigma_{yz} = \sigma_{zy} = 2\mu\epsilon_{yz} = 2\mu\epsilon_{zy}$$

$$(12) \quad \sigma_{zx} = \sigma_{xz} = 2\mu\epsilon_{zx} = 2\mu\epsilon_{xz}$$

$$(13) \quad \sigma_{xy} = \sigma_{yx} = 2\mu\epsilon_{xy} = 2\mu\epsilon_{yx}$$

where positive ϵ_{ij} represents components of strains, σ_{ij} represents components of stresses and λ and μ are Lamé's constants. This form is commonly called *Hooke's law*. Lamé's constants are materials constants related to Young's modulus E and Poisson's ratio ν by the relations:

$$(14) \quad \lambda = \frac{E\nu}{(1 + \nu)(1 - 2\nu)}$$

$$(15) \quad \mu = \frac{E}{2(1 + \nu)}$$

The governing differential equation is the equation of motion for a continuum:

$$(16) \quad \frac{\partial\sigma_{xx}}{\partial x} + \frac{\partial\sigma_{xy}}{\partial y} + \frac{\partial\sigma_{xz}}{\partial z} = \rho\frac{\partial^2 u_x}{\partial^2 t}$$

$$(17) \quad \frac{\partial\sigma_{xy}}{\partial x} + \frac{\partial\sigma_{yy}}{\partial y} + \frac{\partial\sigma_{yz}}{\partial z} = \rho\frac{\partial^2 u_y}{\partial^2 t}$$

$$(18) \quad \frac{\partial\sigma_{xz}}{\partial x} + \frac{\partial\sigma_{yz}}{\partial y} + \frac{\partial\sigma_{zz}}{\partial z} = \rho\frac{\partial^2 u_z}{\partial^2 t}$$

where u_x, u_y and u_z are the components of the particle displacement vector and where body forces are neglected.

Consider a plane wave of the form:

$$(19) \quad u_x = A_x \cos\left(k_x x + k_y y + k_z z - \omega t\right)$$

$$(20) \quad u_y = A_y \cos\left(k_x x + k_y y + k_z z - \omega t\right)$$

$$(21) \quad u_z = A_z \cos\left(k_x x + k_y y + k_z z - \omega t\right)$$

where A_x, A_y and A_z are the components of the amplitude of the displacement; k_x, k_y and k_z are the components of the wave vector; and ω is the angular frequency (radian per second).

These parameters have the same physical and mathematical meaning as the corresponding terms for the one-dimensional case discussed in the introduction. The wave vector, in fact, has a magnitude equal to the wave number k:

$$(22) \quad k = \sqrt{k_x^2 + k_y^2 + k_z^2}$$

where the wave number and the frequency are related to the phase speed of the wave by the relation:

$$(23) \quad v = \frac{k}{\omega}$$

Other physical and mathematical importance is attached to the wave vector. The components (k_x, k_y, k_z) are the components of a vector to the plane of equal phase points. The wave travels through space so that the plane of equal phase points moves so as to remain parallel to itself. For this reason, the wave vector describes the direction of wave propagation. Often, a unit vector **v** is defined by the relation:

$$(24) \quad \mathbf{k} = k\mathbf{v}$$

Here, v is the direction of wave propagation and the magnitude of the k is the wave number, as stated above.

With some mathematical manipulation, the relations between strain and displacements (Eqs. 25 to 30) can be used to obtain the three-dimensional wave equation:

$$(25) \quad \epsilon_{xx} = \frac{\partial u_x}{\partial x}$$

$$(26) \quad \epsilon_{yy} = \frac{\partial u_y}{\partial y}$$

$$(27) \quad \epsilon_{zz} = \frac{\partial u_z}{\partial z}$$

$$(28) \quad \epsilon_{xy} = \frac{1}{2}\left(\frac{\partial u_x}{\partial y} + \frac{\partial u_y}{\partial x}\right)$$

$$(29) \quad \epsilon_{yz} = \frac{1}{2}\left(\frac{\partial u_y}{\partial z} + \frac{\partial u_z}{\partial y}\right)$$

$$(30) \quad \epsilon_{zx} = \frac{1}{2}\left(\frac{\partial u_z}{\partial x} + \frac{\partial u_x}{\partial z}\right)$$

The three-dimensional wave equation governs wave propagation through the prescribed linear, elastic, homogeneous, isotropic material:

$$(31) \quad (\lambda+\mu)\frac{\partial \Delta}{\partial x} + \mu\nabla^2 u_x = \rho\frac{\partial^2 u_x}{\partial t^2}$$

$$(32) \quad (\lambda+\mu)\frac{\partial \Delta}{\partial y} + \mu\nabla^2 u_y = \rho\frac{\partial^2 u_y}{\partial t^2}$$

$$(33) \quad (\lambda+\mu)\frac{\partial \Delta}{\partial z} + \mu\nabla^2 u_z = \rho\frac{\partial^2 u_z}{\partial t^2}$$

where Δ is the volume dilation of the displacements given by the sum of the normal strains:

$$(34) \quad \Delta = \epsilon_{xx} + \epsilon_{yy} + \epsilon_{zz}$$

and ∇^2 is the laplacian operator, defined by the following set of derivatives:

$$(35) \quad \nabla^2 = \frac{\partial^2}{\partial x^2} + \frac{\partial^2}{\partial y^2} + \frac{\partial^2}{\partial z^2}$$

The assumed particle displacements (Eqs. 19 to 21) are substituted into Eqs. 31 to 33. Then, the resulting values of ϵ_{ij} are substituted into Hooke's law (Eqs. 8 to 13) to obtain expressions for the stress components. Finally, these expressions for the stress components are substituted into the differential equations of motion for the material (Eqs. 16 to 18). The resulting equations are algebraic and are known as *Christoffel's equations.*

$$(36) \quad \left[(\lambda+\mu)v_x v_x + \left(\mu-\rho v^2\right)\right]A_x + (\lambda+\mu)v_x v_y A_y + (\lambda+\mu)v_x v_z A_z = 0$$

$$(37) \quad (\lambda+\mu)v_y v_x A_x + \left[(\lambda+\mu)v_y v_y + \left(\mu-\rho v^2\right)A_y\right] + (\lambda+\mu)v_y v_z A_z = 0$$

$$(38) \quad (\lambda+\mu)v_z v_x A_x + (\lambda+\mu)v_z v_y A_y + \left[(\lambda+\mu)v_z v_z + \left(\mu-\rho v^2\right)A_z\right] = 0$$

These equations are homogeneous in the variable v^2. If there is a nontrivial (nonzero) solution for v^2, then the determinant of the coefficients of these equations must be zero. The determinant shown as Eq. 39 (see below) provides the values of wave speeds that can propagate in the given material. Mathematically and physically, it can be shown that Eq. 39 always has real and positive roots, so that there are always three real values of phase speed that are solutions to Christoffel's equations.

$$(39) \quad \begin{vmatrix} Lv_x v_x + (\mu-\rho)v^2 & Lv_x v_y & Lv_x v_z \\ Lv_y v_x & Lv_y v_y + (\mu-\rho)v^2 & Lv_y v_z \\ Lv_z v_x & Lv_z v_y & Lv_z v_z + (\mu-\rho)v^2 \end{vmatrix} = 0$$

where L is the sum of Lamé's constants λ and μ.

For isotropic materials, two of the roots of Eq. 39 are always equal so that there are only two distinct values of wave speeds that can propagate in an isotropic medium. The values of these roots are:

$$(40) \quad v_L = \sqrt{\frac{\lambda + 2\mu}{\rho}}$$

$$(41) \quad v_T = \sqrt{\frac{\mu}{\rho}}$$

If these roots are substituted for phase speed v in the set of homogeneous equations (Eqs. 36 to 38), the corresponding directions of particle displacement vectors that can propagate with the two distinct wave speeds are found. The first root has particle displacements always parallel to the wave vector. This mode is called *longitudinal* (because of the parallel relation between the particle displacement and the direction of propagation), *dilational* (because it is associated with the dilation or volume change that occurs locally as the wave passes through a region) or *irrotational* (because the displacement field has no rotation field).

The second root is the double root of the determinant equation. The corresponding particle displacement vector is a solution to Eq. 35 for this value of phase speed and can be shown to lie in any direction in the plane perpendicular to the wave vector. For this reason, this mode is called the *transverse mode*. Transverse mode is also referred to as *shear* (because the strain field associated with it is pure shear), *distortional* (for the same reason) or *equivoluminal* (because there is no local volume change as the wave propagates through a region).

The longitudinal wave always propagates at a speed faster than the transverse mode because both λ and μ are always positive. Typical wave speed values are given in Table 1.

Surface Waves

Rayleigh Waves

It has been observed experimentally in a variety of applications that large amplitude waves propagate in solid materials along the bounding surfaces. These waves are constrained to lie near the surface and hence expand in only two dimensions. Because of this fact, the effect of these waves can be felt at greater distances from the wave source than the three-dimensional body plane waves in the discussion of wave properties, above.

TABLE 1. Acoustic parameters of typical materials.

Material	Velocity (km·s⁻¹)		Longitudinal Acoustic Impedance (10^6 kg·m⁻²·s)	Wavelength for Longitudinal Wave at 10 MHz (mm)	Density (10^3 kg·m⁻³)
	V_L	V_T			
Metals					
Aluminum uranium alloy	6.35	3.10	17.2	0.635	2.71
Aluminum, galvanized	6.25	3.10	17.5	0.625	2.80
Beryllium	12.80	8.71	23.3	1.28	1.82
Brass (naval)	4.43	2.12	36.1	0.443	8.1
Bronze, phosphor (5 percent)	3.53	2.23	31.2	0.353	8.86
Copper	4.66	2.26	41.8	0.466	8.9
Lead, pure	2.16	0.70	24.6	0.216	11.4
Lead, antimony (6 percent)	2.16	0.81	23.6	0.216	10.90
Magnesium	5.79	3.10	10.1	0.579	1.74
Mercury	1.42	—	18.5	0.142	13.00
Molybdenum	6.29	3.35	63.5	0.629	10.09
Nickel	5.63	2.96	49.5	0.563	8.8
Nickel chromium alloy (wrought)	7.82	3.02	64.5	0.782	8.25
Molybdenum alloy (wrought)	6.02	2.72	53.1	0.602	8.83
Silver nickel (18 percent)	4.62	2.32	40.3	0.462	8.75
Steel	5.85	3.23	45.6	0.585	7.8
Stainless steel, austenitic	5.66	3.12	45.5	0.566	8.03
Stainless steel, martensitic	7.39	2.99	56.7	0.739	7.67
Titanium	6.10	3.12	27.7	0.610	4.54
Tungsten	5.18	2.87	99.8	0.518	19.25
Nonmetals					
Acrylic resin	2.67	1.12	3.2	0.264	1.18
Air	0.33	—	0.00033	0.033	0.001
Fused quartz	5.93	3.75	13.0	0.593	2.20
Ice	3.98	1.99	4.0	0.398	1
Oil (transformer)	1.38	—	1.27	0.138	0.92
Plate glass	5.77	3.43	14.5	0.577	2.51
Heat resistant glass	5.57	3.44	12.4	0.557	2.23
Quartz (natural)	5.73	—	15.2	0.573	2.65
Water	1.49	—	1.49	0.149	1.00

As an example of two-dimensional spreading, it is often observed that the major damage following an earthquake is caused by waves that propagate at velocities slightly slower than the phase speed of the transverse body wave. To model these waves mathematically, Rayleigh suggested that they be represented by the following equations:

$$(42) \quad u_x = A_1 e^{-\alpha z} \cos(ky - \omega t)$$

$$(43) \quad u_y = A_2 e^{-\alpha z} \cos(ky - \omega t)$$

$$(44) \quad u_z = A_3 e^{-\alpha z} \cos(ky - \omega t)$$

where A_1, A_2 and A_3 are the amplitudes of the displacement field associated with the wave and α is an attenuation factor.

The attenuation factor causes the wave amplitude to decay as the observer moves away from the boundary into the interior of the body (that is, in the positive Z direction) and the wave is assumed to be propagating along the boundary of an isotropic material in the direction of the Y axis. The value of alpha must be positive for the wave to be constrained to lie near the surface of the material; otherwise, the wave amplitude increases as the wave enters the material. The meanings of k and ω are the same as for the body waves in the discussion of plane body waves, above.

The wave having displacements given in Eqs. 42 to 44 must satisfy the equations of motion (Eqs. 31 to 33) and must satisfy the boundary conditions along the surface of the material. If the surface is a free surface, a good approximation for ultrasonic work in the laboratory, the stresses on the surface must be zero. At $z = 0$:

$$(45) \quad \sigma_{xz} = \sigma_{yz} = \sigma_{zz} = 0$$

At ultrasonic frequencies in the megahertz region and above, sound waves attenuate rapidly in air. Ultrasonic waves traveling in solid material almost totally reflect at a boundary with air. For all practical purposes, the wave is constrained to remain in the solid and the boundary is considered to be in free space. Thus, the assumption of zero stresses on the boundary is very reasonable.

When the assumed surface wave displacements (Eqs. 42 to 44) are substituted into the equation of motion, it is found that two possible modes may propagate with the following wave characteristics. For mode 1:

$$(46a) \quad \alpha_1 = k\sqrt{1 - \frac{v^2}{v_L^2}}$$

and:

$$(46b) \quad \frac{A_z}{A_y} = \frac{ia_1}{k}$$

and:

$$(46c) \quad A_x = 0$$

For mode 2:

$$(47a) \quad \alpha_2 = k\sqrt{1 - \frac{v^2}{v_T^2}}$$

and:

$$(47b) \quad \frac{A_z}{A_y} = \frac{ik}{\alpha_2}$$

and:

$$(47c) \quad A_x = \text{not set}$$

When a wave with these characteristics is used to attempt to satisfy the stress free boundary equations, it is found that the equations cannot be identically equal to zero unless the amplitude of the wave itself is zero. Because experimental observation says that such waves do indeed exist, the mathematical modeling must be adjusted to find an equation that predicts more of the wave characteristics, particularly the phase speed and particle displacement direction of the wave.

Rayleigh suggested that both mode 1 and mode 2 must be present simultaneously. When they are assumed to be so, the net displacement field is the sum of the two surface wave modes. Then, if the boundary conditions of zero stress are to be satisfied, the following additional characteristics must be true for the surface (rayleigh) waves. That is, on substituting the sum of the particle displacements of the two modes into the boundary equations, the following conditions must be true on the boundary: (1) A_1 must be zero for mode 2 and (2) the phase speed v_R of the rayleigh wave must satisfy the equation:

$$(48) \quad \left[\frac{v_R^2}{v_T^2}\right]^3 - 8\left[\frac{v_R^2}{v_T^2}\right]^2 + 8(3 - 2\gamma^2)\left[\frac{v_R^2}{v_T^2}\right] - 16(1 - \gamma^2) = 0$$

where:

(49) $\gamma = \dfrac{v_T}{v_L} = \dfrac{1-2v}{2(1-v)}$

It can be shown that Eq. 48 must have a solution for $n_R \cdot v_T^{-1}$ that lies between zero and one. Thus, $n_R < v_T < v_L$ and the attenuation coefficients for both modes are therefore real and positive. Hence, the surface wave has the desired characteristics observed experimentally: (1) the phase speed must be less than the transverse body wave speed v_T and (2) the attenuation coefficient is positive, thus constraining the propagating wave to lie in the vicinity of the bounding surface of the solid.

For a material with Poisson's ratio v having a value of 0.25, the phase speed of the rayleigh surface is $0.91940\ n_T$ and the corresponding values of α are:

(50) $\alpha_1 = 0.84754\ k$

(51) $\alpha_2 = 0.3933\ k$

Note that the higher the frequency of the surface wave, the larger is the value of the wave number k (the wave number varies inversely with the wavelength) and the greater is the value of the attenuation coefficients. Physically, this means that higher frequency waves are constrained to lie closer to the surface of the solid than lower frequency waves. Thus, by varying the frequency of the surface wave used in an ultrasonic test, material properties may be determined at varying depths in the material.

The particle displacement associated with the rayleigh wave has components in both the Y and the Z directions. Hence, rayleigh waves cannot be classified as longitudinal or transverse. Rather, rayleigh waves have a combination of the motions associated with longitudinal and transverse waves. Particle displacement on the surface of the test object moves through an elliptical path as one complete cycle of the wave passes a point on the surface (Fig. 4). This motion is similar to the path followed by a buoy floating on the surface of a lake as a water surface wave passes. The normalized longitudinal and transverse displacements for a plane rayleigh surface wave are shown as a function of depth in the material in Fig. 5.

FIGURE 5. Normalized longitudinal $\hat{U}$ and transverse $\hat{W}$ displacements as function of depth for plane rayleigh surface wave. Solid curves indicate poisson ratio of 0.34; dashed curves indicate poisson ratio of 0.25.

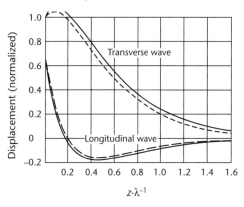

Legend
$\hat{U}_R$ = longitudinal displacement of rayleigh wave
$\hat{W}_R$ = transverse displacement of rayleigh wave
$\hat{W}_{DR}$ = transverse depth
z = depth in Z direction
λ = wavelength

PART 3. Extensions to Other Types of Surface Waves

Leaky Rayleigh Waves

Planar Fluid-to-Solid Geometry

An important extension of the simple geometry analyzed above is the case of a solid half space mechanically coupled to a fluid half space. In this circumstance, the boundary conditions of Eq. 45 must be modified to account for continuity of the normal stress component σ_{zz}. In addition, a wave potential must be introduced for the acoustic wave in the fluid. The text below details the physical behavior of a surface wave under these conditions.

A plane rayleigh surface wave propagating on a half space in contact with a fluid couples its vertical displacements to the fluid medium through the normal stress boundary condition. This periodic particle motion in the fluid can lead, under favorable circumstances, to the excitation of an acoustic wave in the fluid leaving the surface at an angle determined by Snell's law. That is, the X components of the two wave vectors (surface and acoustic wave) are identical. Another way to visualize the situation is to imagine the surface wave crests to be associated with a particular phase point on the acoustic wave. At some instant of time, the phase difference between successive points along the acoustic wave vector is 2π, if the angle at which this wave leaves the solid surface is given by $\sin^{-1}(v_f \cdot v_R^{-1})$, where v_f is the fluid wave speed and the angle is measured from the surface normal.

Time reversal invariance implies the existence of the inverse phenomenon, namely the generation of rayleigh surface waves by means of an acoustic beam incident on the fluid-to-solid interface at the angle indicated above, called the *rayleigh angle*. The two effects combine to produce an apparent displacement and distortion of the reflected beam, characteristic of this type of acoustic surface wave interaction. First reported in 1950,[2] this effect has since been explained in full theoretical detail.[3] Numerous experimental studies have also been carried out.[4-8]

The surface wave is radiation damped by the leakage of energy into the acoustic mode — hence the name *leaky waves*. For elastically soft materials such as plastics (polymethyl methacrylate, for instance), the rayleigh wave speed lies below the acoustic velocity of water. In this case, no radiation damping of a rayleigh wave on the plastic surface occurs and the radiation angle calculated from the expression above is purely imaginary. Although there is particle displacement in the fluid near the interface, the incipient wave is evanescent and carries no energy into the fluid.

The typical behavior observed in such studies is indicated schematically in Fig. 6. An incident beam of ultrasound strikes the fluid-to-solid interface at the rayleigh angle. The ensuing reflected field is characterized by (1) a displacement of the beam weight center along the propagation direction and (2) a redistribution of acoustic energy into two main lobes (Fig. 6). These lobes are separated by a null zone resulting from a phase difference between portions of the reflected field. Beyond this region is a trailing field in which the amplitude decreases exponentially with propagation distance. For comparison, a specular reflection (ignoring diffraction) is shown as dashed lines in Fig. 6.

One approach to solving this problem[3] assumes that the main contribution to the reflected field arises from a simple pole of the reflection coefficient lying in the complex wave vector plane and

FIGURE 6. Typical geometry for leaky wave studies: transducer position or frequency may be varied. Dashed lines indicate specular reflection. When a leaky wave is present, sound energy is concentrated in shaded regions with trailing exponential decay. The null zone is a region of phase cancellation.

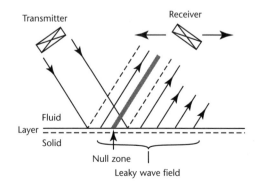

corresponding to the solution of Eq. 48 generalized to include the fluid. By integrating analytically over the product of reflection coefficient and incident beam profile, an expression is obtained for the reflected field in terms of rational and tabulated functions:

$$(52) \quad F = F_{SP} + F_{LW}$$

$$(53) \quad F_{SP}(x,z) = -\Gamma_0 \frac{e^{\left(\frac{-x^2}{a_r^2}\right)}}{\sqrt{\eta}\, a_r \cos\theta}$$
$$\times\; e^{ik_f(x\sin\theta - z\cos\theta)}$$

$$(54) \quad F_{LW}(x,z) = -2F_{SP}\Big[1 - \sqrt{\eta}\, a_r$$
$$\times\; e^{\gamma^2}\frac{erfc(\gamma)}{\Delta_s}\Big]$$

$$(55) \quad \gamma = \frac{a_r}{\Delta_s} - \frac{x}{a_r}$$

where a_r is a factor related to the incident beam width, $erfc(\gamma)$ is the complex complementary error function,[9] F_{LW} is the leaky wave portion of the field, F_{SP} is the specular portion of the field, k_f is the fluid wave vector, Γ_0 is a wave potential amplitude and Δ_s is a parameter depending only on material constants and relating to the degree of coupling between acoustic and surface waves.

The coordinates X and Z have their origin at the intersection of the solid surface and incident beam center. Although complicated, Eqs. 52 to 55 show the only analytical expression calculated so far for the reflected field of a leaky rayleigh wave. In addition, the result of those equations requires the assumption of an incident gaussian beam profile for its derivation.

Absorptive Losses in Solid

Several additional features may now be added to the planar fluid-to-solid geometry to increase its generality. The first feature is absorptive losses in the solid. As the attenuation in the solid medium increases with frequency, the behavior of the reflected field increasingly deviates from that expected on the basis of lossless theory. At angles of incidence higher than the transverse critical angle, all energy is reflected if losses are ignored. As the attenuation in the solid approaches $0.073\ \text{Np·}\lambda_r^{-1}$, there is a rapid onset of energy leakage into the solid, accompanied by a consequent reduction in the acoustic reflected field amplitude.

As observed[10] and modeled,[11] this effect was given a full explanation in 1973 in an analysis of acoustic beam reflection from fluid-to-solid media.[3] In the lossless case, the rayleigh pole zero pair (complex wave vector values where the reflection coefficient approaches infinity or zero, respectively) sits across the real axis in the complex plane with the pole in the first quadrant and the zero in the fourth, each equidistant from the real axis. Rising absorptive losses in the solid cause the pair to migrate to higher imaginary values until the zero eventually crosses the real axis from below. At this point, the plane wave acoustic reflection amplitude at the rayleigh angle vanishes and all wave energy leaks into the solid. The calculated magnitude of the reflection coefficient[11] for a water-to-stainless steel interface is shown in Fig. 7. For losses higher than the critical value, the acoustic reflection increases but the distortion and lateral shift of the beam no longer occur.

Layered Half Space

Another complicating feature on the basic fluid-to-solid geometry is the addition to the half space of a solid isotropic layer. The layer differs from the half space in its elastic properties and may be of any thickness (Fig. 8). In this case, the surface wave speed becomes dispersive or frequency dependent. At low sound frequency, the wavelength of the rayleigh

FIGURE 7. Magnitude of reflection coefficient for a steel to water interface with varying values of transverse wave attenuation in units of nepers per wavelength (Np·λ^{-1}). At critical value of 0.073 Np·λ^{-1}, reflected amplitude falls sharply to zero. Higher or lower attenuation results in partial reflection.[11]

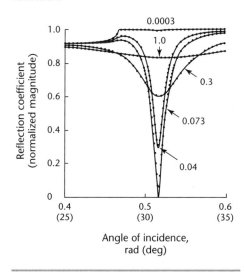

wave is much larger than the layer thickness. The sound wave speed is thereby controlled primarily by the elastic properties of the substrate and the layer may be viewed as a perturbation to the elastic environment of the surface.

At the other frequency extreme, the wavelength is much smaller than the layer thickness and the surface wave is hardly affected by the presence of the substrate. Instead, the layer properties essentially determine the speed of the wave. At intermediate values of the wavelength-to-layer thickness ratio, a proportionate mixing of the elastic constants could be expected. This simple physical representation is not completely accurate, as discussed below.

A complete theoretical exposition of various effects involving the layered half space in vacuum is given in the literature.[12] The elastic wave propagation problem is formulated and solved for a wide variety of cases, including anisotropic and piezoelectric materials. Details of the phenomena are presented graphically and the reader is referred to this and other sources for thorough treatments of the factors complicating surface wave propagation.[3,12-16]

For the layered half space, the wave displacements of Eqs. 42 to 44 and the boundary conditions of Eq. 45 must be generalized to the two elastic media of the layer and half space. Expressing Eq. 45 in terms of wave displacements leads to a set of simultaneous linear equations in the wave potentials. For there to be solutions of these homogeneous equations, the determinant of the coefficients must vanish. The wave vector values that satisfy this requirement are then roots of the suitably generalized secular equation, similar to Eq. 48. In this geometry, the roots are once again real (because no fluid is present) and may be inverted to give the phase velocity of the surface waves.

There are two distinguishable cases: the layer rayleigh wave speed can be either higher or lower than that of the substrate. A higher layer wave speed stiffens the substrate and the velocity dispersion takes the form shown in Fig. 9, calculated for silicon on a zinc oxide substrate. At zero layer thickness, the surface wave speed is indeed that of the substrate and as the thickness or frequency increases, the effective wave speed approaches the value appropriate for the layer. However, near $kd = 0.8$, the mode ceases to propagate when the wave speed reaches the substrate transverse velocity. This effect is connected to the fact that, near the cutoff, the vertical displacement amplitude decays very slowly away from the surface. If the wave does not become leaky into the substrate, it must cease to propagate.

When the layer wave speed is lower than the substrate's, the dispersion follows the intuitive picture constructed above. These results for a zinc oxide layer on silicon are shown in Fig. 10. Here, the two limiting values of the curve are the rayleigh wave speed of the substrate and layer, as expected. This loading case is marked by the existence of higher order modes, not shown in Fig. 10. The first of these is called the *sezawa wave*, with the additional excitations simply being numbered.[13] The higher order modes differ from the rayleigh mode in several respects, including their asymptotic approach to the layer transverse wave speed at large kd. To derive these curves, zeros of complicated transcendental equations must generally be sought, a delicate problem in nonlinear optimization best left to a high speed computer.

FIGURE 8. Layered half space geometry.

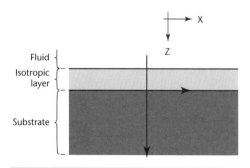

FIGURE 9. Velocity dispersion of rayleigh wave on stiffened half space as function of kd. Phase velocity is bounded by the substrate C_r and transverse wave speed. Materials are silicon on zinc oxide.[12]

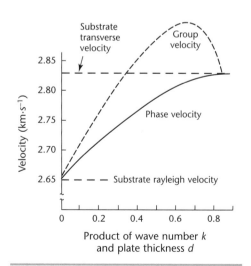

Fluid Coupled Layered Half Space

To a layered half space geometry, an additional feature may be added — a fluid in place of the vacuum. With appropriate modification of the boundary conditions, the wave displacement technique now yields a 7×7 matrix containing all mechanical motion of the layer, half space and fluid. Leaky rayleigh waves have been studied in both loading and stiffening layers and beam profiles have been measured and elicited.[17-21] As in the case of the simple fluid coupled half space, the fluid has little influence on the wave speed dispersion but does cause the wave vector to become complex because the surface wave radiates energy into the fluid as it propagates.

Following the procedures of earlier studies,[3] it has been demonstrated that the influence of the layer on finite beam reflection in the lossless case is isolated in the dispersive rayleigh wave pole.[22] This result implies that the analytical expression of Eqs. 52 to 55 can be generalized to the layered half space by substituting the appropriate incident angle and generalized, frequency dependent values of Δ_s. If the incident angle is different from the rayleigh angle, Δ_s decreases rapidly and specular reflection is soon restored. The analytical connection between Δ_s and the simple half space calculation is straightforward.[3] This parameter is known as the *schoch displacement*[2] and is related to the complex rayleigh wave pole through:

$$(56) \quad \Delta_s = \frac{2}{\mathrm{Im}\left(\xi_p\right)}$$

Examples of experimental data, accompanied by theoretical predictions, for acoustic beam reflection from layered half spaces are shown in Figs. 10 and 11. The material system in both cases is copper on stainless steel. The products of frequency and layer thickness are nearly equal. In Fig. 11, the nonspecular nature of the reflected field is evident whereas the trailing leaky wave field can be seen as a slower decay to zero amplitude on the right side. At an incident angle only 3 mrad (0.2 deg) different from the rayleigh angle in Fig. 12, the deep null expected at this value of frequency and layer thickness has nearly disappeared. In both of these examples, the theoretical model[19-21] extending the original calculation[3] is in good agreement with the measurements.

Transverse Horizontal Waves

Another topic deserves mention because of its applicability to electromagnetic acoustic transducers (EMATs).[23,24] By restricting particle displacements to the Y axis, a different type of wave motion is observed. In this case, Eqs. 42 to 44 are written as:

FIGURE 10. Velocity dispersion of fundamental rayleigh mode on loaded half space as function of kd. Phase velocity is bounded by substrate and layer C_r. Higher order modes are not shown. Materials are zinc oxide on silicon.[12]

FIGURE 11. Reflected field amplitude as function of coordinate for copper layered steel half space at rayleigh angle incidence. Experimental measurements are plotted as discrete points. Solid curve is model calculation. Product of frequency times thickness is 0.34.[20]

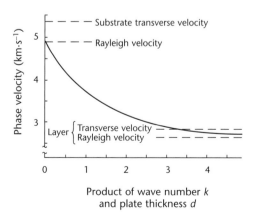

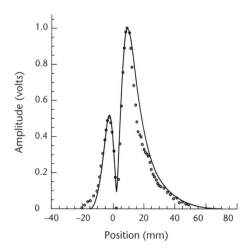

(57) $u_x = u_z = 0$

and:

(58) $u_y = A_y e^{-\alpha z} \cos(ky - \omega t)$

where there is only a single nonzero displacement amplitude. The appropriate stress tensor element is:

(59) $\sigma_{yz} = \pi \left(\dfrac{\partial u_y}{\partial z} + \dfrac{\partial u_z}{\partial y} \right)$

The wave implied by the above conditions is a horizontally polarized transverse wave, also known as a *transverse horizontal wave*. Propagation at the transverse wave speed in the bulk or parallel to the surface of a half space is possible because no displacements are normal to the surface. The wave has convenient properties in reflection at interfaces, making it attractive in certain applications. The addition of a fluid to the solid half space geometry is irrelevant in this case, where the absence of vertical surface displacements means there will be no coupling between transverse horizontal waves and acoustic waves in the fluid.

As a preliminary step to the treatment of a related wave type on a layered half space, note how this wave behaves in a free plate. An analytical dispersion relation[25,26] for this type of wave can be determined by following a line of development similar to that for the rayleigh wave and by noting that the surface tractions σ_{yz} vanish at the top and bottom of the plate of thickness d:

(60) $k^2 = \left(\dfrac{\omega}{v_T} \right)^2 - \left(\dfrac{\pi n}{d} \right)^2$

where d is the thickness (meter) of a free plate in which these waves are propagating (meter); n is a positive integer and n_T is the infinite medium transverse wave speed (meter per second);

Traveling wave modes for this excitation exist for all values of n, such that the right hand side of Eq. 60 is greater than zero. Otherwise, the resulting imaginary wave vector k corresponds to a standing wave solution. Depending on whether the number of particle displacement modes in the plate is even or odd, the transverse horizontal modes will be symmetric or antisymmetric, respectively. From Eq. 60, it can be seen that in the case of the lowest order symmetric mode ($N = 0$) there is dispersionless propagation at the transverse wave speed. All other modes are dispersive. The group velocity, which can be calculated from Eq. 60, is shown for several transverse horizontal plate waves in Fig. 13.

If the free plate in the above example is in welded contact to a half space of differing elastic properties, its wave characteristics, under the assumption of Y axis displacements only, change considerably. The plate still functions as a wave guide, as in the case of transverse

FIGURE 12. Reflected field amplitude distribution for copper on steel with $fd = 0.41$, where f is frequency and d is plate thickness. Open circles are data and solid curve is theory. Incident angle is 3 mrad (0.2 deg) different from rayleigh angle, giving rise to much weaker null zone.[19]

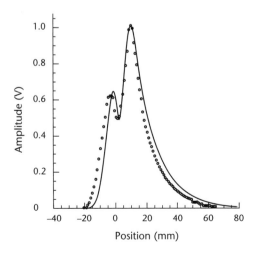

FIGURE 13. Dispersion of group velocity for several transverse horizontal plate waves. Fundamental mode is nondispersive.

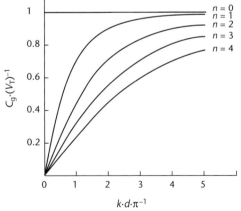

Legend
C_g = group velocity
d = distance
k = wave number
v_T = transverse wave speed

horizontal plate waves, but the cutoff behavior noted for the free plate is replaced by transitions to leaky waves for modes that exceed critical wavelengths. Furthermore, this wave type can propagate only if the layer transverse wave speed is less than that of the substrate. A dispersion relation for these waves has been derived:[14]

$$(61) \quad \tan\left[d\sqrt{\left(\frac{\omega}{\hat{v}_T}\right)^2 - k^2}\right] = \frac{\mu}{\hat{\mu}}\frac{\sqrt{k^2 - \left(\frac{\omega}{\hat{v}_T}\right)^2}}{\sqrt{\left(\frac{\omega}{\hat{v}_T}\right)^2 - k^2}}$$

where k is the wave vector of the disturbance, μ is the transverse modulus (ratio of shearing stress to shearing strain) and ω is the circular frequency (radian per second).

The circumflex ($\wedge$) denotes the layer properties. By way of illustration, Fig. 14 shows transverse displacements for the fundamental wave, known as a *love mode*,[27] for several values of kd. As kd approaches zero, the phase velocity tends to the transverse wave speed of the substrate. At large kd values, the excitation is confined to the layer and propagates at a phase velocity near b for the layer. The presence of the tangent function in Eq. 61 leads to the existence of higher order modes, all of whose phase velocities are bounded by b and $\hat{b}$.

Other Elastic Excitations

There are many more elastic excitations connected with surface wave propagation, including interesting variations in

behavior that occur when the material properties are anisotropic. Various phenomena occur in piezoelectric materials combined with conductors or insulators. New wave types are observed and familiar modes exhibit unusual characteristics.

There are also further possible solutions in the leaky wave case where a slow guided mode at the fluid-to-solid interface (known as the *scholte wave*) can exist.[28] These and other surface wave types are covered in the literature.[25,26,29-33]

FIGURE 14. Transverse displacement as function of depth for fundamental love mode at several values of kd, where k is wave number and d is plate thickness. Materials are gold on fused quartz.[12]

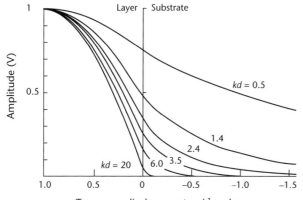

51

PART 4. Reflection at Plane Boundary in Stress Free Media

The simplest problem that can be treated for an ultrasonic wave incident at a material surface is that of a plane wave incident at a free, plane boundary in an isotropic material. Because the material is isotropic, any convenient coordinate system may be used. For the discussion below, the YZ plane is considered the plane of incidence. The incident plane (see Fig. 15 for the coordinate system) contains the normal n to the plane boundary and the wave vector of the incident wave k.

The problem can be considered in three parts: (1) an incident longitudinal wave (called a *pressure wave* in geophysics); (2) an incident transverse wave with particle displacements parallel to the boundary surface (a transverse horizontal wave); and (3) an incident transverse wave with particle displacements lying in the incident plane (a transverse vertical mode). Any incident transverse mode can be resolved into a component parallel and a component perpendicular to the plane of incidence.

Any incident transverse wave also may be resolved into such components and each component can be treated separately (see below). All equations that follow are linear so the complete displacement field is the sum of the displacements found in the incident transverse horizontal mode and the incident transverse vertical mode.

Whatever type of wave is incident on the boundary, consideration of the stress free boundary conditions requires that the phase of each plane wave (both incident and reflected) be equal at all positions along the boundary and for all time. This mathematical statement leads to the important physical principle known as *Snell's law* for reflection or refraction. The condition relates the phase speeds of the incident and reflected (or refracted waves in the situation where the boundary surface separates two different media) to the angles of incidence and reflection, as shown below by Eq. 66.

Incident Longitudinal Wave

An incident longitudinal wave has particle displacements parallel to the direction of the wave vector k. Direction of k is given relative to the normal n of the plane boundary by the incident angle θ_I. Hence, the particle displacements of the incident wave may be written as:

$$(62) \quad u_I = \lfloor j \sin \theta_I + k \cos \theta_I \rfloor A_I$$
$$\times \ e^{\omega t - k_y y + k_z z}$$

where j is unit vector parallel to the Y axis, k is unit vector parallel to the Z axis, $k_y = k_I \sin \theta_I$ and $k_z = k_I \cos \theta$.

This displacement field must satisfy the equations of motion (Eqs. 31 to 33) and must simultaneously satisfy the stress free boundary conditions on the surface of the material. A longitudinal wave with displacements in the form of Eq. 59 satisfies the motion as long as the velocity of the wave is given by Eq. 40. However, this displacement field cannot by itself satisfy the stress free boundary conditions.

To satisfy the conditions of no stress on the reflection boundary, it is necessary to have the reflection of two independent waves because there are two independent boundary conditions — the stress component σ_{zz} and s_{zy} must simultaneously be zero. In fact, the third stress component σ_{zx} on the surface must also be zero. It can be shown that if the incident wave has a wave normal in the YZ plane as assumed, s_{zx} will be identically zero and this condition does not offer any further constraints on the problem solution. Because two types of body waves can satisfy the equation of motion for an isotropic material, consider the possibility that two reflected waves result from the incident longitudinal wave (recall that two independent reflected

FIGURE 15. Definition of terms for longitudinal wave incident on plane stress free boundary.

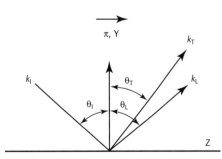

waves are needed to satisfy the boundary conditions). The reflected waves are then a longitudinal wave at angle θ_L:

$$(63) \quad u_L = \left[j \sin\theta_L + k \cos\theta_L \right] A_L$$
$$\times \; e^{\omega t - k_p y + k_p z}$$

and a reflected transverse wave S at the angle θ_T (see Fig. 15):

$$(64) \quad u_T = \left\lfloor j \sin\theta_T + k \cos\theta_T \right\rfloor A_T$$
$$\times \; e^{\omega t - k_p y + k_p z}$$

The quantities involved have the same physical and mathematical meanings as those given for Eq. 67. The subscripts have been changed to indicate different waves of interest. The boundary conditions can now be written as in Eq. 65 at $z = 0$:

$$(65a) \quad \sigma_{zz} = 0$$

and:

$$(65b) \quad \sigma_{zy} = 0$$

When substituting into these equations using the constitutive equations (Eqs. 8 to 13), the strain displacement relations (Eqs. 25 to 30), the displacement fields for the incident longitudinal wave (Eq. 62), the reflected longitudinal wave (Eq. 63) and the reflected S wave (Eq. 64), a system of two algebraic equations is obtained. These equations provide two important mathematical and physical conclusions concerning the nature of the reflected waves. First, in order that the equations be satisfied for all time and position along the boundary, the following set of equations must be satisfied:

$$(66) \quad \frac{v_I}{\sin\theta_I} = \frac{v_L}{\sin\theta_L} = \frac{v_T}{\sin\theta_T}$$

These equations are the mathematical expression for Snell's law. They state that the incident and reflected waves must propagate along the boundary at the same phase speed. Note that the equations state that the component of the phase speed of each wave parallel to the plane boundary is equal.

The second important property obtained from these algebraic equations provides information on the relative size of the amplitude of each reflected wave compared to the incident wave. The amplitude ratios of the reflected longitudinal wave $(A_L \cdot A_I^{-1})$ and the reflected transverse wave $(A_T \cdot A_I^{-1})$ compared to the incident wave amplitude are called the *reflection coefficients*:

$$(67) \quad R = \frac{\sin 2\theta_I \sin 2\theta_T - \kappa\cos^2 2\theta_T}{\sin 2\theta_I \sin 2\theta_T + \kappa\cos^2 2\theta_T}$$

$$(68) \quad T = \frac{2\kappa\sin 2\theta_I \cos^2 2\theta_T}{\sin 2\theta_I \sin 2\theta_T + \kappa\cos^2 2\theta_T}$$

where R is the reflection coefficient for the reflected longitudinal wave, T is the reflection coefficient for the reflected transverse wave, κ is the ratio of the longitudinal wave speed to transverse wave speed and v is Poisson's ratio for the material.

$$(69) \quad \kappa = \frac{v_L^2}{v_T^2} = \frac{2(1-v)}{1-v}$$

Figure 16 provides a typical solution for the reflection coefficients of an incident longitudinal wave in a material having a Poisson's ratio of 0.25.

Incident Transverse Horizontal Mode

An incident transverse mode with particle displacements parallel to the reflecting boundary is considered a transverse horizontal mode. The reflection problem for this mode is comparatively simple. Write the displacement field as:

$$(70) \quad u_{SH} = i \, A_{SH} \, e^{\omega t - k_y y + k_z z}$$

Assume that the reflected waves are a longitudinal wave of the type in Eq. 63 and a transverse wave of the type in Eq. 64 with potentially an additional component in the direction of the X axis:

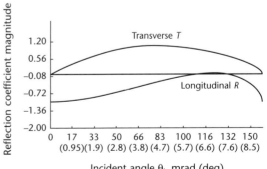

FIGURE 16. Reflection coefficients for longitudinal wave incident on plane stress-free boundary for material with Poisson's ratio of 0.25.

(71) $\quad \boldsymbol{u}_T = \boldsymbol{i}\,A_{T_1} + \left(\boldsymbol{j}\sin\theta_T + \boldsymbol{k}\cos\theta_T\right)A_{T_2}$

$\qquad \times\ e^{\omega t - k_T y + k_T z}$

After substitution into the same stress free boundary conditions, it is found that A_L and A_{T2} must be identically zero, that A_{T1} must be identically equal to A_{SH} and that the angle of the reflected wave must equal the angle of the incident wave. That is, an incident transverse horizontal mode is reflected as a transverse horizontal mode, no mode conversion occurs and the amplitude of the reflected mode equals the amplitude of the incident mode.

Incident Transverse Vertical Mode

This is the most complicated of the three incident wave problems. The problem must be further categorized into the ranges of incident angles smaller than a specific angle called the *critical angle* and incident angles greater than the critical angle. Assume an incident transverse wave with particle displacements lying parallel to the incident plane:

(72) $\quad \boldsymbol{u}_I = \left(\boldsymbol{j}\sin\theta_I + \boldsymbol{k}\cos\theta_I\right)A_{T2}$

$\qquad \times\ e^{\omega t - k_I y + k_I z}$

The critical angle for reflection (and refraction) of a wave is defined by Snell's law as the angle of incidence for which the angle of the reflected longitudinal mode becomes $0.5\,\pi$. For any incidence angles greater than the critical angle, no reflected longitudinal mode can occur. The boundary conditions, still numbering two, cannot be satisfied by the reflection of the two types of body waves and it is necessary, both physically and mathematically, for a nonbody wave to be reflected. The only other possible type of wave is a surface wave similar to the rayleigh wave.

By Snell's law (Eq. 66), the relation between reflected angles, incident angles and phase speeds is:

(73) $\quad \dfrac{v_I}{\sin\theta_I} = \dfrac{v_L}{\sin\theta_L} = \dfrac{v_T}{\sin\theta_T}$

When the incident wave is a transverse wave, this relation becomes:

(74) $\quad \dfrac{v_T}{\sin\theta_T} = \dfrac{v_L}{\sin\theta_L}$

or:

(75) $\quad \sin\theta_L = \sin\theta_T\,\dfrac{v_L}{v_T}$

Because v_L is always greater than v_T, the ratio of the phase speed on the right hand side of Eq. 75 is always greater than 1. There is a real solution for θ_L only for values of $\sin\theta_T$ in which the product of $\sin\theta_T$ and the ratio of the phase speeds $v_L \cdot v_T^{-1}$ is less than 1. In fact, there is a single value of the incident angle θ_T that makes the right hand side of Eq. 75 exactly 1:

(76) $\quad \theta_{TC} = \sin^{-1}\dfrac{v_T}{v_L}$

For all incident angles less than θ_{TC}, there are real solutions for θ_L from Eq. 75. For all incident angles greater than θ_{TC}, no real solution for θ_L exists and there can be no reflected longitudinal body wave. The angle θ_{TC} is called the *critical angle reflection* because it separates the reflection problem for an incident transverse vertical mode into two regions depending on the incident angle. There is a region where both longitudinal and transverse (shear vertical) are reflected and a region where a transverse vertical mode and a surface mode are reflected (for incident angles below and above the critical angle, respectively).

Incident Angles Less than Critical Angle Reflection

For a transverse vertical wave incident at all angles below the critical angle, both a reflected longitudinal mode and a reflected transverse vertical mode generally occur. Depending on the value of Poisson's ratio, there are for some materials specific values of incident angles when the amplitude of the reflected transverse vertical mode is zero. In all cases, there is always a reflected longitudinal mode for this range of incident angles. With stress free boundary conditions, there is a set of reflection coefficients for this problem as follows:

(77) $\quad R = \dfrac{2\kappa\sin 2\theta_T \sin 2\theta_T}{2\sin 2\theta_L \sin 2\theta_T + \kappa\cos^2 2\theta_T}$

(78) $\quad T = \dfrac{2\sin 2\theta_L \sin 2\theta_T - \kappa\cos^2 2\theta_T}{2\sin 2\theta_L \sin 2\theta_T + \kappa\cos^2 2\theta_T}$

All parameters have the same definitions as given above for the reflected longitudinal mode. This problem, with the exception of the appearance of the critical angle phenomenon, is symmetric in results to the reflected longitudinal mode discussed above.

First, there is mode conversion on reflection of a longitudinal mode. Second, note the reciprocity between the values of the reflection coefficients (compare Eqs. 77 and 78 with Eqs. 67 and 68). Finally, note that Snell's law is identical with Eq. 66 as long as the appropriate wave speed and incident angle are used for the incident mode.

Incident Angles Greater than Critical Angle Reflection

For a transverse vertical wave incident on a stress free boundary at incident angles greater than the critical angle given by Eq. 76, a reflected longitudinal mode cannot occur. Because there are still two independent, not identically zero, boundary conditions on the stress components that must be satisfied, it is both physically and mathematically necessary to postulate the reflection of a second mode, in addition to a reflected transverse vertical mode. The governing equation of motion allows only the longitudinal wave and the transverse wave to propagate in a linear elastic medium. There is no physically distinguishable difference between the transverse vertical and transverse horizontal mode as far as the interior of the body is concerned. Hence, the only possible second reflected mode is a mode that cannot propagate into the interior but must be confined to propagation along or near the boundary surface.

By using the displacement fields assumed for the incident and reflected transverse vertical modes (Eqs. 63 and 64, respectively), a surface wave with displacements of the form assumed by Rayleigh (Eqs. 42 to 44) in the equations of motion (Eqs. 31 to 33) and in the boundary conditions for stress (Eq. 45), then a set of algebraic equations is found to characterize the exact forms of the wave displacements. It is found, for example, that the reflected transverse vertical wave has a reflection coefficient equal to –1 in this case. On reflection, the wave also undergoes a change in phase relative to the incident wave by an amount 2ζ that depends on the angle of incidence (see below).

The reflected surface wave is similar in properties to the rayleigh wave but is distinctly different from a rayleigh wave. The surface wave is also phase shifted relative to the incident wave by the amount ζ. The reflection coefficient of the reflected surface wave is:

(79) $S = 2 \sin \zeta \sin \theta_T \tan 2\theta_T$

The phase angle ζ is given by:

(80) $\zeta = \tan^{-1} - \cos^2 2_T$

$$\div \left(2 \sin \theta_T \sin 2\theta_T \sqrt{\sin^2 \theta_T - \frac{1}{k}} \right)$$

One of the major differences between the reflected surface wave and the rayleigh wave is the fact that the phase velocity of the reflected surface wave is not less than that of the transverse mode in the material. In fact, the phase velocity of the reflected wave must vary with the angle of incidence as given by the equation:

(81) $v_S = \dfrac{v_T}{\sin \theta_T}$

The amplitude of the surface wave decreases exponentially with distance away from the surface according to the factor $e^{-\alpha z}$ where the attenuation coefficient α is:

(82) $\alpha = k_2 \sqrt{1 - \dfrac{v_S^2}{v_T^2}}$

Finally, the wave number of the reflected surface wave is found from the relation:

(83) $k_2 = k \sin \theta_T$

The values of α and the wave number k_2 are also distinctively different from the corresponding relations for the rayleigh wave. Note again that all of these relations are mandated by the solution to the equation of motion and the boundary conditions of stress on the reflecting boundary. Figure 17 presents sample

FIGURE 17. Reflection coefficients for transverse vertical wave incident on plane stress free boundary for material with Poisson's ration of 0.25.

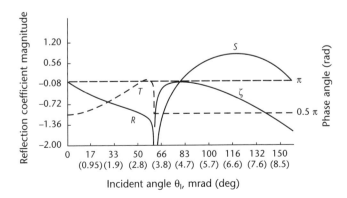

values for the reflection coefficients of incident transverse vertical waves throughout the entire range of incident angles.

Figure 18 shows orientation of several waves. In this schematic, the longitudinal waves are horizontal and the transverse waves are close to the normal. On top are the reflected waves and on bottom are the transmitted waves. The incident wave can be either of two different cases: the incident wave can be a longitudinal wave or a transverse wave. The behavior of these waves is described in standard texts.[34,35]

FIGURE 18. Transmission and reflection of ultrasonic waves.

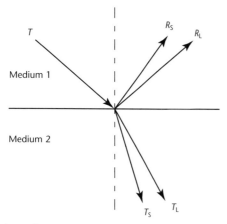

Legend
I = incident wave
R_L = reflected longitudinal (or pressure) wave
R_S = reflected transverse (or shear) wave
T_L = transmitted longitudinal (or pressure) wave
T_S = transmitted transverse (or shear) wave

References

1. Henneke, E.G., II, D.E. Chimenti and E.P. Papadakis. Section 3, "Fundamental Principles of Ultrasonic Wave Propagation." *Nondestructive Testing Handbook,* second edition: Vol. 7, *Ultrasonic Testing.* Columbus, OH: American Society for Nondestructive Testing (1991): p 33-63.
2. Schoch, A. "Schallreflexion, Schallbrechung und Schallbeugung." *Ergebnisse der Exakten Naturwissenschaften.* Vol. 23. Berlin, Germany: Springer (1950): p 127-234.
3. Bertoni, H. and T. Tamir. *Applied Physics.* Vol. 2. Berlin, Germany: Springer-Verlag (1973): p 157.
4. Diachok, O. and W. Mayer. "Conical Reflection of Ultrasound from a Liquid-Solid Interface." *Journal of the Acoustical Society of America.* Vol. 47, No. 1. Melville, NY: American Institute of Physics, for the Acoustical Society of America (1970): p 155.
5. Neubauer, W. and L. Dragonette. "Measurement of Rayleigh Phase Velocity and Estimates of Shear Speed by Schlieren Visualization." *Journal of Applied Physics.* Vol. 45, No. 2. Melville, NY: American Institute of Physics (1974): p 618.
6. Breazeale, M.A., L. Adler and G. Scott. "Interaction of Ultrasonic Waves Incident at the Rayleigh Angle onto a Liquid-Solid Interface. *Journal of Applied Physics.* Vol. 48, No. 2. Melville, NY: American Institute of Physics (1977): p 530.
7. Burlii, P. and I.Y. Kucherov. *Zhurnal Eksperimental'noi i Teoreticheskoi Fiziki, Pis'ma v Redakt.* Vol. 26. Melville, NY: American Institute of Physics (1977): p 490.
8. Bogy, D. and S. Gracewski. "Nonspecular Reflection of Bounded Acoustic Beams from Liquid-Solid Interface of Two Elastic Layers on a Halfspace under Water." *International Journal of Solids and Structures.* Vol. 20, No. 8. New York, NY: Pergamon Press (1984): p 747.
9. Stegun, I. and R. Zucker. "Automatic Computing Methods for Special Functions (Part IV): Complex Error Function, Fresnel Integrals and Other Related Functions." *Journal of Research of the National Bureau of Standards.* Vol. 86, No. 6. Gaithersburg, MD: National Institute of Standards and Technology (1981): p 661.
10. Rollins, F. "Critical Ultrasonic Reflectivity — A Neglected Tool for Material Evaluation." *Materials Evaluation.* Vol. 24, No. 12. Columbus, OH: American Society for Nondestructive Testing (December 1966): p 683.
11. Becker, F.L. and R. Richardson. "Influence of Material Properties on Rayleigh Critical-Angle Reflectivity." *Journal of the Acoustical Society of America.* Vol. 51, No. 5. Melville, NY: American Institute of Physics, for the Acoustical Society of America (1972): p 1609.
12. Farnell, G.W. and E.L. Adler. *Physical Acoustics.* Vol. 9. W.P. Mason and R.N. Thurston, eds. New York, NY: Academic Press (1972).
13. Sezawa, K. and K. Kanai. *Bulletin of the Earthquake Research Institute.* Vol. 13. Tokyo, Japan: University of Tokyo (1935): p 237.
14. Tournois, P. and C. Lardat. "Love Wave-Dispersive Delay Lines for Wide-Band Pulse Compression." *Transactions on Sonics and Ultrasonics.* Vol. 16. New York, NY: Institute of Electrical and Electronics Engineers (1969): p 107.
15. Coldren, L.A. and G.S. Kino. "Monolithic Acoustic Surface-Wave Amplifier." *Applied Physics Letters.* Vol. 18, No. 8. Melville, NY: American Institute of Physics (1971): p 317.
16. Tiersten, H.F. "Elastic Surface Waves Guided by Thin Films." *Journal of Applied Physics.* Vol. 40, No. 2. Melville, NY: American Institute of Physics (1969): p 770.
17. Adler, E.L. "Observation of Leaky Rayleigh Waves on a Layered Half-Space." *Transactions on Sonics and Ultrasonics.* Vol. 18, No. 3. New York, NY: Institute of Electrical and Electronics Engineers (1971): p 181.
18. Hattunen, M. and M. Luukkala. *Applied Physics.* Vol. 2. New York, NY: Springer-Verlag (1973): p 257.

19. Chimenti, D.E., A. Nayfeh and D. Butler. "Leaky Rayleigh Waves on a Layered Halfspace." *Journal of Applied Physics*. Vol. 53, No. 1. Melville, NY: American Institute of Physics (1982): p170.

20. Nayfeh, A. and D.E. Chimenti. "Reflection of Finite Acoustic Beams from Loaded and Stiffened Half-Spaces." *Journal of the Acoustical Society of America*. Vol. 75, No. 5. Melville, NY: American Institute of Physics, for the Acoustical Society of America (1984): p1360.

21. Chimenti, D.E. "Energy Leakage from Rayleigh Waves on a Fluid-Loaded, Layered Half-Space." *Applied Physics Letters*. Vol. 43, No. 1. Melville, NY: American Institute of Physics (1983): p46.

22. Nayfeh, A., D.E. Chimenti, L. Adler and R. Crane. *Journal of Applied Physics*. Vol. 53. Melville, NY: American Institute of Physics (1982): p175.

23. Fortunko, C., R. King and M. Tam. "Nondestructive Evaluation of Planar Defects in Plates Using Low-Frequency Shear Horizontal Waves." *Journal of Applied Physics*. Vol. 53, No. 5. Melville, NY: American Institute of Physics (1982): p3450.

24. Fortunko, C.M. and R.E. Schramm. "An Analysis of Electromagnetic Acoustic Transducer Arrays for Nondestructive Evaluation of Thick Metal Sections and Weldments." *Review of Progress in Quantitative Nondestructive Evaluation*. Vol. 2A. New York, NY: Plenum (1983): p283-307.

25. Beaver, W.L. "Sonic Nearfields of a Pulsed Piston Radiator." *Journal of the Acoustical Society of America*. Vol. 56, No. 4. Melville, NY: American Institute of Physics, for the Acoustical Society of America (1974): p1043-1048.

26. Seki, H., A. Granato and R. Truell. "Diffraction Effects in the Ultrasonic Field of a Piston Source and Their Importance in the Accurate Measurement of Attenuation." *Journal of the Acoustical Society of America*. Vol. 28, No. 2. Melville, NY: American Institute of Physics, for the Acoustical Society of America (1956): p230-238.

27. Love, A.H. *Some Problems in Geodynamics*. London, United Kingdom: Cambridge University Press (1911).

28. Scholte, J. "Geophysics." *Royal Astronomical Society: Monthly Notices*. Supplement 5. Oxford, United Kingdom: Blackwell Scientific Publications (1947): p120.

29. Mansour, T.M. "Evaluation of Ultrasonic Transducers by Cross-Sectional Mapping of the Near Field Using a Point Reflector." *Materials Evaluation*. Vol. 37, No. 7. Columbus, OH: American Society for Nondestructive Testing (June 1979): p50-54.

30. *Nondestructive Testing Handbook,* first edition. Columbus, OH: American Society for Nondestructive Testing (1959).

31. Papadakis, E.P. "Absolute Measurements of Ultrasonic Attenuation Using Damped Nondestructive Testing Transducers." *Journal of Testing and Evaluation*. Vol. 12, No. 5. West Conshohocken, PA: ASTM International (1984): p273-279.

32. Papadakis, E.P. "Diffraction of Ultrasound Radiating into an Elastically Anisotropic Medium." *Journal of the Acoustical Society of America*. Vol. 36, No. 3. Melville, NY: American Institute of Physics, for the Acoustical Society of America (1964): p414-422.

33. Papadakis, E.P. "Ultrasonic Diffraction Loss and Phase Change in Anisotropic Materials." *Journal of the Acoustical Society of America*. Vol. 40, No. 4. Melville, NY: American Institute of Physics, for the Acoustical Society of America (1966): p863-876.

34. Graff, K. *Wave Motion in Elastic Solids*. New York, NY: Dover (1963, 1991).

35. Kolsky, H. *Stress Waves in Solids*. New York, NY: Dover (1975, 2003).

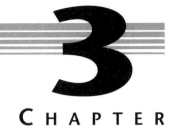

CHAPTER

Generation and Detection of Ultrasound

Gary L. Workman, University of Alabama in Huntsville, Huntsville, Alabama (Part 6)

George A. Alers, San Luis Obispo, California (Part 9)

Theodore L. Allen, Southwest Research Institute, San Antonio, Texas

Yoseph Bar-Cohen, Jet Propulsion Laboratory, Pasadena, California (Part 5)

Frederick A. Bruton, Southwest Research Institute, San Antonio, Texas (Part 2)

Francis H. Chang, Fort Worth, Texas

Butrus Pierre T. Khuri-Yakub, Stanford University, Stanford, California (Part 10)

Michael Moles, Olympus NDT Canada, Toronto, Ontario, Canada (Part 4)

Jean-Pierre Monchalin, National Research Council Canada, Québec (Part 8)

Joseph L. Rose, Pennsylvania State University, University Park, Pennsylvania (Part 7)

Part 1 adapted from *Piezoelectric Technology Data for Designers* (Morgan Matroc, Vernitron Division)

PART 1. Piezoelectricity[1,2]

Piezoelectricity means "pressure electricity" and is a property of certain crystals, including quartz, rochelle salt, tourmaline and barium titanate. As the term suggests, electricity results when pressure is applied to one of these crystals. The reverse effect also is present — when an electric field is applied, the crystal rapidly changes shape.

Piezoelectric Materials

Piezoelectric materials commonly used for electromechanical transducers include barium titanate and ceramics containing lead zirconate and lead titanate. These ceramics are polycrystalline and do not have piezoelectric properties in their original state. Piezoelectric behavior is induced by polarization or so-called *poling* procedures. In addition to the traditional ceramic elements, organic materials such as polyvinyllidene fluoride (PVDF) have been demonstrated to be effective in piezoelectric ultrasound transducers.[3] Polyvinyllidene fluoride transducers are lightweight, low cost and broad band. Transducer manufacturers provide polyvinyllidene fluoride transducers. Other, similar ferroelectric materials have been developed for ultrasonic transducers.

FIGURE 1. Basic deformations of piezoelectric plates: (a) thickness shear; (b) face shear; (c) thickness expansion.

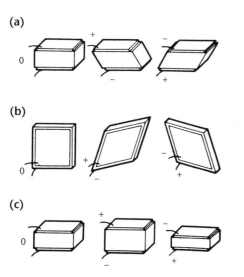

(a)

(b)

(c)

Piezoelectric Actions

The type of piezoelectric material determines the degree of deformation resulting from application of an electric field and, conversely, the nature of the deforming forces needed to develop an electric charge (Fig. 1).

Generally, at least two of these deformations are present simultaneously. In some cases, one type of expansion is accompanied by a contraction that compensates for the expansion and produces no net change in volume. For example, the expansion of plate length may be compensated by an equal contraction of width or thickness. In some materials, the compensating effects are not of equal magnitude and net volume change does occur. In all cases, the deformations are very small when amplification by mechanical resonance is not involved. The maximum displacements are on the order of micrometers.

Piezoelectric Actions from Various Materials

In piezoelectric ceramic materials, the directions of the electrical and mechanical axes depend on the direction of the original direct current polarizing field. During the poling process, a ceramic element undergoes a permanent increase in thickness between poling electrodes and a permanent decrease in length parallel to the electrodes.

When a direct current voltage of the same polarity as the poling voltage but of smaller magnitude is subsequently applied between the poling electrodes, the element experiences further but temporary expansion in the poling direction and contraction parallel to the electrodes. Conversely, when direct current of opposite polarity is applied, the element contracts in the poling direction and expands parallel to the electrodes. In either case, the element returns to the original poled dimensions when the voltage is removed from the electrodes.

These effects are shown greatly exaggerated in Fig. 2. The thickness and transverse effects are not of equal magnitude and there is a small volume change when voltage is applied to the electrodes.

When compressive force is applied in the poling direction or when tensile force is applied parallel to the electrodes, the voltage that results between electrodes has the same polarity as the original poling voltage. Reversing the direction of the applied force reverses the polarity of the resulting voltage between electrodes.

Assume that the poling electrodes are removed from a ceramic element and the element is provided with signal electrodes perpendicular to the poling direction. When a voltage is applied, a deformation takes place transversely, around an axis perpendicular to both the poling and signal directions (Fig. 3). When transverse forces are applied to the element, corresponding voltage appears between the signal electrodes.

FIGURE 2. Basic deformations of piezoelectric ceramic plates: (a) poled but at rest; (b) top electrode positive, bottom negative; (c) top electrode negative, bottom positive.

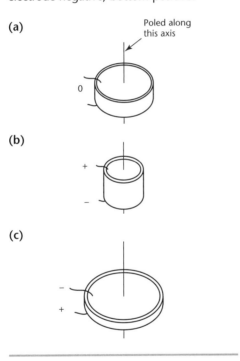

(a)

(b)

(c)

FIGURE 3. Shear action of ceramic plates.

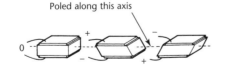

Mechanical and Acoustical Impedance Considerations

The mechanical impedance or acoustical impedance of crystal plates and ceramics are on the same order of magnitude as those of solids or liquids. For this reason, such piezoelectric elements are well suited for underwater sound applications and those mechanical applications involving large forces with small displacements.

Because these impedances are several orders of magnitude greater than those of gases, the transfer of energy to air, for example, is poor. For acoustical applications in air and mechanical applications involving small forces with comparatively large displacements, a system of levers is often used to obtain a better impedance match.

Resonant Devices

To obtain optimum performance from a piezoelectric device, the circuit to which it is connected must have certain characteristics in turn dictated by the design of the device. In discussing this subject, it is convenient to divide piezoelectric devices into two broad categories: nonresonant devices and resonant devices.

Nonresonant devices are so named because they are designed to operate well below resonance or over a relatively large frequency range, usually several octaves. All or most of the operating frequency range typically lies below the resonant frequency of the device. However, in some cases, the useful frequency range includes the frequencies of one or more resonances. In such cases, heavy damping is used. Nonresonant devices include microphones, headphones, accelerometers, high voltage sources and some underwater receiving transducers.

Resonant devices are designed to operate at a single frequency (the mechanical resonance frequency of the device) or over a band of frequencies usually less than an octave (the band includes the resonance frequency of the device). Resonant devices include ultrasonic transducers and underwater power transducers.

The electrical impedance of a piezoelectric device is more complicated than the simple capacitor representation typically used in discussing nonresonant devices. A more appropriate model is a capacitor representing the static capacitance of the piezoelectric element, shunted by an impedance representing the mechanical vibrating system. In most nonresonant devices, the latter impedance may be approximated by a capacitor.

Under these circumstances, there is a capacitor in parallel with a capacitor (a single capacitor representation).

In devices designed for operation at resonance, the impedance representing the mechanical system may at resonance become a resistance of relatively low value, shunted by the same static capacitance.

The shunt static capacitance typically is undesirable, whether the device is designed for operation at resonance or for broad band, below resonance operation. In electrically driven devices, shunt static capacitance shunts the driving amplifier or other signal source requiring that the source be capable of supplying extra current. In the case of mechanically driven piezoelectric devices, the static capacitance acts as a load on the active part of the transducer, reducing the electrical output.

In nonresonant devices, not much can be done about the shunt capacitance, except choosing a piezoelectric material with maximum activity. In resonant devices, the static capacitance may be neutralized by using a shunt or series inductor chosen to resonate with the static capacitance at the operating frequency (Fig. 4).

Properties of Piezoelectric Materials

Figure 5 shows typical symbols used to describe piezoelectric materials. These symbols are used to identify properties of materials and should not be used to describe piezoelectric elements made of

FIGURE 4. Resonant piezoelectric device with static capacitance neutralized by inductor: (a) for low impedance electrical source or load; (b) for high impedance electrical source or load.

(a)

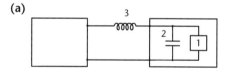

(b)

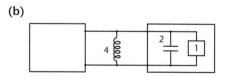

Legend
1. Impedance representing resonant mechanical system.
2. Static capacitance.
3. Series inductor.
4. Shunt inductor.

these materials. Electric boundary conditions are identified by indicating locations and connections of electrodes.

Axes

Piezoelectric materials are anisotropic and their electrical, mechanical and electromechanical properties differ for electrical or mechanical excitation along different directions. For systematic tabulation of properties, a standardized means for identifying directions is required. Where crystals are concerned, the orthogonal axes are referred to by numerals: 1 corresponds to the X axis, 2 corresponds to the Y axis and 3 corresponds to the Z axis.

Piezoelectric ceramics are isotropic and are not piezoelectric before they are polarized. Once they are polarized, they become anisotropic. The direction of the poling field is identified as direction 3. In the plane perpendicular to axis 3, the ceramics are nondirectional. Accordingly, the 1 and 2 axes may be arbitrarily located but must be perpendicular to each other.

Elastic Constants

To identify the directions of stress and strain, two numerical subscripts are added to the symbol S for elastic compliance (strain and stress). The first numeral indicates the direction of stress or strain and the second numeral indicates the direction of strain or stress. The symbol S with appropriate subscripts is used to identify elastic behavior under the specific condition that all external stresses not embraced by the symbol remain constant. Thus S_{13} is the symbol for the ratio of strain in direction 3 to stress in direction 1 provided there is no change in stress in directions 2 and 3. It also is the symbol for the ratio of strain in direction 1 to stress in direction 3 provided there is no change in stress in directions 1 and 2.

The restriction regarding stresses in other directions needs emphasizing. Suppose that a piezoelectric plate is clamped in a vise that applies a load, causing a stress in direction 3. Now, apply the load to cause stress to the plate in direction 1 and calculate the resulting strain in direction 1. If the plate were not clamped in the vise, the stress along axis 1 causes strain in direction 1 equal to S_{11} times the stress. In addition, there is strain in directions 2 and 3. The vise, however, tends to prevent the strain in direction 3 and in so doing, causes stress in direction 3. The development of this stress violates the requirement imposed in the definition that S_{11} cannot be used to calculate the strain in direction 1.

Consider a second example. This time the plate is resting on the table and a weight is placed on top. The weight causes a stress in direction 3. Now, apply the load to cause a stress in direction 1 and calculate the resulting strain in direction 1. As a result of the stress in direction 1, the plate experiences strain in direction 3, lifting the weight slightly. However, stress in direction 3 caused by the weight has not changed (except momentarily while the weight was being lifted) and accordingly the symbol S_{11} is, in this case, appropriate for calculating the strain in direction 1 resulting from application of stress in direction 1.

Shear stress or strain around axis 1 is indicated by the subscript 4, around axis 2 by subscript 5 and around axis 3 by subscript 6. Thus, S_{44} is the ratio of transverse strain around axis 1 to transverse stress around axis 1. A restriction requiring that stresses not embraced by the symbol must remain constant is theoretically applicable here also but, because of symmetry conditions, it is not applicable to transverse compliances of ceramics.

Because piezoelectric materials interchange mechanical (elastic) and electrical energy, the elastic properties depend on electric boundary conditions. For example, when electrodes on a bar of piezoelectric material are connected together, the bar displays higher elastic compliance than when the electrodes are not connected together. Thus, in defining elastic properties, the electric boundary conditions must be identified. This is done by adding a superscript to the symbol.

When the electric field across the piezoelectric body is held constant, for example by short circuiting the electrodes, the superscript E is used. When the electric charge density is held constant, for example by maintaining an open circuit at the electrodes, the superscript D is used. Thus S_{33}^E is the symbol for the ratio of strain to stress along axis 3 if all other external stresses are constant and the electric field is constant.

Dielectric Constants

In piezoelectric materials, the dielectric constant ε (dielectric displacement or

FIGURE 5. Typical symbols used to describe piezoelectric material properties.

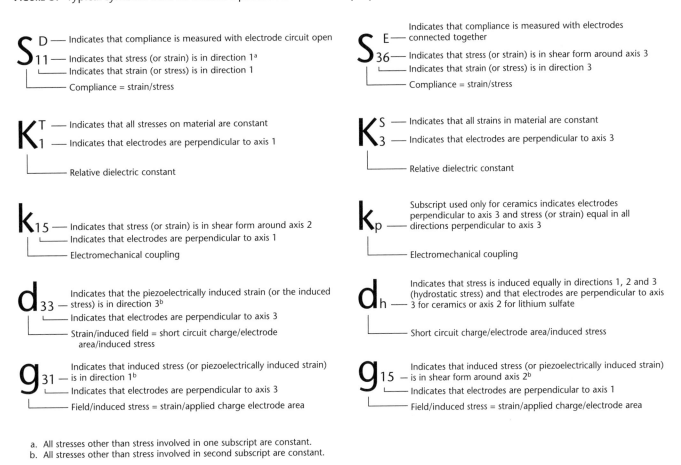

a. All stresses other than stress involved in one subscript are constant.
b. All stresses other than stress involved in second subscript are constant.

charge density per electric field) depends on the directions of field and dielectric displacement. For this reason, subscripts are added to the symbol to indicate the directions. The first subscript denotes the direction of the electric field or dielectric displacement. The second subscript denotes the direction of the dielectric displacement or electric field. Thus ε_{33} is the ratio field applied in direction 3 to the resulting dielectric displacement in direction 3.

In most piezoelectric materials used in ultrasonic transducers, a field along one axis results in dielectric displacement only along the same axis, so that the two subscripts for these materials are always the same. Accordingly, one subscript often is omitted: ε_3 means the same as ε_{33}.

Because piezoelectric materials interchange electrical and mechanical energy, the electrical properties depend on mechanical boundary conditions. When a piezoelectric body is completely free to vibrate, the dielectric constant is higher than when the body is mechanically restrained. Accordingly, superscripts are added to the symbol for dielectric constant to indicate the mechanical boundary conditions. Superscript T denotes the condition of constant stress (no mechanical restraint). Superscript S denotes the condition of constant strain (material completely restrained to prevent any mechanical deformation when field is applied, a condition that can be approached only under very special conditions). Thus ε_{11}^{T} is the dielectric constant for field and dielectric displacement in direction 1 under the condition of constant stress on the body and ε_{11}^{S} is the corresponding dielectric constant under the condition of constant strain in the body.

The relative dielectric constant, sometimes identified by the symbol K, is the ratio of the material dielectric constant ε to the dielectric constant of a vacuum ε_0 ($\varepsilon_0 = 8.85 \times 10^{12}$ F·m^{-1}):

$$(1) \quad K_{11}^{T} = \frac{\epsilon_{11}^{T}}{\epsilon_0}$$

Piezoelectric Constants

The most common electromechanical constants are coupling k, strain constant d and stress constant g. For each of these, the directions of field and stress or strain are indicated by two subscripts.

The first subscript indicates the direction of electric field. The second subscript indicates the direction of stress or strain. As in the case of elastic constants, subscripts 4, 5 and 6 denote stress or strain around axes 1, 2 and 3 respectively.

Coupling

Coupling is an expression for the ability of a piezoelectric material to exchange electrical energy for mechanical energy or vice versa. Coupling squared is equal to the transformed energy divided by the total energy input. The same constant is applied for conversion from electrical to mechanical energy and from mechanical to electrical energy.

Except in one special case noted below, the coupling coefficients typically used and those given here are for the cases where all external stresses (except the input stress considered in the energy transformation) are constant:

$$(2) \quad K_{31}^{2} = \frac{a}{b}$$

where a is transformed electrical energy causing mechanical strain in direction 1 when all external stresses are constant and b is electrical energy input to electrodes on faces perpendicular to axis 3. For example:

$$(3) \quad K_{31}^{2} = \frac{c}{d}$$

where c is transformed mechanical energy causing an electrical charge to flow between connected electrodes on faces perpendicular to axis 3 and d is the mechanical energy input accompanying the stress in direction 1, with all other external stresses constant.

A special case of considerable practical importance involves using thickness vibrations in ceramic plates or disks at frequencies above the resonant frequencies determined by the length and width of the element. Under these conditions, the inertia of the piezoelectric material effectively prevents lateral vibrations. The effect is the same as though infinitely rigid clamps were applied to the plate to prevent length and width vibrations. Such theoretical clamps would cause opposing dynamic stresses as the element tries to vibrate laterally. The qualification that all external stresses are constant is not met and accordingly k_{33} does not define electromechanical coupling under such conditions. The coupling in this special case is identified by the symbol k_{t}.

Another special case involves coupling between electric field in direction 3 in ceramics and mechanical action simultaneously in the 1 and 2 directions. This coupling is identified by the symbol k_{p} (planar coupling). It is important because of the ease with which it may be measured with high accuracy, yielding a simple measure of the effectiveness of poling of ceramic components.

Piezoelectric *d* Constants

The piezoelectric *d* constants express the ratio of strain developed along or around a specified axis to the field applied parallel to a specified axis, when all external stresses are constant. The *d* constants also express the ratio of short circuit charge per unit area of electrode flowing between connected electrodes that are perpendicular to a specified axis to (1) the stress along a specified axis or (2) the stress around a specified axis, when all other external stresses are constant. For example, $d31$ denotes the ratio of strain in direction 1 to the field applied in direction 3 when the piezoelectric material is mechanically free in all directions. It also denotes the ratio of charge (per unit area of electrode) that flows between electrodes perpendicular to axis 3 and connected together to the stress in direction 1 when the material is free of external stresses in all other directions.

A special case applies to piezoelectric ceramics. These materials develop substantial charge when subjected to uniform load along all three axes (hydrostatic pressure). The ratio of short circuit charge per unit area of electrode to the applied hydrostatic pressure is identified by the symbol d_h, the hydrostatic *d* constant. For ceramics, the electrodes are understood to be perpendicular to axis 3. For lithium sulfate, the electrodes are understood to be perpendicular to the Y or 2 axis. A more descriptive symbol is d_{3h} or d_{2h} but such designations are not commonly used.

Piezoelectric *g* Constants

The piezoelectric *g* constants express the ratio of field developed along a specified axis to the stress along or around a specified axis when all other external stresses are constant. The *g* constants also express the ratio of strain developed along or around a specified axis to the electric charge per unit area of electrode applied to electrodes perpendicular to a specified axis.

For example, g_{33} denotes the ratio of field developed in direction 3 to stress in direction 3 when all other external stresses are zero. It also denotes the ratio of strain developed in direction 3 to the charge per unit area of electrode applied to electrodes on faces perpendicular to axis 3.

Frequency Limitations

An important restriction must be observed in the constants discussed above when calculating the behavior of actual bodies of piezoelectric material. If the stress, strain, electric field and dielectric displacement involved in the constants are uniform throughout the body, then the constants may be used directly in simple calculations. For example, when a static or low frequency alternating field is applied, the change in length of a piezoelectric bar equals the product of the appropriate *d* constant, the applied field and the length.

On the other hand, if the stress or field is not uniform throughout the body, then the behavior of the body as a whole may be determined only by integrating the behavior of all the incremental portions of the body. In this case, the constants discussed above are used to relate stress, strain, field and charge density in each increment.

The most common situation where nonuniform distribution of stress is encountered, preventing simple bulk calculation, is when the frequency of the electrical or mechanical excitation of the body is at or close to the mechanical resonance frequency of the body.

Frequency Constant

The frequency constant *N* is the product of the mechanical resonant frequency under specified electrical boundary conditions (short circuit or open circuit) and the dimension that determines that resonant frequency. It is applicable only to specific boundary conditions.

For example, N_1 for piezoelectric ceramics applies only to a long, thin, narrow bar polarized perpendicular to the length and measured with the polarizing electrodes connected together. The same bar poled along the length has a different frequency constant. In this case, the assigned designation N_{3a} applies when measurement is made with the electrodes open circuited.

Electrical Losses

Some piezoelectric materials, including quartz, are high quality dielectrics. Other piezoelectric materials, notably the piezoelectric ceramics, are relatively lossy. The dielectric losses in ceramics may be the limiting factor in the power handling capabilities of transducers. The losses are expressed as a dissipation factor, the ratio of effective series resistance to effective series reactance.

Mechanical Losses

When an elastic body is deformed, most of the mechanical energy applied in causing the deformation is stored as elastic energy. However, a small part of the applied energy is dissipated as heat because of molecular friction.

In some applications of piezoelectric materials, such mechanical losses may become important. Usually they are far outweighed by mechanical losses in other elements of the piezoelectric device — in particular, in cement joints between piezoelectric materials and driving or driven members. Mechanical losses are expressed in terms of mechanical Q, the ratio of mechanical stiffness reactance or mass reactance at resonance to the mechanical resistance.

Aging

Most of the properties of piezoelectric ceramics change gradually. The changes tend to be logarithmic with time after the original polarization. For example, the dielectric constant 1 h after poling may be 1000 and 10 h after poling it may be 990. At 100 h, it is about 980, at 1000 h about 970 and at 10 000 h about 960. In this case, the dielectric constant is said to age about 1 percent per time decade. The aging of various properties depends on the ceramic composition and on the way the ceramic is processed during manufacture. Exact aging rates cannot be specified but it is typical to specify that the aging of a given property is less than some limiting rate.

Because of aging, exact values for various properties such as dielectric constant, coupling and elastic modulus may be specified only at a stated time after poling. The longer the time period after poling, the more stable the material becomes.

High Stress

Most of the properties of piezoelectric ceramics vary with the level of electrical or mechanical stress when such stresses are large. Data commonly presented for piezoelectric ceramics are for stress levels low enough for the results to be independent of stress.

Curie Point

For each piezoelectric material, there is a characteristic temperature called the *curie point*. When a ceramic element is heated above the curie point, it suffers permanent and complete loss of piezoelectric activity. In practice, the operating temperature for a piezoelectric ceramic must be limited to some value substantially below the curie point.

In addition, at elevated temperatures, the aging process is accelerated, electrical losses increase and the maximum safe stress is reduced.

Properties of Piezoelectric Elements

Equivalent Circuits

Equivalent circuit techniques have been used for many years to obtain solutions to electrical and mechanical problems. These same techniques are used to describe the behavior of piezoelectric elements.[4,5] Table 1 shows the electrical and mechanical units used in the construction of equivalent circuits for electromechanical systems.

These equivalent circuits are shown in Fig. 6. If the constants in these two circuits are suitably related, the circuits are

TABLE 1. Analogous electrical and mechanical units for electromechanical systems.

Electrical Unit	Mechanical Unit
Voltage	force
Current	velocity
Charge	displacement
Capacitance	compliance
Inductance	mass
Impedance	impedance

FIGURE 6. Basic equivalent circuits: (a) ratio of N to 1; (b) ratio of 1 to N'.

(a)

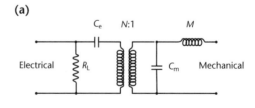

(b)

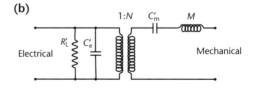

Legend
C = capacitor
M = mechanical inductance
N = voltage output proportional to number of turns
R = resistor

equivalent at all frequencies. The mechanical terminals represent the face or point of mechanical energy transfer to or from the piezoelectric element. The inductance symbol M represents the effective vibrating mass of the element.

The transformer symbol represents an ideal electromechanical transformer, a device that transforms voltage to force and vice versa and current to velocity and vice versa, without loss and without energy storage. The transformation ratio $N{:}1$ in Fig. 6a is the ratio of voltage input to force output of the ideal transformer and also the ratio of velocity input to current output. It is used in purely electrical network calculations. The transformation ratio $1{:}N'$ in Fig. 6b has similar significance. The capacitance symbols on the electrical side represent electrical capacitances. The capacitance symbols on the mechanical side represent mechanical compliances.

The choice of circuit for a particular problem depends on the external circuit elements connected to the piezoelectric element. Because the two circuits are equivalent, either may be used but often one is more convenient than the other. For example, if the electrical terminals are connected to a constant current generator and it is necessary to calculate the force applied to a mechanical load connected to the mechanical terminals of the piezoelectric element, the problem is simplified by selecting the circuit in Fig. 6a to eliminate capacitance C_e from the calculations.

These circuits are useful for most design purposes. However, it should be emphasized that they only approximate the actual behavior of the piezoelectric elements. The approximation is useful up to and slightly above the first resonance frequency of the mounted, unloaded element. At higher frequencies, further resonances typically may be observed in the behavior of a piezoelectric element because of the distributed nature of the mass and compliance, for which only lumped elements are used. Better approximations of the actual performance can be obtained by modifying the equivalent circuits to include additional reactance elements or by allowing some elements of the simple circuits to vary with frequency in a prescribed manner.

Because of the approximate nature of equivalent circuits, the accuracy of representing the piezoelectric element is better at some frequencies than at others. The most accurate frequency range depends on the choice of values assigned to the elements of the circuit.

The effective mass or moment of inertia is chosen so that the equivalent circuit has the same resonant frequency as the actual crystal. The height of the actual measured resonance peak of the element is finite because of mechanical losses. The equivalent circuit data include no mechanical loss element so that the computed response is infinite at resonance.

For most nonresonant electromechanical transducer design problems, this omission is not significant. Introduced losses (usually for control of frequency response) greatly outweigh internal losses.

PART 2. Transduction[1]

The approach to transducer design presented below is aimed at engineered design using computer modeling. Before the design process is addressed, important performance parameters are identified and techniques are selected to measure these parameters. The instrumentation used to characterize transducers must not modify the transducer response. Some of the measurements should be performed under conditions that simulate the actual testing application of the transducer. The transducer's components must be characterized individually and then incorporated into the transducer design.

A computer model has the advantage of predicting the performance of a transducer, allowing fine tuning of the design before committing resources and materials to fabrication.

Instrumentation

Instrumentation and Transducer Characterization

Significant differences have been observed between transducer characterization data from different sources. One investigation revealed that differences in instrumentation and measurement technique could seriously affect the apparent performance of a transducer (Figs. 7 and 8). Figure 7c shows the waveform and frequency data furnished by a manufacturer with its 10 MHz transducer. Figure 8 shows the data acquired from the transducer when tested at the buyer's facility. The waveforms and the spectra are very different: the manufacturer's spectrum peaks at about 10 MHz and the buyer's spectrum peaks at about 6 MHz.

Research showed that the discrepancy was largely a matter of technique. In an effort to duplicate the manufacturer's data, pulser damping and signal gating were adjusted until a close match was achieved (see Figs. 7a and 7b). This exercise strongly emphasizes the need to include the essential elements of test procedures, directly or by specific reference, within a transducer specification.

Transducer Characterization Station

A computerized system for measuring typical ultrasonic transducer parameters has been developed. It can measure waveform and spectrum as well as relative

FIGURE 7. Comparison of performance characteristics from commercial transducer (see Fig. 8): (a) signal waveform with damping and gating; (b) frequency spectrum; (c) data furnished by manufacturer (frequency and waveform).

(a)

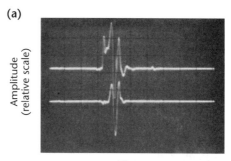

Time
(relative scale)

(b)

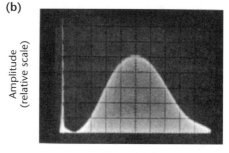

Frequency
(relative scale)

(c)

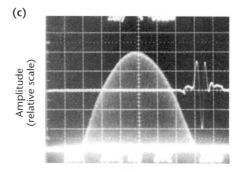

Time
(relative scale)

sensitivity, electrical impedance and sound field beam profiles. Transducer design and optimization software allows for transducer modeling and predicted performance based on the transducer model. Impedance matching software is included for selection of effective impedance matching networks, including component value calculation.

System components and their individual functions are as follows. A pulser is used to pulse the transmitting transducer and initiate overall system timing, including repetition rate. A pulse generator produces a variable width pulse for delayed triggering and the introduction of a time offset between the two pulsers. A second pulser is used for pulsing the transducer being evaluated. Lastly, a commercial receiver is used for amplification and attenuation of the test transducer's received signal.

The catch transducer's received signal is used as a trigger to produce a moving gate while the function trigger select switch box (Fig. 9) is used to differentiate the pulse generator's output. It is also used to switch the correct trigger signal to both the first pulser and the computer oscilloscope. Switching is needed because

the trigger to be used depends on the particular measurement being performed. The computer oscilloscope is used for acquisition of waveform data and an analog oscilloscope is used for setup and monitoring purposes. A jet printer is used to produce hardcopy. A personal computer controls the entire process, including the motor/drive unit used to provide precise positioning capability for sound field measurements.

Differences in Transducer Performance

Several factors contribute to differences between the measured and predicted performance of ultrasonic transducers. The observed differences outside the range of instrument and test error and the contributing factors are discussed below.

Inductance and Resistance

Inductors used in the matching networks contain a resistive element that affects the circuit. However, it is customary to assume that the effect is negligible. To verify this assumption, measurements were taken on the inductive and resistive components of inductors at 5 MHz. The study consisted of measuring the resistance and inductance of a group of five inductors at each of 34 nominal inductor values. Figure 10 shows an example of inductive and resistive components over a frequency range of 1 to 10 MHz for one inductor.

Table 2 reports the measured averages for each inductor grouped by the nominal inductor value. The inductors are specified not to exceed ±10 percent of the nominal

FIGURE 8. Data from research transducer developed to meet specific performance criteria: (a) signal waveforms; (b) frequency spectrum.

(a)

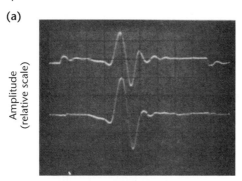

Time
(relative scale)

(b)

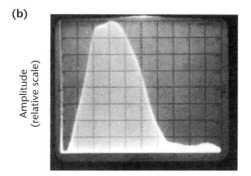

Frequency
(relative scale)

FIGURE 9. Function trigger select switch box (50 Ω cable used throughout, with shields tied to common chassis ground).

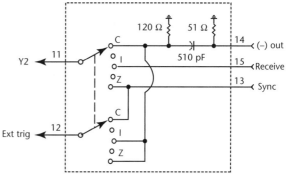

Legend
Z = impedance/pulser characterization
I = Immersion transducers
C = contact transducers

Figure 10. Gain phase analyzer data of 15 μH (nominal) inductor.

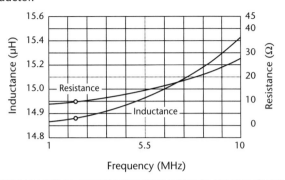

Frequency (MHz)

Table 2. Measured average inductor values.

Nominal Inductor Value (μH)	Average Measured Inductance (μH)	Average Measured Resistance (Ω)
0.10	0.090	0.162
0.15	0.142	0.256
0.18	0.172	0.314
0.22	0.213	0.394
0.27	0.259	0.416
0.33	0.306	0.496
0.39	0.385	0.688
0.47	0.451	0.836
0.56	0.546	0.990
0.68	0.660	1.142
0.62	0.772	1.272
1.0	0.956	1.400
1.5	1.502	1.148
1.8	1.750	1.434
2.2	2.198	1.910
2.7	2.764	1.946
3.3	3.116	1.512
3.9	3.822	1.936
4.7	4.574	2.388
5.6	5.194	2.828
6.8	6.502	2.864
8.2	7.652	3.558
10.0	9.560	4.486
15.0	14.636	7.086
18.0	17.504	9.794
22.0	22.040	15.064
27.0	26.528	14.954
33.0	32.562	18.34
39.0	39.027	23.35
47.0	45.996	27.88
56.0	56.812	25.056
68.0	65.912	48.24
82.0	78.960	38.2
100.0	95. 480	57.22

value. Figure 11 shows plots of inductance versus resistance data taken as illustrated in Fig. 10. This study of transducer fabrication incorporating matching networks has been mostly in the 20 to 30 μH range with inductors that have resistive elements on the order of 8 to 15 Ω. The resistance of the inductors is sufficient to affect transducer performance and should be included in the calculation of the series resistance for the matching network. The series resistance value of the matching network is included as one of the parameters in the transducer modeling software.

Figure 11. Plots of measured inductance versus measured resistance over range of inductors: (a) small nominal inductance; (b) medium nominal inductance; (c) large nominal inductance.

(a)

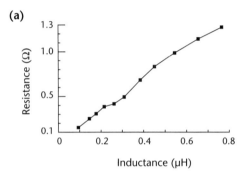

Inductance (μH)

(b)

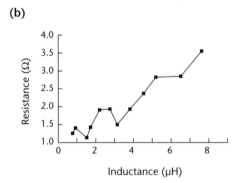

Inductance (μH)

(c)

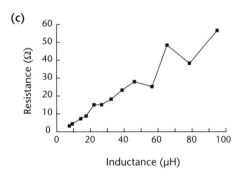

Inductance (μH)

Piezoelectric Element

The piezoelectric element parameter values supplied by the manufacturer are usually based on an average value derived from sampling several batches of piezoelectric materials. The nominal values are not sufficiently precise for use in modeling the performance of transducers. A means of measuring the piezoelectric coupling factor, the damped capacitance, the dielectric constant and the free resonant frequency of piezoelectric elements are a key to transducer modeling.

To measure the damped capacitance C_0 and the electromechanical coupling factor k of piezoelectric transducer elements, a technique consists of the sudden placement of an electronic charge on the plated surfaces of the element and then measuring the variation of the resulting voltage between these surfaces.[6] What is observed is a voltage step followed by a train of triangular waves as shown in Fig. 12. Figure 13 is a simplified illustration of this technique.

FIGURE 12. Wave train during measurement of damped capacitance.

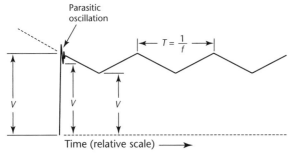

Time (relative scale) ⟶

Legend
f = frequency
T = wave cyclic interval
V = signal amplitude

FIGURE 13. Basic circuit for measuring damped capacitance and electromechanical coupling factor of piezoelectric transducers.

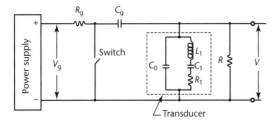

Legend
C = capacitor
g = subscript designating input
R = resistor
L = inductance
V = electric potential

The input capacitor C_g is charged to a voltage V_g through resistors R_g and R_L and then the switch is closed. Following the closure, the voltage V_t across the transducer rises too rapidly to be affected by the mechanical nature of the transducer (represented in the diagram by equivalent series circuit LCR) or by the charging resistors R_g and R_L. The magnitude of this voltage step is used to calculate the value of the damped (constant strain) capacitance of the transducer by using the following equation:

$$(4) \quad C_0 = C_g \frac{V_g - V_{t0}}{V_{t0}}$$

This equation is derived from the equality of Eqs. 5 and 6. After the C_g is fully charged and before the switch is closed, the charge on C_g is given:

$$(5) \quad Q_0 = V_g C_g$$

After the switch is closed, that same quantity of charge is shared by C_g and C_0:

$$(6) \quad Q_0 = V_{t0}\left(C_g + C_0\right)$$

Before the switch is closed, the energy stored in C_g is:

$$(7) \quad W_g = \frac{Q_0^2}{2C_g}$$

After the switch is closed and after the high frequency transients have died out, the stored energy is given by:

$$(8) \quad W_a = \frac{Q_0^2}{2\left(C_g + C_0\right)}$$

Note that W_a is smaller than W_g by the ratio $C_g \cdot (C_g + C_0)^{-1}$. That is, by closing the switch, energy is lost in the amount of $W_g - W_a$. This energy is not recoverable. It is lost either through lossy elements in the circuit or by electromagnetic radiation. Initially, this energy is stored alternately in the parasitic inductances of the circuit and in the circuit capacitances.

During a short period after the switch closure, the high frequency oscillations are observed on the voltage waveform. These oscillations die out as this unavailable energy is dissipated. The oscillations do not significantly affect the measurement of element characteristics when relatively low frequency elements are being evaluated (that is, for elements with characteristic frequencies below 5 MHz). But when element frequencies approach 10 MHz, these oscillations interfere with accurate measurement because they are superimposed on many of the triangular wave's first period.

In a typical circuit configuration, the frequency of these parasitic oscillations is about 100 MHz. The test circuit is laid out and fabricated with care to minimize the parasitic circuit inductance and ensure that the frequencies of the parasitic oscillations are well above the frequencies of the transducers to be tested by the device.

Recall from the analysis above that much energy is contained in the components controlling these oscillations. Therefore, in addition to maximizing the frequency of parasitic oscillations, a means is needed for damping the oscillations so that they die out within a few cycles. Placing resistors in series with the switch provides one means of damping the oscillations but this step is not frequency selective and tends to reduce the effectiveness of the circuit in the frequency range of interest (above 5 MHz). In particular, the severely rounded peaks of the characteristic triangular wave increase the likelihood of significant measurement error.

Ferromagnetic ceramic beads have provided an effective solution for this problem. Two or three of these beads threaded over conductors carrying the high frequency currents provide adequate damping. The effects of the beads decrease with decreasing frequency and the effect on the circuit at the operating frequencies of the transducers is negligible.

A silicon controlled rectifier as the switch makes rise times on the order of 10 ns possible, fast enough to excite the 100 MHz parasitic oscillations discussed above. The design of a piezoelectric element test circuit is shown in Fig. 14.

The electromechanical coupling factor k, when squared, represents the fraction of the electrical energy input to a piezoelectric element — the fraction transformed and available to do mechanical work. Conversely, k^2 also represents the fraction of mechanical energy input to an element, transformed and available to do electrical work. In the test device described above, very little energy is radiated as acoustic energy because of the poor acoustic coupling to the element holding fixture and very little is dissipated in the resistors of the test device.

Therefore, this available energy flows back and forth between electrical storage and mechanical storage for a long time as evidenced by the long triangular wave train that follows the first voltage step. This fortunate circumstance allows precise measurements. The resistor R_1' (Fig. 13) represents the dissipative mechanisms within the piezoelectric element. In high Q elements, R_1 is very small compared to the reactance of either C_1 or L_1 at the element's resonant frequency. When the element is loaded acoustically, the effective value of R_1 is increased and the effective Q of the transducer is reduced.

To determine the electrical energy input to the transducer by this special test circuit and the available mechanical energy, two voltage measurements are made across the terminals of the transducer: (1) the voltage V_{t0} at the first peak and (2) the voltage V_{ti} at the first valley of the triangular wave. As a first step, assume that the input capacitor C_g is very small compared to C_0 and its effect is not included in the following calculations. At the end, a correction factor is added to account for this omission. The voltage at the first peak provides the information needed to compute the input energy W_{t0}:

$$(9) \quad W_{t0} = \left(V_{t0}\right)^2 \left(\frac{C_0}{2}\right)$$

but:

$$(10) \quad Q_0 = V_{t0} C_0$$

FIGURE 14. Diagram of piezoelectric element test circuit.

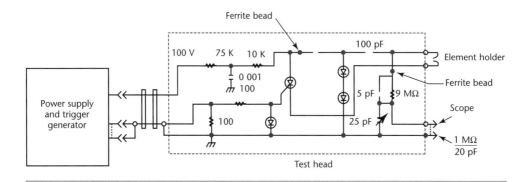

therefore:

$$(11) \quad W_{t0} = \frac{Q_0}{2}(V_{t0})$$

Next, the residual stored energy is computed after all oscillations of the triangular wave of the transducer voltage have died out. Discounting the effects of any direct current paths, the voltage across the transducer settles to a level halfway between the peak and the valley of the triangular wave. The residual energy stored in the transducer is given by:

$$(12) \quad W_{tr} = \frac{Q_0}{2}\left(\frac{V_{t0} + V_{ti}}{2}\right)$$

Now, the energy available for doing mechanical work is computed as the difference between Eqs. 10 and 11:

$$(13) \quad W_{am} = W_{t0} - W_{tr}$$
$$= \frac{Q_0}{2}\left(V_{t0} - \frac{V_{t0} + V_{ti}}{2}\right)$$
$$= \frac{Q_0}{2}\left(\frac{V_{t0} + V_{ti}}{2}\right)$$

The electromechanical coupling factor is determined by the ratio of W_{am} to W_{t0}:

$$(14) \quad k^2 = \frac{W_{am}}{W_{t0}}$$
$$= \frac{V_{2t0} - V_{ti}}{2V_{t0}}$$
$$= \frac{1 - \frac{V_{ti}}{V_{t0}}}{2}$$

This equation is valid when the input capacitor C_g is very small compared to the element's damped capacitance C_0. When this is not the case, the voltage measurements across the element are made in exactly the same way but the input voltage V_g must also be known and used to compute a correction factor. With the correction factor added, the expression for the electromechanical coupling factor becomes:

$$(15) \quad k^2 = \frac{\left(1 - \frac{V_{ti}}{V_{t0}}\right)\left(1 + \frac{V_{t0}}{V_g}\right)}{2}$$

It may be helpful to approach the calculation of k^2 in a different way. This is based on the assumption that the value of C_0 and C_1 are known and Q_0 is shared

according to their relative sizes, so that the total residual energy is given by:

$$(16) \quad W_{t0} = \frac{Q_0^2}{C}C_0$$

After all oscillations have ceased, the voltages across C_0 and C_1 are equal and Q_0 is shared according to their relative sizes, so that the total residual energy is given:

$$(17) \quad W_{tr} = \frac{Q_0^2}{2(C_0 + C_1)}$$

Again, the difference between W_{t0} and W_{tr} is the available mechanical energy W_{am} and k^2 is the ratio of W_{am} to W_{t0}:

$$(18) \quad k^2 = \frac{W_{am}}{W_{t0}} = \frac{W_{t0} - W_{tr}}{W_{t0}}$$
$$= \frac{C_1}{C_0 + C_1}$$

This equation may be confirmed by comparing it with the standard on piezoelectricity.[7] There, the effective electromechanical coupling factor is defined:

$$(19) \quad k_{eff}^2 = \frac{f_p^2 - f_s^2}{f_p^2}$$

where f_s is frequency of maximum conductance and f_p is frequency of maximum resistance. Therefore, k_{eff} can be determined by measuring f_p and f_s with an impedance analyzer. By multiplying both top and bottom of the fraction by $(2\pi)^2$:

$$(20) \quad k_{eff}^2 = \frac{\omega_p^2 - \omega_s^2}{\omega_p^2}$$

where ω_p is radian frequency of maximum resistance and ω_s is radian frequency of maximum conductance.

The characteristic radian frequencies of the equivalent circuit shown in Fig. 13 can be defined in the following ways:

$$(21) \quad \omega_a^2 = \frac{1}{L_1 C_1}$$

and:

$$(22) \quad \omega_0^2 = \frac{1}{L_1 C_0}$$

and:

$$(23) \quad \omega_p^2 = \omega_s^2 + \omega_0^2$$

Substituting these values into Eq. 17, all of the L_1 terms cancel:

$$(24) \quad k_{\text{eff}}^2 = \frac{C_1}{C_1 + C_0}$$

This is identical to Eq. 18 obtained for k^2 by a different analysis.

The period of the triangular wave excited by the test device described above gives a very precise measurement of the piezoelectric element's resonant frequency. Good results can be obtained by measuring period time on high quality oscilloscopes. When the time calibration or linearity of the oscilloscope is not adequate, a comparison technique may be used (the output of a precision signal generator is adjusted to match the frequency of the triangular wave). The test devices discussed here measure three important parameters of piezoelectric elements quickly and with good precision. Those characteristics are the damped capacitance C_0, the electromechanical coupling factor k and the resonant frequency. Experience shows the device to be an important tool for transducer development and fabrication facilities.

Electrode Thickness on Piezoelectric Elements

The effect of the electrode deposited on the piezoelectric element was once considered to have little effect on performance. It was assumed that the two common methods of depositing silver,

fired silver deposit or sputter deposit, resulted in silver layers of uniform thickness on the order of 2.5 µm (0.0001 in.). However, electrode plating on some elements was found to vary from 25 to 75 µm. In this range of thickness, the plating thickness affects the performance of the transducer.

Electrodes are shown in Figs. 15 and 16 (cross section microphotographs of four transducers). The transducers were manufactured using nominal frequency elements from the same manufacturer. The sampling consisted of two groups of transducers: 9.7 mm (0.38 in.) round at 5 MHz and 6.4 mm (0.25 in.) round at 10 MHz. The transducers were characterized, sectioned and photographed at 100× magnification to sample plating thickness and to measure the acoustic impedance of the backing. The variation in electrode thickness is visible in the figures.

The effects of variations in electrode thickness on the performance of transducers can be minimized by using the thinnest electrodes possible. Piezoelectric elements are available with gold alloy electrodes with thicknesses on the order of 5 nm (2×10^{-7} in.), several orders of magnitude less than that of silver plating. Consistency of thickness is not as important when electrodes are less than 2 µm.

Effects of Angle Beam Wedge

With angle beam transducers, plastic wedges are used between a longitudinal

FIGURE 15. Examples of two 9.7 mm (0.38 in.), 5 MHz transducers photographed at 100×: (a) first transducer; (b) second transducer.

(a)

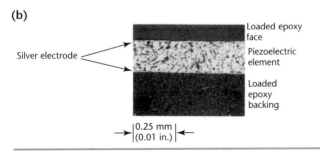

(b)

FIGURE 16. Cross sections of 6.4 mm (0.25 in.) photographed at 100X: (a) 10 MHz transducer; (b) 5 MHz transducer.

(a)

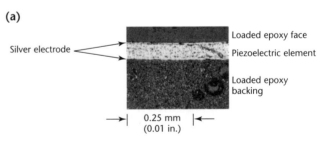

(b)

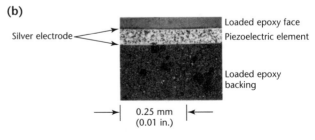

transducer and a test object to generate mode converted transverse waves. The plastics commonly used for the wedges are acrylics such as methyl methacrylate and polymers such as polystyrene. These materials have a strong effect on the frequency response of the pulse emerging from the wedge. A 5 MHz center frequency transducer transmitting a longitudinal wave through the plastic wedge in the angle beam transducer assembly, for example, produced a 3.5 to 4.0 MHz peak frequency, transverse beam in the test object coupled to the wedge.

The effect becomes more acute for frequencies around 10 MHz, when the peak frequency in the transverse beam is shifted to lower values of 6 to 7 MHz. The path length of the ultrasonic wave varies from front to rear as it travels from the transducer through the wedge to the surface in contact with the test object. Different frequencies present in the incident beam suffer different amounts of attenuation. (Attenuation increases with increasing frequency.) The effect is more pronounced at high frequencies for the incident pulse of the broader band width. Therefore, it is important to know the transmission characteristics of ultrasonic pulses through the plastics commonly used for wedges.

Reliable wedge materials are manufactured as acrylics (polymethyl methacrylate) and polymers (polystyrene). Acrylic thermoplastics are products of the homopolymerization of acrylic ester monomers, principally methyl methacrylate. The chemical formula is $[-CH_2(CH_3)(COOCH_3)]$ and is typically amorphous. Many acrylics are copolymers of two monomers. Some of them are linear whereas others are crosslinked. Cast acrylic sheets made of methyl methacrylate monomer are available in linear and crosslinked compositions.

Widely used polystyrene brands are thermoset crosslinked styrene copolymer. Its chemical formula is $[-CH_2CH(C_6H_5)-]$ and it is typically amorphous. Commercial polystyrene typically contains up to 2000 styrene units in the polymer chain. General purpose polystyrene is essentially pure polystyrene with relative molecular mass M_r between 50 000 and 60 000. The relative molecular mass (formerly known as *molecular weight*) is the ratio of the average mass per molecule to 12^{-1} of the mass of an atom of the nuclide carbon-12. Monomers frequently used for copolymerization with styrene are acrylonitril, alphamethyl styrene butadiene, maleic anhydride and methyl methacrylate. Polystyrene is semilinear in structure and amorphous in nature. Impact strength is improved for impact grades by blending with rubbers such as polybutadiene.

Table 3 gives the mechanical properties of an acrylic and a polystyrene wedge material. The attenuation values in Table 4 are from the literature.

Figure 17 is a diagram of experimental equipment used for measuring attenuation at frequencies between 1 MHz and 10 MHz. Attenuation measurements are made at several discrete frequencies over the range of interest (2.25, 5.0, 7.5 and 10 MHz) using narrow band, tuned and undamped transducers. Consistently uniform coupling between each transducer and the test material is important in making all such attenuation measurements. One good procedure is to apply light machine oil between a transducer and a block of the chosen plastic material, wringing the transducer well onto the block to remove air bubbles. A loading device can be designed and used for applying uniform pressure to ensure consistent coupling throughout the measurement.

Plastics have high ultrasonic attenuation coefficients compared to those of metals. In most metals,

TABLE 3. Mechanical properties of two arbitrarily chosen plastic wedge materials — results will vary with other specimens. The acrylic is preshrunk and absorbs ultraviolet radiation.

Property	Acrylic	Polystyrene
Ultrasonic wave velocity (mm·s⁻¹)		
Longitudinal	2.73×10^6	2.36×10^6
Transverse	1.43×10^6	1.45×10^6
Longitudinal wavelength (mm)		
10 MHz	0.273	0.236
5 MHz	0.546	0.472
1 MHz	2.730	2.360
Transverse wavelength (mm)		
10 MHz	0.143	0.145
5 MHz	0.286	0.286
1 MHz	1.430	1.450
Other		
Density (g·cm⁻³)	1.180	1.050
Young's modulus (N·m⁻²)	4.15×10^9	3.2×10^9
Acoustic impedance (g·cm⁻²·s)	3.20×10^5	2.47×10^5
Hardness (rockwell)	M 85	M 65

TABLE 4. Ultrasonic attenuation factor for two plastic materials at various frequencies.

Material	Ultrasonic Attenuation Factor (dB·mm⁻¹)			
	1 MHz	2.5 MHz	5 MHz	10 MHz
Acrylic	1.5	3.5	7	—
Polystyrene	0.8	1.6	3.5	—

attenuation measurements may be made over a wide range of frequencies (using a block of constant thickness and the pulse echo technique) by observing the decay in amplitude of successive echoes. This same technique may be used to measure ultrasonic attenuation in plastics. However, to cover the frequency range of interest, it is usually necessary to use blocks of different thicknesses for different frequencies. These different thicknesses may be provided by steps in a single block.

A block of dimensions of $100 \times 50 \times 50$ mm ($4 \times 2 \times 2$ in.) with four steps of heights 13, 25, 38 and 50 mm (0.5, 1.0, 1.5 and 2 in.), for example, is a useful design for measuring attenuation in polystyrene and methyl methacrylate at frequencies ranging from 1 to 10 MHz. The top and bottom surfaces must be highly finished (typically 0.8 µm) and parallel to each other within 17 mrad (1 deg). For reliable attenuation measurements, the number of echoes obtained in a given material for a given frequency must exceed two.

In Fig. 17, the functions of the pulse modulator and receiver are to generate and receive radiofrequency pulses (tone burst or wave train). The pulse width, the pulse repetition rate, the pulse amplitude and the receiver gain must be carefully adjusted to maintain the narrow band width of the wave train pulse and to avoid saturation of the receiver. It is advisable to obtain as many equally spaced pulse echoes of exponentially decreasing heights as possible on the oscilloscope screen. The attenuation recorder provides a measure of the total

attenuation in decibels based on the first two echoes in the pulse echo train, according to Eq. 25:

$$(25) \quad \alpha = 20 \log \frac{V_1}{V_2}$$

Equation 25 is based on the assumption that no energy is lost at the front and back interfaces, by beam spread or by nonparallel reflecting surfaces. Under such ideal conditions, the pulse echo train produces:

$$(26) \quad \frac{V_1}{V_2} = \frac{V_2}{V_3} = \frac{V_3}{V_4}$$

where V_x is the amplitude in volts of the first through the fourth echoes in the train. However, the sources of error mentioned above do cause Eq. 25 to indicate values that are higher than the true attenuation attributable to internal loss mechanisms. A portion of ultrasonic energy is lost in the bond between the transducer and the test object on successive round trips of the ultrasonic pulse. Effects of these factors must be minimized or accounted for.

The effect of divergence of the sound beam can be minimized by making measurements with all multiple echoes appearing in the near field. In this respect, the stepped blocks are useful for shifting measurements to the step of the most practical height. Tables 5 and 6 show the data needed to make such a shift. When proper care is taken to minimize losses from beam divergence, surface finish and nonparallelism of the step faces, the measured attenuation can be attributed primarily to internal losses such as scattering and absorption.

Figure 18 shows the attenuation versus frequency for methyl methacrylate and styrene polymer. The vertical bar at each point indicates the spread (maximum to minimum) in measured values. At low frequency, the spread is about 0.05 dB, rising to 0.1 dB at high frequency. The overall accuracy of the measurement is 5 to 7 percent. The ultrasonic attenuation coefficient plotted in Fig. 18 was obtained from total measured attenuation divided by twice the height of the step chosen in the test object.

Attenuation coefficients in the acrylic are higher than those of polystyrene at all ultrasonic frequencies between 1 and 10 MHz. At high frequencies, the differences in ultrasonic attenuation coefficients for two plastics is higher than that for low frequencies. This behavior can be explained by those characteristics of polymeric structure important for determining its mechanical response to the elastic stress. These characteristics are

FIGURE 17. Diagram of test setup for attenuation measurement.

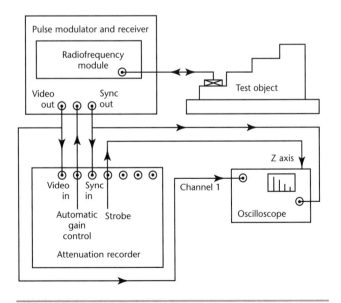

TABLE 5. Calculated values of near field length and half-angle of main lobe to point of zero energy for commercial acrylic, having longitudinal velocity of 2.73×10^6 mm·s^{-1} ($1.0^7 \times 10^5$ in.·s^{-1}), and for ultrasonic transducer, having diameter of 13 mm (0.5 in.).

Frequency (MHz)	Wavelength (mm)	Transducer Diameter to Wavelength (ratio)	Near Field		Half Angle	
			mm	(in.)	mrad	(deg)
10.0	0.27	47	148	(5.84)	26	(1.5)
7.5	0.36	35	111	(4.37)	35	(2.0)
5.0	0.54	23	74	(2.92)	52	(3.0)
2.25	1.09	11	33	(1.31)	117	(6.7)
1.0	2.72	5	15	(0.58)	264	(15.13)

TABLE 6. Calculated values of near field length and half angle of main lobe to point of zero energy for polystyrene, having longitudinal velocity of 2.39×10^6 mm·s^{-1} (9.4×10^4 in.·s^{-1}), and for ultrasonic transducer, having diameter of 13 mm (0.5 in.).

Frequency (MHz)	Wavelength (mm)	Transducer Diameter to Wavelength (ratio)	Near Field		Half Angle	
			mm	(in.)	mrad	(deg)
10.0	0.24	54	171	(6.72)	23	(1.30)
7.5	0.31	40	128	(5.04)	30	(1.73)
5.0	0.47	27	85	(3.36)	45	(2.60)
2.25	1.01	12	38	(1.51)	101	(5.78)
1.0	2.36	5	17	(0.67)	229	(13.12)

FIGURE 18. Ultrasonic attenuation versus frequency for two plastics: (a) methyl methacrylate (acrylic) and (b) styrene polymer (polystyrene).

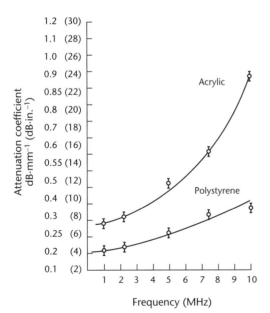

its relative molecular mass, crystallinity, crosslinking and chain stiffening.

The polystyrene shown in Fig. 18 is the thermoset crosslinked styrene polymer. The crosslinking involves the formation of strong covalent bonds between individual polymer chains. The crosslinking increases the mechanical strength and decreases the ability of individual chains to slide past one another. This, in turn, enhances the elastic response and reduces the viscous response of the polymer to the induced stress. Polystyrene, crosslinked, therefore shows less ultrasonic attenuation than does acrylic, not crosslinked.

Part 3. Generation and Reception of Ultrasound[8]

For optimum operation, it is important to understand the effect of the front panel controls on the internal functions of an ultrasonic testing instrument. Described below are the principles of operation for key components in a typical ultrasonic test instrument.

Transducer Excitation

Most transducers used for ultrasonic testing incorporate a thin plate of piezoelectric material to convert electrical energy, typically stored in a capacitor, into an ultrasonic signal that is radiated away. In most discontinuity detection and thickness gaging, it is advantageous to generate a compact ultrasonic waveform. This is best accomplished by exciting the transducer with a short, unipolar voltage waveform whose rise time is shorter than the time required for an ultrasonic impulse to move through the piezoelectric plate.

FIGURE 19. Waveforms used by ultrasonic testing systems: (a) spike pulse; (b) square wave pulse; (c) bipolar tone burst; (d) step pulse.

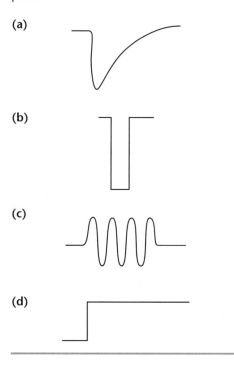

(a)

(b)

(c)

(d)

The influence of transmitter parameters on the shape of the ultrasonic signal has been extensively explored experimentally[9] and theoretically.[10] The effects of transducer parameters on the shape of the emitted ultrasonic signal are also well understood.[11] Figure 19 shows the two waveforms most often used in ultrasonic test instruments: spike and square wave pulses. The less popular bipolar tone burst and step waveforms are also shown.

Bipolar waveforms that have higher energy content are preferred in certain specialized testing applications, particularly to penetrate thick, highly attenuating materials. The use of bipolar signals to excite the transducer can result in significant improvement in signal amplitude but at the expense of a reduction in resolution. This tradeoff is often acceptable, particularly in through-transmission testing.

An alternative method of exciting ultrasonic transducers uses the step pulse. Under certain circumstances, this pulse shape is preferred, because it can cause a piezoelectric transducer to emit a compact, unipolar ultrasonic waveform.[12] Unipolar waveforms generated with step pulse excitation are sometimes used in thickness gages and high resolution pulse echo discontinuity detectors. They can also yield information about gradual changes in material properties. However, because of diffraction effects, which cause the transmitted ultrasonic waveforms to become bipolar at relatively short distances from the transducer, step pulsers are not used in general purpose ultrasonic test instrumentation.[13]

Spike Pulsers

Spike pulsers are among the earliest electronic circuits used to excite piezoelectric transducers. Efficient spike pulsers are relatively simple to construct. The essential components of a spike pulser are shown in Fig. 20a and associated pulse shapes are shown in Fig. 20b.

The spike pulser operates as follows. First, the charging capacitor is charged to a high voltage (typically 250 to 400 V) through the charging resistor and the damping resistor. In most portable instruments, the value of the charging capacitor is 1 to 4 nF while the charging resistor and the damping resistor seldom exceed 200 and 10 kΩ, respectively. These values permit charging the capacitor to the full value of the direct current power supply in less than 1 ms. Thus, pulse repetition frequencies of 1000 Hz can be sustained.

After applying voltage, the switch is abruptly closed, causing the voltage of the fully charged capacitor to appear across the terminals of the transducer. The abrupt voltage change causes the piezoelectric material of the transducer to respond in the form of an emitted ultrasonic wave. The exciting voltage then rapidly decays because of the damping resistor, connected in parallel with the transducer. The value of the damping resistor is typically 10 to 100 Ω. This value can be adjusted by the operator to accommodate different transducer impedances. Proper adjustment of the damping resistor is important because it directly determines transducer ringdown times and the resulting near surface resolution.

Because the acoustic pressure at the front face of the transducer is directly proportional to the time derivative of the applied voltage $dV \cdot dt^{-1}$, it is important to minimize the rise time of the applied pulse. The rise time is affected primarily by the speed at which the switch can be fully closed and by the presence of parasitic inductances in series with the capacitor, switch and transducer (parasitic inductances are not shown in Fig. 20).

Historically, fast switching avalanche transistors have been used in very fast circuits. Spike pulsers, using avalanche transistors, are still frequently used in thickness gages and high resolution discontinuity detectors.

In the past, gas filled thermionic tubes, principally thyratrons, have been favored in applications requiring very high pulse voltages. Silicon controlled rectifiers were used in many general purpose instruments but their switching is not fast enough for high resolution. In general, avalanche transistor circuits should not be used to generate pulse voltages in excess of 200 V. Pulses of 1 kV can be achieved using silicon controlled rectifier switches while thyratrons can control pulses with voltages on the order of 10 kV. Thyratrons and silicon controlled rectifiers exhibit fundamental limitations as fast switching devices.

Ultrasonic transducers are typically connected to the pulser with a length of coaxial cable whose capacitance increases at a rate of about 100 pF·m⁻¹. Therefore, the capacitance of several meters of cable can easily equal or exceed the capacitance of many transducers. In such cases, a significant portion of the pulse energy can be shunted away from the transducer.

The efficiency of excitation can also be degraded by the series inductances and other parasitic impedances. Series inductances tend to increase rise times and prevent the high frequency portion of the pulse energy from reaching the transducer. These effects may severely affect the ability of a spike pulser efficiently to excite thin film transducers, typically 50 mm (2 in.) thick and exhibiting capacitances of only a few picofarads.

Because the electrical operating points of devices used as switches in spike pulsers cannot generally be controlled, impedance matching networks are not recommended. Square wave and tone burst pulsers are better suited for this purpose.

Square Wave Pulsers

Semiconductor switching technology has led to the proliferation of square wave pulsers in ultrasonic instruments. The principal disadvantages of square wave pulsers (high component count and appreciable power consumption) are offset by important operational advantages. In particular, the use of a square wave pulse increases the ability of the operator to control and stabilize important test parameters, including the harmonic content (spectrum) of the transmitted ultrasonic pulses. In addition, the use of a square wave pulse may result in higher pulse amplitudes.

Figure 21a shows the operation of a square wave pulser and Figs. 21b and 21c show its typical pulse shapes. Although the circuit in Fig. 21a is topologically identical to that in Fig. 20, note that the shape of the pulse used to excite the transducer is significantly different. This difference arises from the use of a switching device known as the *metal*

FIGURE 20. Spike pulser: (a) circuit diagram; (b) pulse shape.

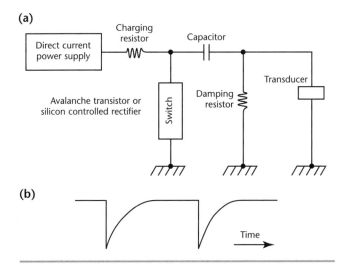

(a)

(b)

oxide *s*uperconductor *f*ield *e*ffect transducer, or *mosfet.*

High power mosfet devices are widely used in square wave pulsers intended to operate between 0.1 and 10 MHz.[14] Mosfet transistor switches permit the application of 1000 V excitations in less than 10 ns. In addition, they can safely handle pulse currents of 30 A and higher. Consequently, square wave pulsers are well suited for driving large, low frequency transducers, which frequently exhibit high capacitances.

Initially, the square wave pulser operates as a spike pulser. The sharp transition associated with the closing of the switch causes the generation of an ultrasonic signal by the transducer. However, because the charging capacitor C is much larger than that used in the spike pulser (typically 1 mF compared to 1 nF), the pulse voltage is not allowed to decay while the switch remains in the closed position. When the switch is finally restored to its original open position, the pulse voltage is returned to zero. This second abrupt transition also causes the generation of an ultrasonic signal. Because the second transition is opposite to the first, the second excited signal is inverted with respect to the first excited signal.

The time duration of the square wave pulse must be carefully adjusted to produce a positive interference between the ultrasonic signals excited by the positive going and negative going transitions of the transducer. If the pulse is too long, then a distorted ultrasonic

waveform is observed. If the pulse is too short, then the ultrasonic pulse amplitude is significantly smaller than that achieved with an equivalent spike pulser. In practice, the pulse duration is adjusted empirically by the operator from the front panel or an external computer.

A properly adjusted square wave pulser can generate twice as much signal voltage as a spike pulser charged to the same voltage. This effect is illustrated in Figs. 22 and 23 and using 2.25 and 5 MHz broad band transducers.[15] Even larger improvements in signal strength are possible when a suitable impedance matching device is interposed between the transducer and the pulser.

The theoretical and practical advantages of square wave pulsers are well understood.[16] Except for specialized applications, such as thickness gages and high resolution discontinuity detectors, square wave pulsers offer better performance than spike pulsers. However, to optimize the performance of a square wave pulser, the damping resistor and pulse duration must be adjusted independently for each transducer. In the

FIGURE 22. Comparison of ultrasonic signal voltages with 2.25 MHz broad band transducer: (a) spike pulser; (b) properly adjusted square wave pulser.

(a)

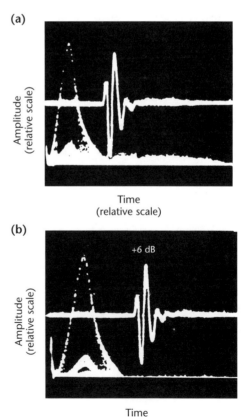

(b)

FIGURE 21. Square wave pulser: (a) circuit diagram; (b) open switch pulse shape; (c) transducer voltage pulse shape.

(a)

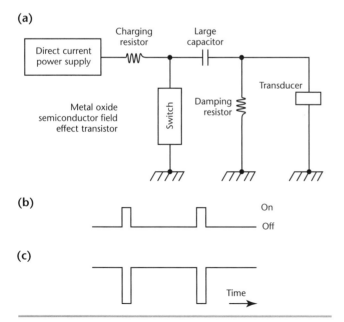

(b)

(c)

spike pulser, only the value of damping resistor is operator adjustable.

Tone Burst Pulsers

Tone burst operation can be achieved by repetitively closing the switch S of the square wave pulser shown in Fig. 21a. The main advantage of operating the square wave pulser in this mode is that it allows the operator to maximize the energy of the transmitted signal at a specific frequency.

Tone burst operation can also be achieved when a spike pulser is used to drive an inductively tuned transducer. In this case, however, frequency control can only be realized by altering the value of the tuning inductor.

Tone burst pulsers are often designed for compatibility with impedance matching networks required to maximize the output of unconventional transducers: electromagnetic acoustic transducers, air coupled elements, dry coupled and roller probes. Pulsers capable of generating 200 A, 450 V tone bursts at frequencies of several megahertz are available. Tone burst excitation is often used in special instruments, including acoustic microscopes, where frequencies of several gigahertz have been demonstrated.[17] Also,

tone burst signals are used in many ultrasonic interferometers for material velocity measurement.[18]

Step Pulsers

The excitation of ultrasonic transducers with step pulses requires circuits that are topologically more complex than those discussed previously. Figure 24a shows a circuit that can impose a step shaped excitation on a piezoelectric transducer. The spike pulser and square wave pulser use one switching device but the step pulser requires two separate switching devices.

Figure 24b shows the timing diagram for the step pulser in Fig. 24a. First, switch 1 is closed to allow the transducer to charge to a high voltage. Next, switch 1 is restored to the open position and switch 2 causes the transducer voltage to decay rapidly to zero. This rapid transition causes the generation of the unipolar ultrasonic waveform.

Figure 25 shows the effect of pulse shape on waveforms observed at the front face of a broad band, thin film ferroelectric polymer transducer. In this case, the same transducer is excited in turn by different step and spike pulsers.[19] The unipolar pulse is more compact than the bipolar pulse produced by a spike pulser. In this case, an external damping resistor was not required because a transducer with high internal damping was used.

Auxiliary Devices

The capabilities of many instruments can sometimes be significantly extended by

FIGURE 23. Comparison of signal voltage with 5 MHz broad band transducer: (a) spike pulser; (b) square wave pulser.

(a)

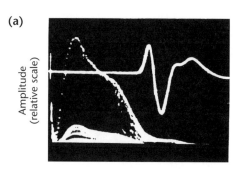

Time
(relative scale)

(b)

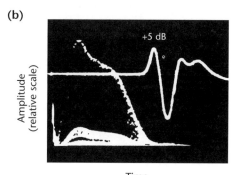

Time
(relative scale)

FIGURE 24. Step pulser: (a) circuit; (b) timing diagram.

(a)

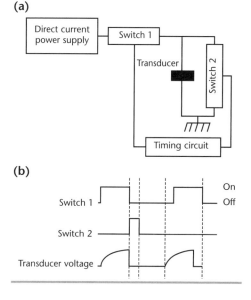

(b)

auxiliary devices. These are typically connected between the transducer and the instrument and include diplexers (transmit/receive switches), multiplexers, impedance matching networks, external power amplifiers and low noise preamplifiers. With the exception of multiplexers, which allow the use of multiple transducers, auxiliary devices are needed to improve electrical compatibility between special purpose transducers and general purpose test instruments.

Diplexers and Transmit/Receive Switches

All pulse echo instruments provide an internal diplexer or transmit/receive switch function. This function can be activated by a front panel switch. With the switch disabled, the instrument is set to operate in the pitch catch mode.

Transmit/receive switches may be used to protect sensitive internal receiver circuitry from the effects of high voltage transmitter pulses. External switches are needed mainly to facilitate the use of external power amplifiers or low noise preamplifiers on portable or laboratory instruments.

To operate a system with an external transmit/receive switch, the internal diplexer must first be disabled to permit the instrument to operate in the pitch catch mode. The output of the switch can then be connected directly to the receiver input. Typical uses of an external switch with a general purpose instrument are shown in Fig. 26.

Multiplexers

External multiplexers are generally used to permit connection of multiple transducers to general purpose, portable or laboratory instruments. The capabilities of most modular equipment can be expanded by adding specialized modules. Multiplexing modules are also available for such instruments. Typically, 2:1, 4:1, 8:1 and higher signal multiplexing is possible. However, care must be used to ensure that transducer mechanical scanning rates are compatible with the instrument pulse repetition frequency setting. Figure 27 shows a multiplexer setup with a general purpose ultrasonic instrument. Possible applications of this configuration include plate, pipe and laminate testing.

FIGURE 26. Typical configurations of external transmit/receive switch and general purpose ultrasonic test instrument: (a) output signal amplification; (b) preamplified input signal.

(a)

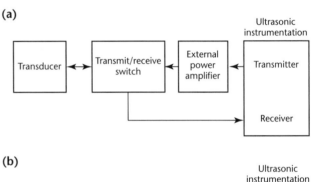

(b)

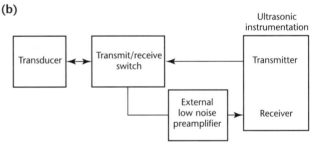

FIGURE 25. Ultrasonic waveforms observed at front face of broad band, thin film ferroelectric polymer transducer: (a) unipolar pulse; (b) bipolar pulse.

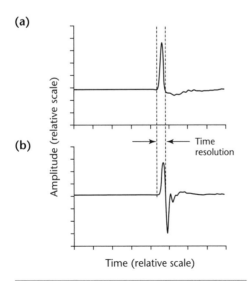

FIGURE 27. Test setup for multiplexer with general purpose ultrasonic test instrument.

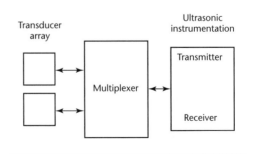

Impedance Matching Devices

Impedance matching networks are used primarily to improve the ratio of signal to noise and to facilitate special purpose transducers. Ultrasonic test equipment is generally designed for compatibility with transducers operating between 1 and 10 MHz. However, poor signal-to-noise performance can result when an attempt is made to use piezoelectric transducers operating at lower frequencies or unconventional transducers such as electromagnetic acoustic transducers, air coupled transducers and many dry coupled probes.

Generally, it is difficult to improve the performance of spike pulsers by using impedance matching devices. On the other hand, such devices can greatly improve the power output of many square wave pulsers and most tone burst pulser designs. On reception, significant improvements in signal to noise can also be achieved by using such networks to match the impedances of the transducer and the input preamplifier.[20]

Because the electrical impedances of piezoelectric transducers are dominated by a large static capacitance, inductors, air cored tapped inductors[8,21] and broad band transformers[22] can be used for matching. Reactive transformers[23] and ladder networks of inductors and capacitors are also effective. Generally, computer modeling is required to achieve optimum results.[24] In broad band matching, a tradeoff between band width and mismatch loss must be accepted.[25] Examples of useful impedance matching networks are shown in Fig. 28.

Figure 29 shows a broad band step-up transformer used to increase the outputs of a high power pulser capable of operating in the square wave and tone burst modes. In the case of the square wave pulser, a 22 dB gain in output power was observed relative to that produced by a spike pulser charged to the same voltage. The low output impedance of the pulser (2 to 3Ω) improved the quality of the match.

Figure 30 shows a simple series inductor used as an impedance matching element. Otherwise, this experimental configuration is identical to that used in Fig. 29 and a 23 dB gain was observed for single pulse excitation. Use of the tone burst signal resulted in a 29 dB improvement in the ratio of signal to noise.

External Power Amplifiers and Pulsers

External power amplifiers are generally used to drive unconventional transducers. For example, thin film transducers exhibit low capacitances that can be easily dominated by cable inductance and capacitance and must be excited using sharp spike pulses. External power amplifiers are also required to drive most low frequency transducers, air coupled transducers and most electromagnetic acoustic transducers.

Such transducers generally exhibit low electrical impedances and often require square wave and tone burst pulsers that can supply peak currents above 100 A. The efficiency of square wave and tone

FIGURE 28. Typical impedance matching networks: (a) series inductor; (b) tapped inductor or autotransformer (step down); (c) tapped inductor or autotransformer (step up); (d) transformer; (e) low pass; (f) high pass.

(a)
From pulser
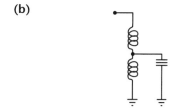

(b)

(c)

(d)
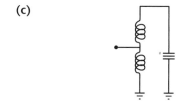
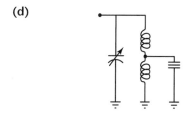

(e)
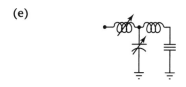

(f)
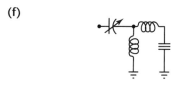

FIGURE 29. Broad band, step up transformer
to increase power outputs of pulser capable
of operating in square wave and tone burst
modes: (a) system configuration; (b) square
wave input; (c) square wave output;
(d) tone burst input; (e) tone burst output.

(a)

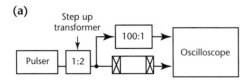

(b)

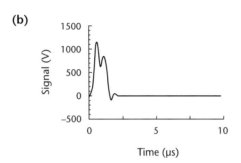

(c)

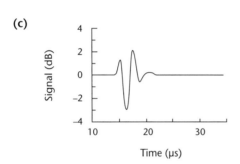

(d)

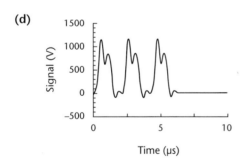

(e)

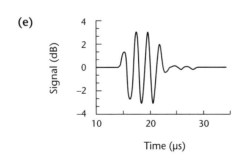

External Receiver Preamplifiers

External preamplifiers are often justified
to improve signal to noise in critical
situations, particularly when operating in
a through-transmission or pitch catch
mode. In such cases, a properly selected
preamplifier can increase the received
signal to noise by 30 dB or more.
However, considerable care must be

FIGURE 30. Simple series inductor used as
impedance matching element: (a) system
configuration; (b) single-pulse input;
(c) single-pulse output; (d) tone burst input;
(e) tone burst output.

(a)

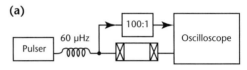

(b)

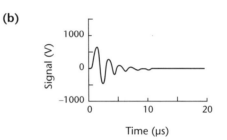

(c)

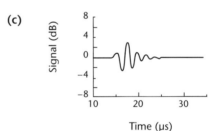

(d)

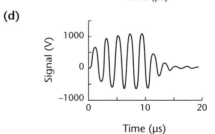

(e)

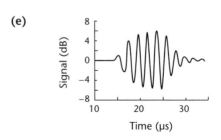

exercised when selecting a preamplifier for a particular application.

Generally, bipolar transistor preamplifiers are preferred in applications where the magnitude of the transducer input impedance is less than 500 Ω. For input impedance between 500 Ω and 10 kΩ, preamplifiers with either bipolar transistor or junction field effect transistors are recommended. For transducers with exceptionally high input impedances, the preamplifier should use either a junction field effect transistor or another field effect transistor as the input device.[26]

Preamplifiers using bipolar transistors as input devices can generally be operated in the 218 to 398 K (–55 to 25 °C; –67 to +257 °F) temperature range. Preamplifiers equipped with field effect transistor front ends can be operated at low temperatures but should not be operated at temperatures higher than 373 K (212 °F).

Because broad band film transducers often exhibit low capacitances, the preamplifier input capacitance should be about 1 pF while the input resistance must be in excess of 4 MΩ. To maximize the signal-to-noise ratio of signals received from low frequency piezoelectric transducers and electromagnetic acoustic transducers, one preamplifier design uses a low noise bipolar transistor as the input device. Such devices generally achieve a higher ratio of signal to noise when used with low impedance transducers between 0.1 and 5.0 MHz. As in the previous example, this design also incorporates a line driver circuit that suits it for driving long cable lengths.

Generally, the band width of the preamplifier has little effect on the final signal-to-noise ratio, except in the case of thin film ferroelectric polymer transducers.[27] Because the signal band width is generally adjustable within the receiver, most preamplifiers are not equipped with frequency controls. The voltage gains of most preamplifiers are in the 20 to 40 dB range. These gain levels are generally sufficient to override the internal noise of most receivers and compensate for cable transmission losses.

Signal Reception and Conditioning

Ultrasonic transducers are typically excited with pulse amplitudes from 100 to 1000 V. The voltages of the received signals can range from microvolts to several volts. The received signals may also exhibit frequency characteristics much different from the pulses used to excite the transmitting transducers.

Because most signal processing devices (signal gates, video detectors, level comparators, analog-to-digital converters)

require input signals with amplitudes between 1 and 10 V, most received signals must be amplified. To establish the best ratio of signal to noise, they must also be preamplified immediately after reception and then filtered. These fundamental signal transformations are performed in the instrument's receiver.

The block diagram in Fig. 31 shows the arrangement of the four signal conditioning stages in the receiver section of an ultrasonic discontinuity detector or thickness gage. After reception by the transducer, the signals are successively filtered and preamplified, attenuated and again amplified and filtered. The band width and gain parameters of the receiver are adjusted by the operator using front panel controls. An inconsistent selection of signal band width and gain parameters can lead to unrepeatable test results.

The repeatability of the ultrasonic testing process is strongly influenced by the frequency dependent gain characteristics of the receiver.[28] For this reason, ultrasonic test procedures that prescribe initial instrument adjustments generally stipulate ways to adjust the gain and frequency response of the instrument.

The best band width and gain settings are also influenced by transducer, discontinuity and pulser frequency response characteristics.[29,30] The wide

FIGURE 31. Signal conditioning stages in receiver section of ultrasonic discontinuity detector or thickness gage.

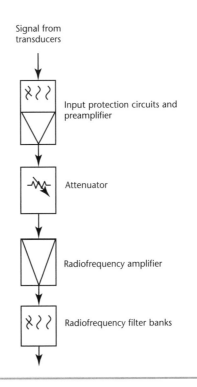

Signal from transducers

Input protection circuits and preamplifier

Attenuator

Radiofrequency amplifier

Radiofrequency filter banks

variability of the pulser, receiver and transducer frequency responses is illustrated in Fig. 32. Because the characteristics of the individual components are so widely variable, appropriately damped ultrasonic reference standards are needed to ensure the repeatability of test results.

Input Circuits

Typical input circuits for discontinuity detectors and thickness gages provide two essential functions: (1) rapid recovery from the transmitter pulses (input protection circuits) and (2) establishment of the signal-to-noise performance of the instrument (preamplifiers).

FIGURE 32. Variability of pulser, receiver and transducer frequency responses: (a) square wave pulser, broad band receiver spectral response; (b) tuned pulser, narrow band receiver spectral response; (c) broad band pulser, narrow band receiver spectral response.

(a)

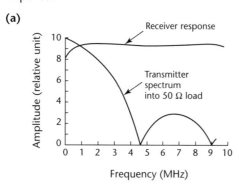

(b)

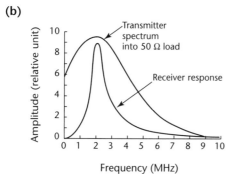

(c)

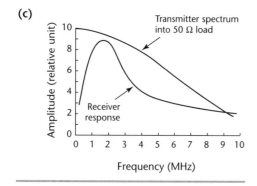

In addition, the input circuits may incorporate features such as special high pass frequency filters for eliminating undesirable responses of some transducers and reducing power line interferences. Properly designed input filters can significantly reduce the effects of transducer radial modes and improve recovery times.

In some modern instrument designs, input circuits incorporate features that facilitate automatic recognition of the transducer type. In such instruments, the gain and filter settings are established automatically by an internal microprocessor. This feature can improve test reliability.

Input preamplifiers are typically broad band, low gain devices that can linearly amplify the full amplitude range of the ultrasonic signals. Preamplifiers are needed for boosting the signals to levels high enough to overcome the noise levels of ensuing amplification and filtering. Their band width and gain characteristics are generally not adjustable. Some laboratory and modular instruments allow for the selection of different preamplifiers to accommodate low and high impedance transducers.

The band widths of the receiver sections of most portable and modular instruments usually extend from 1 to 15 MHz. In some cases, the frequency responses of such instruments can be extended down to 100 kHz by external broad band preamplifiers with sufficient gain to overcome the low frequency filtering of the input protection circuits.

Attenuators

Attenuators are broad band calibrated devices used for two reasons. First, they are needed to reduce the amplitudes of strong signals to prevent them from saturating the receiver gain stages that follow. Second, they are needed to compare accurately the amplitudes of signals with a signal from a known reflector or calibration block.

Attenuators are typically calibrated in decibels to allow quantitative measurements of signal amplitudes over the entire dynamic range of an ultrasonic instrument. Generally, coarse (10 dB) and fine (1 or 2 dB) front panel attenuator controls are provided. In many instruments, the attenuators can also be remotely controlled using a digital signal generated by external computers.

Typically, attenuators permit gain adjustments in the 30 to 50 dB range. This range generally exceeds the linear range of the following analog radiofrequency amplifier. In some designs using nonlinear radiofrequency amplification stages, a much larger attenuator adjustment is provided.

Radiofrequency Amplifiers

Radiofrequency amplifiers are used to raise the amplitudes of ultrasonic signals to a level that permits signal processing circuits to operate properly. For example, the correct gain of the radiofrequency amplification stages is needed to directly display the received signals on a cathode ray tube or similar display device. The internal design of the instrument then ensures the proper operation of the signal processing circuits, including signal gates, video detectors, alarm level comparators and analog-to-digital converters.

Generally, radiofrequency amplifiers are arranged as two or three blocks of fixed gain linear amplification that can be switched in or out using front panel controls. As a rule, the band widths of radiofrequency gain blocks are not individually adjustable using front panel controls. Typical radiofrequency gain blocks provide amplification in 20 dB steps. Because the gain of typical preamplifiers is 20 dB and an additional 30 to 50 dB gain adjustment is possible using attenuators, the instruments can typically be adjusted to process ultrasonic signals over a 100 dB range.

Special purpose instruments may use a logarithmic rather than linear radiofrequency amplifier. The use of such amplifiers allows processing of signals with large dynamic range. The dynamic range of instruments using linear amplification is normally less than 30 dB; the dynamic range of instruments using logarithmic amplification can exceed 100 dB.

Frequency Filters

The frequency characteristics of the signals are established by filters after radiofrequency amplification. Ultrasonic discontinuity detectors must be compatible with a variety of piezoelectric transducers. Typically, transducers with nominal frequencies of 1.0, 2.25, 5.0 MHz and higher must be accommodated. Transducer sizes are also widely variable. To ensure correct operation over the maximum range of transducer parameters, it is desirable to limit the band width of the received signals after radiofrequency amplification. This limit helps maximize the ratio of signal to noise. Bandpass radiofrequency filter banks are provided for this purpose.

The center frequency of radiofrequency filter banks is selectable using front panel controls. Typically, the center frequencies of the filter banks are established to correspond with the nominal frequencies of standard transducers: 1.0, 2.25 and 5.0 MHz. Often, a wideband setting is also selected.

Signal Processing

In traditional discontinuity detectors, signal processing was accomplished with simple analog circuits. The time domain amplitudes of the signals were first recovered from the radiofrequency signals using a video detection process and then were further amplified using low frequency (video) amplifiers. Typically, the resulting signals were then time gated

FIGURE 33. Block diagrams for signal processing: (a) analog; (b) digital, where accept/reject decisions are made by external computer.

(a)

(b)

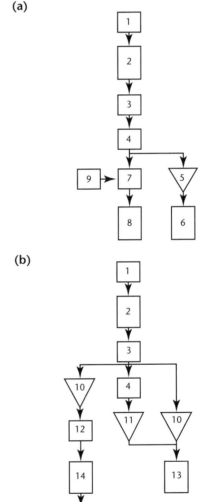

To computer

Legend
1. Transducer
2. Receiver
3. Signal gate
4. Video detector
5. Video amplifier
6. Cathode ray tube
7. Comparator
8. Alarm
9. Threshold level
10. Wideband amplifier
11. Video amplifier
12. Flash analog-to-digital converter
13. Cathode ray tube
14. Buffer

and compared against threshold levels to permit accept/reject decisions.

Advances in digital signal processing make it possible to apply processing techniques directly to the radiofrequency signals. However, the signals must first be converted to a digital format using an analog-to-digital converter. Alternatively, signals can be digitized following peak detection and video amplification. This approach offers practical advantages at the expense of the signal phase information.

Figure 33 illustrates the essential differences between the analog and digital approaches to signal processing. Figure 33a shows the traditional analog approach. The approach in Figure 33b allows accept/reject decisions to be made by an internal microprocessor or an external digital computer.

Signal Gates

Ultrasonic discontinuity detectors are usually equipped with one or more signal gates. The signal gates are used to isolate a time domain region of the received ultrasonic pulse train. The selected region can then be processed by the following signal processing stages. The signal gates are designed to process the selected region of the signal train and reject the other regions.

The width and position of the signal gates can usually be adjusted by the operator. In addition, the timing of each gate can either be synchronized with the transmitted pulse or with the arrival of a selected ultrasonic signal such as an interface echo. The latter feature allows automatic tracking of the gate with a particular portion of the signal train.

Video and Peak Detectors

The video detector is essentially a rectifier circuit with low pass filtering that eliminates signals at twice the highest frequency of the ultrasonic signal. The band width of the video detector is adjustable using controls that adjust the resistive capacitive time constant. Figure 34 shows the transformation of the radiofrequency signal as it is passed through the video detector. The effects of positive and negative half-wave rectification on the same input waveform (three half cycles) are clearly shown in Figs. 34b and 34c.

Most discontinuity detectors use full-wave rectification (see Fig. 34d). Consequently, the operator cannot select the shorter of the two rectified waveforms. However, some laboratory and production instruments allow the selection of either positive, negative or full-wave rectification. The ability to choose the polarity of the rectification is only important for broad band transducers.

A peak detector is basically a half-wave rectifier with a narrow band width. This effect is achieved by choosing a long time constant. Peak detectors are often used with signal gates in discontinuity alarm circuits. The signal gate is needed to

FIGURE 34. Transformation of radiofrequency signal as it passes through video detector: (a) input waveform; (b) after positive half-wave rectification; (c) after negative half-wave rectification; (d) full-wave rectification.

(a)

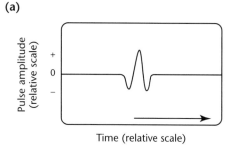

Time (relative scale)

(b)

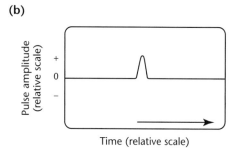

Time (relative scale)

(c)

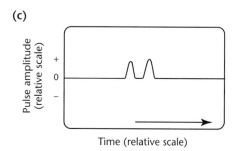

Time (relative scale)

(d)

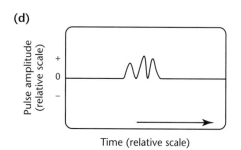

Time (relative scale)

permit processing of later signals. The associated waveforms are shown in Fig. 35.

Video Amplifiers

Video amplifiers are usually needed to boost the amplitude of the signal after video detection so that they are large enough to drive the vertical plates of a cathode ray tube. Video amplifiers are also used as buffer amplifiers to drive sample-and-hold circuits.

Generally, the gains of video amplifiers in portable ultrasonic test equipment cannot be adjusted using front panel controls. However, video amplifiers can be followed by low pass filter circuits that allow the operator to change the appearance of the demodulated ultrasonic signals by using front panel controls.

Sample and Hold Circuits

Figure 36a shows the principle of a sample-and-hold circuit. The basic circuit uses two switches. When closed, the input switch allows the storage capacitor to charge to the output voltage of the peak detector. This voltage can then be sampled by the analog-to-digital converter. The capacitor is then fully discharged using the second switch. The associated waveforms are shown in Figs. 36b and 36c.

Sample-and-hold circuits are often used for interfacing to slow analog-to-digital circuits and external display devices, including strip chart recorders and plotters. They can also be used to compare the amplitudes of different portions of the same ultrasonic signal.

Analog-to-Digital Converters

Analog-to-digital converters are circuits that typically allow the conversion of a voltage signal to a digital word. In the case of direct conversion of radiofrequency signals to digital format, flash analog-to-digital converters are available. Currently, waveforms with frequencies up to 50 MHz can be sampled with eight-bit precision. Peak detected waveforms do not contain high frequency components. Currently, such waveforms can be converted using the more precise 12-bit converters.

FIGURE 36. Sample-and-hold circuit: (a) circuit diagram; (b) input signal; (c) output signal.

(a)

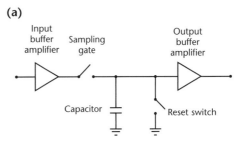

(b)

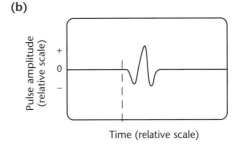

(c)

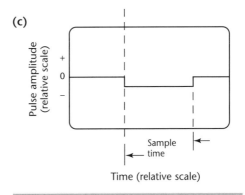

FIGURE 35. Peak detector waveforms: (a) input pulse; (b) output pulse.

(a)

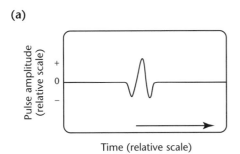

(b)

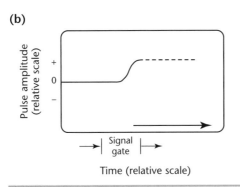

Part 4. Phased Arrays

Introduction

Ultrasonic phased arrays use multiple ultrasonic elements and electronic time delays to generate and receive ultrasound, creating beams by constructive and destructive interference. As such, phased arrays offer significant technical advantages over conventional single-probe ultrasonic testing: the phased array beams can be steered, scanned, swept and focused electronically.

Electronic scanning permits very rapid coverage of the components, typically an order of magnitude faster than a single-probe mechanical system.

Beam forming permits the selected beam angles to be optimized ultrasonically by orienting them perpendicular to the discontinuities of interest — for example, lack of fusion in welds.

Beam steering (usually called sectorial scanning) can be used for mapping components at appropriate angles to optimize probability of detection. Sectorial scanning is also useful for inspections where only a minimal footprint is possible.

Electronic focusing permits optimizing the beam shape and size at the expected discontinuity location, as well as optimizing probability of detection. Focusing improves signal-to-noise ratio significantly, which also permits operating at lower pulser voltages.

Overall, phased arrays optimize discontinuity detection while minimizing test time.

Operation

Ultrasonic phased arrays are similar in principle to phased array radar, sonar and other wave physics applications. However, ultrasonic development is behind the other applications because of a smaller market, shorter wavelengths, mode conversions and more complex components. Industrial applications of ultrasonic phased arrays have increased in the twenty-first century.[31-36]

Phased arrays use an array of elements, all individually wired, pulsed and time shifted. These elements can be a linear array, a two-dimensional matrix array, a circular array or some more complex form (see Fig. 37). Most applications use linear arrays, because these are the easiest to program and are significantly cheaper than more complex arrays because of fewer elements. As costs decline and experience increases, greater use of the more complex arrays can be predicted.

The elements are ultrasonically isolated from each other and packaged in normal probe housings. The cabling usually consists of a bundle of well shielded micro coaxial cables. Wireless systems have increased since 2005. Commercial multiple-channel connectors are used with the instrument cabling.

Elements are typically pulsed in groups from 4 to 32, typically 16 elements for welds. With a user friendly system, the computer and software calculate the time delays for a setup by using either operator input on interrogation angle, focal

FIGURE 37. Array types: (a) one-dimensional linear array of 16 sensors; (b) two-dimensional matrix array of 32 sensors; (c) sectorial annular array of 61 sensors.

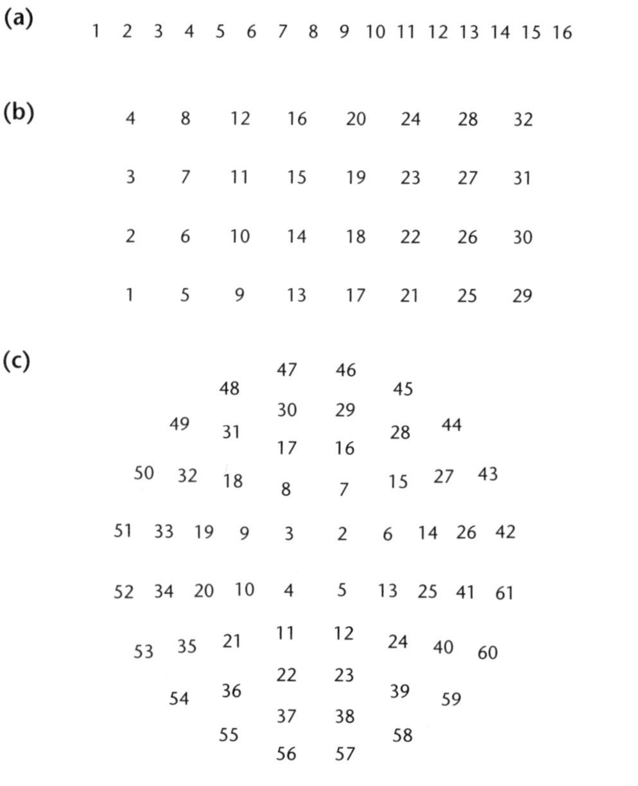

(a)
1 2 3 4 5 6 7 8 9 10 11 12 13 14 15 16
(b)
4 8 12 16 20 24 28 32
3 7 11 15 19 23 27 31
2 6 10 14 18 22 26 30
1 5 9 13 17 21 25 29
(c)
47 46
48 45
30 29
49 31 28 44
17 16
50 32 18 8 7 15 27 43
51 33 19 9 3 2 6 14 26 42
52 34 20 10 4 5 13 25 41 61
53 35 21 11 12 24 40 60
22 23
54 36 39 59
37 38
55 58
56 57

distance, scan pattern and other test circumstances or by using a predefined file (see Fig. 38). The time delays are back calculated using time-of-flight from the focal spot, and the scan assembled from individual focal laws. Time delay circuits must be accurate to around 2 ns to provide the phasing accuracy required.

Each element generates a beam when pulsed; these beams constructively and destructively interfere to form a wave front. (This interference can be seen, for example, with photoelastic imaging.[37] The phased array instrumentation pulses the individual channels with time delays as specified to form a pre-calculated wave front. For receiving, the instrumentation effectively performs the reverse, i.e. it receives with precalculated time delays, then sums the time shifted signal and displays it. This is shown in Fig. 39.

The summed waveform is effectively identical to a single-channel discontinuity detector using a probe with the same angle, frequency, focusing, aperture and other settings. Figure 39 shows typical time delays for a focused normal beam and transverse wave. Sample scan patterns are shown in Fig. 40 and are discussed below.

Implementation

From a practical viewpoint, ultrasonic phased arrays are merely a means of generating and receiving ultrasound; once the ultrasound is in the material, it is independent of generation method, whether generated by piezoelectric, electromagnetic, laser or phased arrays. Consequently, many of the details of ultrasonic testing remain unchanged; for example, if 5 MHz is the optimum test frequency with conventional ultrasonic

testing, then phased arrays would typically start by using the same frequency, aperture size, focal length and incident angle.

While phased arrays require well developed instrumentation, one of the key requirements is good, user-friendly software. Besides calculating the focal laws, the software saves and displays the results, so good data manipulation is essential. As phased arrays offer considerable application flexibility, software versatility is highly desirable. Phased array inspections can be manual, semiautomated (that is, encoded) or fully automated, depending on the application, speed, budget and other considerations. Encoder capability and full data storage are usually required.

Although it can be time consuming to prepare the first setup, the information is recorded in a file and only takes seconds

FIGURE 39. Beam: (a) emitting; (b) receiving.

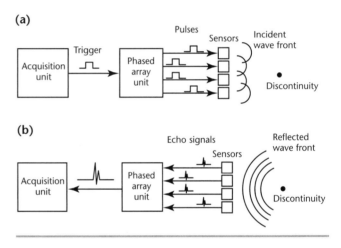

(a)

(b)

FIGURE 38. Generation of scans using phased arrays: (a) linear focusing; (b) sectorial focusing; (c) depth focusing.

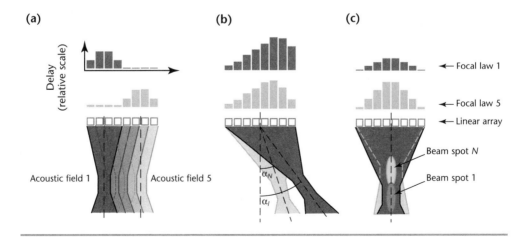

(a)

(b)

(c)

to reload. Also, modifying a prepared setup is quick in comparison with physically adjusting conventional probes.

Scan Types

Electronic pulsing and receiving provide significant opportunities for a variety of scan patterns, as shown in Fig. 40 and below.

Electronic Scans

Electronic scans are performed by multiplexing the same focal law (time delays) along an array (see Fig. 41). Typical arrays have up to 128 elements. Electronic scanning permits rapid coverage with a tight focal spot. If the array is flat and linear, then the scan pattern is a simple B-scan. If the array is curved, then the scan pattern will be curved. Electronic scans are straightforward to program. For example, a phased array can be readily programmed to perform corrosion mapping, or to test a weld using 0.8 rad (45 deg) and 1 rad (60 deg) transverse waves, which mimics conventional manual inspections.

Sectorial Scans (S Scans)

Sectorial scanning is unique to phased arrays. Sectorial scans use the same set of elements but alter the time delays to sweep the beam through a series of angles (see Fig. 42). Again, this is a straightforward scan to program. Applications for sectorial scanning typically involve a stationary array, sweeping across a relatively inaccessible component like a turbine blade root,[38] to map out the features and discontinuities. Depending primarily on the array frequency and element spacing, the sweep angles can vary from ±0.3 rad (±20 deg) up to ±1.4 rad (±80 deg).

Combined Scans

Combining linear scanning, sectorial scanning and precision focusing leads to a practical combination of displays (Fig. 43). Optimum angles can be selected for welds and other components whereas electronic scanning permits fast and functional tests. For example, combining linear and longitudinal wave sectorial scanning permits full ultrasonic testing of components over a given angle range, such as ±0.3 rad (±20 deg). This type of test is useful when simple normal beam tests are inadequate, such as titanium castings in aerospace where discontinuities can have random orientations. A related approach applies to weld inspections, where specific angles are often required for weld geometries; for

FIGURE 40. Schematic time delays (histograms): (a) focused normal beam; (b) focused transverse wave.

(a)

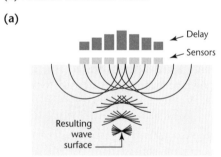

(b)

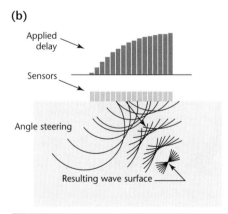

FIGURE 41. Electronic scanning.

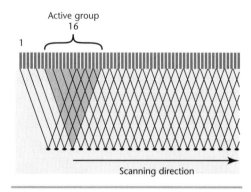

FIGURE 42. Sectorial scanning on turbine rotor for sequence of *N* scans.

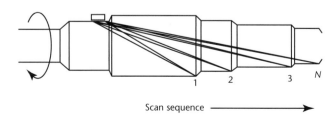

these applications, specific beam angles are programmed for specific weld bevel angles at specific locations.

Linear Scanning of Welds

Manual ultrasonic weld inspections are performed using a single probe, which the operator rasters back and forth to cover the weld area. Many automated weld test systems use a similar approach (see Fig. 44a), with a single probe scanned back and forth over the weld area. Rastering is time consuming because the system has dead zones at the start and finish of the raster.

In contrast, most multiple-probe systems and phased arrays use a linear scanning approach (see Fig. 44b). Here the

probe pan is scanned linearly round or along the weld, while each probe sweeps out a specific area of the weld. The simplest approach to linear scanning is found in pipe mills, where a limited number of probes test electric resistance welded pipe.[39]

Phased arrays for linear weld tests operate on the same principle as the multiprobe approach; however, phased arrays offer considerably greater flexibility than conventional automated ultrasonic testing. Typically, it is much easier to change the setup electronically, either by modifying the setup or reloading another; often it is possible to use many more beams (equivalent to individual conventional probes) with phased arrays; special inspections can be implemented simply by loading a setup file.

FIGURE 43. Phased array imaging patterns: (a) scanning pattern using sectorial and linear scanning; (b) image using all data merged together.

(a)

(b)

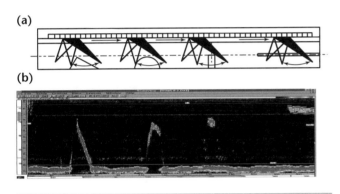

FIGURE 44. Scanning: (a) conventional raster; (b) linear.

(a)

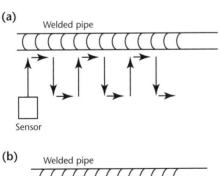

(b)

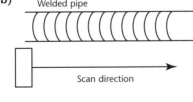

Legend
▲ = Data collection step
➤ = Raster step

Applications

Ultrasonic phased arrays are flexible and can address many types of problems. Consequently, they are used in a wide variety of industries where the technology has inherent advantages. These industries include aerospace, nuclear power, steel mills, pipe mills, petrochemical plants, pipeline construction, general manufacturing and construction, plus a selection of special applications. All these applications take advantage of one or more of the dominant features of phased arrays:

1. Speed — scanning with phased arrays is much faster than single probe conventional mechanical systems, with better coverage.
2. Flexibility — setups can be changed in a few minutes, and typically a lot more component dimensional flexibility is available.
3. Test angles — a wide variety of test angles can be used, depending on the requirements and the array.
4. Small footprint — small matrix arrays can give significantly more flexibility for testing restricted areas than conventional probes.
5. Imaging — an image (enhanced to simulate three dimensions) of discontinuities is much easier to interpret than a waveform. The data can be saved and redisplayed as needed.

Each feature generates its own applications. For example, speed is important for pipe mills and pipelines, plus some high volume applications. Flexibility is important in pressure vessels and pipeline welds due to geometry changes. Test angle is key for pipelines, some pressure vessel and nuclear applications. Small footprint is applicable to some turbine applications. Imaging is useful for weld tests.

Phased array nondestructive testing is relatively new and still requires some setup effort, especially for complex three-dimensional applications. Two-dimensional setups are generally straightforward, provided the software is user friendly. For example, automated setup procedures have been developed for weld tests. Phased array systems have sometimes been more costly than single-channel systems; however, the higher speed, data storage and display, smaller footprint and greater flexibility can often offset the higher costs, especially with the newer portable instruments.

PART 5. Focused Beam Immersion Techniques[40]

Focused Transducers

Sound can be focused by lenses in a manner analogous to focusing light. The basic difference between the two is the ratio of the lens thickness to the wavelength. In optics, the lens thickness is 10^4 to 10^5 times the wavelength. In ultrasonic testing, the lens thickness is about 10 times the wavelength. As a result, sound waves with opposite phases are emitted from the surface of an acoustic lens in concentric rings several millimeters apart and interfere at the focal plane.

Acoustic lenses can improve testing reliability by reducing and controlling certain energy losses. They are usually an integral part of the transducer assembly. In most applications, the lens concentrates the energy into a long and narrow beam, increasing its intensity. Special sharp focused transducers can be made with a usable test range less than 6.4 mm (0.25 in.). Such a focused transducer can resolve a 0.4 mm (0.015 in.) flat bottom hole located 1 mm (0.04 in.) beneath the surface of a steel block. These transducers are particularly useful for tests of thin materials, high resolution C-scan imaging and the determination of bond quality in sandwich structures.

Generally, focused transducers allow the highest possible resolving power with standard equipment because the front surface is not in the focal zone and the concentration of energy at the discontinuity makes its reflection very high, providing a ratio up 10^4 to 1 between the front surface and the discontinuity echo.

Using a cylindrical lens, an improvement in resolving power can be achieved to a lesser degree without decreasing the horizontal width of the beam. With this construction, a 75 mm (3 in.) wide beam can provide clear resolution of discontinuities from about 2.0 mm (0.08 in.) below the surface to a depth of 13 mm (0.5 in.). For standard ultrasonic equipment operating at 10 MHz, such transducers are produced for tests of thin airframe aluminum extrusions.

Focused beams reduce the effect of surface roughness and the effect of multiple minute discontinuities such as

FIGURE 45. Improvement with focused transducer on curved test surface: (a) distorted A-scan image with flat transducer; (b) elimination of distortion with focused transducer.

(a)

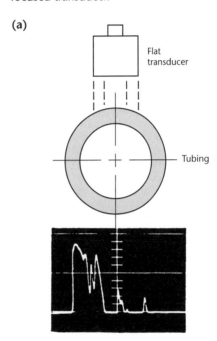

Flat transducer

Tubing

(b)

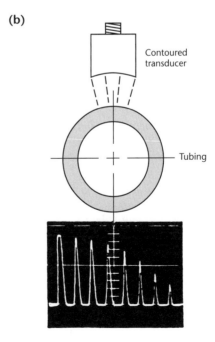

Contoured transducer

Tubing

grain boundaries and porosity. In addition, these transducers produce plane wave behavior at the focal spot and are used in appropriate experimental studies.[41]

Focused transducers are more commonly used in the immersion environment where they are not exposed to wear or erosive conditions. Such transducers are also preferable for tests of curved surfaces. When an ultrasonic beam encounters divergence at a curved surface, a flat transducer is used. A focused beam maintains a circular or cylindrical wave front and is not distorted by a curved surface (see Fig. 45).

Ultrasonic Lenses

Ultrasonic beams are focused using three basic techniques: (1) a curved, ground piezoelectric material, (2) a plano concave lens cemented to a flat piezoelectric crystal and (3) a biconcave lens placed in front of the transducer. Curved transducers provide a well defined acoustic field with limited noise and energy losses. The need to fix a damper on the back of the crystal (to obtain broad band characteristics) makes the use of curved crystals less practical. Lenses glued to crystals are more common.

Spherical lenses are used in most nondestructive testing applications. When a line focus is needed, cylindrical transducers are used. In some special applications, an external lens is attached in front of a flat transducer to focus its beam and improve test sensitivity. Such lenses produce a certain amount of disturbance and absorption because some materials, such as vulcanized rubber, contain fillers.

Lens Design Criteria[42]

Lenses can be made of solids or liquids. For most nondestructive test applications, the lens is a solid and the host or the conducting medium is fluid. If so, the acoustic velocity is higher in the lens than in the host medium. This produces a converging lens that is concave (the reverse of optic lenses).

When designing an ultrasonic lens, there are several necessary considerations, including acoustic impedance, acoustic velocity, attenuation, fabrication and nonhazardous materials.

Matching acoustic impedances is required to minimize energy loss from reflections in the lens. This condition is expressed in Eq. 27.

(27) $\rho_1 V_1 = \rho_2 V_2$

where V is acoustic velocity (meter per second) and ρ is density. The index 1 values are for the water medium. Index 2 values are for the lens medium. A high index of refraction $(V_2 \cdot V_1^{-1})$ is required to allow a small radius of curvature. The energy absorption and scattering must be as small as possible.

It is difficult to find materials that completely meet lens design requirements. Lenses undergo specific and, in some ways, unique fabrication processes, demanding particular material characteristics within limited tolerances. In addition, when a fluid lens is used, the fluid must not be harmful to personnel and must be inert to the materials it contacts.

The reflection coefficient for most host and lens combinations is significantly high unless a fluid or a lithium lens is used in a fluid host. Note that air has a very low acoustic impedance and cannot be present in any form in an ultrasonic focusing system.

Biconcave Lenses[43]

When a lens is immersed in front of a transducer, the lens must be concave on both surfaces to accommodate beam divergence from the transducer. The half angle of divergence r is:

(28) $\sin \theta = \dfrac{1.22\,\lambda}{d}$

FIGURE 46. Attachment of acoustic lens to transducer: (a) transducer separated from lens induces transverse wave in lens because of angular incidence; (b) bonded lens has near zone longer than focal length of lens.

(a)

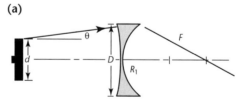

(b)

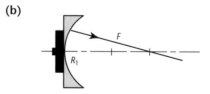

Legend
D = lens diameter
d = sensor diameter
F = focal length
R = refractive concavity
θ = angle of diffraction

where d is the diameter (millimeter) of the transducer and λ is the ultrasonic wavelength (millimeter) in the lens.

As shown in Fig. 46a, the acoustic beam impinges on the solid lens at an angle. This angular incidence on the fluid-to-solid interface of the lens produces a transverse wave in addition to the longitudinal wave. These two waves have different velocities and generate a double focus.

The radius of curvature R_1 of the first surface of the lens is:

$$(29) \quad R_1 = \frac{Dd}{2.44\,\lambda}$$

where D is the diameter of the lens aperture in millimeters. The focal length of a biconcave lens can be determined from the following expressions.

$$(30) \quad F = \frac{R_2}{1-\dfrac{V_1}{V_2}} \times \frac{R_1}{d\left(\dfrac{V_1}{V_2}-1\right)+R_1-R_2}$$

where d is the thickness of the lens (millimeter), R_1 and R_2 are the radii of curvature (millimeter), V_1 is the acoustic velocity in the host (meter per second), V_2 is acoustic velocity in the lens (meter per second) and $V_1 \cdot V_2^{-1}$ is the index of refraction of the lens material relative to the host medium.

Plano Concave Lenses

When an ultrasonic lens is glued directly to a transducer (see Fig. 46b), then the near field is usually longer than the focal length of the lens and no clear focus can be produced.[44] To determine the focal length F for a plano concave lens, Eq. 31 can be used. The equation contains a correction term for large angles of aperture.

$$(31) \quad F = \frac{R}{1-\dfrac{V_1}{V_2}} \times \frac{d\left(\dfrac{V_1}{V_2}\right)}{2\left(\dfrac{V_2}{V_1}-1\right)}$$

where R is the radius of curvature in millimeters. For small apertures, d is effectively 0. With the increase of the angle of aperture, the focus moves toward the lens and the focal area is widened. This reduces the concentration of energy and the accuracy of the focal position.

Focused Beam Profile and Intensity

At the focal plane, the normalized amplitude distribution is expressed as follows:

$$(32) \quad \frac{P}{P_{max}} = \frac{2J_1(ka_m r)}{ka_m r}$$

where k is $2\pi \cdot \lambda^{-1}$ (wave number), a_m is $\arcsin(R \cdot F^{-1})$, F is focal length (millimeter), J_1 is the bessel function of the first kind and first order, R is radius of the lens aperture (millimeter), r is cylindrical coordinate in the focal plane and λ is wavelength (millimeter);

For small angles, where $a_m < 0.5$ rad (30 deg), $a_m = R \cdot F^{-1}$. Figure 47 shows the distribution of $P \cdot P_{max}^{-1}$ as a function of the parameter ka_m^r. The first lobe of the described distribution also defines the diffraction limit for a given frequency, namely the smallest focal spot diameter. This diffraction limit D_L is also known as an *airy disk of the first order*.

FIGURE 47. Normalized acoustic pressure distribution on focal plane for radius $R = 10$ mm and $R = 8.5$ mm: (a) frequency $f = 5$ MHz and focal length $F = 60$ mm; (b) $f = 2.5$ MHz and $F = 60$ mm; (c) $f = 2.5$ MHz and $F = 40$ mm.

(a)

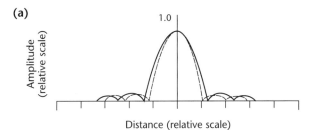

Distance (relative scale)

(b)

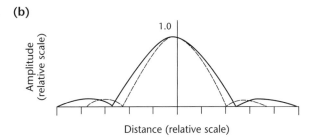

Distance (relative scale)

(c)

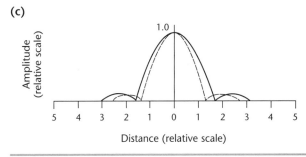

Distance (relative scale)

(33) $\quad D_L = \dfrac{1.22 \lambda F}{r}$

where F is the lens focal length (millimeter) and r is the radius of aperture of the lens (millimeter).

The theory is discussed in further detail elsewhere.[45]

For a 10 MHz wave in water, the wavelength is 0.148 mm. With a lens of 13 mm diameter and 25 mm focus, the diffraction limit is 0.35 mm. Effectively, this is also the smallest focus that can be obtained. This limit value can be a constraint on the effective use of an acoustic lens at low frequencies. At 1 MHz, the diffraction limit becomes 3.5 mm.

The gain of lenses has been derived as follows:[43]

(34) $\quad G_p = \dfrac{\pi D^2}{2 \lambda F} \dfrac{T}{2}$

and:

(35) $\quad T = \dfrac{4 Z_1 Z_2}{\left(Z_1 + Z_2 \right)^2}$

where T is the transmission coefficient, Z_1 is $\rho_1 V_1$ (acoustic impedance of the host medium) and Z_2 is $\rho_2 V_2$ (acoustic impedance of the lens material).

The main disadvantages of acoustic lenses are aberrations and the energy loss from reflections and attenuation. Most lenses are made from plastics for a low reflection coefficient. Unfortunately, plastics are highly attenuative. To reduce attenuation, ultrasonic applications use so called *zone lenses,* the acoustic equivalent of fresnel lenses in optics. In a zone lens, rings are scribed on a plate so that every second ring is in phase, generating constructive interference at a predetermined point. This point is dependent on the frequency and is regarded as the focal spot. The rings that are out of phase are covered to eliminate their contribution. Zone lenses have found very limited application in nondestructive testing.

Focal Distance

The focal distance of a transducer is measured experimentally with a small ball target from which its reflection is examined. It is assumed that a spherical wave front is produced and the surface of the ball behaves as an equal phase reflector. The focal point is inferred to be at the geometric center of the ball. When the ball diameter is larger than the diffraction limit, then it is common to add the radius of the ball to the water path. This path is measured by a pulse echo time-of-flight test. The transducer is moved back and forth with the sphere along its axis, until maximum amplitude is measured.

The focal distance becomes shorter when the ultrasonic beam propagates from a fluid to a solid material. The reduction of the focal distance can be determined from a geometrical analysis of the position of the front surface of the material along the beam path (Fig. 48):

(36) $\quad R = \dfrac{X_w + \left(F_L - X_w \right) \dfrac{V_w}{V_{tm}}}{F}$

where R is the ratio of the focal length change, V_{tm} is acoustic velocity in the test object (meter per second), V_w is acoustic velocity in water (1485 m·s⁻¹) and X_w is the one-way water path between the transducer and the front surface of the solid material (millimeter).

The focal depth inside the solid is:

(37) $\quad X_{tm} = F_L - \left(F_L - X_w \right) \dfrac{V_w}{V_{tm}}$

Because of the difference in velocities for metal and water, changes of the water path have a relatively small effect on the focal depth in the metal. The metal surface forms a second lens much more powerful than the acoustical lens itself. This effect pulls the focal spot very close to the metal surface, compared to the focal length of a transducer in water.

FIGURE 48. Ultrasonic focus effect in metals, demonstrating effect of second lens as result of immersion in water.

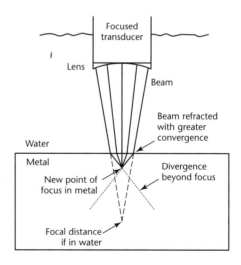

The second lens has three other important effects: it sharpens the beam, increases the sensitivity to objects in the focal zone and makes the transducer act as a very directional and distance sensitive receiver. Large increases in sensitivity are produced by these complex interactions. This makes it possible to locate minute discontinuities and to study areas that produce very low amplitude reflections, including the bond juncture between stainless steel and electroformed copper, for example.

Pencil Shape Focus

In many ultrasonic applications, a long focused beam is required to test a large depth range. Two lens configurations produce such a focused beam,[21] as shown in Fig. 49. The long axial test ranges are limited mainly by the rate at which signal amplitude falls off in the far field of the beam.

Acoustic Microscopy

An acoustic microscope uses acoustic waves and a set of one or more lenses to obtain information about the elastic microstructural properties of test objects. The finest detail resolvable by an acoustic microscope is determined by the diffraction limit of the system. Such

microscopes are available commercially for tests of thin structures such as integrated circuits.[47] The acoustic microscope can also be used to study bond integrity, microstructure formation and material stress effects.

In scanning acoustic microscopes (SAM), a piezoelectric crystal is bonded to a sapphire or quartz substrate to which it transmits plane waves. At the back of the substrate is a spherical lens machined with a low reflection coating. The lens produces a highly focused beam in water allowing the pair — transducer and lens — to operate as a focused transducer in a pulse echo mode. A shallow region close to the surface of the test material is examined.

The scanning procedure is similar to an ultrasonic C-scan and produces an image of the test area on the monitor. The contrast of the image is determined by the surface reflectivity of the test object and the phase of the reflected wave.

Closing

Ultrasonic techniques are implemented primarily in the pulse echo and through-transmission modes, with contact or immersion coupling. Pulse echo immersion is a coupling technique not commonly used in field applications because of the complexity associated with maintaining the couplant. Several means are commercially available to overcome the limitations of immersion coupling, including wheels and boots.

Pulse echo techniques provide very detailed information about test objects. This capability is attributed to the various parameters that can be analyzed, including time of flight, amplitude of back surface reflection and amplitude of extraneous reflections. The 1990s saw significant improvements in the capability of the technique with the introduction of microprocessor controlled pulser/receivers, signal analyzers and computerized C-scan controllers. Tests became more reliable; data, easier to interpret; systems, capable of testing complex object shapes.

Pulse echo immersion may be used with materials made of metal, plastic, composites and ceramics — the raw materials for most engineering structures. A wide variety of discontinuities can be detected and characterized with pulse echo techniques: the location, depth, size and discontinuity type can be determined.

FIGURE 49. Acoustic field where $d_F \cdot d_N^{-1} \cong F \cdot N^{-1}$ for: (a) concave lens; (b) angled concave lens.[46]

(a)

(b)

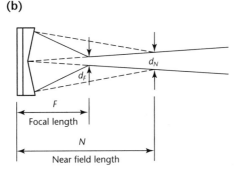

PART 6. Lamb Waves

The theory of lamb waves was originally developed by Horace Lamb in 1916 to describe the characteristics of waves propagating in plates.[48] Frequently, they are also referred to as plate waves. Lamb waves can be generated in a plate with free boundaries with an infinite number of modes for both symmetric and antisymmetric displacements within the layer. The symmetric modes are also called longitudinal modes because the average displacement over the thickness of the plate or layer is in the longitudinal direction. The antisymmetric modes are observed to exhibit average displacement in the transverse direction and these modes are also called flexural modes.[49,50] The infinite number of modes exists for a specific plate thickness and acoustic frequency which are identified by their respective phase velocities. Figure 50 shows a typical example of generating lamb waves in a solid plate using an angle wedge. The normal way to describe the propagation characteristics is by the use of dispersion curves based on the plate mode phase velocity as a function of the product of frequency times thickness. The dispersion curves are normally labeled as S0, A0, S1, A1 and so forth, depending on whether the mode is symmetric or antisymmetric.

Although the dispersion diagrams are very complex, they can be simplified by using the incidence angle of the exciting wave to determine which mode is to be dominant. A particular lamb wave can be excited if the phase velocity of the incident longitudinal wave is equal to phase velocity for the particular mode.

The phase velocity of the incident longitudinal wave is then given by:

$$(38) \quad V_p = \frac{V_L}{\sin \varphi}$$

where V_L is the group velocity of the incident longitudinal wave, V_p is the phase velocity of the incident longitudinal wave and φ is the angle of incidence of the incident longitudinal wave.

Lamb waves are extremely useful for detection of cracks in thin sheet materials and tubular products. Extensive developments in the applications of lamb waves provides a foundation for the inspection of many industrial products in aerospace, pipe and transportation. The generation of lamb waves can be performed using contact transducers, optical, electromagnetic, magnetostrictive, and air coupled transducers.

Magnetostrictive transducers operate by producing a small change in the physical dimensions of ferromagnetic materials, resulting in a deformation of crystalline parameters.[51] Applying high frequency power to the transducers then produces ultrasonic waves in the material. Lamb waves are produced when thin or tubular materials are excited by high frequency oscillations. The technique also works with nonferromagnetic samples: a ferromagnetic sheet, such as nickel, is bonded to the nonferromagnetic sample being tested. The lamb waves generated in this manner can be used to detect cracks or other material characteristics in areas away from the excitation source because the waves propagate along the sample for long distances. When used this way, the ultrasonic waves are also called *guided waves*. Technology using guided waves developed into a very useful ultrasonic test technique in the 1990s and is expected to continue to develop in the twenty-first century.[52] For example, new sensor development introduces smaller transducers, such as capacitive micromachined devices,[53] air coupling[54] and new characterization studies on the lamb wave modes propagating in plate structures.[55]

FIGURE 50. Lamb wave propagating in plate: (a) symmetric; (b) antisymmetric.

(a)

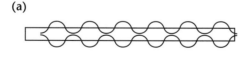

(b)

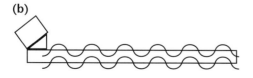

Part 7. Ultrasonic Guided Waves

Introduction

Ultrasonic guided waves are well documented in the technical literature.[56-62] Compared to ultrasonic bulk waves that travel in infinite media with no boundary influence, guided waves require a structural boundary for propagation. As an example, some guided wave possibilities are illustrated in Fig. 51 for a rayleigh surface wave, a lamb wave and a stonely wave at an interface between two materials. There are many other guided wave possibilities, of course, as long as a boundary on either one or two sides of the wave is considered. Natural waveguides include plates (such as aircraft skin), rods (rails, cylinders, square rods), hollow cylinder (pipes, tubing), multilayer structures, curved or flat surfaces on a half space and one or more layers on a half space.

Most structures are natural wave guides provided the wavelengths are large enough with respect to dimensions in the wave guide. If the wavelengths are very small, then bulk wave propagation can be considered, those waves used traditionally for many years in ultrasonic nondestructive pulse echo and through-transmission testing. One very interesting difference, of many, associated with guided waves, is that many different wave velocity values can be obtained as a function of frequency whereas, for most practical bulk wave propagation, wave velocity is independent of frequency. In fact, tables of wave velocities are available from most manufacturers of ultrasonic equipment — tables applicable to bulk wave propagation in materials, showing just a single wave velocity value for longitudinal waves and one additional value for transverse waves.

To get some idea of how guided waves are developed in a wave guide, imagine many bulk waves bouncing back and forth inside a wave guide with mode conversions between longitudinal and transverse constantly taking place at each boundary. The resulting superimposed wave form traveling along the wave guide is just a sum of all of these waves including amplitude and phase information. The outcome can strongly depend on frequency and introductory wave angles of propagation inside the structure. The strongly superimposed

results are actually points that end up on the phase velocity dispersion curve for the structure. Elsewhere is strong cancellation. To solve for the points on the dispersion curve, either a partial wave summation process could account for all reflections and mode conversions or an appropriate boundary value problem in wave propagation can be solved.

The use of ultrasonic guided waves increased tremendously after 1990 for various reasons, especially because of improved analytic techniques. The principal benefits of guided waves can be summarized as follows.

1. Inspection over long distances from a single probe position is possible, giving complete volumetric coverage of the test object.
2. There is no need for scanning: all of the data are acquired from a single probe position. Often, greater sensitivity than that obtained in conventional normal beam ultrasonic testing or other nondestructive techniques can be obtained, even with low frequency ultrasonic guided wave test techniques.

FIGURE 51. Guided wave types: (a) rayleigh (surface) waves; (b) lamb waves; (c) stonely waves.

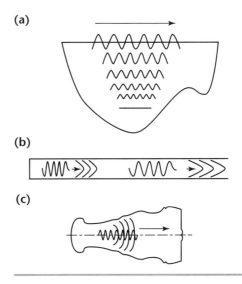

(a)

(b)

(c)

3. There is also an ability to inspect hidden structures, structures under water, coatings, insulations and concrete because of the ability to test from a single probe position via wave structure change and controlled mode sensitivity along with an ability to propagate over long distances.
4. There is also a tremendous cost effectiveness associated with guided waves because of the test simplicity and speed.

Dispersion

The subject of dispersion and the propagation of either dispersive or nondispersive modes is very critical to understand when dealing with ultrasonic guided waves. Figure 52 shows an example of dispersive and nondispersive guided wave propagation. For nondispersive wave propagation, the pulse duration remains constant as the wave travels through the structure. On the other hand, for dispersive wave propagation, because wave velocity is a function of frequency, the pulse duration changes from point to point inside the structure. The change is because each harmonic of the particular input pulse packet travels at a different wave velocity. There's a decrease in amplitude of the waveform and an increase in pulse duration but energy is still conserved — unless of course lossy media are considered.

Consider the development of a phase velocity computation in a wave guide, such as a plate having boundary conditions with traction free upper and lower surfaces. If we now consider some form of a governing wave equation and

an assumed harmonic solution for displacement, elasticity permits derivation of equations to satisfy the boundary conditions. This leads to a transcendental equation, or a characteristic equation. In extracting the roots from the characteristic equation, associated with a system of homogeneous equations, the determinant of the coefficient matrix must be set equal to zero. In this case, the roots extracted determine the values of phase velocity versus frequency that can be plotted. Figure 53 shows the phase velocity dispersion curves and group velocity dispersion curves for a particular traction free aluminum plate. The modes are labeled as antisymmetric A0, A1 and so on, or symmetric S0, S1 and so on. The particular limits in the diagram as plate velocity, surface wave velocity, transverse wave velocity and cutoff frequencies are all shown in the figure. Details on the development and the nomenclature considered here can be found in references.[15] Derivable from the phase velocity dispersion curves are sets of group velocity dispersion curves. The values of the group velocity dispersion curves depend on the ordinate and slope values of the phase velocity dispersion curves. The group velocity is defined as the velocity measured in a wave guide of a packet of waves of similar frequency. This group velocity is what you actually measure in an experiment.

If an aluminum plate is under water, there will be energy leakage as the wave travels along the plate, because of an out-of-plane displacement component that would load the liquid. The in-plane displacement components would not travel into the liquid medium because this would be like shear loading on the fluid. If you solve this wave propagation problem — or, as another example, the wave propagation associated with bitumen coating on a pipe — there would also be leakage of ultrasonic energy as the wave propagates along the plate. Following the phase and group velocity dispersion curves, the complex roots from the characteristic equation would then lead to a set of attenuation dispersion curves.

A sample set of these attenuation dispersion curves for bitumen coating on a pipe structure is illustrated in Fig. 54. A pipe sample problem is used here. For the plate problem the modes would be labeled as A0, A1, A2, S0, S1, S2 and so on because of their symmetric and antisymmetric character (see Fig. 53). In the case of guided wave in pipes, the axisymmetric longitudinal waves may be labeled as L(0,1), L(0,2), L(0,3) and so on and the axisymmetric torsional waves as T(0,1), T(0,2), T(0,3) and so on. Flexural modes are also possible because of partial

FIGURE 52. A0 nondispersive and S0 dispersive waves: (a) S0 dispersive, time = 10.0 s; (b) S0 dispersive, time = 20.0 s; (c) A0 non-dispersive, time = 10.0 s; (d) A0 non-dispersive, time = 14.0 s.

(a)

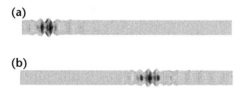

(b)

(c)

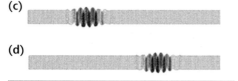

(d)

loading around the circumference of a pipe. See elsewhere[63] for more details on flexural modes. Note in Fig. 54 that attenuation does not always increase as frequency is increased as in a usual bulk wave problem. Some modes attenuate more quickly than others. Note the dotted curve for the L(0,3) mode in this case. One of the mode's attenuations improved significantly with higher frequency but this is the surface wave on the uncoated side of the pipe. For other modes, for higher frequency, the wave amplitudes are significantly reduced.

All guided wave problems have associated with them the development of appropriate dispersion curves and corresponding wave structures. Of thousands of points on a dispersion curve, only certain ones lead to a valid test — for example, those with greatest penetration power; with maximum displacement on

the outer, center or inner surface; with only in-plane vibration on the surface to avoid leakage into a fluid; or with minimum power at an interface between a pipe and a coating. A sample set of wave structure curves are illustrated in Fig. 55 to illustrate this point. In this case, the S0 mode propagation in an aluminum plate is considered. Notice the in-plane vibration behavior across the thickness compared to the out-of-plane motion. The wave structure changes from point to point along every mode on a dispersion curve. The characteristics of every point on each dispersion curve are different, primarily with respect to wave structure, a critical feature for the development of an efficient test technique for a particular structure. Notice that for an $f \cdot d$ value (value of frequency f times thickness d) of 0.5, the in-plane displacement is totally dominant across the thickness with

FIGURE 53. Dispersion curves for traction free aluminum plate: (a) phase velocity dispersion curves; (b) group velocity dispersion curves.

(a)

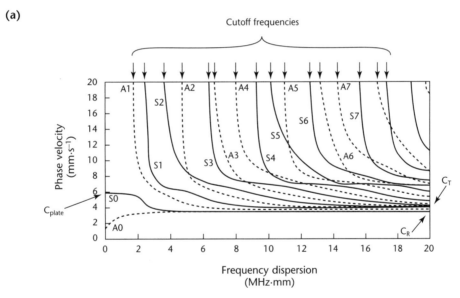

Frequency dispersion
(MHz·mm)

(b)

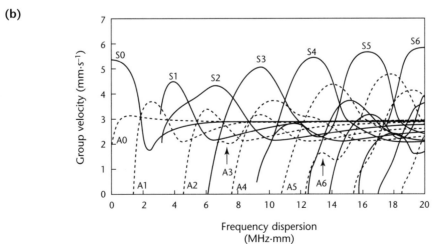

Frequency dispersion
(MHz·mm)

almost no out-of-plane vibration. This mode, as an example, would travel very far even if the aluminum plate were under water. If we now move forward and consider the product of frequency times thickness equal to 2.0, the in-plane displacement on the outer surface of the plate is almost zero whereas the out-of-plane vibration is a maximum on the upper and lower surfaces. If this S0 mode were to propagate at an $f \cdot d$ value of 2.0, the leakage would be substantial and waves under water would not propagate very far along the plate.

In addition to the lamb waves illustrated so far in Figs. 53 to 55, there could be transverse horizontal guided wave propagation in the plate as well, depending on the sensor loading situation. In this case, the transverse horizontal wave produces an in-plane component perpendicular to the wave propagation or wave vector direction but still in the plane of the plate. For the transverse horizontal mode, there is no out of plane displacement. The leakage into a fluid media from an aluminum plate would be nonexistent as far as wave propagation is concerned. Keep in mind, however, that mode conversion at a discontinuity could create some leaky reflected waves.

Source Influence

The development of the dispersion curves discussed so far uses harmonic plane wave excitation in the wave guide. Because of a bounded transducer problem, however, it is necessary to study a source influence problem for a particular size sensor. The finite size of a transducer and various vibration characteristics give rise to a phase velocity spectrum in addition to the

ordinary frequency spectrum. These two spectral band widths, frequency and phase velocity, make it difficult to excite a specific point on a dispersion curve. Some interesting discussion on the source influence problem can be found elsewhere.[15,64,65] Mode separation in the dispersion curve then becomes useful for single-mode excitation potential.

Guided wave energy can be induced into a wave guide by various techniques. The challenge is to excite a particular mode at a specific frequency. Normal

FIGURE 55. Wave structure for various points on S0 mode of aluminum plate: (a) frequency $f \times$ thickness $d = 0.5$; (b) $f \times d = 1.0$; (c) $f \times d = 1.5$; (d) $f \times d = 2.0$.

(a)
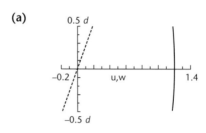

(b)
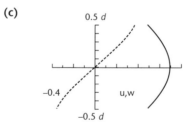

(c)
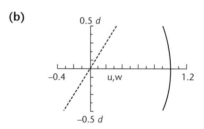

FIGURE 54. Attenuation dispersion curves for a 100 mm (4 in.) schedule 40 steel pipe with a 125 µm (0.005 in.) bitumen coating.

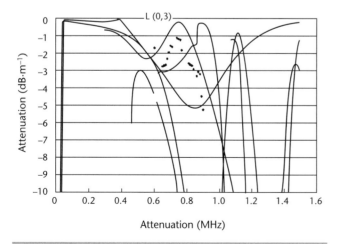

(d)
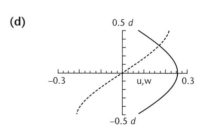

Legend
—— = u, in-plane
------ = w, out-of-plane

beam probes can be used. Angle beam sensors can also be used to impart beams that lead to desired kinds of guided waves in a pipe or plate. A comb transducer (a number of different elements at a specific spacing) can be used to pump ultrasonic energy into the plate, causing wave propagation of a certain wavelength in the wave guide. The excitation zones in the phase velocity dispersion curve can be evaluated by the source being considered in the problem. Again, references[15,64,65] provide details in this exercise. A comb transducer, as an example, could be wrapped completely around a pipe or laid out as fingers or an interdigital transducer design on a plate.

Pipeline Inspection

Guided wave inspection of pipeline materials is particularly useful because a large area can be tested from a single transducer position.[66,67,68] Some of the initial work done in this area was for steam generator tube testing. It was discovered that these waves could go far and still be able to evaluate discontinuities at a long distance from the transducer position.[66] In looking at pipeline inspection over long distances,

phased array focusing techniques are reported.[68,69] Beam focusing is possible, although a different computation technique to achieve focusing is necessary being different than the computations required in phased arrays for bulk wave focusing.

A sample configuration of pipeline testing with a typical wraparound guided wave sensor arrangement is illustrated in Fig. 56. There are a number of arrangements for this application via normal beam sensors, angle beam sensors, electromagnetic acoustic transducers, magnetostrictive sensors and others at frequencies ranging from 20 to 800 kHz, depending on the distance of propagation and the discontinuities sought. Typically, low frequency test systems find discontinuities that have a 5 percent cross sectional area or more. Higher frequencies can go down to 1 percent cross sectional area or less.

Aircraft Inspection

A variety of different problems can be tackled in the aircraft industry.[70] Aircraft skins are well suited to guided wave testing. Note in Fig. 57 a possibility of guided wave testing. In Fig. 57a, if ultrasonic energy can be passed from a transmitter to a receiver across a lap splice joint, the integrity of the bond line can be evaluated. Nevertheless, the problem is not as simple as it looks because the wave structure has to be adjusted to have sufficient energy at the interface to allow propagation into medium 2. The wave structure variation and the kind of energy obtained can result from calculations of wave structure for a particular mode and frequency in a phase velocity dispersion curve. Once the technique is developed,

FIGURE 56. Representative wraparound ultrasonic guided wave array for long range ultrasonic guided wave inspection of piping: (a) attached; (b) detached.

(a)

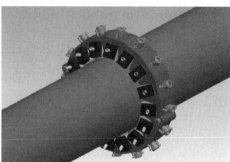

(b)

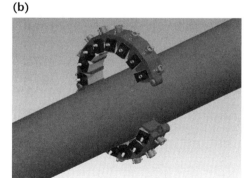

FIGURE 57. Lap splice test sample problem: (a) through-transmission; (b) double-spring hopping probe.

(a)

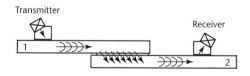

(b)

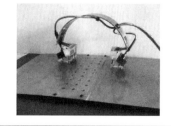

tools can be used as illustrated in Fig. 57b, as an example, the double spring hopping probe illustrated here can be placed on a material quite easily and at the appropriate mode and frequency can evaluate the integrity of the lap splice joint.

Closing

Because of tremendous advances in the understanding of guided wave propagation and the superb computational ability by mathematical and finite element analysis, guided wave testing is a practical test option. The technique can be used to solve many problems using guided wave analysis in nondestructive testing and structural health monitoring is very bright.

PART 8. Optical Generation and Detection of Ultrasound[71]

Generation and detection of ultrasound by optical means, which together are known as *laser ultrasonics* or *laser based ultrasound,* represent an area of intensive research and development which was until the twenty-first century limited to the laboratory and pilot demonstrations.[72] The technology has matured and applications have been transitioned to industry. It is also commercially available. Laser ultrasonic techniques are also useful for material characterization and optical detection can be used to characterize piezoelectric transducers.

Advantages of Optical Ultrasound Generation and Detection

Noncontact Tests

A major advantage of optical techniques is that there is no mechanical contact made with the test object surface. In fact, these techniques are not simply noncontacting but may be used for remote sensing — a clear distinction and potential advantage over electromagnetic acoustic transducer and capacitance transducer techniques.

Because transduction of light energy to acoustic energy is performed by the test material, no intervening couplant is needed. Likewise, material surface vibrations are directly encoded onto a light beam, also without couplant. These techniques make possible ultrasonic testing in conditions difficult for other techniques — probing hot materials, testing in vacuum (in space) and probing moving objects either transversely or toward the transducer. Important for industrial applications is the ease of testing objects with contoured surfaces and nonplanar shapes.

With laser ultrasonic techniques, there is no requirement for precise transducer orientation, such as that found in conventional piezoelectric techniques.

Other Advantages

Also notable is the optical resolution obtained with laser ultrasonics. For example, detection spot diameters down to 10 µm (4×10^{-4} in.) are used routinely in experimental systems. Because laser beams can be easily scanned, array of small generation sources or detection spots can be realized. In addition, the spectral content of laser generated elastic waves may be extremely broad band. Using optical pulses of picosecond duration, acoustic signals of only 2 ns have been generated. This provides a potential for discontinuity detection in materials as thin as a razor blade. Narrow band signals can be generated as well by delaying in time or separating in space an array of sources.

Optical generation and detection of ultrasound does have some limitations that primarily affect detection sensitivity. Elastic waves generated by optical sources often have relatively low amplitude. Using higher laser intensities to increase acoustic amplitude may damage to the test object surface. High intensity is often prohibited but in many applications invasive marking by the generation laser does not matter, such as probing of hot metals during processing.

Optical Generation of Elastic Waves

When light radiation is absorbed by the irradiated portion of a test object, thermal expansion results, producing elastic ultrasonic waves. A contribution might also come from the momentum transfer of the reflected light but these radiation pressure effects are extremely small compared to those associated with light absorption.

With increasing incident optical intensity, the temperature rise at the object surface can be so great that vaporization of the material may occur. The momentum transfer of the ablated material leaving the surface and the pressure of the produced plasma result in a force normal to the surface that also gives rise to elastic waves. This subject has been reviewed in the literature and its main features are outlined below.[72,73]

Waves from Free Surface

Optical absorption produces two mechanisms for elastic wave generation and these may be used to generate ultrasound in at least three ways.

FIGURE 58. Types of laser generated ultrasound: (a) thermoelastic or free surface; (b) constrained surface; (c) ablated surface.

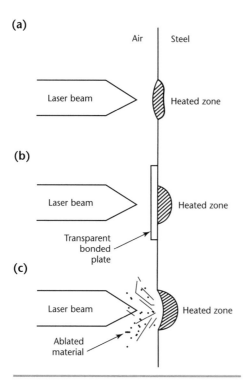

(a)

(b)

(c)

FIGURE 59. Radiation patterns of laser generated ultrasound for surface conditions shown in Fig. 58 (longitudinal wave directivity for a source smaller than the ultrasonic wavelength): (a) thermoelastic surface; (b) constrained surface or ablated surface.

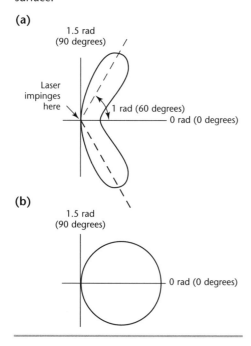

(a)

(b)

Figures 58a and 59a illustrate what happens when light is absorbed near the free surface of a material at a power density below that which causes material ablation (about 10^5 W·mm^{-2} for aluminum). Note that the thermoelastic expansion of the source volume is not constrained by the surface. As a result, thermoelastic generation on the free surface gives rise to little compressional energy directed along the axis perpendicular to the surface. Instead, longitudinal (compressional) waves are directed in a pattern that takes the form of a hollow cone with an apex half angle of about 1 rad (60 deg).

This conical radiation pattern is observed for sources smaller than the ultrasonic wavelength. The pattern was predicted theoretically by early models that assumed point sources of radiating force vectors acting in the plane of the surface.[73,74] Experimental results using an aluminum hemisphere as a test object substantially confirm these predictions. In fact, epicentral measurements (measurements on axis) show a significant retraction of the test object surface opposite the source following the arrival of the longitudinal wave (Fig. 60).

Figure 60 shows a small outward deflection of the object's back surface immediately after arrival of the longitudinal wave. Early models for the thermoelastic source did not predict this leading spike because they assumed the source had no thickness. More recently, investigators have developed models without heuristic assumptions that show the spike.[75,76] Other developments have linked its origin to thermal-to-acoustic

FIGURE 60. Epicentral displacement caused by point laser source in thermoelastic mode.

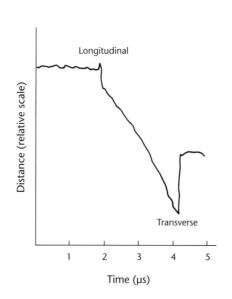

mode conversion at the test object surface.[77]

In addition to longitudinal waves, both transverse and rayleigh waves are generated in the free surface thermoelastic mode. Rayleigh wave directivity has been demonstrated using focused line sources.[78] An annular illumination pattern has also been demonstrated, giving rise to convergent rayleigh waves and very strong amplitude at the center of the annulus.[79] Other generation patterns can also be used with various advantages, such as an array of lines that gives narrow band emission and minimizes surface damage by distributing laser energy. Generation can also be enhanced by sweeping the line or array of lines source.[80] For samples of thickness smaller than the rayleigh wavelength, plates (lamb) waves can be similarly generated.

Waves from Constrained Surface

Acoustic waves also may be optically generated as illustrated in Fig. 58b, where the surface of the test object is constrained by a transparent material. Constraint may be obtained by bonding a glass plate to the surface or more simply by coating the surface with a thin layer of water, oil or grease.

The displacement out of the surface is redirected into the bulk of the test object. As a result, the directivity pattern for longitudinal waves is altered so that most of the longitudinal wave energy is directed on axis (Fig. 59b).[74] Enhancement of the longitudinal and transverse waves is observed as high as 30 dB over free surface generation, depending on the test object material and the type of surface constraint. Similar effects occur when light penetrates deeper into the test object, producing a buried ultrasonic source.[72,81] This effect is found particularly important for testing polymer materials, in particular polymer matrix materials.[72]

Waves from Ablated Surface

A third way for generating acoustic waves optically occurs when the source energy density is sufficiently high to cause ablation of material from the test object surface (Fig. 38c).[82,83] The ablated material may be the base material or it may be a coating ablated after absorbing the light energy. The momentum transferred to the surface during ablation produces a greatly increased normal force on the surface. As is the case with a constrained surface, both the directivity and the amplitude of the longitudinal wave energy are changed. Owing to the large normal force, longitudinal waves are directed most strongly along the axis normal to the surface.

Although the ablative technique is destructive, it may be used when surface finish is not critical during early stages of material processing. Also note that in this case, the displacements are comparable to those produced by conventional piezoelectric transducers excited by a few hundred volts. The displacements are weaker in the thermoelastic and free surface mode.

To generate ultrasound in these three modes, a pulsed laser is used. Many reported studies have been performed with quantum based switched solid lasers such as the neodymium yttrium-aluminum-garnet laser with pulse lengths from 5 to 30 ns. Pulsed gas lasers also may be used, such as the transversely excited atmospheric pressure carbon dioxide laser, used for inspecting polymer matrix composites.[72]

Optical Detection of Ultrasound

Optical techniques for ultrasonic wave detection can be divided into two classes. The first includes techniques that permit real time detection of ultrasonic disturbances at a single point or over a single zone on a test object surface. The second category includes full field techniques that provide maps of the acoustic energy distribution over an entire field of view at one instant in time.[84]

Full field techniques have insufficient sensitivity and are not used, so the present discussion focuses on single-spot detection techniques. Such techniques have been widely reviewed in the literature[85] except for the variants described below. Generally, in the case of laser generated ultrasound, the ultrasonic displacements (on the surface of generation and any other surface) have a nonvanishing normal component. Therefore, it is generally sufficient to detect this component, although in-plane motion can be detected by optical techniques.[86] For detecting normal displacement, two interferometric techniques and two variants of them have found application.

Simple Interferometric Detection

A technique called *optical heterodyning* or *simple interferometric detection* uses a wave scattered by the surface to interfere with a reference wave directly derived from the laser (Fig. 61). Such a technique is sensitive to optical speckle and the best sensitivity is obtained when one speckle is effectively detected. This means that the mean speckle size on the focusing lens has to be about the size of the incoming beam and that this beam should be focused onto the surface. This technique generally allows the measurement of ultrasonic displacement over a small spot and provides point detection, except at high frequencies.

Compensation for vibrations can be performed by an electromechanical feedback loop that generally uses a piezoelectric translator for path length compensation. For more severe vibration environments, the heterodyne configuration is preferred. In this setup, the optical frequency in one arm is shifted by a radiofrequency and the detector receives a signal at this shift frequency, phase modulated by ultrasound and vibrations. Electronic circuits can be devised to retrieve the ultrasonic displacement independently of vibrations.

Velocity Interferometry, or Time Delay Interferometry

The second detection method, called *velocity interferometry* or *time delay interferometry*,[85] is based on the doppler frequency shift produced by surface motion and its demodulation by an interferometer having a filter response (Fig. 62). This technique is primarily sensitive to the velocity of the surface and is insensitive to low frequencies. The filter response is obtained by giving a path delay between the interfering waves within the interferometer. Two-wave interferometers (michelson, mach-zehnder) or multiple-wave interferometers (fabry-perot) can be used.

Unlike optical heterodyning, this technique permits reception of many speckles. A large detecting spot (several millimeters or more) is obtained when known modifications are used to increase throughput and field of view (field widened michelson interferometer,

confocal fabry-perot interferometer). This interferometer is made simply with two concave mirrors separated by a distance equal to their radius of curvature and is widely used for industrial applications.[85]

Interferometric Technique Variants

Velocity interferometry does not have a flat detection response but generally has a large throughput corresponding to its large detection area. Simple interferometric detection, on the other hand, has a flat response (limited by the detector cutoff frequency or the shift frequency) but also has a small throughput corresponding to its small detection area. Variants of these techniques have however been developed that provide both broad detection band width and large throughput.

A first variant consists in using the confocal fabry-perot interferometer in reflection.[87] In this case, there is interference between the light directly reflected by the front mirror and light reflected and leaked out of the fabry-perot cavity, both having wavefronts substantially matched. The light leaked out in reflection is stripped from its sidebands for frequencies above Δv (as defined in Fig. 62) and acts as a reference wave. This system has a response

FIGURE 62. Ultrasound detection with time delay velocity interferometer: (a) test setup; (b) principle of detection.

(a)

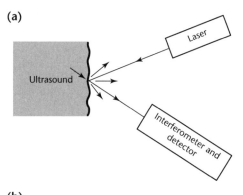

(b)

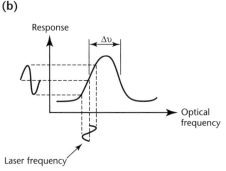

FIGURE 61. Configuration for optical heterodyning or simple interferometric detection. A frequency shifter such as a bragg cell can be introduced in either arm (heterodyne michelson interferometer).

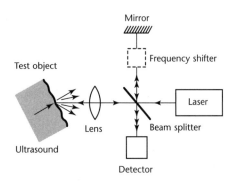

essentially flat above Δν (which means in practice a few megahertz).

A second variant consists in using an adaptive beam splitter/mixer. By two-wave mixing in a photorefractive crystal, the wave reflected by the surface beats with a pump wave directly derived from the laser to produce a real time hologram in the crystal.[88,89] This hologram diffracts a reference wave matched to the transmitted wave, as sketched in Fig. 63. This system has a flat response from very low frequencies (1 kHz to 100 kHz depending on the pump wave power) to the detector cutoff frequency and a large throughput.

Note that the flexibility of such interferometric detection systems is greatly increased by including an optical fiber link between the interferometer and the test surface. In the case of optical heterodyning, single mode fibers must be used. Velocity interferometry and the two variants mentioned above may use large core fibers that make application simpler.

Finally, despite the diversity of interferometric detection system designs, their sensitivities to ultrasonic surface motion are generally of the same order of magnitude. In the case of shot noise limited detection, the sensitivity is on order of 0.01 nm for an electronic band width of 10 MHz and an intensity received by the interferometer of about 1 mW.

Applications

Ultrasonic Metrology

Optical probes for detection of ultrasound can be used to map ultrasonic fields at the surface of test objects or at the surface of ultrasonic transducers. Probes based on optical heterodyning are preferred for this purpose because they can be easily calibrated and allow the measurement of the absolute value of ultrasonic displacements.

Optical probes can be used for detection of ultrasonic transducer malfunctions resulting from improper manufacture or aging. Optical probes can also be used to clarify complicated ultrasonic testing procedures by mapping the ultrasonic displacement field over the surfaces of a test object.[90]

Gaging

Laser ultrasonic testing, like any other ultrasonic technique, can be used for measuring thickness. Because it operates at a distance, however, it allows gaging parts at elevated temperature. As with conventional ultrasonic testing, this application is based on measuring the time-of-flight between consecutive echoes and then, by using the value of the acoustic velocity in the material, to relate time-of-flight to thickness. This velocity has to be calibrated by independent measurements because it depends on temperature.

The technique has been particularly developed for wall thickness gaging of seamless tubes at elevated temperature on a production line and is now commercially available.[91] Figure 64 shows the measuring head of a system installed on line above a hot and rotating tube in a seamless tube production plant. This head is linked by optical fibers to the lasers and the interferometer, located remotely in an environmentally controlled enclosure. This arrangement allows adequate servicing of the lasers (for example, change of the flash lamps) away from the hot and dusty environment of the plant.

FIGURE 63. Ultrasound detection with two-wave mixing photorefractive interferometer.

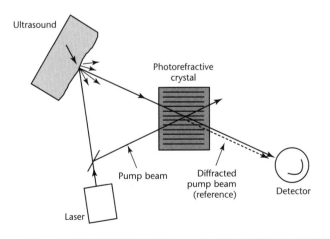

FIGURE 64. Wall thickness gaging and austenite grain size determination on seamless tubes: view of measuring head on top of hot tube.

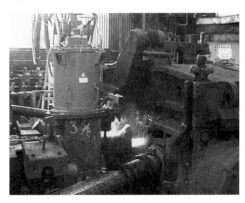

The system includes also a pyrometer to measure the temperature from which the proper velocity can be found from the previous calibration. Such a system allows controlling the tube making process and has demonstrated significant productivity gain. It has also the advantage compared to gamma-ray tomography, another technology that could be used for determining the wall thickness of tubes, to permit measurement with a piercing mandrel inside the tube.

Discontinuity Detection

Laser ultrasonics produces an ultrasonic source at the surface of a test object and allows detection from the object surface, independently of shape and orientation. Curved and complex geometries such as pipes, rotor blades and the edges of aircraft wings can then be tested.

In particular, delaminations in flat or curved graphite epoxy laminates can be easily detected.[92] Figure 65 shows the results (C-scan and B-scans) obtained by raster scanning a U shaped specimen with delaminations on the flat surfaces and along a corner. These results are made possible by using a generation laser that provides adequate penetration and absorption of light in the top epoxy layer and contributes to the constraining effect mentioned above. The generated longitudinal wave is always essentially normal to the surface, independently of the direction of the laser beams. Therefore, there is no need to know or to follow the part contour as with conventional ultrasonic testing.

This application to polymer matrix composite inspection has been extensively developed and is now routinely used for part inspection by a major military aircraft manufacturer.[93] A turnkey system has been built for the United States Air Force.[94] The technology has also been used at the validation and production stages by aerospace companies in Europe[95] This technology could be used not only for inspecting fabricated parts but also for inspecting an aircraft during maintenance.[96] Unlike conventional water jet ultrasonics, laser ultrasonics allows scanning to the very edge of the part. For the C-scan of a horizontal stabilizer, a transversely excited atmospheric pressure pulsed carbon dioxide laser operating at 10.6 μm has been used to generate ultrasound. For detection, a long pulse, high stability neodymium yttrium-aluminum-garnet laser specially developed for laser ultrasonics is used and coupled to a confocal fabry-perot interferometer. Photorefractive interferometers with better low frequencies sensitivity could be advantageously used for thick part testing, more than 12 mm (0.5 in.).

On metallic parts, the detection of surface breaking cracks has been demonstrated by using laser generated surface acoustic waves. When the generation laser beam passes over the crack, the signal detected at some distance from generation is very different from the one encountered from a crack free region and allows reliable detection of surface cracking.[97] By using the filtering effect of the crack (low frequencies go through, high frequencies are blocked), these discontinuities can also be sized. In metallic parts, because the acoustic source is at the surface and can be made very small, the technique can easily generate by scanning an array of ultrasonic A-scans and is advantageously coupled to a numerical focusing technique such as the synthetic aperture focusing technique (SAFT).[98] In combination with such a technique, high resolution imaging can be

FIGURE 65. Laser ultrasonic test of U shaped graphite epoxy composite showing time-of-flight C-scan above B-scans at indicated locations.

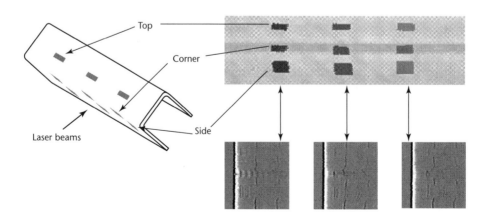

obtained throughout the part volume. Fourier domain processing has been developed to minimize computer processing time.[99] Figure 66 shows an example in which a test specimen with stress corrosion cracks was imaged from the surface opposite to cracking.[98] The C-scan at the crack opening surface is compared with an image obtained by liquid penetrants. The amplitude of the crack indication obtained after numerical reconstruction provides also some information on crack depth. One will note that in this combined technique, longitudinal or transverse waves can either be used for imaging because they are both generated by the laser.

Materials Characterization

The approaches for material characterization by laser ultrasonic testing

FIGURE 66. Stress corrosion cracks on stainless steel sample: (a) laser ultrasonic image; (b) liquid penetrant test.

(a)

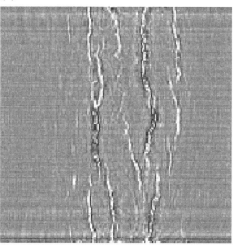

(b)

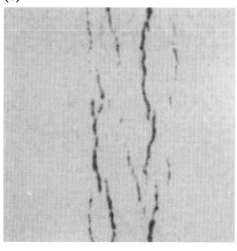

are essentially the same as the ones used with conventional ultrasonics and are based on the monitoring of ultrasonic velocity, ultrasonic attenuation and backscattered microstructure noise. Optical detection is particularly advantageous for measuring backscattered noise, which relates to grain size in metals, because a small detection spot is readily obtained.

A first type of application consists in using the velocity information for the determination of elastic constants. Because a laser generates longitudinal and transverse waves at the same time, both velocities can be deduced from the measurement of the two propagation times. Assuming there is a suitable model to link velocities and elastic constants, these constants also can be determined. Ultrasonic velocity measurements have been reported in numerous research contributions for this purpose. The materials include metals (aluminum and steel), ceramics and metal ceramic composites, at room temperature and at elevated temperatures.[100-103] These experiments were performed by generating ultrasound with a short pulse laser (generally a Q switched, neodymium yttrium-aluminum-garnet laser) on one side of the test object and detection from the other side. Different approaches have been considered to improve the accuracy of the time interval determination, including the use of ablation to produce strong spike pulses,[100,102] off epicenter probing[100] to enhance transverse features, modeling of the source[101] and cross correlation between consecutive echoes.[103]

Velocity measurements can also be used to measure material anisotropy, or texture. Two approaches can be used for plate samples. A first one consists in generating rayleigh or lamb waves propagating in a given direction using line source generation.[104] Wave arrival is detected at some distance from generation. A second approach is based on normally propagating bulk waves (longitudinal and transverse) and the frequency analysis of the multiple echoes. If there is anisotropy, resonance will occur at different frequencies for the transverse waves according to their polarization.[105] This has been demonstrated to be applicable for monitoring annealing of steel and aluminum alloys because during this process the new grains grow usually with a different orientation.[105-107] Velocity monitoring can also be used to monitor phase change or to determine phase composition.[108] In particular, the retained austenite fraction in steel can be determined (Fig. 67).

It is known that materials can also be characterized by measuring ultrasonic attenuation. Such a measurement made with conventional piezoelectric techniques is generally difficult because it requires a test object with parallel surfaces, a precise orientation of the transducer (immersion technique) or a uniform bond. Furthermore, to apply diffraction corrections, the transducer should satisfy to a good approximation the assumption of a piston source and of a uniform baffled receiver.[109] Laser ultrasonic testing requires test objects of sufficiently uniform thickness but is free of orientation and bond problems because the source and the receiver are on the surface of the test object.

It has been shown that sufficiently accurate measurements can be performed by operating in two cases: (1) the spherical wave limit corresponding to point generation and detection and (2) the plane wave limit corresponding to large generation and detection spots.[110] On steel, good correlation was observed between measured attenuation and grain size.[111] More recently this application has been extended to the measurement of austenite grain size on line.[112,113]

Further Developments

Since the 1990s, laser ultrasonic testing has made the transition from the laboratory to industry in two important areas: (1) polymer-matrix composite testing and (2) gaging and microstructure determination in the steel industry, specifically for seamless tubes. The technique is also used in microelectronics for characterizing very thin layers or measuring their thickness.[114,115]

It is reasonable to expect that the use of the technology in the areas for which the transition to industry had already

occurred will increase. One promising area of application is the steel industry as an on-line sensing technology for microstructure and phase transformations. Other industries that use laser based manufacturing techniques, such as the automotive industry, can benefit from laser ultrasonic testing. The nuclear industry because of the radiation environment could also benefit from remote sensing with lasers.

Among the barriers preventing a wider use of laser ultrasonics is the possible damage to the material surface, laser ocular safety and beyond these aspects, some complexity of the technology. This complexity leads to a relatively high cost, usually higher than conventional means. Therefore the hybrid approaches that use laser generation, electromagnetic acoustic transducers or air coupled detection may find use in special cases. However, electromagnetic acoustic transducers are limited to metals and proximity sensing and transmission through air suffers high losses increasing with frequency. There have also been efforts to make the laser ultrasonic technology more affordable.[116]

In conclusion, although the principles of the technology are not expected to change, its industrial application is expected to grow in the twenty-first century.

FIGURE 67. Austenite grain growth monitoring by laser ultrasonic testing versus metallography.

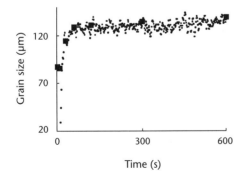

Legend
■ = Metallography
• = Laser ultrasonics

Part 9. Electromagnetic Acoustic Transduction[117]

The electromagnetic acoustic transducer (EMAT) is a device for the excitation and detection of ultrasonic waves in conductive or magnetic materials. No physical contact is required with the test object because the coupling occurs through electromagnetic forces. The working distances are typically less than a millimeter and the probe often is allowed to rest on the surface of the test object. This ability to provide reproducible signals with no couplant is often more important than noncontact operation.

Physical Principles

The physical principles of electromagnetic acoustic transducer transduction[118] are shown in Fig. 68. Suppose that a wire is put next to a metal surface and driven by a current at the desired ultrasonic frequency. Eddy currents $\bar{J}_w$ are induced within the metal and, if a static magnetic bias induction $\bar{B}_0$ is also present, the eddy currents experience periodic lorentz forces $\bar{F}_L$ given by:

$$(39) \quad \bar{F}_L = \bar{J}_w \times \bar{B}_0$$

The lorentz forces on the eddy currents are transmitted to the solid by collisions with the lattice or other microscopic processes. These forces on the solid are alternating at the frequency of the driving current and act as a source of ultrasonic waves. The process is in many ways similar to that which creates motion in an electrical motor. Reciprocal mechanisms also exist whereby waves can be detected, a process analogous to operation of an electrical generator.

If the material is ferromagnetic, additional coupling mechanisms are found. Direct interactions occur between the magnetization of the material and the dynamic magnetic fields associated with the eddy currents. Magnetostrictive processes are the tendency of a material to change length when magnetized. These processes can also play a major role in generating ultrasound. Again, reciprocal processes exist whereby these mechanisms can contribute to detection.

Probe Configurations

Practical electromagnetic probes consist of much more than a single wire. It is usually necessary to wind a coil and design a bias magnet structure so that the distribution of forces predicted by Eq. 39 couples to a particular wave type. Figure 69 shows the cross sections of five coil types.

Included are probes that couple to (1) radially polarized transverse beams, (2) longitudinal or (3) transverse plane polarized beams propagating normal to the surface and (4) longitudinal or vertically polarized transverse beams or (5) horizontally polarized transverse horizontal beams propagating at oblique angles. By virtue of the spatially periodic stresses that it excites, the meander coil electromagnetic acoustic transducer shown in Fig. 69d can also excite rayleigh waves on surfaces or lamb modes in plates. The periodic permanent magnet transducer in Fig. 69e can also excite horizontally polarized transverse modes in plates.

Advantages of Electromagnetic Acoustic Transducers

The major motivation for using electromagnetic acoustic transducers is their ability to operate without couplant

FIGURE 68. Single element of electromagnetic acoustic transducer.

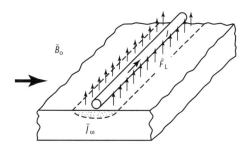

Legend
$\bar{B}_0$ = magnetic bias induction
$\bar{F}_L$ = body forces
I = applied current
$\bar{J}_\omega$ = eddy current

or contact. Important consequences of this include operation on moving objects, in remote or hazardous locations, at elevated temperatures, in vacuum and on oily or rough surfaces. Moreover, alignment problems may be reduced because the direction in which the wave is launched is primarily determined by the orientation of the test object surface rather than the probe. Finally, electromagnetic acoustic transducers have the ability to conveniently excite horizontally polarized transverse waves or other special wave types that provide test advantages in certain applications.

It must be noted that the cost of realizing these advantages is a relatively low operating efficiency. This inefficiency is overcome by high transmitter currents, low noise receivers and careful electrical matching. In ferromagnetic materials, the magnetization or magnetostrictive mechanisms of coupling can often be used to enhance signal levels.

Modeling of Electromagnetic Acoustic Transducer Measurements

Because the coupling of electromagnetic acoustic transducers is very reproducible, it is possible to model them with high accuracy. This is important for three reasons.

1. First, it allows the design of measurement systems that fully exploit the ability of the transducers to excite special wave types and radiation patterns.
2. It provides a tool for optimizing system performance and counteracting low sensitivity problems.
3. In ferromagnetic materials, it allows full use of the magnetization and magnetostriction mechanisms for optimized transduction efficiency.

As an example, a physical transducer model based on the theory of electromagnetic ultrasonic transduction in ferromagnetic metals is described below.[119] Its predictions have been analyzed to derive essential rules of transducer behavior and these have been

FIGURE 69. Cross sectional view of practical electromagnetic acoustic transducer configurations: (a) spiral coil exciting radially polarized transverse wave propagating normal to surface; (b) tangential field electromagnetic acoustic transducer for exciting plane polarized longitudinal waves propagating normal to surface; (c) normal field transducer for exciting plane polarized transverse waves propagating normal to surface; (d) meander coil transducer for exciting oblique longitudinal or vertically polarized transverse waves, rayleigh waves or guided modes of plates; (e) periodic permanent magnet for exciting obliquely propagating horizontally polarized transverse waves or guided horizontally polarized shear modes of plates.

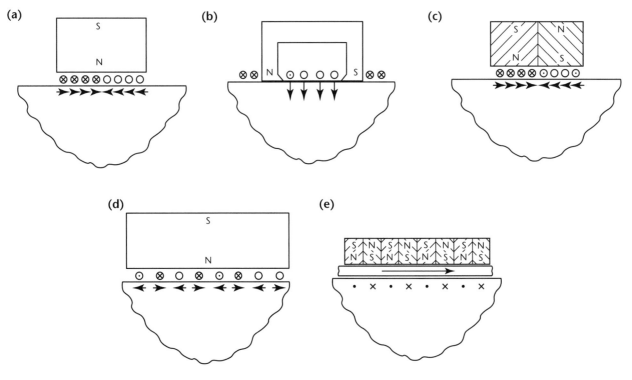

systematically checked in a series of experiments.

For generating ultrasound, the transducer is modeled through a two-dimensional pattern of radiofrequency currents distributed in the space above the material surface and a homogeneous magnetic bias field. For this configuration, the displacements in the ultrasonic wave field generated in the material are calculated. For ultrasonic reception, the model gives the electrical voltage induced in the coil winding pattern during the incidence of an ultrasonic wave. To obtain these results, the coupled dynamic equations of the electromagnetic field and of elastic stress and strain have been solved.[119]

Results of Theoretical Studies

Theoretical results have been checked systematically in experimental studies of transverse wave transduction using a semicylindrical block of soft iron. As a measure of transduction efficiency, the transfer impedance of a transducer pair is used, a quantity that can readily be measured and is also straightforwardly obtained from the theoretical treatment. The model gives directly the sensitivities of the transmitter and receiver. The multiplication of both yields the transfer impedance, that is, the ratio of the receiving voltage to the transmitting current. Losses from attenuation and diffraction must also be properly included in these calculations.

The theoretical and experimental directivity pattern of vertically polarized transverse waves can be generated by a meander coil designed to enhance the radiated intensity at an angle of $\theta = \sin^{-1}(\lambda D)$ with respect to the surface normal (where D is coil period and λ is wavelength). The experiments were conducted on a half cylinder of soft iron with a magnetic bias field normal to the surface. The ordinate is the transfer impedance (drawn to a logarithmic scale) occurring when the line probe receiver is moved along the cylindrical surface of the test object. The transmitter coil has a dolph-chebychev tapering to obtain lowest side lobe levels. The transfer impedance measured at the main lobe maximum is about 20 percent lower and the measured side lobe level is somewhat higher than the calculated values. Through the dependence on wavelength, the main lobe's angle of incidence depends on the frequency. The largest discrepancy between experimental and theoretical values is about 20 percent. These results demonstrate the usefulness of the applied model in calculating absolute transducer efficiencies and directivity patterns.

The numerical model is a strong engineering tool for optimizing transducers. In addition, careful impedance matching and proper electronic design are necessary to overcome insertion losses.

Thickness Gaging with Electromagnetic Acoustic Transducers

Ultrasonic techniques are widely used for thickness gaging and electromagnetic acoustic transducers expand the possible range of applications. Because of the electromagnetic acoustic transducer's ability to operate at high speed and elevated temperatures, thickness gaging is well suited for online measurements during materials processing. With these transducers, it is also particularly easy to generate transverse waves. This has advantages when measuring thin materials because the transverse velocity is roughly half the longitudinal wave velocity. For a given thickness, the echo occurs later, is more easily resolved from electrical leakage and the change in arrival time per unit change in thickness is greater.

Beams Propagating Normal to Surfaces

Delay lines are commonly used with fluid coupled transducers to measure thin material. They cannot be used with electromagnetic acoustic transducers (later reflections can often be used to circumvent problems with system recovery time). Although electromagnetic acoustic transducers can operate as high as 12 MHz, a more practical limitation at present is the 5 to 7.5 MHz range (even at 5 MHz, cable lengths must be kept short). This limits measuring thicknesses to those greater than about 1 mm (0.04 in.).

Measurements in thick materials are eventually limited by the ratio of signal to noise. In practice, beam spread losses (that decrease as the transducer coil gets larger) must be balanced with available drive currents (that usually increase as the coil gets smaller).

In most situations, any coil can operate reliably over a 3:1 thickness range and still accommodate a coil liftoff variation of at least 0.5 mm (0.02 in.). Smaller liftoff variation often allows a coil to operate over a 10:1 thickness range.

The most efficient electromagnetic acoustic transducer for thickness measurements with normally propagating bulk transverse waves uses a planar coil. If separate transmit and receive coils are used, then they should be of nearly identical geometry. Figure 70 shows a particularly simple configuration with a single spiral coil (Fig. 69a). The coil diameter, wire size and magnet size depend on the application and the current source available for driving the transducer.

Angle Beams

Online monitoring of wall thickness is desirable but the technique must be able to operate on rough, scale covered surfaces that are not only moving rapidly past the testing station but may be at temperatures above the boiling point of water. By using electromagnetic acoustic transducers, the sensitivity to surface speed, temperature and cleanliness can be minimized. Furthermore, the sensors can be mounted on simple carriages that track the surface as it bounces through the testing station.

Seamless steel tubing is manufactured at speeds that approach 1 m·s^{-1} (200 ft·min^{-1}). Abnormal variations in wall thickness are the major cause for rejection. Figure 71 shows a plot of the thickness profile measured by an electromagnetic acoustic gage positioned to record a thickness value every 3 mm (0.125 in.) along a longitudinal path on a

13 m (42 ft) tube moving past the sensor at 0.9 m·s^{-1} (3 ft·s^{-1}) in an operating steel mill.[120] The transducer introduces transverse waves into the pipe wall at an angle that allows the transmitter and receiver to be physically separated, lengthening the transit time for thin walled tubes.[121]

An accuracy better than ±1 percent was obtained from the installed unit. The system has eight electromagnetic acoustic transducers around the circumference to yield eight thickness profile graphs like the one in Fig. 71. All these data are processed in real time by a dedicated computer so that the operator is given a display of the test results immediately after the pipe passes through the station.

This report provides the average wall thickness, the length of the tube, its weight per unit length, the minimum wall thickness detected and the maximum eccentricity of the center bore hole. In addition, the display shows the standard deviation in thickness and eccentricity as well as the location and thickness values of any points thinner than the limit set for rejection.

A paint system is activated by the computer to mark the location of critically thin spots so that they can be verified with subsequent manual scanning. All of the data, including the eight individual thickness profiles, are stored in computer memory for later analysis and for statistical summaries of production runs.

FIGURE 70. Permanent magnet transverse wave electromagnetic acoustic transducer about 25 mm (1 in.) in diameter and 38 mm (1.5 in.) high. Magnet pole diameter should be about twice coil diameter.

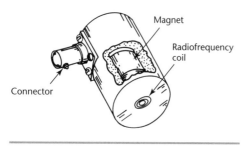

Weld and Cladding Tests

The testing of austenitic welds can be strongly influenced by wave speeds in the weld metal that generally differ from those in the base metal. Because of the strong elastic anisotropy of weld materials, the difference in base metal and weld metal acoustical impedance leads to reflection and refraction of the ultrasonic wave at the interface. These phenomena have been studied in detail for vertically polarized transverse and longitudinal waves. For horizontally polarized transverse waves, most of the existing work covers propagation in austenitic weld metal.[122-126]

Horizontally Polarized Waves

Compared to vertically polarized transverse and longitudinal waves, horizontally polarized transverse waves have a number of advantages for testing welds. When reflecting from surfaces parallel to the polarization direction, transverse horizontal waves do not mode convert to other types of waves and less clutter is observed. When passing through

FIGURE 71. Plot of wall thickness profile produced by automatic thickness gage using electromagnetic acoustic transducer on 350 mm (14 in.) diameter, 9.5 mm (0.375 in.) wall seamless steel tube at production line speed of 0.9 m·s^{-1} (3 ft·s^{-1}) in operating steel mill.

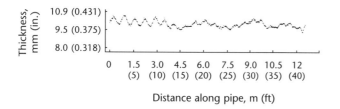

interfaces with surfaces parallel to the polarization direction, transmission coefficients are often higher than for other wave types.

Furthermore, these waves can be excited over a wide range of angles. With electromagnetic acoustic transducers, an angle range from 0.3 to 1.5 rad (20 to 90 deg) can be covered. In contrast, transverse horizontal waves can only be excited with difficulty[125] when using conventional piezoelectric transducers (transmission of a transverse wave with a steel wedge and highly viscous coupling). For practical applications, the transverse horizontal method has not been extensively used. Because transverse horizontal waves can be excited and detected in electrically conductive materials without contact using electromagnetic acoustic transducers, more applications are possible.[127,128]

Tests of Austenitic Welds

The potential of transverse horizontal waves for austenitic weld testing has been investigated in detail.[127] It has been demonstrated that such waves are almost totally transmitted into the weld metal in a wide range of incidence angles between 0.8 and 1.5 rad (48 and 90 deg). Figure 72 shows the computed coefficients of reflection and transmission at the interface between base metal and weld metal as a function of incidence angle. It is assumed that the columnar grains are oriented perpendicular to the material surface and parallel to the interface between the base metal and the weld.

These theoretical values have been confirmed by measurement (Fig. 73). Two electromagnetic acoustic transducers were used to transmit through the base metal (Fig. 73b) and through the base metal with the weld metal (Fig. 73c) at different angles of incidence. The received ultrasonic amplitudes were measured and recorded for comparison. For incidence angles between 0.9 and 1.5 rad (55 and 90 deg), the amplitude values are the same (Fig. 73a). For angles smaller than 0.9 rad (55 deg), an increasing part of the incident energy is reflected at the interface between the base metal and the weld metal, and the transmitted signal amplitude diminishes in the test object.

FIGURE 72. Horizontally polarized transverse waves at base metal weld interface:
(a) diagram of austenitic weld;
(b) computed reflection and transmission coefficients.

(a)

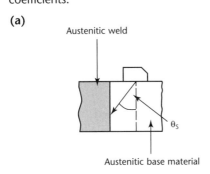

(b)

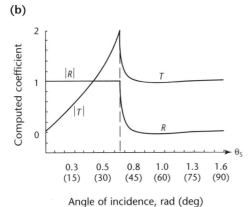

Angle of incidence, rad (deg)

Legend
R = reflection coefficient
T = transmission coefficient
θ_S = shear incidence angle

FIGURE 73. Experimental measurements of ultrasonic transmission of horizontally polarized transverse waves: (a) plot of amplitude versus incidence angle;
(b) diagram of transmission through base metal; (c) diagram of transmission through base metal, welds and interfaces.

(a)

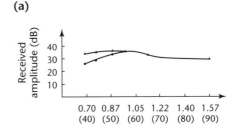

Angle of incidence, rad (deg)

(b)

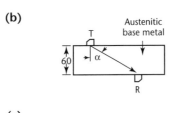

(c)

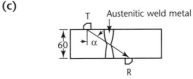

Another important aspect of wave propagation in austenitic materials is beam skewing. Beam skewing has been extensively studied in austenitic and dissimilar metal welds with a ray tracing model.[126] According to these studies, the smallest skewing is observed for transverse horizontal waves and longitudinal waves.

Tests of Austenitic Cladding

Reflection and transmission at the interface between a ferritic base metal and austenitic cladding have been studied as further examples of the interactions of transverse horizontal waves at an interface between an anisotropic and isotropic medium.

It is assumed that the columnar grains in the cladding are directed perpendicular to the surface. The incidence angle with respect to the material surface corresponds to the incidence angle θ_s at the interface. Figure 74 shows the computed reflection

and transmission coefficient of the transverse horizontal wave at the interface of the austenitic cladding and the ferritic base metal as a function of incident transverse horizontal wave θ_s in the cladding.

The transverse horizontal wave is transmitted almost completely in an angle range of θ_s from 0 to 1.2 rad (0 to 70 deg). Between 0 and 0.3 rad (0 and 20 deg), the reflected amplitude is about 11 percent of the incident amplitude. Between 0.3 and 0.8 rad (20 and 47 deg), the value of the reflected amplitude decreases until it vanishes. It subsequently rises to an amplitude of 2.5 percent of the incident amplitude before passing through 0 percent again. Above 1.1 rad (68 deg), the reflected portion increases rapidly up to 1.2 rad (76 deg). For higher angles, the reflection and transmission coefficients become complex. The reflection coefficient $|R|$ is equal to 1 (the incident wave is totally reflected in this angle range).

Because of the additional reflection of the transverse horizontal wave at the stress free outer surface of the cladding, a guided transverse horizontal wave can propagate at flat incidence angles in the cladding by zigzag reflection Z (Fig. 75). At the clad side of a test object, an electromagnetic acoustic transducer with a period of 5 mm (0.2 in.) is transmitting a transverse horizontal wave with a frequency of 572 kHz at grazing incidence — a 6 dB drop of the main lobe is about 1.1 rad (65 deg).

At the front surface of the test object, an ultrasonic signal is received with a piezoelectric transducer (Y quartz, 1 MHz,

---

FIGURE 74. Horizontally polarized transverse waves at interface of ferritic base metal and an austenitic weld: (a) diagram of weld; (b) computed reflection and transmission coefficients.

(a)

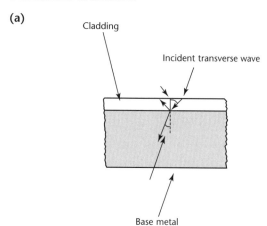

(b)

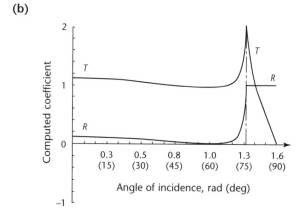

Legend
R = reflection coefficient
T = transmission coefficient

FIGURE 75. Guided horizontally polarized transverse waves in austenitic cladding: (a) received signal in range of cladding (love wave); (b) received signal in base metal.

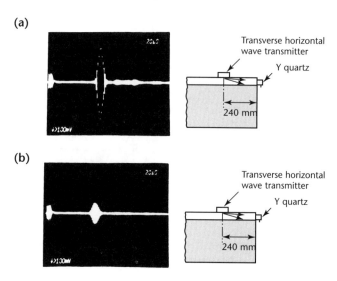

polarization direction parallel to clad surface). Figure 75a shows the received signal propagating in the cladding. This sort of signal is called a *love wave,* with a group velocity lower than the phase velocity of a bulk transverse horizontal wave in the base metal. Figure 75b shows the received signal propagating in the base metal. The velocity inferred from Fig. 75b corresponds nearly to the velocity of a bulk transverse horizontal wave in the base metal. The amplitude of the transverse horizontal wave guided in the cladding is 3.4× the amplitude of the bulk transverse horizontal wave in the base metal.

This has important consequences for testing austenitic cladding with transverse horizontal waves from the clad side. Because of the guidance of the wave in the cladding, the beam divergence losses are small and large distances can be tested. It is also possible to test curved geometries like the corner range of a pressure vessel nozzle with waves propagating in the circumferential direction.

The general advantages of transverse horizontal waves include surface test, corner reflection independent of the incidence angle and no mode conversion. These features open new possibilities for the nondestructive testing of austenitic and dissimilar welds in hazardous environments.[128]

High Temperature Tests

Electromagnetic acoustic transducers are well suited for high temperature measurements because no fluid coupling is required. In general, there are three options available for designing these transducers for high temperature environments: (1) cool both the radiofrequency coil and the magnet, (2) cool only the magnet or (3) cool neither the magnet nor radiofrequency coil. In practice, all three approaches have been used successfully.

High Temperature Material Considerations

High temperature interferes with the operation of electromagnetic acoustic transducers in several ways. The insulation on standard copper magnet wire for electric motor windings is seldom rated above 220 °C (430 °F). Polyimide insulators can be used to higher temperatures and in some cases, where low voltage insulation is adequate protection, long term operation to 350 °C (660 °F) is possible.

Ceramic insulation can be applied to copper wire as well as high temperature metals such as platinum and certain nickel-chromium alloys (these materials are only available in small quantities and are not yet available commercially). Many materials used for high temperature insulation are thick compared to normal insulation and surface adhesion tends to be poor. It is possible to produce electromagnetic acoustic transducer drive and receive coils that operate up to 1500 °C (2800 °F).

Most magnetic steels cannot be used as magnet pole materials above 550 °C (1000 °F) but some cobalt alloys function as magnet poles up to 820 °C (1500 °F). Most permanent magnet materials cannot be used above 120 °C (250 °F) and some high field materials degrade rapidly above 100 °C (212 °F). Consequently, these magnets require some cooling for operation near surfaces such as hot aluminum or steel.

Cooling Procedures for High Temperature Tests

Studies show the success of cooling both the magnet and the radiofrequency coil for high temperature tests. One compact approach uses a pulsed bias magnetic field that is practical when a low duty factor is satisfactory.[129]

Another effective system is designed for continuous wall thickness measurements on hot seamless steel pipe at 980 °C (1800 °F) at six positions equally spaced around the circumference. For this application, both the radiofrequency coils and the magnet poles are cooled.[130] Because an electromagnet is used, the system is massive but this is not typically a problem in a steel mill.

A second alternative is to cool the magnet (incidental cooling of the radiofrequency coil may also occur). When small uncooled or slightly cooled radiofrequency coils are used, a smaller liftoff is of significant value for achieving an acceptable signal-to-noise ratio.

Figure 76 shows an electromagnetic acoustic transducer made with high temperature insulation on a high temperature wire. This unit can receive either longitudinal or transverse waves.[131] Using metal enameling or ceramic glazing techniques, the radiofrequency coil is bonded to a copper cooling plate. Care must be taken not to have the electrically conducting cooling plate too close to the radiofrequency coil. The cooling plate prevents the permanent magnet from heating above 40 °C (104 °F), even when the radiofrequency coil is immediately above a surface at 1090 °C (2000 °F). One transducer of this design had a noise threshold of 0.03 nm, with an output sensitivity of 0.5 mV·nm^{-1} at 1 MHz. A band width of 10 MHz and a spatial resolution of 4×6 mm (0.15×0.2 in.) were also achieved.

Testing Metals in Fabrication

One of the most important applications of high temperature electromagnetic acoustic transducers is for testing metal products at the fabrication mill. The transducers must not only be made of materials that withstand high temperatures but also be powerful enough to overcome the high attenuation in metals near their melting points.

Laboratory studies of sound propagation in steel show that longitudinal waves at a frequency near 1 MHz can penetrate hot steel[132] and this information was used to design a compact transmitter and receiver pair of electromagnetic acoustic transducers[133] on each side of a 100 mm (4 in.) square block of stainless steel.[134]

For both of these transducers, the magnetic field is supplied by flat, circular coils of heavy copper wire oriented with their planes parallel to the surface of the steel. The coils are positioned in heat exchangers less than 2.5 mm (0.1 in.) from the steel.[129] A pulse of high current (about 1.5 kA) through these coils applies a magnetic field of 0.5 T (5 kG) to the steel. Separate, spiral coils sandwiched between the heat exchanger and a ceramic cover plate form the coils that induce or detect eddy currents in the steel surface. All of the coils and heat exchangers are surrounded by ceramic tubes about 300 mm (12 in.) in length to protect the wires and coaxial cables from the radiant heat generated by the nearby hot ingots.

In one application of such an electromagnetic acoustic transducer system, the transit time of the sound through a steel billet is measured to determine its internal temperature.[120] This measurement is made on billets as they emerge from a continuous casting furnace located about 6 m (20 ft) upstream from the ultrasonic testing station.

Tests with Moving Transducers

Pipeline Tests

To achieve electromagnetic coupling, an electromagnetic acoustic transducer coil and magnet need only be brought close to a metal surface. There is no need for an operator to adjust the transducer alignment or to optimize the thickness of the coupling fluid layer. In-line tests of buried gas pipelines are possible without interrupting the flow of the gas (Figs. 77 and 78). In such an application, no coupling liquid is available and the test device must move unattended through many kilometers of moderate diameter pipe at speeds averaging 6.7 m·s⁻¹ (22 ft·s⁻¹ or 15 mi·h⁻¹). An inline testing robot (called a *pig*) is suited for performing this test. The device is designed to test 750 mm (30 in.) diameter pipelines using eight electromagnetic acoustic transducers distributed around its circumference.[135] Because these transducers can excite and detect lamb waves in plates, the system can locate corrosion in the walls of a pipeline. This location is done by detecting echoes reflected from areas of irregular pitting in the path of a lamb

FIGURE 76. Diagram of permanent magnet, longitudinal wave, high temperature electromagnetic acoustic transducer that is also sensitive to transverse waves. Not shown is cooled shield on the four open sides.

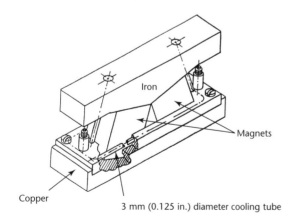

FIGURE 77. Pipe and tube testing with electromagnetic acoustic transduction.

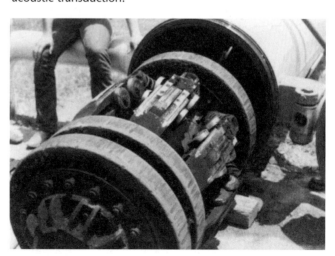

wave propagating around the pipe's circumference.[136]

Eight sensors ensure adequate sensitivity in those areas where coal tar coatings on the outside of the pipe cause high attenuation of the waves. Because the device must withstand the pressure of gas in the line, its central structure comprises a heavy walled tube containing batteries, signal processing electronics and data recording devices. The magnetic field required by the electromagnetic acoustic transducers is generated by special permanent magnets mounted on wheels. These magnetize only the region around each of the eight transducer coils. Acquired test data are recorded as the pig is transported along the pipe. After a test, offline computers analyze the test data recorded by an onboard computer to produce a map, showing the location of suspect areas.

Pipe and Tube Testing

Electromagnetic acoustic transducers can be mounted on wheels so that they can move through the inside of pipes or tubes in a wide variety of industrial settings. Figure 78 shows a crawler motor designed to pull an electromagnetic acoustic transducer package through a small diameter pipe in a natural gas distribution system. Ultrasonic guided waves are sent from the probe around the pipe circumference to detect corrosion pits or cracks by both pulse echo and through-transmission techniques. In either case, the signals are generated and detected by tiny circuits inside the probe and sent through cables to external signal processing systems far outside the pipe.

When the inside of the pipe is unavailable, a hand or motor propelled carriage can be used to drive a wheeled electromagnetic acoustic transducer probe along the length of long, above-ground pipes such as those found in refineries or chemical processing plants. Here, again, the inspecting ultrasonic waves are guided wave modes that propagate around the circumference. This technique is particularly useful for detecting corrosion under pipe supports from a transducer placed on the easily accessible top of the pipe.

If the operator can steer the wheels of the probe, guided wave inspection techniques can be applied to the inspection of large areas such as the bottom and sides of liquid storage tanks. Figure 79 shows a mobile electromagnetic acoustic transducer probe held against the side of a large storage tank by magnetic wheels. In this configuration, the operator can control the path of the probe up, down and around the tank surface. Because the area tested is the rectangular area under the probe itself, anomalous areas can be established and mapped by guiding the probe along a well defined scanning pattern over the outer surface of the tank.

Moving Tests in Steel Mills

Another important application of moving electromagnetic acoustic transducers is found in steel mills. One example is the thickness measurement discussed above. Another application is based on rayleigh waves, surface acoustic waves easily

FIGURE 78. Small tractor motor pulls electromagnetic acoustic transducer test probe into small diameter pipe. Guided waves propagate around circumference to inspect pipe wall.

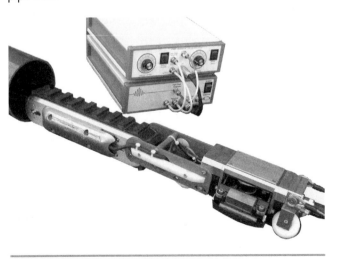

FIGURE 79. Mobile electromagnetic acoustic transducer test probe held in place by magnetic wheels is being driven around surface of large liquid storage tank. Corrosion anywhere in rectangular area under probe is detected.

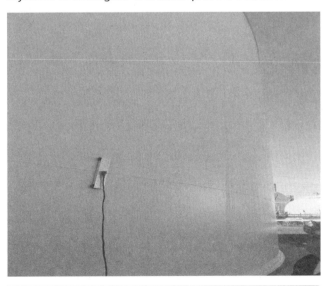

excited by electromagnetic acoustic transducers using a meander coil.[137]

By directing these waves around the circumference of tubular products, common discontinuities such as laps, seams and pits can be detected. More important, simple signal processing techniques can be used to obtain a quantitative measure of the depth of laps and seams[138] at production line speeds so that the manufacturer can immediately segregate materials according to the amount of rework needed for specified quality.

Sheet metal is supplied to rolling mills in the form of individual coils that have to be welded together to form a continuous strip to support the continuous processing of useful products. The weld must be of high quality to maintain the integrity of the strip along the entire production line because a failure will shut down the line and can harm the machines and personnel in the immediate vicinity of the break. Therefore, it is imperative that the weld be tested for discontinuities as soon as it is formed and before it begins its journey down the production line.

Electromagnetic acoustic transducers are well suited to performing this test because they can interrogate the weld line with guided waves produced and detected from a point downstream from the weld using a pulse echo technique. Figure 80 shows a drawing of the butt weld that joins the tail of one coil to the head of the next coil. Two clamps hold the head and tail sections in contact while the weld is made and while a transmitter/receiver pair of electromagnetic acoustic transducers scans across the width dimension looking for echo signals emanating from discontinuities in the weld. The transmitter and receiver ride on wheels so that they can be driven across the width of the sheet by a screw mechanism attached to a stationary bridge that spans the production line.

Phased Arrays for Testing of Seamless Tube

Given the ability to operate when the metal test object is moving past the electromagnetic acoustic transducer at production speeds, it would be helpful to be able to rapidly change the characteristics of the interrogating radiation, to obtain as much information as possible. One approach uses phased arrays whose ability to excite and detect ultrasonic beams with electronically controlled angles of propagation and focusing is familiar from piezoelectric applications. Electromagnetic acoustic transducers have been used in a similar way. These arrays consist of several small,

discrete elements rather than the series connected meander, multiple-period radiofrequency coils that excite narrowband, obliquely propagating bulk waves and guided modes when driven by gated bursts of radiofrequency current. When the discrete elements are appropriately driven, the electromagnetic acoustic phased arrays exhibit a unidirectional directivity pattern and produce broad band signals of controlled direction and focusing.[139] These provide

FIGURE 80. Coil configurations of electromagnetic acoustic transducer arrays: (a) nonsegmented meander coil; (b) segmented coil; (c) staggered, segmented coil.

(a)

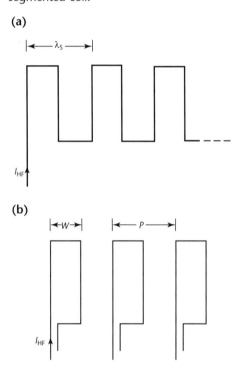

(b)

(c)

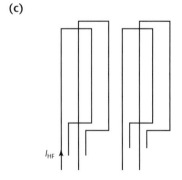

Legend
I_{HF} = high frequency current
P = segmented transducer period
W = transducer width
λ_S = nonsegmented transducer period

great flexibility in both the selection of wave mode and angles of propagation. One important application of the latter is the need to interrogate inclined discontinuities from both sides to ensure that the largest possible signal is obtained.

The meanderlike multiple-period coil (Fig. 80a) is segmented into several elements (Fig. 80b), each with a dipole radiation pattern. The radiofrequency pulses energizing the different elements are time shifted by electronic delay lines

FIGURE 81. Echoes from 5 percent calibration discontinuity as observed with phased array: (a) angle incidence for inside diameter discontinuity; (b) angle incidence for outside diameter discontinuity; (c) rayleigh wave.

(a)

Discontinuity echo

(b)

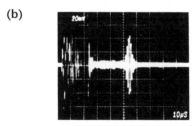

Discontinuity echo

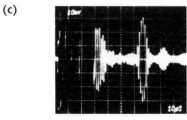

(c)

Discontinuity echo

(charge coupled devices). For guided modes, this delay corresponds to the time of flight that the ultrasonic wave requires to propagate from one element to the other. For obliquely propagating bulk waves, it corresponds to the time of propagation to an equiphase plane inclined at the desired angle. The signals received by the receiver elements are time shifted analogously. If a second set of staggered coils is added (Fig. 80c) and driven with the appropriate phase, radiation in the desired direction can be further enhanced. The advantage of the phased array technique is that the incident angle and the direction of radiation (backward or forward) can be switched rapidly following computer controlled settings of the time delays.

A system that can generate and detect signals under a selectable angle promises high testing speed (because no couplant is needed) and easy automation (because no mechanical adjustments are needed to obtain the required beam pattern and direction). Such systems have been designed for industrial applications for ultrasonic testing of seamless ferritic tubes with outer diameters ranging from 185 to 650 mm (7 to 25 in.) and wall thicknesses between 6 and 50 mm (0.25 and 2.0 in.).[140-142] The sensitivity is that needed to satisfy European standards. This means that longitudinal notches must be detected that reach a depth of 5 percent wall thickness or 1.5 mm (0.03 in.). Transverse notches must be detected that reach a depth of 10 percent of the wall thickness or 3 mm (0.1 in.), where again, the minimum of both has to be chosen.

Figure 81 shows echo signals of these calibration discontinuities obtained by the system in a static experiment. These exhibit the signal-to-noise ratio of 20 dB achieved with the phased array transducer at a circumferential speed of 2 m·s⁻¹ (6.5 ft·s⁻¹). To distinguish echoes from discontinuities on the outer tube surface from those on the inner tube surface, the electromagnetic acoustic transducer can be switched to another mode of operation where only surface waves are generated. The system was tested online in a tube mill up to circumferential tube speeds of 2.2 m·s⁻¹ (7.2 ft·s⁻¹).

Moving Tests of Railroad Rail

Further applications of moving tests are found in the railroad industry. Modern railroads realize significant fuel savings by applying a lubricant onto their rails to reduce friction. Unfortunately, this complicates conventional ultrasonic tests because the liquid layer needed for coupling the piezoelectric transducer with the rail no longer wets the surface sufficiently for transmitting the acoustic energy. Electromagnetic acoustic transducers can excite and detect ultrasonic vibrations through the lubricant layer without difficulty and high speed scanning of rails can be done without removal of the lubricant or interruption of normal train schedules. Figure 82 shows a prototype testing trailer[143] on a section of track at the Transportation Test Center, Pueblo, Colorado, where the Association of American Railroads is conducting tests on the wear rate of lubricated rail under severe loads.

This system has two electromagnetic acoustic transducers supported on individual carriages in front of and behind the automobile tire in the center of the trailer. The front unit tests the head of the rail by sending transverse horizontal waves fore and aft, so that a discontinuity is detected twice as it passes under the carriage. The transducers in the rear send a normal beam transverse wave directly to the base of the rail where it is reflected back to the transducer. This wave is used with a pulse echo procedure to detect discontinuities in the rail web.

Both of these units use small, high efficiency electromagnets mounted on their carriages to supply the magnetic fields required by the electromagnetic transduction process. For transverse horizontal waves, a magnetostrictive coupling mechanism[144,145] requires high tangential magnetic fields. These fields are obtained by pulsing a large current through the electromagnet whenever a test of the rail head is required.

Because the transverse horizontal waves can be directed at an angle near grazing along the surface[146] a region in front of and behind the transducer can be tested with each pulse. Power for these electromagnets is supplied as direct current from the motor and generator mounted in the center of the trailer. The power unit also provides alternating current for the instrumentation housed in the box on the front of the trailer. Motive power comes from a towing vehicle that houses the operator and the recording equipment.

Moving Tests of Railroad Wheels

In wheel rail systems, the undercarriage and the wheels are also exposed to high loads. Through dynamic working, cracks (thermal and fatigue) occur and sometimes result in total wheel failure. There is no simple way to predict how these discontinuities evolve and their timely detection is instrumental for safety. In such applications, visual tests are time consuming and do not allow detection of critical discontinuities in time, particularly subsurface discontinuities.

An ultrasonic system has been developed for the German Railway Society to provide in-service tests of the wheel treads on its high speed trains.[147,148] This system can detect and classify critical discontinuities *in motion* using an ultrasonic rayleigh wave, a surface wave excited by electromagnetic acoustic transducers integrated with the rail when the wheel is in contact with the transducer. The wave pulse travels along the surface of the wheel with little attenuation. The wheel's response to the pulse is detected by a receiving transducer either as a discontinuity echo in the pulse echo mode or as a through-transmission signal after several round trips.

The transducer shown in Fig. 83 consists of an electromagnet in the lower part of a housing mounted in a mechanical support fixed at the rail. The magnet produces a magnetic field normal to the wheel surface. A meander radiofrequency coil is located on top of the central pole piece. The transducer period is 7 mm (0.3 in.), selected to equal

FIGURE 82. Trailer supporting electromagnetic acoustic transducers for testing head and web of installed railroad rail. The rubber tire in the center of the vehicle can be lowered for highway towing.

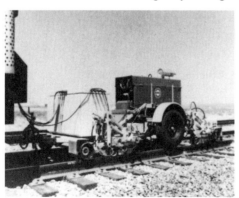

FIGURE 83. Schematic diagram of electromagnetic acoustic transducer installed in railroad rail for wheel tread testing.

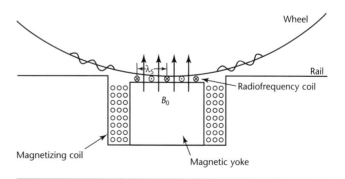

the wavelength of a rayleigh wave at about 430 kHz.

The complete system, which operated for two years in the field, was fully automatic, including a microcomputer for system control and for storing and evaluating test data. Two probes are attached to each rail (see Fig. 84), one covering the dead zone of the other. The probe support is slightly flexible and allows the probe to touch the wheel as it passes. The test is done in the pulse echo mode.

The ultrasonic frequency has been optimized for sensitivity of discontinuity detection and attenuation, so that the wave examines a distance of two circumferences of the wheel tread during testing. The lab trials have shown that a 1 mm (0.04 in.) deep transverse saw cut in the center of the tread can be detected with a signal-to-noise ratio of 15 dB, independent of the distance of the saw cut from the probe.

An optimized sizing algorithm distinguishes discontinuities up to a depth of 3 mm (0.1 in.) and cross sections larger than 10 mm^2 (0.02 in.^{2}) into three classes based on cross section. The classes are used to specify subsequent action for the tested wheels.

Ultrasonic Testing in Vacuum

Many special alloys used for rocket engines can only be welded in a vacuum chamber with electron beams or high power lasers. Like all welds, the full thickness of these joints must be tested with radiographic or ultrasonic techniques. This requires removal of the test object from the chamber, testing at a special facility and returning to the chamber if a reweld is necessary. This slow process has been eliminated by using electromagnetic acoustic transducers to perform the test inside the vacuum

chamber immediately after the weld is formed. This is possible because the electromagnetic coupling mechanism can operate across a vacuum and because the transducer can be made of materials that withstand the temperature immediately after a weld — as high as 350 °C (660 °F).

The mechanical system scans a pair of high frequency electromagnetic acoustic transducers around the weld line on a test object as it sits inside a vacuum chamber.[149] The object is a cylinder with a circumferential weld line near its top. Two electromagnetic acoustic transducers straddle the weld and test it with angle beam transverse waves, from both above and below the weld, using a pulse echo technique.[150] Because the wall thickness of the cylinder is only about 5 mm (0.2 in.) and the sensitivity specification requires detection of a 0.75 mm (0.03 in.) diameter flat bottom hole, the electromagnetic acoustic transducer wires were curved and positioned to focus 7 MHz ultrasonic waves at the center of the wall thickness dimension.[151]

This focal spot is scanned over the total weld volume by translating the transducers perpendicularly to the weld line while the cylinder is rotated. A personal computer controls the operation and takes about 300 s to collect the echo amplitude and position data and to make an accept/reject decision. Hardcopy C-scan images of the joint can be prepared offline from data in the computer's memory.

High Speed Self-Aligning Probes

To test small objects produced at rates approaching one per second, the ultrasonic transducer and the object must be accurately positioned relative to one another and then a 100 percent scan must be performed in a fraction of a second. By using electromagnetic acoustic transducers in air instead of piezoelectric transducers in water, the test object can be kept dry and the positioning mechanism does not have to be as precise (there is no refraction of the ultrasonic beam at the surface of the test object). An example of these simplifications is a system for testing machine gun projectiles as they are produced.[152]

The system consists of a rotating drum that picks up each projectile from a feed line and delivers it rotating to the gap between the pole pieces of a direct current electromagnet. Three electromagnetic acoustic transducer coils mounted on compliant substrates slide into light contact with the projectile surface as it enters the gap. Because the compliance of

FIGURE 84. Detail of electromagnetic acoustic transducer test probes for wheel tests.

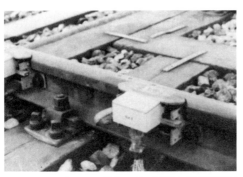

the substrate allows the coils to conform to the curved surface, the ultrasonic waves enter the test object over a well defined profile inside the object. Each sound beam interrogates a different, critical area of the projectile with a pulse echo technique while the rotation ensures that every part of the circumference is inspected several times during a test cycle.

If any one of the transducers detects an echo larger than a preset limit for its channel, the object is rejected and the control computer records the event so that at the end of a production run, a printout of the number of rejections in each channel is available.

Stress Measurements

Several ultrasonic velocity or transit time techniques have been used to determine both applied and residual stresses in metals. The basis for these techniques is a stress induced shift in the velocity. The major source of error in most methods lies in determining the contribution of texture (material anisotropy) to the elastic velocities being measured. This contribution is a result of the polycrystalline character of the material. The individual grains are essentially small, single crystals and the ultrasonic velocity in each depends on its orientation. If the grains have a preferred orientation (texture), the velocity in the metal depends on propagation direction. The problem is to differentiate velocity shifts due to this effect from those due to stress. In one solution, it has been found that if two transverse velocities can be measured where the polarization and propagation directions are interchanged, then a texture

independent velocity difference directly proportional to the stress is obtained. The theory behind this approach and its experimental confirmation demonstrates that the procedure produces reliable numbers for applied stresses.[153]

Most practical ultrasonic stress and texture measurements have been made using electromagnetic acoustic transducers because the errors associated with transducer coupling are much smaller in such a system. A small transducer that has been used successfully for stress and texture measurements is shown in Fig. 85. The travel time for a transverse horizontal plate wave propagating between the two receivers can be obtained within 1 ns by calculating the cross correlation function of the two receiver signals.

Measurement repeatability is within ±3 ns with most of the error coming from lack of reproducibility in the transducer coupling to the surface. For a 30 mm (1.2 in.) propagation distance, this corresponds to an error of about 1 m·s⁻¹ (200 ft·min⁻¹) in the velocity or an error in stress measurements of about ±10 MPa. In other words, at 3 mm·μs⁻¹, 30 mm is covered in 10 μs. If the error is 30 ns or 3000 μs, the error is 300× the reading.

Conclusion

Among the desirable capabilities demonstrated for electromagnetic acoustic transducers are operation in vacuums or high temperature; high speed or moving tests; self-alignment; phased array compatibility; and the excitation of horizontally polarized transverse waves for the measurement of stress or tests of anisotropic weldments. The major drawback is lower efficiency than piezoelectric transducers. Careful modeling is sometimes required to design an optimum ultrasonic electromagnetic acoustic transducer test. Considerable knowledge about the principles and engineering characteristics of these devices is available to draw on in designing custom applications.[118,131,154-156]

FIGURE 85. Horizontally polarized transverse wave, periodic permanent magnet transmitter and two horizontally polarized transverse wave line receivers used for velocity measurements to determine stress and texture.

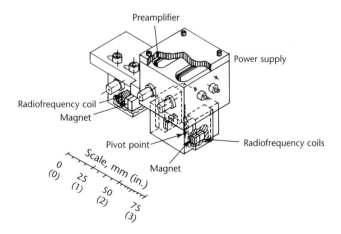

PART 10. Air Coupled Transducers[157]

Ultrasonic transducers operating in liquids and solids have many applications in signal processing devices such as delay lines, resonators, convolvers and correlators and in systems for medical imaging, nondestructive testing and underwater sensing. In air, ultrasonic transducers are used for robotic and metrology applications. They have a more limited potential at high frequencies (over 500 kHz) because of the low impedance of air and the high attenuation of sound waves.

The physics of sound propagation in air is reviewed below and the parameters that control the design and implementation of air coupled transducers are highlighted. Examples are given for the most popular transducer designs and there is discussion of the requirements that could increase the usefulness of air coupled ultrasonics.

Physical Principles of Air Coupling

The theoretical framework for the propagation of sound waves in air has been known for centuries and the fundamental thermodynamic principles explaining the physics of sound propagation in air are widely detailed in the literature.[158-161] The discussion below sketches the basic principles for sound propagation in air and gives examples of transducers, their performance and limitations. In addition, novel materials such as silica aerogels are considered and their impact on the performance of air transducers is discussed.

Sound Velocity in Air

Assume that air is a classical newtonian fluid. Euler's equation of motion and mass conservation is used to set up the wave equation:

$$(40) \quad \nabla^2 P = \frac{1}{v^2} \frac{\delta^2 P}{\delta t^2}$$

where P is the air pressure (pascal) and v is the wave velocity in air (meter per second). The P term is related to the density by Laplace's adiabatic assumption for an ideal gas:

$$(41) \quad P = K_\gamma^q$$

where K is a constant representing the ratio of ambient pressure to density, γ is the ratio of the specific heat coefficients at constant pressure and volume (1.4 for air) and ρ is the total density (kilograms per cubic meter).

An expression is derived for the velocity v by substituting Eq. 41:

$$(42) \quad v^2 = \frac{dP}{d\rho}$$

Using the ideal gas equation:

$$(43) \quad P = \rho RT$$

It is found that:

$$(44) \quad v^2 = \gamma RT$$

where R is a constant (value dependent on the gas) and T is temperature of the gas (kelvin).

Using the above equation for dry air at 0 °C (32 °F), $v = 331$ m·s^{-1}. From Eq. 44, it was found by simple taylor expansion around 0 °C (32 °F) that:

$$(45) \quad v = 331 + 0.1 T_c$$

where T_c is the temperature in celsius. Measurements of the speed of sound in air and its temperature dependence agree well with these calculations. The low velocity of sound in air results in a smaller wavelength at a given frequency compared to sound waves in water or solids. The smaller wavelength provides improved test resolution for metrology and imaging systems.

Mechanical Impedance of Air

The mechanical impedance Z of a material is defined as the ratio of the sound wave stress or pressure to its velocity. This leads to the more simple and useful expression:[162,163]

$$(46) \quad Z_0 = pv$$

For air at 0 °C (32 °F), $Z_0 = 400$ kg·m^{-2}·s^{-1}. For comparison, the impedance of water is 1.5×10^6 kg·m^{-2}·s^{-1}

and for most solids it is in the range of 3 to $100 \times 10^6 \ kg \cdot m^{-2} \cdot s^{-1}$. This value for the impedance of air is the source of the difficulty in coupling and exciting high frequency waves in air. This difficulty can be explained by noting that the power excited by a transducer is proportional to the product of the impedance of the medium, the square of the frequency and the square of the displacement on the surface of the transducer.

One way to overcome this difficulty is to use what is known as *matching layers* between the transducer and the air. For instance, if a piezoelectric ceramic with an impedance of $35 \times 10^6 \ kg \cdot m^{-2} \cdot s^{-1}$ is to excite waves in air, a matching layer with $0.1 \times 10^6 \ kg \cdot m^{-2} \cdot s^{-1}$ is nearly ideal for coupling into the air at a single frequency, because it is halfway between 35×10^6 and 400.

Sound Attenuation in Air

There are three sources of sound attenuation in air: viscous, thermal and vibrational losses. Viscous losses are caused by frictional damping and are proportional to the coefficient of viscosity and the square of the frequency. Thermal losses result from the conversion to heat of some energy in the sound wave and its conduction from elevated temperature (high pressure) gases to low temperature (low pressure) gases. This loss depends on the thermal conductivity and the square of the frequency. Vibrational losses are caused by coupling the sound wave into resonances of the constituent molecules of air. These losses occur at specific frequencies and are negligible elsewhere in the frequency domain.[158,159]

Attenuation can be plotted as a function of frequency for air at a temperature of $20 \ ^\circ C$ ($68 \ ^\circ F$), at atmospheric pressure and relative humidity of 20 percent, corresponding to a water volume fraction of 4.7×10^{-3}. Relaxation frequencies correspond to resonances in the molecules of oxygen and nitrogen, at 12.5 kHz and 173 Hz respectively.

At frequencies over 20 kHz, this loss mechanism is not important and viscous and thermal losses dominate with their frequency square dependence. At a frequency of 1 MHz, the attenuation is calculated to be $101 \ dB \cdot m^{-1}$ but actual measurements yield $165 \ dB \cdot m^{-1}$.[161] This loss limits a pulse echo measurement in air at a frequency of 1 MHz to about 250 mm (10 in.) for a system with a reasonable signal-to-noise ratio. It is useful to compare the attenuation in air to that of water ($0.22 \ dB \cdot m^{-1}$ at 1 MHz) to understand the difficulty in using high frequency ultrasonics in air. It is also important to remember that because of the lower velocity and resulting shorter wavelength, a $5\times$ better resolution occurs while operating in air at the same frequency.

Low Frequency Transducers

The earliest air transducers operated under 100 kHz and typically belonged to one of the following classes: modulated airflow units, mechanical vibrating sources (whistles), electroacoustic transducers (a piezoelectric tube operating in its length resonant mode), flexurally vibrating transducers (cantilevers clamped on one or two ends), electrostatic transducers (including the automatic focus transducer described below) and microphones.[160] All these devices operate at low frequency with large displacements to generate large power density in the air.

Figure 86 is a schematic diagram of a low frequency (under 500 kHz) bimorphic

FIGURE 86. Details of ultrasonic transducer: (a) piezoelectric layering; (b) poling; (c) mode of displacement; (d) final device assembly.

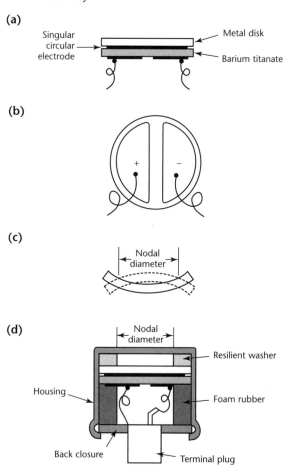

ultrasonic transducer. With proper electrical tuning, good band width characteristics are obtained in both transmitting and receiving modes.

Electrostatic Transducer

An electrostatic transducer has been developed and is widely used in the range finder of an autofocusing commercial film camera.[164] The transducer is shown in Fig. 87 and operates as a conventional electrostatic transducer. A special foil is stretched over a grooved plate, forming a moving element that transforms electrical energy into sound waves. The returning echo is transformed into electrical energy.

A grooved metallic back plate is in contact with the foil and forms a capacitor. When charged, the capacitor exerts electrostatic force on the foil.[164] The frequency response of the transducer is shown in Fig. 88, highlighting the broad band width essential for operation of the range finder.

Air Coupled System

A 250 kHz air coupled ultrasonic system has been used for robotic range sensing and wind velocity measurements.[165,166] The transducer for this work is similar to conventional immersion transducers and consists of a resonant disk of piezoelectric ceramic. Because of the small diameter-to-thickness ratio (2:1) used for the piezoelectric ceramic, particular care must be taken to dampen the lateral modes that interact with the casing and reduce the band width of the transducer.

A matching layer of epoxy resin is used to improve coupling into the air. Though the impedance of the matching layer is not ideal, the device is functional and a successful metrology system has been demonstrated. Such devices are typically narrow band and their two-way insertion loss is in the range of 40 to 50 dB.

Ceramic Transducer

A device has been developed that operates at 200 kHz but with good band width.[167] The transducer has a compact impulse response that reflects the large band width at the center frequency of 200 kHz. This good performance is the result of two novel ideas in the design of the transducer. First, it uses a composite material with a ceramic volume fraction of about 1 percent. Second, it uses ceramics resonant in the cross polarization direction.

Composite ceramics are popular for water immersion applications because it is possible to tailor their impedance, dielectric constant and coupling coefficient for the application. In present applications, a reduction in the impedance improves the match into air with no decrease in the electromechanical coupling coefficient. The ceramic is damped along its length in the resonant direction and this also improves the band width of the transducer. A focused, higher frequency, version of this device is of use in imaging and nondestructive testing.

High Frequency Transducers

High frequency transducers operate above 500 kHz and are limited to short distances

FIGURE 87. Construction details of an electrostatic acoustic transducer.

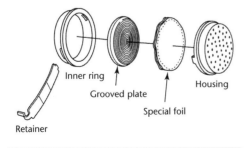

FIGURE 88. Transmit and receive frequency responses of electrostatic acoustic transducer shown in Fig. 87: (a) typical transmit response; (b) typical free field receive response.

(a)

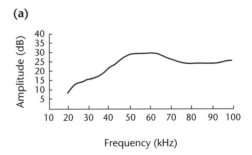

(b)

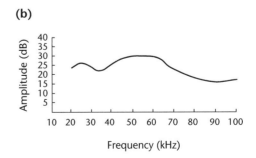

because of the high attenuation of sound waves in air. The traditional plane piston, water immersion transducer for air applications has been well documented.[168,169] In this design, the main problem is that of matching the impedances of the ceramic and air, which differ by six orders of magnitude. Conventional design rules require matching layers with impedances on the order of 1×10^4 kg·m^{-2}·s^{-1}.

Impedance Matching Layers

In one high frequency application, a silicone rubber matching layer with an impedance of 1×10^6 kg·m^{-2}·s^{-1} is used to match a ceramic transducer to air.[168] The two-way insertion loss of the device is about 35 dB with a fractional band width of 3 percent. In another application, a mixture of silicone rubber and glass microbubbles is used to obtain a matching layer with an impedance of 0.3×10^6 kg·m^{-2}·s^{-1}. This material is used in transducers with single and double matching layers for the purpose of imaging threads in cloth.[169]

The insertion loss of a device with two matching layers is 50 dB, with a large 6 dB fractional band width of 38 percent at a center frequency of 1 MHz. The insertion loss is 15 dB higher than expected because of errors in controlling the thickness of the matching layer and, more importantly, because of attenuation in the second matching layer.

Mismatch and Attenuation

A study of mismatch and attenuation in matching layers has demonstrated that attenuation controls the insertion loss and the band width of the device.[170] The limit on the band width is set because the mechanical band width (due to attenuation) is far narrower than the electrical band width caused by the impedance mismatch between air and the ceramic.

Attenuation also controls the insertion loss — because of the impedance mismatch, large stresses are set up in the matching layer leading to large attenuation. A design with multiple matching layers is preferred because the stress fields set up in the matching layers are weaker and the influence of attenuation in each matching layer is reduced.

Matching Layer Materials

A design criterion optimizes two matching layers when the lowest impedance layer is not optimum.[170] Not having the necessary low impedance is a common problem with such transducers — to obtain low insertion losses and large band width, it is necessary to have materials with low impedance *and* low attenuation.

One such material is silica aerogel.[171,172] Samples of silica aerogels have a measured impedance of 0.01×10^6 kg·m^{-2}·s^{-1} and a mechanical Q of 50.

(47) $\quad Q \;=\; \dfrac{k}{2\alpha}$

where k is the wave number and α is the attenuation (neper per unit length).

With this material, it is possible to make devices that have low two-way insertion loss (less than 20 dB) and broad 3 dB band width (greater than 30 percent).[170] Unfortunately, silica aerogels are difficult to work with — they disintegrate when exposed to water and are difficult to machine to small thicknesses. It is possible that such layers may be cast to final thickness over a piezoelectric ceramic.

Ligneous materials such as cork and balsa wood have been studied as possible matching layer materials.[172] The impedance of cork is 1.5×10^5 kg·m^{-2}·s^{-1} and the impedance of balsa wood is 8×10^4 kg·m^{-2}·s^{-1}. Cork and balsa wood are ideal for matching lead zirconate titanate ceramics to air (these ceramics have impedances around 3.5×10^6 kg·m^{-2}·s^{-1}). However, the advantage is compromised when it is noted that the attenuation expressed by the mechanical Q is 1.98 for cork and 1.52 for balsa wood. For high frequency devices, the search continues for better matching layer materials.

References

1. Allen, T.L., F.A. Bruton, D. Jolly and R. Roch. Section 4, "Ultrasonic Transducers and Piezoelectric Characteristics." *Nondestructive Testing Handbook,* second edition: Vol. 7, *Ultrasonic Testing.* Columbus, OH: American Society for Nondestructive Testing (1991): p 65-100.

2. *Piezoelectric Technology Data for Designers.* Bedford, OH: Morgan Matroc, Vernitron Division (1965).

3. Brown, L.F. and J.L. Mason. "Disposable PVDF Ultrasonic Transducers for Nondestructive Testing Applications." *IEEE Transactions on Ultrasonics, Ferroelectrics, and Frequency Control.* Vol. 43, No. 4. New York, NY: Institute of Electrical and Electronics Engineers (1996): p 560-568.

4. Mason, W.P. "An Electromechanical Representation of a Piezoelectrical Crystal Used As a Transducer." *Proceedings of the IRE.* New York, NY: Institute of Radio Engineers (October 1935): p 1252-1263.

5. Mason, W.P. *Electromechanical Transducers and Wave Filters,* second edition. New York, NY: Van Nostrand (1948).

6. Struetzer, O.M. "Impulse Response Measurement Technique for Piezoelectric Transducer Arrangements." *IEEE Transactions on Sonics and Ultrasonics.* Vol. SU-15, No. 1. New York, NY: Institute of Electrical and Electronics Engineers (January 1968): p 13-17.

7. IEEE 176, *IEEE Standard on Piezoelectricity.* New York, NY: Institute of Electrical and Electronics Engineers (1987).

8. Fortunko, C.M. Section 5, "Ultrasonic Testing Equipment." *Nondestructive Testing Handbook,* second edition: Vol. 7, *Ultrasonic Testing.* Columbus, OH: American Society for Nondestructive Testing (1991): p 101-129.

9. Posakony, G.J. "Influence of the Pulser Parameters on the Ultrasonic Spectrum." *Materials Evaluation.* Vol. 43, No. 4. Columbus, OH: American Society for Nondestructive Testing (March 1985): p 413-419.

10. Hayward, G. "The Influence of Pulser Parameters on the Transmission Response of Piezoelectric Transducers." *Ultrasonics.* Vol. 23, No. 3. Saint Louis, MO: Elsevier (1985): p 103-112.

11. DeSilets, C.S., J.D. Frasier and G.S. Kino. "The Design of Efficient Broadband Piezoelectric Transducers." *Transactions on Sonics and Ultrasonics.* SU-25, No. 3. New York, NY: Institute of Electrical and Electronics Engineers (1978): p 115-125.

12. Hazony, D. and T. Kocher. "Finite-Response Ultrasonic Transducers." *Journal of the Acoustical Society of America.* Vol. 71, No. 1. New York, NY: Acoustical Society of America (1982): p 203-206.

13. Buchler, J., M. Platte and H. Schmidt. "Electronic Circuit for High Frequency and Broadband Ultrasonic Pulse-Echo Operation." *Ultrasonics.* Vol. 25, No. 2. Saint Louis, MO: Elsevier (1987): p 112-114.

14. Mattila, P. and M. Luukkala. "FET Pulse Generator for Ultrasonic Pulse-Echo Applications." *Ultrasonics.* Vol. 19, No. 5. Saint Louis, MO: Elsevier (1981): p 235-236.

15. Rose, J.L. *Ultrasonic Waves in Solid Media.* London, United Kingdom: Cambridge University Press (1999).

16. MacDonald, D. Private communication. Palo Alto, CA: Electric Power Research Institute (1989).

17. Wickramasinghe, H.K. "Acoustic Microscopy: Present and Future." *IEE Proceedings.* Vol. 131, Part A, No. 4. London, United Kingdom: Institution of Electrical Engineers (June 1984): p 282.

18. Ilic, D.B., G.S. Kino and A.R. Selfridge. "Computer Controlled System for Measuring Two Dimensional Acoustic Velocity Fields." *Review of Scientific Instruments.* Vol. 50, No. 12. Woodbury, NY: American Institute of Physics (1979): p 1527-1531.

19. Hughes, M.S., D.K. Hsu and D.O. Thompson. "Characteristics of a Prototype Unipolar Pulse-Echo Instrument for NDE Applications." *Review of Progress in Quantitative Nondestructive Evaluation* [Brunswick, ME, July 1989]. Vol. 9A. New York, NY: Plenum Press (1990): p 917-925.
20. Motchenbacher, C.D. and F.C. Fitchen. *Low-Noise Electronic Design.* New York, NY: Wiley Interscience (1973): p 47-59.
21. Krautkrämer, J. and H. Krautkrämer. *Ultrasonic Testing of Materials,* fourth edition. Berlin, Federal Republic of Germany: Springer-Verlag (1990): p 204-205.
22. Sevick, J. *Transmission Line Transformers.* Newington, CT: American Radio League (1987).
23. Clarke, K.K. and D.T. Hess. *Communication Circuits: Analysis and Design.* Reading, MA: Addison-Wesley Publishing Company (1971): p 16-64.
24. Selfridge, A.R., R. Baer, B.T. Khuri-Yakub and G.S. Kino. "Computer-Optimized Design of Quarter-Wave Acoustic Matching and Electrical Matching Networks for Acoustic Transducers." *Ultrasonics Symposium Proceedings.* New York, NY: Institute of Electrical and Electronics Engineers (1982): p 644-648.
25. Cuthbert, T.R. *Circuit Design Using Personal Computers.* New York, NY: Wiley-Interscience (1983): p 189-194.
26. Sloan, W.W. "Detector-Associated Electronics." *Infrared Handbook.* Ann Arbor, MI: Environmental Research Institute of Michigan (1989): p 16.2-16.33.
27. Lewin, P.A. and A.S. DeReggi. "Short Range Applications." *The Applications of Ferroelectric Polymers.* New York, NY: Chapman Hall Publishing (1988): p 165-167.
28. Green, E.R. "The Effect of Equipment Bandwidth and Center Frequency Changes on Ultrasonic Inspection Reliability: Modeling and Experimental Results." *Review of Progress in Quantitative Nondestructive Evaluation* [Brunswick, ME, July 1989]. Vol. 9A. New York, NY: Plenum Press (1990): p 901-908.
29. Posakony, G.J. "Experimental Analysis of Ultrasonic Responses from Artificial Defects." *Materials Evaluation.* Vol. 44, No. 13. Columbus, OH: American Society for Nondestructive Testing (December 1986): p 1567-1572.
30. Green, E.R. "Worst-Case Defects Affecting Ultrasonic Inspection Reliability." *Materials Evaluation.* Vol. 47, No. 12. Columbus, OH: American Society for Nondestructive Testing (December 1989): p 1401-1407.
31. *Introduction to Phased Array Ultrasonic Technology Applications.* Waltham, MA: R/D Tech [Olympus NDT Canada] (2004).
32. Wüstenberg, H., A. Erhard and G. Schenk, "Some Characteristic Parameters of Ultrasonic Phased Array Probes and Equipments." *NDT.net.* Vol. 4, No. 4. Kirchwald, Germany: NDT.net (April 1999).
33. Clay A.C., S.-C. Wooh, L. Azar and J.-Y. Wang. "Experimental Study of Phased Array Beam Characteristics." *Journal of NDE.* Vol. 18, No. 2. New York, NY: Plenum (June 1999): p 59.
34. Lafontaine, G. and F. Cancre. "Potential of Ultrasonic Phased Arrays for Faster, Better and Cheaper Inspections." *NDT.net.* Vol. 5, No. 10. Kirchwald, Germany: NDT.net (October 2000).
35. Lareau, J.P and R.M. Plis. "Phased Array Imaging First Use Qualification Effort: BWR Feedwater Nozzle Inner Radius Inspection from Vessel OD for a US Nuclear Power Plant." *NDT.net.* Vol. 7, No. 5. Kirchwald, Germany: NDT.net (May 2002).
36. Whittle, A.C. "Phased Arrays — Panacea or Gimmick?" *Insight.* Vol. 46, No. 11. Northhampton, United Kingdom: British Institute of Nondestructive Inspection (November 2004): p 674-676.
37. Ginzel, E.A. and D. Stewart. "Photo-Elastic Visualisation of Phased Array Ultrasonic Pulses In Solids." *16th World Conference on Nondestructive Testing* [Montreal, Canada, August-September 2004]. Hamilton, Ontario, Canada: Canadian Institute for Nondestructive Evaluation (2004).
38. Ciorau, P., D. MacGillivray, T. Hazelton, L. Gilham, D. Craig and J. Poguet. "In-Situ Examination of ABB 1-0 Blade Roots and Rotor Steeple of Low-Pressure Steam Turbine, Using Phased Array Technology." *15th World Conference on NDT* [Rome, Italy, October 2000]. Brescia, Italy: Associazione Italiana Prove non Distruttive [Italian Society for Nondestructive Testing and Monitoring Diagnostics] (2000).

39. Dubé, N. "Electric Resistance Welding Inspection." *15th World Conference on NDT* [Rome, Italy, October 2000]. Brescia, Italy: Associazione Italiana Prove non Distruttive [Italian Society for Nondestructive Testing and Monitoring Diagnostics] (2000).

40. Bar-Cohen, Y. Section 8, "Ultrasonic Pulse Echo Immersion Techniques." *Nondestructive Testing Handbook,* second edition: Vol. 7, *Ultrasonic Testing.* Columbus, OH: American Society for Nondestructive Testing (1991): p 219-266.

41. Born, M. and E. Wolf. *Principles of Optics.* Oxford, United Kingdom: Pergamon Press (1970).

42. Lees, S. "Useful Criteria in Describing the Field Pattern of Focusing Transducers." *Ultrasonics.* Vol. 16, No. 5. Saint Louis, MO: Elsevier (1978): p 219-436.

43. Tarnoczy, T. "Sound Focusing Lenses and Waveguides." *Ultrasonics.* Vol. 3. Saint Louis, MO: Elsevier (July 1965): p 115-127.

44. Madsen, E., M. Goodsitt and J. Zagzebski. "Continuous Waves Generated by Focusing Radiators." *Journal of the Acoustical Society of America.* Vol. 70, No. 5. Melville, NY: American Institute of Physics, for the Acoustical Society of America (1981): p 1508-1517.

45. O'Neil, H. "Theory of Focusing Radiators." *Journal of the Acoustical Society of America.* Vol. 21, No. 5. Melville, NY: American Institute of Physics, for the Acoustical Society of America (1949): p 516-526.

46. Turner, J. *Development of Novel Focused Ultrasonic Transducers for NDT.* Report No. 313/1986. Cambridge, United Kingdom: The Welding Institute (1986).

47. Lemons, P. and C. Quate. "Acoustic Microscope." *Physical Acoustics: Principles and Methods.* Vol. 14. New York, NY: Academic Press (1979): p 1-92.

48. Lamb, H. "On Waves in an Elastic Plate." *Proceedings of the Royal Society of London.* Series A, Vol. 93. London, United Kingdom: Royal Society (1917): p 114-128.

49 Achenbach, J.D. *Wave Propagation in Elastic Solids: With Applications to Scattering by Cracks.* Amsterdam, Netherlands: North-Holland/Elsevier (1973).

50. Achenbach, J.D. "Theory of Ultrasound Propagation in Solids." *Topics on Nondestructive Evaluation:* Vol. 1, *Sensing for Materials Characterization, Processing, and Manufacturing.* Columbus, OH: American Society for Nondestructive Testing (1998): p 3-21.

51. Kwun, H. and K.A. Bartels. "Magnetostrictive Sensor Technology and Its Applications." *Ultrasonics 36.* Guildford, Surrey, United Kingdom: Elsevier (1998): p 171-178.

52. Rose, J.L. and X. Zhao. "Anomaly Throughwall Depth Measurement Potential with Shear Horizontal Guided Waves." *Materials Evaluation.* Vol. 59, No. 10. Columbus, OH: American Society for Nondestructive Testing (October 2001): p 1234-1238.

53. Badi, M.H., G.G. Yaralioglu, A.S. Ergun, S.T. Hansen and B.T. Khuri-Yakub. "Capacitive Micromachined Ultrasonic Lamb Wave Transducers Using Rectangular Membranes." *IEEE Transactions on Ultrasonics, Ferroelectrics, and Frequency Control.* Vol. 50, No. 9. New York, NY: Institute of Electrical and Electronics Engineers (2003): p 1191-1203.

54. Holland, S.D. and D.E. Chimenti. "Air-Coupled Acoustic Imaging with Zero-Group-Velocity Lamb Modes." *Applied Physics Letters.* Vol. 83, No. 13. Melville, NY: American Institute of Physics (2003): p 2704-2706.

55. Telschow, K.L., V.A. Deason, R.S. Schley and S.M. Watson. *Journal of the Acoustical Society of America.* Vol. 106. Melville, NY: American Institute of Physics (1999) p 2578-2587.

56. Viktorov, I.A. *Rayleigh and Lamb Waves — Physical Theory and Applications.* New York, NY: Plenum (1967).

57. Achenbach, J.D. *Wave Propagation in Elastic Solids.* Amsterdam, Netherlands: North-Holland/Elsevier (1984).

58. Auld, B.A. *Acoustic Fields and Waves in Solids,* second edition. Malabar, FL: R.E. Krieger (1990).

59. Graff, K.F. *Wave Motion in Elastic Solids.* New York, NY: Dover (1963, 1991).

60. Nayfeh, A.H. *Wave Propagation in Layered Anisotropic Media with Applications to Composites.* Netherlands: North-Holland/Elsevier (1995).

61. Shull, P.J. *Nondestructive Evaluation: Theory, Techniques and Applications.* New York, NY: Marcel Dekker (1999).

62. Rose, J.L. "A Baseline and Vision of Ultrasonic Guided Wave Inspection Potential." *Transactions of the ASME: Journal of Pressure Vessel Technology.* Vol. 124. New York, NY: ASME International (2002): p 273-282.
63. Sun, Z., L. Zhang and J.L. Rose. "Flexural Torsional Guided Wave Mechanics and Focusing in Pipe." *ASME Transactions Journal of Pressure Vessel Technology.* Vol. 127, No. 4. New York, NY: ASME International (2005): p 471-478.
64. Ditri, J.J., J.L. Rose and A. Pilarski. "Generation of Guided Waves in Hollow Cylinders by Wedge and Comb Type Transducers." *Review of Progress in Quantitative Nondestructive Evaluation* [La Jolla, CA: July 1992]. Vol. 12A. New York, NY: Plenum (1993): p 211-218.
65. Rose, J.L., J. Ditri and A. Pilarski. "Wave Mechanics in Acousto-Ultrasonic Nondestructive Evaluation." *Journal of Acoustic Emission.* Vol. 12. Los Angeles, CA: Acoustic Emission Group (1994): p 23-26.
66. Rose, J.L., K.M. Rajana and F.T. Carr. "Ultrasonic Guided Wave Inspection Concepts for Steam Generator Tubing," *Materials Evaluation.* Vol. 52, No. 2. Columbus, OH: American Society for Nondestructive Testing (February 1994): p 307-311.
67. Alleyne, D.N. and P. Cawley. "Long Range Propagation of Lamb Waves in Chemical Plant Pipework." *Materials Evaluation.* Vol. 55, No. 4. Columbus, OH: American Society for Nondestructive Testing (April 1997): p 504-508.
68. Rose, J.L., Z. Sun, P.J. Mudge and M.J. Avioli. "Guided Wave Flexural Mode Tuning and Focusing for Pipe Inspection." *Materials Evaluation.* Vol. 61, No. 2. Columbus, OH: American Society for Nondestructive Testing (February 2003): p 162-167.
69. Li, J. and J.L. Rose. "Implementing Guided Wave Mode Control by Use of a Phased Transducer Array." *IEEE Transactions on Ultrasonics, Ferroelectrics, and Frequency Control.* Vol. 48. New York, NY: Institute of Electrical and Electronics Engineers (2001): p 761-768.
70. Rose, J.L. and L.E. Soley. "Ultrasonic Guided Waves for the Detection of Anomalies in Aircraft Components." *Materials Evaluation.* Vol. 59, No. 10. Columbus, OH: American Society for Nondestructive Testing (September 2000): p 1080-1086.
71. Monchalin, J.-P. and J.W. Wagner. "Optical Generation and Detection of Ultrasound." *Nondestructive Testing Handbook,* second edition: Vol. 7, *Ultrasonic Testing.* Columbus, OH: American Society for Nondestructive Testing (1991): p 313-325.
72. Monchalin, J.-P. "Laser-Ultrasonics: From the Laboratory to Industry." *Review of Progress in Quantitative Nondestructive Evaluation.* Vol. 23A. New York, NY: American Institute of Physics (2004): p 3-31.
73. Scruby, C.B., R.J. Dewhurst, D.A. Hutchins and S.B. Palmer. *Research Techniques in Nondestructive Testing.* Vol. 5. New York, NY: Academic Press (1982): p 281-327.
74. Hutchins, D.A. "Ultrasonic Generation by Pulsed Lasers." *Physical Acoustics.* Vol. 18. New York, NY: Academic Press (1988): p 21-23.
75. Doyle, P.A. "On Epicentral Waveforms for Laser-Generated Ultrasound." *Journal of Physics D: Applied Physics.* Vol. 19. Melville, NY: American Institute of Physics (1986): p 1613-1623.
76. Schleichert, U., K.J. Langenberg, W. Arnold and S. Fassbender. "A Quantitative Theory of Laser-Generated Ultrasound." *Review of Progress in Quantitative Nondestructive Evaluation* [La Jolla, CA, July-August 1988]. Vol. 8A. New York, NY: Plenum Press (1989): p 489-496.
77. McDonald, F.A. "On the Precursor in Laser-Generated Ultrasound Waveforms in Metals." *Applied Physics Letters.* Vol. 56, No. 3. Melville, NY: American Institute of Physics (1990): p 230-232.
78. Aindow, A.M., R.J. Dewhurst and S.B. Palmer. "Laser Generation of Directional Surface Acoustic Wave Pulses in Metals." *Optics Communications.* Vol. 42. Amsterdam, Netherlands: Elsevier (1982): p 116-120.
79. Cielo, P., F. Nadeau and M. Lamontagne. "Laser Generation of Convergent Acoustic Waves for Material Inspection." *Ultrasonics.* Vol. 23. Saint Louis, MO: Elsevier (1985): p 55-62.
80. Yamanaka, K., O.V. Kolosov, Y. Nagata, T. Koda, H. Nishino and Y. Tsukahara. "Analysis of Excitation and Coherent Amplitude Enhancement of Surface Acoustic Waves by Phase Velocity Scanning Method." *Journal of Applied Physics.* Vol. 74. Amsterdam, Netherlands: Elsevier (1993): p 6511-6522.

81. Conant, R.J. and K.L. Telschow. "Longitudinal Wave Precursor Signal from an Optically Penetrating Thermoelastic Laser Source." *Review of Progress in Quantitative Nondestructive Evaluation* [La Jolla, CA, July-August 1988]. Vol. 8A. New York, NY: Plenum Press (1989): p 497-504.

82. Hoffman, A. and W. Arnold. "Modeling of the Ablation Source in Laser-Ultrasonics." *Review of Progress in Quantitative Nondestructive Evaluation* [Montréal, Canada, July 1999]. Vol 19A. Melville, NY: American Institute of Physics (2000): p 279-286.

83. Hébert, H., F. Vidal, F. Martin, J.-C. Kieffer, A. Nadeau, T.W. Johnston, A. Blouin, A. Moreau and J.-P. Monchalin. "Ultrasound Generated by a Femtosecond and a Picosecond Laser Pulse near the Ablation Threshold." *Journal of Applied Physics*. Vol. 98, Paper 033104. Amsterdam, Netherlands: Elsevier (2005).

84. Wagner, J.W. "High Resolution Holographic Techniques for Visualization of Surface Acoustic Waves." *Materials Evaluation*. Vol. 44, No. 10. Columbus, OH: American Society for Nondestructive Testing (September 1986): p 1238-1243.

85. Monchalin, J.-P. "Optical Detection of Ultrasound." *Transactions on Ultrasonics, Ferroelectrics and Frequency Control*. UFFC-33. New York, NY: Institute of Electrical and Electronics Engineers (1986): p 485-499.

86. Monchalin, J.-P., J.D. Aussel, R. Héon, C.K. Jen, A. Boudreault and R. Bernier. "Measurement of In-Plane and Out-of-Plane Ultrasonic Displacements by Optical Heterodyne Interferometry." *Journal of Nondestructive Evaluation*. Vol. 8, No. 2. New York, NY: Plenum (1989): p 121-133.

87. Monchalin, J.-P., R. Héon, P. Bouchard and C. Padioleau. "Broadband Optical Detection of Ultrasound by Optical Sideband Stripping with a Confocal Fabry-Perot." *Applied Physics Letters*. Vol. 55. Melville, NY: American Institute of Physics (1989): p 1612-1614.

88. Blouin, A. and J.-P. Monchalin. "Detection of Ultrasonic Motion of a Scattering Surface by Two-Wave Mixing in a Photorefractive GaAs Crystal." *Applied Physics Letters*. Vol. 65. Melville, NY: American Institute of Physics (1994): p 932-934.

89. Delaye, P., A. Blouin, D. Drolet, L.-A. de Montmorillon, G. Roosen and J.-P. Monchalin. "Detection of an Ultrasonic Motion of a Scattering Surface by Photorefractive InP:Fe under an Applied DC Field." *Journal of the Optical Society of America*. Vol. 14. Washington, DC: Optical Society of America (1997): p 1723-1734.

90. Monchalin, J.P., R. Héon and N. Muzak. "Evaluation of Ultrasonic Inspection Procedures by Field Mapping with an Optical Probe." *Canadian Metallurgical Quarterly*. Vol. 25. Willowdale, Ontario, Canada: Pergamon of Canada (1986): p 247-252.

91. Monchalin, J.-P., M. Choquet, C. Padioleau, C. Néron, D. Lévesque, A. Blouin, C. Corbeil, R. Talbot, A. Bendada, M. Lamontagne, R.V. Kolarik II, G.V. Jeskey, E.D. Dominik, L.J. Duly, K.J. Samblanet, S.E. Agger, K.J. Roush and M.L. Mester. "Laser Ultrasonic System for On-Line Steel Tube Gauging." *Review of Progress in Quantitative Nondestructive Evaluation* [Bellingham, WA, July 2002]. Vol. 22A. Melville, NY: American Institute of Physics (2003): p 264-272.

92. Monchalin, J.-P., J.-D. Aussel, P. Bouchard and R. Héon. "Laser-Ultrasonics for Industrial Applications." *Review of Progress in Quantitative Nondestructive Evaluation* [Williamsburg, VA, June 1987]. Vol. 7B. New York, NY: Plenum (1988): p 1607-1614.

93. Turner, W., T. Drake, M. Osterkamp, D. Kaiser, J. Miller, P. Tu and C. Wilson. "Using Computer Vision to Map Laser Ultrasound onto CAD Geometries." *Review of Progress in Quantitative Nondestructive Evaluation* [Bellingham, WA, July 2002]. Vol. 22A. Melville, NY: American Institute of Physics (2003): p 340-347.

94. Fiedler, C.J., T. Ducharme and J. Kwan. "The Laser-Ultrasonic Inspection System (LUIS) at the Sacramento Air Logistics Center." *Review of Progress in Quantitative Nondestructive Evaluation* [Brunswick, ME, July-August 1996]. Vol. 16A. Vol. 16A, New-York, NY: Plenum Press (1997): p 515-522.

95. Pétillon, O., J.-P. Dupuis, H. Voillaume and H. Trétout. "Applications of Laser Based Ultrasonics to Aerospace Industry." *Proceedings: 7th European Conference on Non-Destructive Testing* [Copenhagen, Denmark, May 1998]. Vol. 1. Broendby, Denmark: 7th ECNDT: p 27-33.

96. Choquet, M., R. Héon, C. Padioleau, P. Bouchard, C. Néron and J.-P. Monchalin. " Laser-Ultrasonic Inspection of the Composite Structure of an Aircraft in a Maintenance Hangar." *Review of Progress in Quantitative Nondestructive Evaluation* [Snowmass Village, CO, July-August 1994]. Vol. 14A. New York, NY: Plenum (1995): p 545-552.

97. Fomitchov, P.A., A.K. Kromine, S. Krishnaswamy and J.D. Achenbach. "Ultrasonic Imaging of Small Surface-Breaking Defects Using Scanning Laser Source Technique." *Review of Progress in Quantitative Nondestructive Evaluation* [Brunswick, ME, July-August 2001]. Vol. 21A. Melville, NY: American Institute of Physics (2002): p 356-362.

98. Ochiai, M., D. Lévesque, R. Talbot, A. Blouin, A. Fukumoto and J.-P. Monchalin. "Visualization of Surface-Breaking Tight Cracks by Laser-Ultrasonic F-SAFT." *Review of Progress in Quantitative Nondestructive Evaluation* [Bellingham, WA, July 2002]. Vol. 22A. Melville, NY: American Institute of Physics (2003): p 1497-1503.

99. Lévesque, D., A. Blouin, C. Néron and J.-P. Monchalin. "Performance of Laser-Ultrasonic F-SAFT Imaging." *Ultrasonics.* Vol. 40. Saint Louis, MO: Elsevier (2002): p 1057-1063.

100. Monchalin, J.-P., R. Héon, J.F. Bussière and B. Farahbakhsh. "Laser-Ultrasonic Determination of Elastic Constants at Ambient and Elevated Temperatures." *Nondestructive Characterization of Materials II.* J.F. Bussière, J.P. Monchalin, C.O. Ruud and R.E. Green, Jr., eds. New York, NY: Plenum Press (1987): p 717-723.

101. Bresse, L.F., D.A. Hutchins and K. Lundgren. "Elastic Constant Determination Using Ultrasonic Generation by Pulsed Lasers." *Journal of the Acoustical Society of America.* Vol. 84, No. 5. Melville, NY: American Institute of Physics, for the Acoustical Society of America (1988): p 1751-1757.

102. Dewhurst, R.J., C. Edwards, A.D.W. McKie and S.B. Palmer. "A Remote Laser System for Ultrasonic Velocity Measurement at High Temperatures." *Journal of Applied Physics.* Melville, NY: American Institute of Physics (1988): p 1225-1227.

103. Aussel, J.D. and J.-P. Monchalin. "Precision Laser-Ultrasonic Velocity Measurement and Elastic Constant Determination." *Ultrasonics.* Vol. 27, No. 3. Saint Louis, MO: Elsevier (1989): p 165-177.

104. Lindh-Ulmgren, E., M. Ericsson, D. Artymowicz and B. Hutchinson. "Laser-Ultrasonics As a Technique to Study Recrystallisation and Grain Growth." *Materials Science Forum.* Vol. 467-470. Zurich, Switzerland: Ütikon, Trans Tech Publications (2004): p 1353-1362.

105. Moreau, A., D. Lévesque, M. Lord, M. Dubois, J.-P. Monchalin, C. Padioleau and J.F. Bussière. "On-Line Measurement of Texture, Thickness and Plastic Strain Ratio Using Laser-Ultrasound Resonance Spectroscopy." *Ultrasonics.* Vol. 40. Saint Louis, MO: Elsevier (2002): p 1047-1056.

106. Kruger, S.E., G. Lamouche, A. Moreau and M. Militzer. "Laser Ultrasonic Monitoring of Recrystallization of Steels." *Materials Science and Technology 2004 Conference Proceedings* [New Orleans, LA, September 2004]. Warrendale, MI: Association for Iron and Steel Technology (2004): p 809-812.

107. Kruger, S.E., A. Moreau, M. Militzer and T. Biggs. "In-Situ, Laser-Ultrasonic Monitoring of the Recrystallization of Aluminum Alloys." *Thermec 2003 International Conference on Processing & Manufacturing of Advanced Materials.* Part 1. Zurich, Switzerland: Ütikon, Trans Tech Publications (2003): p 483-488.

108. Dubois, M., A. Moreau and J.F. Bussière. "Ultrasonic Velocity Measurements during Phase Transformations in Steels Using Laser-Ultrasonics." *Journal of Applied Physics.* Vol. 89, 11. Melville, NY: American Institute of Physics (2001): p 6487-6495.

109. Truell, R., C. Elbaum and B.B. Chick. *Ultrasonic Methods in Solid State Physics.* New York, NY: Academic Press (1969).

110. Aussel, J.D. and J.P. Monchalin. "Measurement of Ultrasound Attenuation by Laser Ultrasonics." *Journal of Applied Physics*. Vol. 65, No. 8. Melville, NY: American Institute of Physics (1989): p2918-2922.

111. Dubois, M., M. Militzer, A. Moreau and J.F. Bussière. "A New Technique for the Quantitative Real-Time Monitoring of Austenite Grain Growth in Steel." *Scripta Materialia*. Vol. 42, No. 9. Oxford, United Kingdom: Elsevier (2000): p867-874.

112. Jeskey, G., R. Kolarik II, E. Damm, J.-P. Monchalin, G. Lamouche, S.E. Kruger and M. Choquet. "Laser Ultrasonic Sensor for On-Line Seamless Steel Tubing Process Control." *Proceedings of the 16th World Conference on Nondestructive Testing* [Montreal, Canada, August-September 2004] Hamilton, Ontario, Canada: Canadian Institute for NDE (2004).

113. Kruger, S.E., G. Lamouche, J.-P. Monchalin, R.V. Kolarik II, G.V. Jeskey and M. Choquet. "On-Line Monitoring of Wall Thickness and Austenite Grain Size on a Seamless Tubing Production Line at the Timken Co." *Iron and Steel Technology*. Vol. 2, No. 10. Warrendale, PA: Association for Iron and Steel Technology (2005): p25-31.

114. Maris, H.J. "Picosecond Ultrasonics." *Scientific American*. New York, NY: Scientific American (1998): p 86-89.

115. Rogers, J.A., A.A. Maznev, M.J. Banet and K.A. Nelson. "Optical Generation and Characterization of Acoustic Waves in Thin Films." *Annual Review of Material Science*. Vol. 30. Palo Alto, CA: Annual Reviews (2000): p 117-157.

116. Carrion, L., A. Blouin, C. Padioleau, P. Bouchard and J.-P. Monchalin. "Single-Frequency Pulsed Laser Oscillator and System for Laser-Ultrasonics." *Measurement Science and Technology*. Vol. 15. Bristol, United Kingdom: Institute of Physics (2004): p 1939-1946.

117. Alers, G.A. and B.W. Maxfield. "Electromagnetic Acoustic Transducers." *Nondestructive Testing Handbook,* second edition: Vol. 7, *Ultrasonic Testing*. Columbus, OH: American Society for Nondestructive Testing (1991): p 326-340.

118. Thompson, R.B. "Physical Principles of Measurements with EMAT Transducers." *Physical Acoustics*. Vol. 19. New York, NY: Academic Press (1990): p 157-200.

119. Wilbrand, A. "Quantitative Modeling and Experimental Analysis of the Physical Properties of Electromagnetic-Ultrasonic Transducers." *Review of Progress in Quantitative Nondestructive Evaluation* [Williamsburg, VA, June 1987]. Vol. 7A. New York, NY: Plenum (1988): p 671-680.

120. Alers, G.A. and H.G.N. Wadley. "Monitoring Pipe and Tube Wall Properties during Fabrication in a Steel Mill." *Intelligent Processing of Materials and Advanced Sensors*. Warrendale, PA: American Institute of Metallurgical Engineers (1987): p17-27.

121. Alers, G.A. "Electromagnetic Induction of Ultrasonic Waves: EMAT, EMUS, EMAR." *16th World Conference on Nondestructive Testing* [Montreal, Canada, August-September 2004]. Hamilton, Ontario, Canada: Canadian Institute for Nondestructive Evaluation (2004).

122. Kupperman, D.S. and K.J. Reimann. "Ultrasonic Wave Propagation in Austenitic Stainless Steel Weld Metal." *Transactions on Sonics and Ultrasonics*. Vol. SU-27, No. 1. New York, NY: Institute of Electrical and Electronics Engineers (January 1980): p 7-15.

123. Hirsekorn, S. "Directional Dependence of Ultrasonic Propagation in Textured Polycrystals." *Journal of the Acoustical Society of America*. Vol. 79, No. 5. Melville, NY: American Institute of Physics, for the Acoustical Society of America (May 1986): p 1269-1279.

124. Hubschen, G. "Results for Testing Austenitic Welds and Cladding Using Electromagnetically Excited SH-Waves." *Proceedings of the Sixth International Conference on Nondestructive Evaluation in the Nuclear Industry*. Materials Park, OH: ASM International (1984): p238-289.

125. Silk, M.G.A. "A Computer Model for Ultrasonic Propagation in Complex Orthotropic Structures." *Ultrasonics*. Vol. 19, No. 9. Saint Louis, MO: Elsevier (September 1981): p208-212.

126. Ogilvy, J.A. "Ultrasonic Beam Profiles and Beam Propagation in an Austenitic Weld Using a Theoretical Ray Tracing Model." *Ultrasonics*. Vol. 24, No. 11. Saint Louis, MO: Elsevier (November 1986): p337-347.

127. Hübschen, G. and H.J. Salzburger. "UT of Austenitic Welds and Cladding Using Electromagnetically Excited SH-Waves." *Review of Progress in Quantitative Nondestructive Evaluation* [Williamsburg, VA, June 1985]. Vol. 5B. New York, NY: Plenum (1986): p 1687-1695.

128. Hubschen, G. and H.J. Salzburger. "Inspection of Dissimilar Metal Welds Using Horizontally Polarized Shear Waves and Electromagnetic Ultrasonic (EMUS) Probes." *Proceedings of the International Atomic Energy Agency Specialists Meeting on Inspection of Austenitic Dissimilar Materials and Welds.* Vienna, Austria: International Atomic Energy Agency (1988).

129. Burns, L.R., G.A. Alers and D.T. MacLauchlan. "A Compact Electromagnetic Acoustic Transducer Receiver for Ultrasonic Testing at Elevated Temperatures." *Review of Progress in Quantitative Nondestructive Evaluation* [Williamsburg, VA, June 1987]. Vol. 7B. New York, NY: Plenum (1988): p 1677-1683.

130. Sato, I., K. Miyagawa, Y. Sasaki, K. Kawamura, S. Sato, S. Sasaki, J. Kubota and S. Susumu. United States Patent 4 348 903, *Electromagnetic Ultrasonic Apparatus* (September 1982).

131. Maxfield, B.W., A. Kuramoto and J.K. Hulbert. "Evaluating EMAT Designs for Selected Applications." *Materials Evaluation.* Vol. 45, No. 10. Columbus, OH: American Society for Nondestructive Testing (September 1987): p 1166-1183.

132. Papadakis, E.P., L.C. Lynnworth, K.A. Fowler and E.H. Carnevale. "Ultrasonic Attenuation and Velocity in Hot Specimens by the Momentary Contact Method with Pressure Coupling and Some Results on Steel to 1200° C." *Journal of the Acoustical Society of America.* Vol. 52, No. 3. New York, NY: Acoustical Society of America (1972): p 850.

133. Alers, G.A., D.T. MacLauchlan and L.R. Burns, Jr. United States Patent 4 777 824, *A Compact Ultrasonic Transducer for Hostile Environments.* (October 1988).

134. Boyd, D.M. and P.D. Sperline. "Noncontact Temperature Measurement of Hot Steel Bodies Using an Electromagnetic Acoustic Transducer (EMAT)." *Review of Progress in Quantitative Nondestructive Evaluation* [Williamsburg, VA, June 1987]. Vol. 7B. New York, NY: Plenum (1988): p 1669-1676.

135. Gwartney, W.R., Jr. Private communication. Tulsa, OK: T.D. Williamson, Incorporated (1984).

136. Thompson, R.B., G.A. Alers and M.A. Tennison. "Application of Direct Electromagnetic Lamb Wave Generation to Gas Pipeline Inspection." *Ultrasonics Symposium Proceedings.* 72-CHO-708-8SU. New York, NY: Institute of Electrical and Electronics Engineers (1972): p 91.

137. Thompson, R.B. "A Model for the Electromagnetic Generation and Detection of Rayleigh and Lamb Waves." *Transactions on Sonics and Ultrasonics.* Vol. SU-20. New York, NY: Institute of Electrical and Electronics Engineers (October 1973): p 340.

138. Palanisamy, R., C.J. Morris, D.M. Keener and M.N. Curran. "On the Accuracy of A.C. Flux Leakage, Eddy Current, EMAT and Ultrasonic Methods of Measuring Surface Connecting Flaws in Seamless Steel Tubing." *Review of Progress in Quantitative Nondestructive Evaluation* [Williamsburg, VA, June 1985]. Vol. 5A. New York, NY: Plenum (1986): p 215-223.

139. Repplinger, W. and H.J. Salzburger. "A Broadband Electromagnetic UT System." *Proceedings of the Sixth International Conference on Nondestructive Evaluation in the Nuclear Industry.* Materials Park, OH: ASM International (1984): p 585-591.

140. Repplinger, W., A. Wilbrand, W. Bottger and W. Weingarten. "Verfahren und Gerat für die Electromagnetische Ultraschallprüfung von Mittlerohren." *Annual Conference.* Vol. 10, Part 1. Berlin, Germany: Deutsche Gesellschaft für Zerstörungsfreie Prüfung (1987): p 508-515.

141. Bottger, W., W. Weingarten, A. Wilbrand and W. Repplinger. "Verfahren und Gerat für die Elecktromagnetische Ultraschallprüfung von Mittelrohren." *Annual Conference.* Vol. 10, Part 1. Berlin, Germany: Deutsche Gesellschaft für Zerstörungsfreie Prüfung (1987): p 116-121.

142. Bottger, W., W. Repplinger, W. Weingarten and A. Wilbrand. "EMA Angle-Probe Prototype Tests Steel Tubes On-Line." *Steel Times.* Vol. 215, No. 8. Redhill, Surrey, United Kingdom: DMG World Media (UK) (August 1987): p 402.

143. Alers, G.A. "EMAT Rail Flaw Detection System." Contract Report DTFR-53-86-C00015. Washington, DC: United States Department of Transportation (November 1988).

144. Thompson, R.B. "A New Configuration for the Electromagnetic Generation of SH Waves in Ferromagnetic Materials." *Ultrasonic Symposium Proceedings.* No. 78CH-1344-1SU. New York, NY: Institute of Electrical and Electronics Engineers (1978): p 374-378.

145. Repplinger, W., G. Hubschen and H.-J. J. Salzburger. United States Patent 4 466 287, *Non-Destructive, Non-Contact Ultrasonic Material.* (1984).

146. Vasile, C.F. and R.B. Thompson. "Periodic Magnet, Noncontact EMAT-Theory and Application." *Ultrasonic Symposium Proceedings.* No. 77-CH1264-1SU. New York, NY: Institute of Electrical and Electronics Engineers (1977): p 84-88.

147. Salzburger, H.J. and W. Repplinger. "Automatic In-Motion Inspection of the Head of Railway Wheels by E.M.A. Excited Rayleigh Waves." *Conference Proceedings of Ultrasonics International.* London, United Kingdom: Butterworth Scientific (1983): p 497-501.

148. Salzburger, H.J., W. Repplinger and W. Schmidt. "Entwicklung, Betriebstest und Einsatz eines Automatischen Systems zür Wiederkehrenden. Prüfung der Laufflachen von Eisenbahn-Radern." *Materialprüfung.* Vol. 10, Part 1. Berlin, Germany: Deutsche Gesellschaft für Zerstörungsfreie Prüfung (1987): p 253-264.

149. Prati, J. and C. Bird. *Electron Beam Welding System Based on EMATs.* Toledo, OH: Teledyne CAE (1989).

150. Alers, G.A. and L.R. Burns. "EMAT Designs for Special Applications." *Materials Evaluation.* Vol. 45, No. 10. Columbus, OH: American Society for Nondestructive Testing (September 1987): p 1184-1189.

151. Alers, G.A. *Electromagnetic Transducers for Weld Inspection.* MEA-8212868. Washington, DC: National Science Foundation (May 1987).

152. Thompson, R.B. and C.M. Fortunko. United States Patent 4 184 374, *Ultrasonic Inspection of a Cylindrical Object.* (January 1980).

153. Thompson, R.B., S.S. Lee and J.F. Smith. "Angular Dependence of Ultrasonic Wave Propagation in a Stressed, Orthorhombic Continuum: Theory and Application to Measurement of Stress and Texture." *Journal of the Acoustical Society of America.* Vol. 80, No. 3. Melville, NY: American Institute of Physics, for the Acoustical Society of America (1986): p 921-931.

154. Dobbs, E.R. "Electromagnetic Generation of Ultrasonic Waves." *Physical Acoustics.* Vol. 10. New York, NY: Academic Press (1976): p 127-193.

155. Frost, H.M. "Electromagnetic-Ultrasound Transducers: Principles, Practice and Applications." *Physical Acoustics.* Vol. 14. New York, NY: Academic Press (1979): p 179-276.

156. Maxfield, B.W. and C.M. Fortunko. "The Design and Use of Electromagnetic Acoustic Wave Transducers (EMATs)." *Materials Evaluation.* Vol. 41, No. 12. Columbus, OH: American Society for Nondestructive Testing (November 1983): p 1399-1408.

157. Khuri-Yakub, B.T. "Air Coupled Transducers." *Nondestructive Testing Handbook,* second edition: Vol. 7, *Ultrasonic Testing.* Columbus, OH: American Society for Nondestructive Testing (1991): p 320-325.

158. Malecki, I. *Physical Foundations of Technical Acoustics.* Oxford, United Kingdom: Pergamon (1969).

159. Pierce, A.D. *Acoustics: An Introduction to Its Physical Principles and Applications.* New York, NY: McGraw-Hill (1981).

160. Massa, F. "Ultrasonic Transducers for Use in Air." *Proceedings of the IEEE.* Vol. 53, No. 10. New York, NY: Institute of Electrical and Electronics Engineers (October 1965).

161. Fox, J.D. *Sensing with High-Frequency Ultrasound in Air.* Dissertation. Stanford, CA: Stanford University (December 1985).

162. Auld, B.A. *Acoustic Waves and Fields in Solids.* New York, NY: Wiley (1973).

163. Kino, G.S. *Acoustic Waves: Devices, Imaging and Analog Signal Processing.* Englewood Cliffs, NJ: Prentice-Hall (1987).

164. *Ultrasonic Ranging System.* Document P1834B. Cambridge, MA: Polaroid (1981).

165. Canali, C., G. DeCicco, B. Morten, M. Prudenziati and T. Taroni. "An Ultrasonic Proximity Sensor Operating in Air." *Sensors and Actuators.* Vol. 2, No. 1. Lausanne, Switzerland: Elsevier Sequoia (1981-1982): p 97-103.

166. Canali, C., G. DeCicco, B. Morten, M. Prudenziati and T. Taroni. "A Temperature Compensated Ultrasonic Sensor Operating in Air for Distance and Proximity Measurements." *Transactions on Industrial Electronics.* IE-29, No. 4. New York, NY: Institute of Electrical and Electronics Engineers (November 1982): p 336-341.

167. Klenschmidt, P. and V. Magori. "Ultrasonic Robotic Sensors for Exact Short Range Distance Measurement and Object Identification." *Proceedings of the Ultrasonics Symposium.* Vol. 1, Paper 85CH2209-5SU. New York, NY: Institute of Electrical and Electronics Engineers (1985).

168. Fox, J.D., B.T. Khuri-Yakub and G.S. Kino. "High-Frequency Acoustic Wave Measurements in Air." *Proceedings of the Ultrasonics Symposium.* 83CH1947-1SU. New York, NY: Institute of Electrical and Electronics Engineers (1983): p 581-584.

169. Tone, M., T. Yano and A. Fukomoto. "High Frequency Ultrasonic Transducers Operating in Air." *Japanese Journal of Applied Physics.* Vol. 23, No. 6. Tokyo, Japan: Oyo Butsurigaku Obunshi Kankokai (June 1984): p L436-L438.

170. Khuri-Yakub, B.T., J.H. Kim, C.H. Chou, P. Parent and G.S. Kino. "A New Design for Air Transducers." *Proceedings of the Ultrasonics Symposium.* Vol. 1. New York, NY: Institute of Electrical and Electronics Engineers (1988): p 503-506.

171. *Aerogels: Proceedings of the First International Symposium. Proceedings in Physics.* Vol. 6. Berlin, Germany: Springer-Verlag (1986).

172. Schiller, S., C.K. Hsieh, C.H. Chou and B.T. Khuri-Yakub. "Novel High-Frequency Air Transducers." *Review of Progress in Quantitative Nondestructive Evaluation* [Brunswick, ME, July 1989]. Vol. 9A. New York, NY: Plenum (1990): p 795-798.

CHAPTER

Ultrasonic Signal Processing[1]

Doron Kishoni, Aurora, Colorado

Laszlo Adler, Ohio State University, Columbus, Ohio

Alain Jungman, University of Paris, Paris, France

Peter B. Nagy, University of Cincinnati, Cincinnati, Ohio

Joseph L. Rose, Penn State University, University Park, Pennsylvania

Part 1. Signal Acquisition and Processing

Introduction

Signal processing and data analysis techniques are common tools for research and industrial development. They also have become a valuable addition to the ultrasonic nondestructive test method. The purpose of signal processing and data analysis is to enhance certain features of received signals in order to extract information about the test object. Such data may remain completely hidden or too distorted to interpret with conventional techniques.

For instance, signal processing can improve the detectability of small discontinuities embedded in heterogeneous structures (weldments, composites, ceramics) as well as those near disturbing geometrical features (surfaces, interfaces, corners or edges) that can produce strong artifact signals. Similarly, data processing might be needed to assess bond quality from ultrasonic signals transmitted through or reflected from interfaces in adhesive joints, solid state welds or thin coatings.

This text introduces techniques of ultrasonic signal processing and gives examples. Some mathematics helps explain the techniques. For more detailed information about mathematical definitions, concepts and proofs, the reader is referred to the extensive literature on signal processing and data analysis.[2-11]

Definition of Signal

In its most general sense, the term *signal* is understood to be a physical phenomenon whose presence or change provides information. In ultrasonic testing, the variation of pressure or the particle displacement in a material conveys information about the test object. To transport, analyze or store this information, it is convenient to convert it from its original, mechanical form to a related electrical quality (potential, current or power). For instance, in pulse echo discontinuity detectors, the reflected ultrasonic wave is converted into an electrical pulse that can be displayed on the screen of an oscilloscope as an A-scan, electrical potential versus time.

Although some basic features of this signal (amplitude, delay time, length) can be directly evaluated to obtain the location and approximate size of a discontinuity, further analysis of the signal may provide additional information on the physical nature, shape, orientation and dimensions of the reflector. To achieve this goal, ultrasonic tests require sophisticated processing to select the signal of interest, to improve the signal-to-noise ratio, to compare the signal to a reference, to identify specific features of the signal, to present it in an appropriate form and to store it for further analysis and interpretation.

Signal Classification

There are three classes of signals: (1) deterministic signals versus random signals, (2) periodic signals versus transient signals, (3) analog signals versus digital signals.

Deterministic versus Random Signals

A signal caused by preceding events and physical laws is called *deterministic*. This signal can be reproduced exactly and repeatedly. For example, when a pulse propagating through an elastic medium encounters a discontinuity such as a void or an inclusion, the resulting material and wave interaction produces a deterministic echo signal. Wave propagation, reflection, transmission and scattering are generally solved analytically or numerically using equations of elasticity.[12-16]

Random signals cannot be predicted precisely or reproduced exactly because they are determined only in a statistical sense. Information on the random process producing such signals can be obtained only by statistics. It is necessary to distinguish between two different types of random process.

1. Time based random signals, such as electrical noise, can be reduced by using higher quality electronic components, increased transmitter power or signal averaging. Signal averaging is done simply in digital systems where noise rejection on the order of 10 to 40 dB can be achieved by averaging 10 to 10 000 waveforms.

2. Spatially random signals such as grain scattering in polycrystalline materials and ceramics or fiber scattering in reinforced composites cannot be reduced by simple (time) averaging because they are coherent in the time domain (they are equally present in subsequent waveforms). The only way to reduce such random signals is to use spatial averaging (to repeat the measurements at slightly different locations or in different directions and to then average the detected waveforms).

Spatial averaging is more difficult, more time consuming and less effective than time averaging because the number of waveforms that can be averaged in this way is rather low. It is also very important to recognize that spatial noise is not necessarily an adverse effect. The source of this random signal is the heterogeneity of the test object and very often this signal conveys useful information on important material properties such as grain size, porosity or fiber orientation.

Information deduced from random ultrasonic signals can be interpreted only in terms of statistics. For instance, the average pore size and volume fraction can be determined for porous castings. Similarly, surface parameters, such as the root mean square roughness or the correlation length of the surface profile, can be determined as statistical averages. Examples of such spectroscopic applications are presented elsewhere.

Periodic versus Transient Signals

A deterministic signal is described as periodic if it repeats at regular time intervals of T_0. A signal is transient if it appears and then disappears within a short time period. Mathematically, a periodic signal $s(t)$ can be defined as:

$$(1) \quad s(t) = s(t - T_0)$$

that is, the amplitude of the signal at time t is the same as the amplitude at time $(t - T_0)$. A periodic signal can be written as a fourier series:

$$(2) \quad s(t) = \sum_{n=1}^{\infty} A_n \cos(n\omega_0 t + \phi_n)$$

where A_n is the amplitude of the nth harmonic, $n = 1, 2 \ldots$ and ϕ_n is the phase of the nth harmonic component.

The frequency content of a periodic signal is made of discrete individual frequencies nf_0 (Fig. 1b). The simplest form is a pure sine function whose frequency content is reduced to a single

frequency. The spectral representation of a transient signal is given by its fourier integral:

$$(3) \quad S(f) = \int_{-\infty}^{+\infty} s(t) e^{-j(2\pi f t)} dt$$

The variable f in the complex exponential exp $(-j2\pi ft)$ denotes the frequency and $S(f)$ is known as the *continuous time fourier transform*. This is a complex quantity that involves both amplitude and phase. As a result, the frequency content of a transient signal is expressed by a continuous spectrum (Fig. 1d) rather than a series of discrete spectrum lines (Fig. 1b). In a similar way, the time domain signal can be calculated from the spectral

FIGURE 1. Comparison of periodic square wave and square pulse: (a) square wave in time domain; (b) its frequency spectrum; (c) square pulse in time domain; (d) its frequency spectrum.

(a)

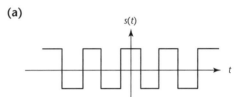

(b)

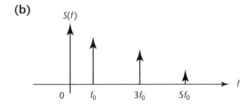

(c)

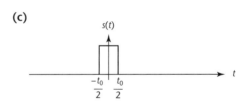

(d)

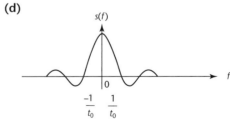

Legend
f = frequency
S = square wave
s = signal
t = time

representation by using the inverse fourier transform:

$$(4) \quad s(t) = \int_{-\infty}^{+\infty} S(f) e^{j(2\pi f t)} df$$

The $s(t)$ and $S(f)$ terms form the continuous time fourier transform pair. One of the most important features of this relation is that the duration of the transient signal t_0 is inversely proportional to the bandwidth of its spectrum. Generally, a short ultrasonic pulse contains a wide range of frequencies whereas a long pulse has a narrow spectrum. In this respect, the limiting case is called the *dirac impulse*. Here, the time duration t_0 of the pulse approaches zero while the amplitude approaches infinity. The spectrum of this function is flat, infinitely wide and independent of the

FIGURE 2. Comparison of delta function and sine wave: (a) dirac delta function; (b) its frequency spectrum; (c) continuous harmonic (sine) wave; (d) its frequency spectrum.

(a)

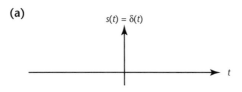

(b)

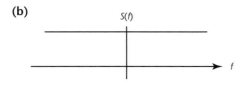

(c)

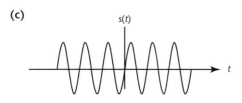

(d)

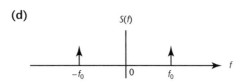

Legend
f = frequency
S = frequency spectrum
s = temporal signal
t = time

actual original pulse shape (rectangular, triangular, rounded). On the other hand, there is the pure harmonic sine wave of infinite duration (t_0 approaching infinite) whose spectrum is limited to a single frequency (Fig. 2).

Ultrasonic spectroscopy is the study of ultrasonic pulses through their fourier transforms. It is important to distinguish between broad band and narrow band techniques. Short ultrasonic pulses are needed to obtain continuous spectral information over a wide frequency range. Continuous or quasicontinuous, long tone bursts bring information over a narrow frequency band which has to be tuned over a wider range to obtain spectral characteristics. Ultrasonic spectroscopy based on broad band ultrasonic pulses takes advantage of the fact that the spectrum of the echo contains quantitative information about the target.[17]

The narrow band technique is advantageous for increasing the sensitivity of the system at one given frequency. However, the narrow band technique can be used to test frequency dependent properties only by (1) additional tuning of the transmitter and/or receiver frequencies and (2) repeating the same measurement over and over at different frequencies. This somewhat troublesome operation has to be used in situations where maximum sensitivity is required. For example, the narrow band technique is used during detection of lamb modes in heterogeneous plates by varying the angle of incidence at a single frequency[18] or during surface roughness tests by plotting the backscattered radiation pattern of a narrow band ultrasonic signal at different discrete frequencies.[19]

The major disadvantage of the narrow band technique is the extensive time consumed by collecting data at many frequencies. Broad band techniques bring information over a wide frequency range but at a loss of sensitivity.

Analog versus Digital Signals

An analog signal $s(t)$ is defined as a continuous function of time t. A digital signal $s[n]$ is a sequence of real or complex numbers defined for every integer n (discrete time signal), whose amplitude can take only a finite number of values. Therefore, digital signal processing deals with transformations of signals that are discrete in both amplitude and time. Because only such digital signals can be processed by a digital computer, it is important to know how they arise and what their features are with respect to the original physical phenomenon of interest.

Data Acquisition and Analog-to-Digital Conversion

Data in ultrasonic testing equipment are acquired by capturing the electric signals generated by transducers when detecting mechanical energies of the ultrasonic vibrations. The signal has a continuous form: conversion of an analog signal into a digital form is required for it to be processed by a computer. The conversion of an analog signal into a digital number is obtained by sampling the signal at discrete instants of time and digitizing the amplitudes in digital words (Fig. 3).

Sampling Procedures

Theoretically, the amplitude is sampled instantaneously at every point and the digital representation is infinitely accurate. In reality, however, the sampling is performed only at time intervals T and the amplitude is converted into binary codes of a limited number of digits. For a real valued, band limited signal $s(t)$ with maximum frequency f_M, the continuous time fourier transform is a symmetrical function with a total frequency bandwidth $2f_M$ (Fig. 4a). The sampled signal $s[n]$ can be described by multiplication of $s(t)$ with the sampling function $d(t)$:

$$(5) \quad d(t) = \sum_{n=-\infty}^{\infty} \delta(t - nT)$$

where T is the sampling interval and δ is the discrete delta function.

The discrete delta function is also known as the *kronecker delta function*:

$$(6) \quad \delta(t - nT) = \begin{cases} 1 & \text{when } t = nT \\ 0 & \text{when } t \neq nT \end{cases}$$

The fourier transform $D(f)$ of the sampling function $d(t)$ is also a sampling function:

$$(7) \quad D(f) = \frac{1}{T} \sum_{k=-\infty}^{\infty} \delta(f - kF)$$

where $F = T^{-1}$. The sampled signal $s[n]$ can be described as a weighted sum of discrete impulse functions:

$$(8) \quad s[n] = \sum_{n=-\infty}^{\infty} s(t) \delta(t - nT)$$

where $s(t)$ indicates the original continuous signal, and $s[n]$ indicates the sampled signal, noted by the rectangular brackets instead of the parentheses used for continuous functions.

By using the convolution theorem, the fourier transform of $s[n]$ can be written as the product of the fourier transforms of $s(t)$ and $\delta(t - nT)$:

$$(9) \quad S[k] = S(f) * D(f)$$
$$= \frac{1}{T} \sum_{k=-\infty}^{\infty} S(f - kF)$$

FIGURE 4. Effect of sampling in frequency domain: (a) original spectrum; (b) sampled spectrum when $F > 2f_M$; (c) sampled spectrum when $F < 2f_M$.

(a)
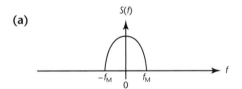

(b)
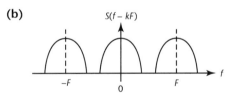

(c)
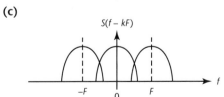

Legend
F = frequency separation
f = frequency
k = kronecker function
S = signal sample

FIGURE 3. Analog-to-digital conversion.

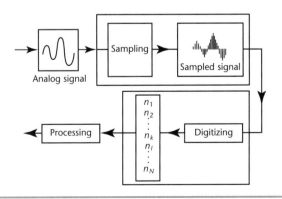

The discrete fourier transform $S[k]$ is a periodic replication of $S(f)$ with a frequency separation $F = T^{-1}$ (Fig. 4). Two special cases can be considered: for $F > 2f_M$ (Fig. 4b), there is no overlap and for $F < 2f_M$ (Fig. 4c), there is overlap between adjacent spectra, a phenomenon known as *aliasing*. The sampling frequency limit $F_N = 2f_M$, above which no overlap occurs, is known as the *nyquist frequency*. If the sampling frequency is higher than the nyquist frequency, the spectrum of the original signal can be easily recovered from its sampled form by a rectangular low pass filter (sampling theorem) as shown in Fig. 5. For lower values of the sampling frequency, the continuous signal cannot be recovered from its sampled form without distortions.

As a consequence of the sampling theorem, digital techniques cannot be applied rigorously to signals not band limited, because aliasing occurs no matter how small the sampling periods. In this case, however, a limited frequency range $(-f_M, f_M)$ is selected with a low pass filter so that most of the signal energy is included and the sampling frequency of F is at least $2f_M$ (Fig. 6). In practice, the digital-to-analog converter holds a value constant until receiving the next value. As a consequence, the resulting signal exhibits strong discontinuities that can be eliminated by a low pass filter (Fig. 7).

Digitization Procedures

The process that converts the series of sample amplitudes into a series of discrete numbers is known as *digitization* or *quantization*. The analog-to-digital converter is basically a quantizer that creates a binary code for each input sample. For an *n*-bit converter, there are 2^n discrete output codes. The conversion is an approximation because the value of the analog voltage has to be rounded to the nearest quantizer level.

The analog-to-digital conversion takes more time when higher resolution is

FIGURE 5. Recovering of original spectrum from its sampled form: (a) sampled spectrum; (b) transfer function of ideal low pass filter; (c) recovered spectrum.

(a)

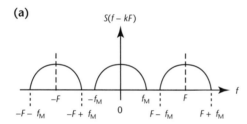

(b)

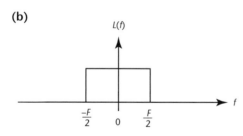

(c)

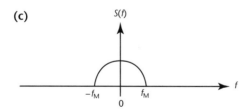

Legend
F = frequency separation
f = frequency
f_M = limited frequency
k = integer
L = lowpass filter
S = signal

FIGURE 6. Effect of antialiasing filter: (a) spectrum of original signal; (b) transfer function of antialiasing filter; (c) spectrum of filtered signal; (d) spectrum of sampled filter.

(a)

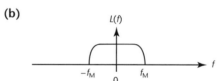

(b)

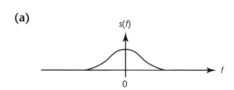

(c)

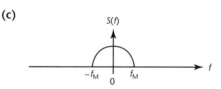

(d)

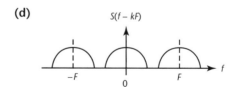

Legend
F = frequency separation
f = frequency
f_M = limited frequency
k = integer
L = lowpass filter
S = signal

required. Instruments can reach 12-bit to 14-bit resolution at 100 to 400 MHz sampling frequencies and higher. When working with nonrepetitive signals (in acoustic emission tests, for example), a compromise must be made between amplitude resolution and frequency bandwidth. In the case of repetitive signals (either periodic or transient), sampling of the waveform can be done over many periods by taking a different sample point from each repetition and then combining them into one sample series, a process called *interleaving*.

Gating Procedures

If several individual signals are present in the output of an ultrasonic system, one signal can be separated with a gate. This technique is used in the case of multiple reflections from a plate (Fig. 8) where only the reflection off the back face of the test object (face 2) has to be spectrum analyzed. Echo 2 is the only one selected for further signal processing.

The amplitude spectrum of a single complex waveform may change dramatically according to the specific part of the signal selected with a gate for data analysis.

According to the convolution theorem, the spectrum $S_g(f)$ of the gated signal $s(t)g(t)$ is the convolution of the fourier transform $S(f)$ of the time domain signal $s(t)$ and the fourier transform $G(f)$ of the gate function $g(t)$. That is, if:

$$(10) \quad s_g(t) = s(t) \cdot g(t)$$

then:

$$(11) \quad S_g(f) = S(f) * G(f)$$

Note that convolution is more complicated than multiplication and the gated spectrum $S_g(f)$ can be very different from $S(f)$. As an example, Fig. 9 shows the measured spectra of an ultrasonic echo at different gate positions. The most commonly used gate function is the square or rectangular function:

$$(12) \quad g_s(t) = \begin{cases} 1 & \text{at } t_0 - T < t < t_0 + T \\ 0 & \text{otherwise} \end{cases}$$

The fourier spectrum of this gate function is:

$$(13) \quad G_s(f) = 2T \frac{\sin 2\pi f T}{2\pi f T} e^{j(2\pi ft)}$$

FIGURE 7. Recovering the original signal from its sample form: (a) digital data; (b) sample-and-hold output of digital-to-analog converter; (c) filtered signal.

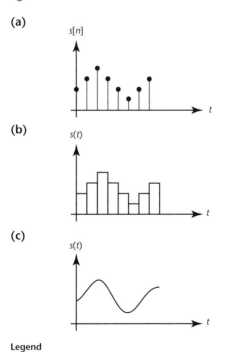

Legend
$s[n]$ = sampled signal
$s(t)$ = time domain signal
t = time

FIGURE 8. Multiple ultrasonic reflections from plate: (a) reflection diagram; (b) corresponding waveforms. Only echo 2 is selected for further signal processing.

(a)

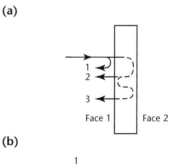

(b)

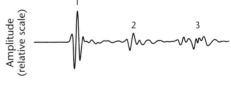

The square gate function and its fourier transform are shown in Fig. 10. For a very long gate (T approaching infinity), $G_s(f)$ becomes very narrow and the spectral distortion of the gating is negligible. On the other hand, short gating significantly modifies the detected spectrum. This effect can be substantially reduced by appropriate weighting techniques called *apodization*. Such options (von hann, hamming, flat top and blackman-harris) are available in most digital data acquisition systems as alternatives to the standard rectangular window.

The gating function can be realized by both analog and digital means. Analog gates are typically stepless. They offer continuously adjustable gating position and width in a number of ranges (see Table 1 for typical specifications). An analog gate often uses a double balanced mixer to turn the signal on and off. Switching times are on the order of 1 to 10 ns. Digital computers can similarly select only a well defined part of the digitized time signal, multiplying all the signal by zero except the part of interest. This time domain filter is sometimes called a *window*.

Signal Processing

To get relevant information from raw ultrasonic data, some transformations of the selected signal must be carried out. This so-called *signal processing* comprises many kinds of operations, including simple techniques commonly used in everyday nondestructive test practice, as well as more sophisticated techniques developed for research applications.

The first category includes the simple signal processing options available on many conventional ultrasonic discontinuity detectors: (1) analog filtering to match the spectrum of the detected ultrasonic signals to that of the receiving electronics so that the optimum signal-to-noise ratio can be ensured, (2) transducer damping to modify the transfer properties, especially the resonant

FIGURE 9. Different spectra of ultrasonic echo at different gate positions: (a) time domain; (b) frequency spectrum at gate 1; (c) frequency spectrum at gate 2.

(a)

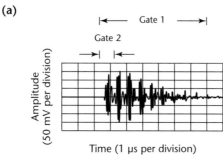

(b)

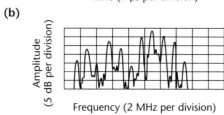

(c)

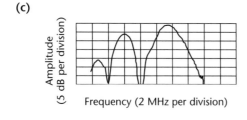

FIGURE 10. Gating: (a) signal; (b) frequency spectrum.

(a)

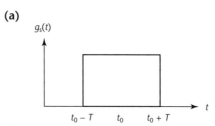

(b)

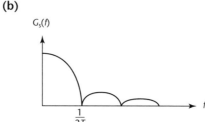

Legend
$G_s(f)$ = fourier spectrum of gate function
$g_s(t)$ = gate function
T = time increment
t = time

TABLE 1. Specifications of typical stepless gate.

Characteristic	Quantity
Gate delay	0.1 to 200 μs
Gate width	0.1 to 200 μs
Blanking delay	3 to 100 μs
Gate input level	± 0.6 V peak
Gate bandwidth	0.5 to 50 MHz
Isolation	46 dB at 30 MHz

behavior, of the transducer, (3) pulse shaping and smoothing of the demodulated signal to optimize the detectability of discontinuities, (4) clipping the signal below a certain threshold value to eliminate noise and (5) automatic volume control to compensate for loss of sensitivity at increasing depth caused by beam divergence or attenuation in the material.

The text below discusses some of the signal processing techniques made available by the advances in microelectronics and the hardware and software components of digital computers. These processing techniques include data averaging, autocorrelation and cross correlation, convolution and deconvolution. Such capabilities offer significant improvements in the test results.

Averaging Procedures

The ensemble average (or mean value) $\bar{x}$ of a series of observations is a weighted sum over all N individual values $x_i(t)$ of these observations:

$$(14) \quad \bar{x} \;=\; \sum_{i=1}^{N} P_i \, x_i(t)$$

where P_i denotes the probability of occurrence of the particular value $x_i(t)$:

$$(15) \quad P_i \;=\; \frac{n_i}{N}$$

For repetitive stationary signals, summed averaging consists of repeated addition with equal weights ($P_i = N^{-1}$) of recurrence of the source waveform. Both time domain and frequency domain averaging are used to improve the received signal. Averaging reinforces the significant signal while random noise is smoothed. Time dependent electrical noise is reduced by averaging several signals taken at the same location. Spatial noise produced by scattering heterogeneities in the test object (roughness, coarse grains and so on) is reduced by scanning the object and averaging signals coming from different locations. Spatial averaging, because it involves part of the surface larger than the acoustic beam, causes a loss of spatial resolution. In some cases, angular scanning can be used.

Autocorrelation and Cross Correlation

Autocorrelation is a process that compares the function $x(t)$ at the time t with its value at the time $t - \tau$. The mathematical expression that relates the data at two different times for a large number N of observations is known as the *coefficient of correlation*. For a stationary process, the autocorrelation coefficient is:

$$(16) \quad C_{xx}(\tau) \;=\; \frac{1}{N} \sum_{k=1}^{N} x(t_k) x(t_k - \tau)$$

The autocorrelation coefficient reaches its local maxima at particular τ values when the analyzed signal $x(t)$ is strongly correlated, that is, very similar to its shifted form $x(t - \tau)$ delayed by τ. Measuring the autocorrelation function is especially useful for determining the periodicity of distorted or noisy quasiperiodic signals where conventional overlapping is too uncertain. Principal applications include precision velocity and dimension measurements, especially in heterogeneous objects.

Unlike autocorrelation, which involves the same signal at two different times, cross correlation characterizes the relationship of one signal at instant t with another signal at instant $t - \tau$. The cross correlation coefficient is:

$$(17) \quad C_{xy}(\tau) \;=\; \frac{1}{N} \sum_{k=1}^{N} x(t_k) y(t_k - \tau)$$

The cross correlation coefficient reaches its local maxima at particular values needed to shift $y(t)$ so that it is similar to $x(t)$. Measuring the cross correlation function is especially useful in determining the exact time delay between similar, but distorted, noisy signals. In particular, cross correlation is often used to eliminate jitter (random time uncertainty in the arrival of quasiperiodic signals) before averaging these signals. This adverse jitter effect can be eliminated by determining the shift of each waveform, with respect to a reference, from the maximum of their cross correlation and compensating for this random delay so that each signal can be added at the right position.[20]

Another application of correlation measurement is found in the ultrasonic characterization of surface topography. Periodic machine marks and other surface corrugations may be hidden in the dominantly random surface roughness so that even a precise profilometer is unable to reveal the regular feature. The autocorrelation function of the recorded profile exhibits maxima regularly spaced with the period of the profile whereas random background is smoothed.[21]

On the other hand, autocorrelation functions of backscattered signals from coarse grains in stainless steel do not show any particular peaks.[22] Grain size assessment based on the possible periodicity of the grain structure fails because the polycrystalline microstructure is irregular. Several spectroscopic techniques can measure grain size accurately.

Signal Filtering

Filtering is the process of modifying the frequency spectrum of the signal by suppressing certain frequency components. The filter can be low pass, high pass, bandpass, bandstop or may have some other more specific transfer function. In a mathematical sense, filtering is equivalent to the multiplication of the frequency spectrum $S(f)$ by $H(f)$ (Fig. 11):

$$(18) \quad S_h(f) = S(f) \cdot H(f)$$

An important consequence of frequency filtering is the modification of the filtered time domain signal $s_h(t)$. According to the convolution theorem, multiplication in the frequency domain is the same as convolution in the time domain:

$$(19) \quad s_h(t) = s(t) * h(t)$$
$$= \int_0^t s(\tau) h(t - \tau) d\tau$$

Where $h(t)$ is the inverse fourier transform of the filter's transfer function $H(f)$ and $s(t)$ is the unfiltered signal. The inverse fourier transform $h(t)$ is also called the *impulse function* because it corresponds to the output signal of the filter when it is driven by a very sharp input pulse of a flat frequency spectrum. Figure 12 shows the impulse function of the rectangular bandpass filter of Fig. 11. The mathematical form of this signal is:

$$(20) \quad h(t) = 2f_1 \frac{\sin(2\pi f_1 t)}{2\pi f_1 t} e^{j(2\pi f_0 t)}$$

This impulse function is not physically feasible because it exists for $t < 0$ (it violates the law of causality by producing an output signal before the appearance of the input excitation). Real filters have smooth transitions between passbands and stopbands and their impulse functions are time limited. Figure 13 shows the transfer and impulse functions of a typical bandpass filter used in nondestructive test applications to optimize detection sensitivity.

FIGURE 11. Steps of signal filtering: (a) input spectrum; (b) transfer function of ideal bandpass filter; (c) filtered spectrum.

(a)

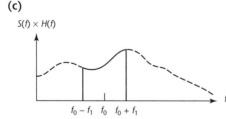

(b)

(c)

Legend
f = frequency
$H(f)$ = filter
S = frequency spectrum

FIGURE 12. Impulse function of ideal bandpass filter with center frequency f_0.

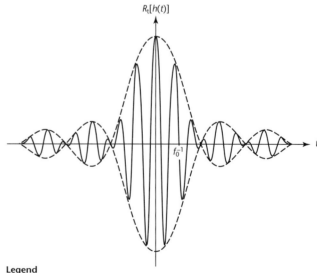

Legend
f = frequency
$h(t)$ = filter
R_t = impulse function
t = time

In ultrasonic testing, the frequency dependence of the attenuation in some materials can also be regarded as a filtering effect. The transfer function of the material is used to evaluate physical and geometrical properties of the medium. Ultrasonic spectroscopy has proven effective in a wide range of applications, including grain size measurement in polycrystalline materials,[23] characterization of surface breaking cracks,[24] surface roughness,[21] porosity assessment in castings[25] and composites.[26]

Convolution and Deconvolution

A typical ultrasonic system includes a great number of components, most notably the test object, the transmitting and receiving transducers, the pulser, the receiver amplifier, matching and coupling elements and some sort of signal processing and display. Figure 14 shows a linear, time invariant system made from these components.

Although this system can be described by the convolution of the individual impulse functions in the time domain, it is much more convenient to deal with the product of the individual transfer functions in the frequency domain, which can be easily determined by spectrum analysis. Notice that for most of the components the signal of interest is an electrical waveform. However, for an important section of the system, the relevant signal is an ultrasonic wave propagating through a coupling medium and the test material.

The detected signal $s(t)$ is the convolution of the input signal $e(t)$ and the impulse function of the system, which includes the test instrument $h(t)$ and the test medium $p(t)$:

$$(21) \quad s(t) = e(t) * h(t) * p(t)$$

Although $s(t)$ is the measured quantity, the information of interest is included in $p(t)$. The aim of deconvolution is to remove the nonideal system characteristics from the significant part needed for further evaluation of the test object. To achieve this, the output signal $s_0(t)$ of the same system must be recorded without the test object. This signal is called the *reference signal* and establishing it as a fundamental requirement before using such systems. A diagram of this procedure is shown in Fig. 14:

$$(22) \quad s_0(t) = e(t) * h(t)$$

By taking advantage of the associative property of the convolution product:

$$(23) \quad s(t) = s_0(t) * p(t)$$

The mathematical process that gives $p(t)$ from $s_0(t)$ and $s(t)$ is called the *operation of deconvolution*. The operation can be done much more easily in the frequency domain than in the time domain because Eq. 23 can be rewritten as the simple product of the corresponding fourier spectra:

$$(24) \quad S(f) = S_0(f) \cdot P(f)$$

FIGURE 13. Bandpass filter typical in ultrasonic testing: (a) transfer function; (b) impulse function.

(a)

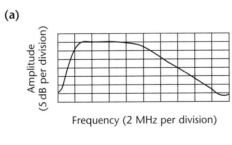

Frequency (2 MHz per division)

(b)

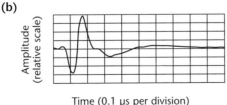

Time (0.1 μs per division)

FIGURE 14. Response of ultrasonic test system: (a) medium tested with instrument; (b) medium replaced by reference response of system; (c) rearranging; (d) impulse response of system.

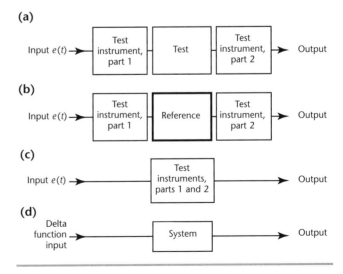

Deconvolution then can be achieved by simple division:

$$(25) \quad P(f) = \frac{S(f)}{S_0(f)}$$

Most often, the spectra of the detected signals are calculated in logarithmic scale and deconvolution is carried out in the frequency domain by subtracting $S_0(f)$ from $S(f)$. Such an operation is commonly used in ultrasonic spectrum analysis to eliminate the response of the transducer and the associated electronics. This so-called *normalization* of the spectrum is a simplified and very effective means of deconvolution because the logarithmic scale is applied only to the amplitude; the phase information is lost.

A typical example of such normalization is shown in Fig. 15. The spectrum of the normally reflected signal from a perfectly smooth surface made of the same material as the test object is taken as a reference (Fig. 15a). The amplitude spectrum of a reflected signal from a periodic profile at the interface between solid and air is shown in Fig. 15b. The deconvolution or normalization procedure (the ratio between the spectra of Figs. 15a and 15b) removes the nonideal system characteristics from the reflected amplitude spectrum. Deconvolved, the amplitude spectrum (Fig. 15c) is suitable for comparison with analytical results.

Smoothing

Smoothing of a waveform reduces the high frequency noise superimposed on the signal. This simple technique can effectively suppress both time based and spatial noise at the cost of reduced resolution. Each sample point in the raw data $\ell(k)$ is replaced by $\ell'(k)$ in the smoothed waveform:

$$(26) \quad \ell'k = \sum_{p=-\frac{N-1}{2}}^{\frac{N-1}{2}} \alpha(p)\,\ell(k+p)$$

where $\alpha(p)$ is a weighting factor dependent on the particular smoothing algorithm used. The N term is an even integer denoting the total number of

FIGURE 15. Primary steps in deconvolution process: (a) reference spectrum; (b) reflection spectrum from periodic surface; (c) normalized spectrum.

FIGURE 16. Ultrasonic tests of fiber reinforced composite plate: (a) backscattering spectrum at 0.42 rad (24 deg) angle of incidence and 1.5 rad (90 deg) azimuthal angle; (b) superimposition of seventeen spectra taken at different locations.[27]

(a)

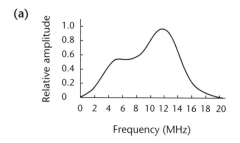

(b)

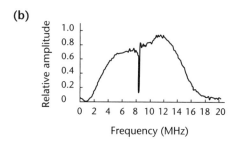

(c)

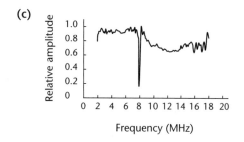

(a)

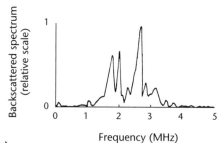

(b)

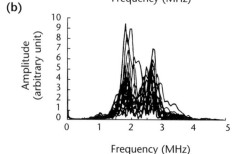

averaged sample points (the length of the smoothing). The weighting factor must always be chosen to satisfy Eq. 27 so that smoothing can be done without gain or loss to signal amplitude:

$$(27) \quad \sum_{p=-\frac{N-1}{2}}^{\frac{N-1}{2}} \alpha(p) = 1$$

The simplest version is the one with constant weighting, when $\alpha = N^{-1}$.

For an example of using smoothing as part of a complex signal processing program, consider the measurement of elastic properties in thin composite plate from backscattered signals.[27] Figure 16a shows the frequency spectrum of the backscattered signal from a fiber reinforced epoxy composite laminate at a single point. Apparently, the sharp peaks are caused by scattering from inherent heterogeneities rather than by lamb modes sought in the plate.

Figure 16b verifies this by showing the superposition of seventeen spectra taken at different locations. In the first step, spatial averaging is applied to reduce this strong scattering background, then smoothing is used to get rid of the remaining noise. Figure 17a shows the processed signal after averaging the

spectra shown in Fig. 16b and normalization by the transducer's response. Finally, Fig. 17b shows the smoothed signal exhibiting well defined maxima corresponding to lamb resonances in the composite plate. These resonances can be used for quantitative assessment of elasticity.

Storage and Presentation

The last step in data analysis is to save the information arising from signal processing for further analysis and archiving. Data are generally stored with computers. For short term storage and a limited amount of data, random access memory is the fastest. It is used for intermediate calculations and quick comparisons such as normalization. Long term storage has to be done on tape, optical disk or other storage medium that saves more data. This information can be used later in other environments with compatible systems.

The purpose of data presentation is to display the final test results in a way that illustrates the behavior of the parameters of interest. The display can be a table of numerical values printed on paper or a curve from a terminal plotter or an oscilloscope monitor. Because the data to be displayed are available in digital form, the computer's display and hard copy capabilities are typically used.

FIGURE 17. Backscattered ultrasonic spectra of Fig. 16: (a) after spatial averaging; (b) after smoothening.[27]

(a)

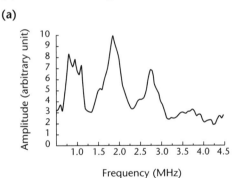

(b)

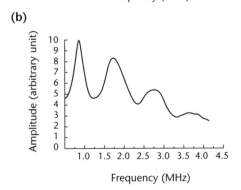

Part 2. Ultrasonic Spectroscopy

The purpose of ultrasonic spectroscopy is to determine the frequency dependent properties of a test object. These might be of geometrical origin (layer thickness, discontinuity size, shape, orientation) or inherently frequency dependent material properties (attenuation and velocity dispersion). The frequency dependent quantity is usually connected to some microscopic geometrical property, such as grain size in polycrystalline materials or fiber diameter and ply thickness in composite plates but exceptions can occur. For instance, frequency dependent absorption depends on nongeometrical material properties such as viscosity, thermal conductivity and relaxation.

Presented below are the components used to build an ultrasonic spectroscopy system. Each element of the system is treated separately, examples of a complete instrument are given and overall system performance is discussed.[28]

System Model

Although there are many possible designs for an ultrasonic spectrum analysis system, each contains provision for (1) generating ultrasound, (2) receiving a portion of the ultrasound that has interacted with the test material and (3) analyzing the received wave to determine its magnitude (and sometimes phase) at a number of frequencies. Figure 18 shows the components of a typical spectroscopic system.

FIGURE 18. Main components of typical ultrasonic spectroscopy system.[17]

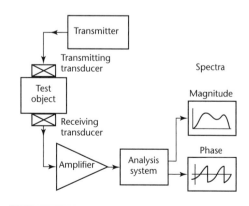

In this system configuration, an electrical waveform generated by the transmitter is applied to the transmitting transducer. Conversion of the electrical energy into mechanical energy occurs within the transducer, producing an ultrasonic wave. As the wave propagates through the test material, interactions of the ultrasonic energy with the material alter the amplitude, phase and direction of the wave. A receiving transducer intercepts a portion of the ultrasonic energy and converts it from mechanical to electrical energy. Because the electrical signal is usually small, an amplifier is used to increase its amplitude. The purpose of the analysis system, which follows the amplifier, is to sort out the signals

FIGURE 19. Elements of ultrasonic spectroscopic system modeled as linear, time invariant system.[17]

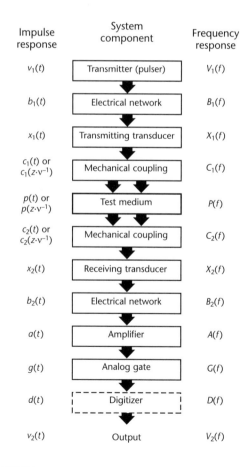

Impulse response	System component	Frequency response
$v_1(t)$	Transmitter (pulser)	$V_1(f)$
$b_1(t)$	Electrical network	$B_1(f)$
$x_1(t)$	Transmitting transducer	$X_1(f)$
$c_1(t)$ or $c_1(z \cdot v^{-1})$	Mechanical coupling	$C_1(f)$
$p(t)$ or $p(z \cdot v^{-1})$	Test medium	$P(f)$
$c_2(t)$ or $c_2(z \cdot v^{-1})$	Mechanical coupling	$C_2(f)$
$x_2(t)$	Receiving transducer	$X_2(f)$
$b_2(t)$	Electrical network	$B_2(f)$
$a(t)$	Amplifier	$A(f)$
$g(t)$	Analog gate	$G(f)$
$d(t)$	Digitizer	$D(f)$
$v_2(t)$	Output	$V_2(f)$

characteristic to the ultrasonic interactions within the material and to present their amplitude and phase spectra.

The behavior of a linear, time invariant system is completely described by its impulse response (in the time domain) or its frequency response (in the frequency domain). The two descriptions of system response are equivalent and are linked by the continuous time fourier transform pair (Eqs. 3 and 4). Figure 19 shows the block diagram of an ultrasonic spectroscope modeled as a linear, time invariant system. Although the impulse response is important, ultrasonic tests deal almost entirely with frequency responses because frequency is the relevant parameter in spectral analysis.

In general, the time domain representation of the signal is monitored. The analysis subsystem provides the transformation to the frequency domain. Distance is the natural selection of the independent variable through system components where an ultrasonic wave propagates. Distance can be used instead of units of time if wave velocity is known. System components in which ultrasonic waves propagate are shown with impulse responses in terms of time varying quantities and distance.

Transmitter

The ultrasonic system transmitter produces an electrical waveform of sufficient amplitude to excite the transmitting transducer. The wave shape (and frequency content) produced by the transmitter in an ultrasonic spectroscopic system is controlled by the electrical circuitry. The time and frequency domain representations of several ideal and realizable transmitter wave shapes are given in Figs. 20 and 21.

Pulsed systems require an electrical waveform containing a wide range of frequencies. An instantaneous voltage spike of infinite amplitude contains uniform magnitude of all frequencies. Such a waveform (called the *dirac delta function*) cannot be realized but pulses

FIGURE 20. Representations of commonly used waveforms: (a) sine wave; (b) rectangle waveform; (c) triangle waveform; (d) cosine.

(a)

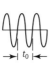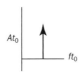

(b)

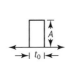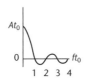

(c)

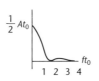

(d)

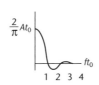

Legend
A = amplitude
f = frequency
t = time

FIGURE 21. Representations of commonly used waveforms: (a) cosine squared; (b) exponential; (c) unit step; (d) dirac delta; (e) sine burst.

(a)

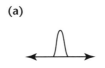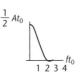

(b)

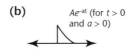

(c)

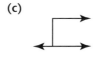

(d)

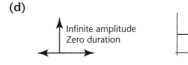

(e)

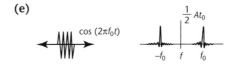

having very short duration and large amplitudes can be produced.

A cosine squared pulse has a bandwidth greater than that of a rectangular pulse with the same duration t_0. However, the circuitry required to produce this signal is more complex. A step pulse with a single transition is attractive because of superior range resolution and the large bandwidth. The bandwidth and transition time of the step are related:

$$(28) \quad B \approx \frac{1}{2t_r}$$

where B is the signal bandwidth (megahertz) and t_r is the transition time of the step (microsecond). For instance, for a transition time of 5 ns, the pulse has a bandwidth of 100 MHz.

A common procedure for pulsing an ultrasonic transducer is to momentarily connect it to a high voltage supply and then let it return to zero. This type of pulse is a unit step with an exponential decay. Transducer excitation occurs only during the transition of the excitation pulse with no appreciable excitation during the exponential decay.

In the continuous wave system, the transmitter ideally produces a single frequency. For cases in which the sinusoid exists for a finite length of time, the frequency domain representation includes more than a single frequency. This type of waveform is represented as a sine wave modulated by a rectangular envelope. In those spectroscopic systems that emit tone bursts, the effect of varying the width of the rectangular envelope should be examined. Figure 22 and Table 2 show the effect of width variation on the frequency content of a sinusoidal burst. The width of the main frequency lobe increases as the length of the rectangular modulating waveform decreases and is independent of the sine wave frequency. The advantages of a narrow frequency output have to be considered against the poor range resolution of a pulse with long time duration.

Pulser waveforms of shapes other than sinusoids (square waves or step transitions) can be obtained by a digital pulse generator. The arbitrary shape of the pulse can be designed by a computer.

Electrical Coupling Network

The electrical waveform produced by the transmitter must be coupled from the transmitter to the transducer. Whether this coupling is as simple as a coaxial cable or as complex as a compensating filter, it has a substantial effect on the ultrasonic spectrum. The main purpose of electrical coupling is to provide good electrical matching between the transmitter electronics and the ultrasonic transducer. In spectroscopic applications, matching is either used to obtain a wider bandwidth or to optimize the sensitivity in a particular frequency range.

TABLE 2. Effect of sinusoid pulse duration on spectrum (see Fig. 22).

Cycles in Burst (quantity)	Main Lobe Width (f_0)
1	2.0
2	1.0
3	0.667
4	0.5
5	0.4
6	0.333
7	0.286
8	0.25
9	0.222
10	0.2
11	0.182
12	0.167
13	0.154
14	0.143
15	0.133
16	0.125
20	0.1
50	0.04
100	0.02

FIGURE 22. Effect of sinusoid pulse duration on ultrasonic spectrum: (a) sine burst; (b) pulsed.[17]

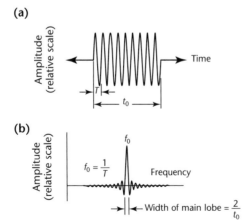

(a)

(b)

Legend
f = frequency
T = time period
t = temporal variable

Ultrasonic Coupling

The effect of a material intervening between the transducer face and the region of interest in the test object is considered below. The important mechanisms of ultrasonic interaction with the material include those giving rise to frequency dependent phase changes (dispersion) and amplitude losses (attenuation). For ultrasonic testing of bulk material properties, such as attenuation or velocity, there is usually a single coupling layer between the transmitting transducer and the material. When a region is tested for discontinuities, the effects of the material between the transducer and the region of interest must be considered as part of the transducer coupling.

In the case of contact testing, a thin layer of liquid is interposed between the transducer and the test object. Immersion testing, on the other hand, is carried out with a much longer ultrasonic path in the liquid coupling medium. The analysis of this complex problem (transducer, coupling medium, test object) must take into account (1) the reflections at both boundaries, (2) attenuation in the coupling layer, (3) delay time of the pulse traveling through the liquid medium and (4) the effect of possible reverberations in the couplant.

System Amplifier

Electrical signals produced by a receiving transducer are low in amplitude. Signal processing electronics require higher voltages so an amplifier is often incorporated into an ultrasonic test system. The gain of the device is given by:

$$(29) \quad A(f) = \frac{V_o}{V_i}$$

Where V_i is the input voltage and V_o is the output voltage. The gain is a complex quantity having a frequency response with phase and amplitude variations.

In addition to the importance of gain and bandwidth, several other characteristics of the amplifier should be considered, including the dynamic range. This is the range of signal amplitudes (from the equivalent noise to the largest signal at the input) that may be amplified without distortion. The dynamic range must be sufficiently wide to cover all anticipated signals.

Consideration should be given to the possibility of using a logarithmic stage for dynamic range compression. Additionally, the output voltage swing of the amplifier should be within the linear range of the following system components. Also, linearity of the amplifier should be stringent enough to ensure that, for a given frequency, the gain is independent of the amplitude of the signal input from the receiving transducer.

Analog Gate

Spectrum analyzers operate on the entire signal input to them. If several discrete pulses are present in the waveform, the spectrum presented by the analyzer is that of the complete ensemble. The spectrum of an individual pulse or a certain part of the waveform can be determined after appropriate gating. Whenever the separation is not distinct enough, gating the waveform cuts into the useful signal and significant distortion of the measured spectrum might occur.

Spectrum Analyzer

Analog Spectrum Analyzers

The simplest analog device for extracting the amplitude of a frequency component is a bandpass filter tuned to the frequency of interest. Ideally, only the center frequency passes through the filter but such an ideal bandpass filter cannot be manufactured. Real devices made of passive or active components have a passband spreading over a small range of frequencies. If the measured signal contains other frequencies adjacent to the center frequency (within the passband), the filter output includes contributions of these nearby frequencies. Although not ideal, very selective filters are available. If there is interest in more than a single frequency, a bank of bandpass filters could be used, each tuned to a different frequency. An alternative is to use a single filter whose center frequency can be swept over a range of frequencies.

Network Analyzers

Spectrum analyzers are used to measure the frequency content of the detected signal to determine the transfer function of the system under study. This is done by applying a given, preferably broad band, excitation to the system and analyzing the changes in its spectrum resulting from interactions with the system.

The same purpose can be achieved by using a narrow band harmonic excitation such as continuous or quasicontinuous tone bursts and then measuring the amplitude (and possibly the phase) of the output signal as the transmitter frequency is swept over the desired frequency range.

Often, the receiver is also tuned parallel to the transmitter to further increase the signal-to-noise ratio. Such so-called *network analyzers* are especially useful in characterizing highly attenuative materials where their superior sensitivity is most needed.

Digital Spectrum Analyzers

Digital techniques are used in spectrum analysis. The fast fourier transform algorithm is used almost exclusively for performing the fourier transformation. It combines high resolution with high computational speed by eliminating the repeated calculation of redundant coefficients.[29-31] The main steps of transforming the received signal $v_2(t)$ into its frequency domain equivalent $V_2(f)$ are shown in Fig. 23. Signal $v_2(t)$ is sampled at intervals t_s forming the series $v_2[n]$. The N data points in this array are processed by the fast fourier transform algorithm to yield a set of N complex numbers that are the real and imaginary parts of the frequency components $V_2[nf_s]$. The magnitude and phase spectra are then calculated from these complex numbers.

Notice that the spectrum from $(N/2)f_s$ to $(N-1)f_s$ is a mirror image of the spectrum in the range f_s to $(N/2)f_s$. That is, the spectrum is folded about the point $(N/2)f_s$. Spectral folding arises from sampling of the signal. To avoid spectral distortions caused by overlapping of different parts of the spectrum, antialiasing filters are used to ensure that the sampled signal has no significant spectral components above half of the sampling frequency. The nyquist frequency is discussed elsewhere.

A useful way to increase frequency domain resolution without changing the sampling rate is to increase the sample size N. The sampled data occupy part of the array while the remaining positions in the array are filled with zeroes. It is easiest to let the actual data occupy the first part of the array (Fig. 24). Shifting the data points in the array leaves the magnitude of the spectrum unchanged but adds a linear term to the frequency dependent phase. To eliminate the disturbing variation of the phase spectrum caused by this effect, the relative delay of the signal with respect to the window should be minimal.

The most common solution is to center the signal around the beginning of the window where the relative time delay is zero. The left part of the signal is cut off in this way but appears in the right end of the window (Fig. 25). It is important to remember that the effect of the technique just described to increase the resolution by padding the array with zeros is merely a process of interpolation: it does not add data to the plot.

Most digital spectrum analyzers facilitate further signal processing operations to determine the transfer

FIGURE 23. Determination of frequency spectrum of time domain signal by using fast fourier transform.[17]

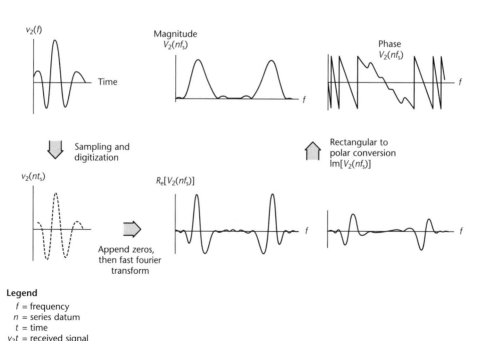

Legend
f = frequency
n = series datum
t = time
v_2t = received signal
V_2f = signal equivalent in frequency domain

function and impulse response of linear, time invariant systems. Fast fourier transforms convert the measured time series into frequency components where convolution becomes a multiplication operation and deconvolution becomes a division operation.

Additional Analysis Techniques

Multiple Signals

Several other techniques have been found useful for analyzing ultrasonic testing signals. One involves analysis of two separate signals (two ultrasonic echoes) fourier transformed as an ensemble.[32,33] The magnitude spectrum of two identical signals separated in time by Δt is:

$$(30) \quad \left|S(f)\right| = \left|2\cos\left(\pi f \Delta t\right)\right|\left|Y(f)\right|$$

where $Y(f)$ is the fourier transform of one echo. If the two echoes are gated into a spectrum analyzer, the envelope of the spectrum is identical to that for a single echo but the spectrum is modulated. The spacing of the frequency minima Δf may

be used to determine the time separation of the ultrasonic echoes Δt:

$$(31) \quad \Delta f = \frac{1}{\Delta t}$$

If the ultrasonic velocity is known, the thickness of the material between the reflectors can be found. When Δt is small, the signals overlap and a wide bandwidth spectrum analyzer is needed because Δf is large.

For two ultrasonic echoes, one modified by frequency dependent attenuation $k(f)$, the spectrum is given by:

$$(32) \quad \left|S(f)\right| = \left\{\left[1-k(f)\right]^2 \right.$$
$$\left. + \; 4k(f)\cos^2\left(\pi f \Delta t\right)\right\}^{\frac{1}{2}}$$
$$\times \; \left|Y(f)\right|$$

The spectrum is similar to that for the two identical echoes except the minima do not reach zero. Equating the modulation in a measured spectrum to that predicted from Eq. 32 allows the attenuation to be determined. In addition to measurement of $k(f)$, acoustic

---

FIGURE 24. Signal at beginning of data record: (a) time domain signal; (b) magnitude spectrum; (c) phase spectrum.[17]

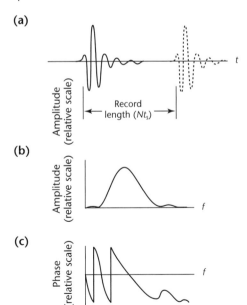

(a)

(b)

(c)

Legend
----- = assumed periodicity outside data record
f = frequency
N = sample size
t = signal duration

FIGURE 25. Signal split between beginning and end of data record: (a) time domain signal; (b) magnitude spectrum; (c) phase spectrum.[17]

(a)

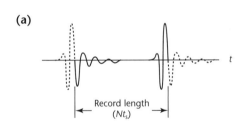

(b)

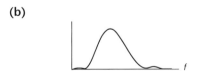

(c)

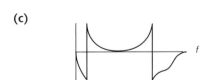

Legend
----- = assumed periodicity outside data record
f = frequency
N = sample size
t = signal duration

impedance measurement through analysis of phase shift at boundaries has also been verified.[33]

Cepstrum Processing

Returning to the spectral modulation produced as a result of placing two signals within the data window, note that the variation is periodic. The modulation frequency can be determined by performing a fourier transform on the logarithm of the amplitude spectrum, which is called a *power cepstrum.*

The cepstrum of repeated (quasiperiodic) signals exhibits distinct maxima corresponding to the time separation between the individual pulses.[34] In some cases, transforming the linear amplitude spectrum instead of the logarithmic spectrum results in better noise rejection.[35] Cepstral processing can be carried out by analog techniques.[36] An analog implementation requires two spectrum analyzers. The first forms the logarithmic spectrum while the second measures the cepstrum from the vertical output of the first.

Maximum Entropy and Maximum Likelihood Spectrum Analysis

When performing analysis using the fast fourier transform, the frequency domain resolution may be improved by appending zeros to the data record before transformation. However, processing time increases as the record is lengthened. Several alternate techniques have been developed for spectral estimation to achieve improved frequency resolution.

These techniques, maximum entropy and maximum likelihood, are useful when the available data record is short and the signal is contaminated by noise. The methods are data adaptive — when an estimate is being made at one frequency, the methods adjust themselves to be least affected by all other frequencies.

Short Time Fourier Transform

The standard fourier transform is only localized in frequency, not in time. It does not give information on the time at which a frequency component occurred.

The short time fourier transform (also known as *short term fourier transform*) addresses the localization issue by multiplying the signal by a window function that is nonzero only in its middle. This window is being moved along the signal, and at each point another fourier transform is calculated. The result is a two-dimension representation of signal, time and frequency.

The continuous short term fourier transform can be expressed as:

$$(33) \quad S_{STFT}(\tau, f) = \int_{-\infty}^{\infty} s(t) w(t - \tau) \times e^{-j(2\pi f t)} dt$$

where $w(t)$ is the window function, $s(t)$ is the signal to be transformed and τ is the shift of the window function. See Eq. 3 for comparison with the simple fourier transform. There is of course a matching inverse, short time fourier transform as well as a discrete short term fourier transform. The magnitude squared of the short term fourier transform gives the spectrogram of the function.

A limitation of the short term fourier transform is its fixed resolution. Selecting the width of the window function influence the results of the transform. A narrow window yields good time resolution but poor frequency resolution and vice verse.[37]

Wavelet Transform

Spectrum analysis involves representing the signal in terms of its harmonic components. The fourier transform is used to calculate these components. The continuous fourier transform is used to calculate the continuous spectrum of a continuous signal. When signal is digitized, the discrete fourier transform is used, usually with an effective algorithm known as *fast fourier transform.* It was noted earlier that when analyzing transient signals, as the case in most ultrasonic tests, the bandwidth of the spectrum is inversely proportional to the duration of the signal because a transient signal is being described as a sum of infinitely long harmonic waves. Furthermore, as noted above. the standard fourier transform is only localized in frequency, not in time. It does not give information on the time at which a frequency component occurred.

The wavelet transform addresses both issues. Instead of being represented in term of harmonic components, the signal is represented in term of assembly of a finite length waves. The base wave is called the *mother wavelet*, and a series of waves (daughter wavelets) is constructed from it by scaling (sometimes called the *father wavelet*) and translation. These components can be constructed to be orthonormal to each other as with a fourier series. The terms *continuous wavelet transform, discrete wavelet transform* and *fast wavelet transform* are used here too, as with the fourier transform.

One of the basic sets of wavelets was defined by Daubechies.[38] Daubechies orthogonal wavelets D2 to D20, where the number represents the number of coefficients, are commonly used. An example of the D20 wavelet function and scaling function is shown in Fig. 26. Extensive mathematical discussion is beyond the scope of this handbook.[39] Ultrasonic applications of the wavelet transform has been demonstrated.[40,41] In one case,[41] three types of mother wavelets were tested: daubechies D40, symlet wavelet of order 8, and coiflet wavelet of order 1 (Fig. 27). It was found that better success was achieved when the mother wavelet resembled the original ultrasonic wave. The symlet wavelet of order 8 was appropriate when single pulse generated the ultrasonic wave, while the daubechies D40 was appropriate when the ultrasonic waves were generated by a burst. The wavelet transform has been used for filtering, improving the ratio of signal to noise, as well as to extract features from complex signals.[40-42]

FIGURE 26. Daubechies D20 wavelet.

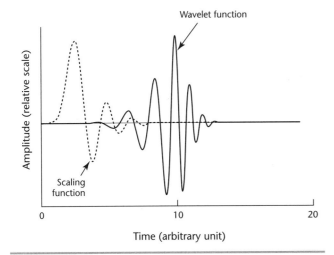

FIGURE 27. Mother wavelets: (a) daubechies wavelet of order 40; (b) symlet wavelet of order 8; (c) coiflet wavelet of order 1 amplitude given in arbitrary unit.[41]

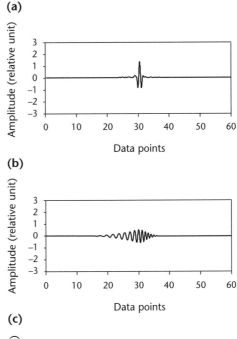

(a)

(b)

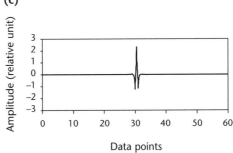

(c)

Part 3. Recognition Principles in Ultrasonic Testing

Defining Pattern Recognition

Automatic pattern recognition presents a challenge to the development of signal classification and image analysis in ultrasonic testing. Mimicking an experienced ultrasonic weld inspector, for example, is more difficult and more detailed than first imagined. The human eye perceives many facts simultaneously and by feedback moves a transducer in infinite increments in three dimensions over time to seek out additional, necessary information — the mind sorts and processes the accumulated real time facts and combines them with empirical data from experience and case history before making a final decision about a specific situation. It is knowledge of this complex procedure that leads to the development of an expert automated testing system. Specialized procedures and software are used to implement data collection and decision protocol so that operators anywhere can use the expertise of the industry's best operators.

Image analysis is another surprisingly complex procedure — a trained and experienced operator perceives many things and draws many conclusions from a radiograph or a B-scan ultrasonic image. Other operators can be trained to achieve the same results but it is much more difficult to establish automated image analysis procedures.

First, the visual data must be converted by specialized hardware or software to establish effective decision criteria. A fundamental concern is to establish what is known as a *good feature,* a particular observation of some critical signal or image characteristic.

Once good features are selected, a choice must be made for various data manipulation and analysis procedures that are based on adaptive learning networks, pattern recognition procedures or neural networks. These procedures mimic the decision mechanisms associated with the human brain. Some very basic pattern recognition techniques are outlined below to illustrate the kind of thinking and analysis needed to implement a decision rule for ultrasonic testing. Detailed treatments of pattern recognition are available in the literature.[43,44]

Early Signature Techniques

Ultrasonic signature analysis has been studied since the early 1960s.[45,46] Pattern recognition is the discipline that attempts to objectively evaluate ultrasonic test signatures. A signature can be obtained as a time domain profile or a frequency profile and the concept can be used in unique applications. In one novel technique, ultrasonic signatures of various structures were used to identify test objects.[47]

During the 1970s, another signature analysis study made use of 23 simulated discontinuities in stainless steel.[48] Using specially designed data collection procedures along with digital signal processing and pattern recognition, a discontinuity characterization algorithm was developed that could identify all the discontinuities 100 percent of the time. Compared to later advances, this study may seem elementary but up to that time ultrasonic analysis could identify and differentiate only the most basic planar versus volumetric discontinuities and then only with very special training for specific applications.

Pattern recognition was used to solve this problem, along with the development of a physical model of mode conversion related to discontinuity sharpness. Some signal averaging was also needed and the early, theoretical work was followed by tests of real discontinuities in a variety of structures.

Another early study of pattern recognition in discontinuity characterization selected special features of the radio frequency waveform. Using a two-space scatter diagram, the study established a decision surface that provided a useful discontinuity classification algorithm for separating critical from noncritical reflectors in stainless steel piping.[49] Even though feature selection was the most critical step, the value of pattern recognition was clearly demonstrated in learning and implementation.

Other pioneering work in conversion of an ultrasonic signature into a decision algorithm used adaptive learning networks. Initial learning machine analysis illustrates the analytical process of decision algorithm development.[50,51]

Role of Pattern Recognition

There is no substitute for good data acquisition based on the physics and the mechanics of wave propagation. Early work in pattern recognition fully exploited the normal beam longitudinal wave procedure for composite material or adhesive bond testing. Sometimes, angle beam radio frequency waveforms were selected from an area of interest with emphasis on beam coverage or accessibility from geometrical constraints. Little concern was placed on different sensitivities of the various mode possibilities or on the physics of wave propagation.

It was found that a combination of features, either physically or statistically based, could lead to failure or the development of an unreliable decision algorithm. Simple solutions could come from using higher frequencies or a different wave mode; from understanding the possible anisotropy, heterogeneity or the stressed state of the structure; or from using oblique incidence to alter the particle velocity vibration direction to an interface.

Once a promising procedure is discovered and refined in the laboratory, pattern recognition is a research aid and an implementation device for practical ultrasonic testing. Pattern recognition can also help clarify or categorize data and can indicate the need for improved data acquisition.

Feature Vectors

A *feature* is the characteristic of a waveform that causes dimensional reduction of an original data set but still preserves significant information about the data set. A feature can be physically based, a physical model of a reflector, for example, that points out special reflection characteristics of pulse preservation, pulse spreading, reduction in pulse rise time, a gradient of reflection factor as a function of angle, a reflected amplitude ratio, arrival time of a particular mode, shifting of a dispersion curve and so on.

A feature can also be statistically based when formulated as the area under a video envelope of a radio frequency waveform, a mean value, the center frequency of a power spectrum, skewness of a waveform or kurtosis. All features must have carefully prepared definitions

and thresholds so that automated feature extraction and pattern recognition can take place. All features are defined from feature sources.

Feature Sources

Many feature sources can be taken from normal beam incidence longitudinal or transverse wave response functions as well as from oblique incidence longitudinal, vertical or horizontal transverse waves or from surface or lamb waves. Wave velocities, skewing angles and a multitude of features can be defined and extracted from these feature sources. Imagination and physical or statistical insights can generate additional feature sources and produce carefully defined, useful features.

Selection of the feature list is one of the most critical elements in pattern recognition. A short, carefully selected list

FIGURE 28. Possible features used in ultrasonic tests of welds: (a) acquired radiofrequency waveform; (b) rectified waveform; (c) video envelope and feature definition.

(a)

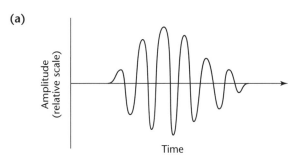

(b)

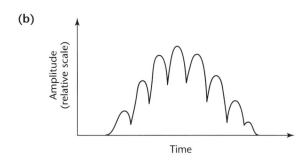

(c)

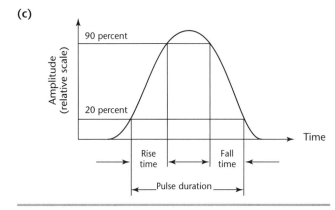

can easily outperform a long random list of features.

For clarification, consider two feature sources and a few possible feature definitions. The first is a radio frequency waveform feature source in the time domain (Fig. 28). Specific features of rise time, pulse duration and fall time can be easily defined once a reasonable video envelope computation procedure is selected. Threshold selection of 20 percent and 90 percent should be based on experience, the amounts of random and material noise and so on. The second feature source is an experimentally generated dispersion profile (Fig. 29). Theoretical modeling of porosity in this case predicted mode shifting as a function of porosity. A reasonable feature for this application is to take an average fd value over the phase velocity range of 6 to 8 mm·μs^{-1} for modes 1, 2 and 3 and also for other porosity values. This feature alone can solve the porosity problem.

Image analysis feature sources include the following: time domain profiles of a radiofrequency waveform; power spectrum in the frequency domain of the signal; analytical spectrum in the frequency domain of the signal; phase angle in the frequency domain of the radiofrequency signal; echo dynamic profiles obtained through motion of the transducer toward and away from the discontinuity; transfer function domain using the initial pulse of the transducer as the reference; reflection factor profiles as a function of angle; dispersion curve profiles; B-scan image; C-scan image; F-scan image. Of these image analysis feature sources, a variety of techniques

can be used in feature definition. One of the most popular is a histogram profile of the gray scale levels in a certain area or along a certain straight line through the image. Note that a feature source in scene or image analysis could be a feature itself, something other than the popular amplitude or amplitude ratio in what might be called a *feature map*. The feature map could be of velocities, areas under certain portions of a power spectrum profile and so on.

Feature Dependence

From a theoretical modeling point of view, it may appear that features selected from a feature source could actually depend on each other. For ultrasonic testing applications, the goal is to first find as many independent features as possible for solving a particular problem. Because precise physical modeling of a reflector and a structure is never possible, feature selection pointing to feature redundancy can be useful.

Theoretical modeling establishes a guideline for data collection, possible feature analysis and thresholds. Variations in feature definition and selection applied to realistic experimental data helps account for multiple discontinuities, material noise and nonlinearities.

Data Structure

Hundreds of techniques are available for examining natural data clustering and modifications for decision rule development. A few of the most popular procedures are outlined below.

Probability Density Function Analysis

Probability density function curves are widely used in feature selection and decision algorithm development.[43-53] There are many possibilities based on histogram distributions of the number of occurrences versus a particular feature bin value.

In the parzen window approach, the beginning operation is an arrangement of the feature data into numerical order. The statistics of minimum, maximum, range, mean, median, mode and variance are then calculated and used as a basis for judgment parameters that might occur.

There is a probability P that a feature assumes a value f between f_1 and f_2:

$$(34) \quad P(f_1 \leq f \leq f_2) = \int_{f_1}^{f_2} p(f) df$$

FIGURE 29. Porosity studies of graphite epoxy composite, showing experimental confirmation of sensitivity to porosity change from 0 to 2 percent along fibers using 1 MHz broad band transducer. Plate modes shift to the left and sensitivity increases with the fd value.

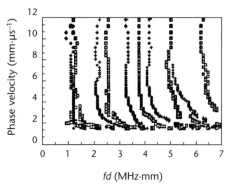

Legend
▫ = porosity change of 0 percent
✦ = porosity change of 2 percent

where $p(f)$ is the probability density function for f. Assuming that $p(f)$ does not change appreciably between f_1 and f_2 (that is, if $f_1 - f_2$ is small):

(35) $\quad P(f_1 \leq f \leq f_2) \cong (f_2 - f_1) p(f)$

Defining Δf as $f_{i+1} - f_i$, Eq. 35 may be written as:

(36) $\quad P(f_1 \leq f \leq f_2) \sim \Delta f\, p(f)$

One way to estimate $P(f_1 \leq f \leq f_2)$ is to count k, the number of samples falling within Δf, and to divide this by the total number n of samples:

(37) $\quad P(f_1 \leq f \leq f_2) \sim \left(\dfrac{k}{n}\right), \epsilon\left[f_i, f_{i+1}\right]$

This leads to:

(38) $\quad \dfrac{k}{n} \sim \Delta f\, p(f)$

or:

(39) $\quad p(f) \sim \dfrac{k_n}{n \Delta f}$

The relationship shows $p(f)$ to be a function of n, the number of samples. Note that k is also a function of n, as is the interval length Δf. The following considerations make this clear. If Δf is too wide, too many values appear in it, producing a smoothed or averaged version of $p(f)$. On the other hand, if Δf is too small, the estimate of $p(f)$ is uncertain. The number of samples counted as belonging to a particular interval depends on the interval size Δf. Therefore, $p(f)$ can be written as:

(40) $\quad p_n(f) = \dfrac{k}{n \Delta f_n}$

The interval Δf_n should decrease as n gets larger. The desired behavior is:

(41) $\quad \lim_{n \to \infty} \Delta f_n = 0$

where:

(42) $\quad \lim_{n \to \infty} k_n = \infty$

and:

(43) $\quad \lim_{n \to \infty} \dfrac{k_n}{n} = 0$

The parzen window approach replaces k_n with a window function $\phi(f)$ that depends on the sample data and on the interval size.

When $|y| \leq 0.5$, the function used is:

(44) $\quad \phi(y) = 1$

otherwise:

(45) $\quad \phi(y) = 0$

where:

(46) $\quad y = \dfrac{f - f_i}{\Delta f_n} = \dfrac{f - f_i}{h_1}$

The h_1 term is a parameter estimated on the basis of the previously calculated statistics (range, mean and so on).

Now $P_n(f)$ may be written as:

(47) $\quad P_n(f) = \dfrac{1}{n \Delta f_n} \sum_{i=1}^{1} \phi \dfrac{f - f_i}{\Delta f_n}$

and:

(48) $\quad k_n = \sum_{i=1}^{n} \phi \dfrac{f - f_i}{\Delta f_n}$

Suppose that substantial amounts of test data are available, providing a long list of radio frequency signals versus some classification value, the classification value being related to either a class 1 or class 2 characteristic. Features should now be extracted from the ultrasonic radio frequency display. As many as a hundred features, for instance, could be studied for their use in correlating a combination of signal features with a classification value.

Each feature could be examined on a probability density function curve such as the one in Fig. 30. Feature 1, for example, is useless in this sample problem (there is no differentiation capability of that feature). Features 2 and 3 are limited in their capability for classifying the problem as either class 1 or 2. Note that feature 4, possibly the center frequency of the reflected signal, provides a clearer differentiation between class 1 and 2. Feature 5 provides an excellent feature for differentiating the two classes with 100 percent reliability.

The probability density function curves provide insight into the difficulties associated with classification problems in pattern recognition. If results similar to those for feature 5 occur, the solution to the problem is complete. If different results occur, it is often desirable to examine space scattering diagrams or even sorting logic procedures based on feature values in the probability density function curves.

Space Scattering Diagrams

After probability density function analysis, it is often useful to plot one feature against another. The result is known as a *two-space scatter diagram or a two-space plot*. The purpose of the plot is to determine if there is any natural clustering of the data. Often, solutions to the decision surface formulation problems can be found by estimating a curve that separates the clusters in a desired fashion, with the selection based on the desired algorithm index of performance. The performance of two-space scatter diagram analysis can be represented by characteristics known as *sensitivity,*

FIGURE 30. Sample probability density function curves for typical two-class classification problem: (a) feature 1 (poor feature); (b) feature 2; (c) feature 3; (d) feature 4; (e) feature 5 (excellent feature).

Number
of times

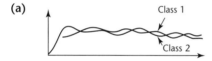
(a)

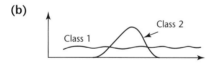
(b)

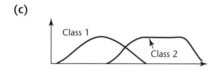
(c)

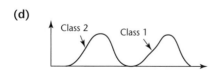
(d)

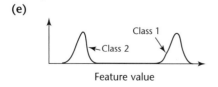
(e)

Feature value

specificity and *false alarm*. Sensitivity is defined as the ability to detect class 1 population. Specificity is defined as the ability to detect class 2 population. False alarm is the indication of a false percentage of critical discontinuities.

A feature space with N dimensions has $0.5\ N(N-1)$ two-space plots associated with it. Even when a decision surface cannot be reliably derived from these plots, they are useful as guides for the selection of useful features. The N space feature data can be projected into a two-space plot by premultiplying the feature vectors by a $2 \times N$ weight matrix:

$$(49) \quad [W]_{2\times N} \cdot [f]_N = [X]_2$$

The components of [W] scale the coordinates of the feature vector, allowing manipulation of the projected values. There are ways to find that [W], in a sense, optimizes the cluster characteristics of the projected two-space plot.

By plotting feature 1 versus feature 2 in two-dimensional space, the promise for obtaining a reasonable solution exists if data clustering occurs. A cluster may be shaped like a ball, ring or string. Combinations of two-dimensional profiles should be plotted for all promising feature types, as indicated by the probability density function analysis. If the cluster situation in two-dimensional feature space is not useful, it is then necessary to use more sophisticated algorithm analyses from pattern recognition.

Clustering

Clustering is a process in which a set of data is organized into groups that have strong internal similarity. The object of clustering procedures is to find natural groupings of the data under study. Many of the algorithms used to perform clustering are intuitive. When a clustering procedure is first considered, particular attention must be given to the goal of finding the natural structure of the data rather than imposing a structure on the data.

Necessary to all algorithms for clustering are measures of likeness or similarity, topics contained in standard textbooks on pattern recognition. Also required is a criterion for defining a cluster. This may be a heuristic method or a minimization (maximization) concept based on a performance index. One of the most popular criteria is the minimization of the sum of squared errors:

$$(50) \quad C = \sum_{j=1}^{N_c} \sum_{X \in S_j} \|x - m_j\|^2$$

where m_j is the mean of the vectors in the jth cluster, N_C is the number of clusters and S_j is the set of vectors in the cluster j. By varying the number of clusters and their membership, a combination is sought that minimizes C.

An example of a heuristic algorithm is the maximum distance algorithm. The first step in this algorithm is to find those two points that are farthest apart. These are defined as cluster centers, say C_1 and C_2. As in most heuristic clustering algorithms, a decision threshold must define cluster inclusion. If a point whose distance from a particular cluster center exceeds this threshold, it is defined as a new cluster center. If not, it is added to that cluster from which its distance is most below the threshold. The threshold used here is a percentage of the average distances between existing cluster centers. The illustration here uses 0.5 as the intercluster average distance:

$$(51) \quad T_1 = 0.5 \frac{D_{C_1, C_2}}{2}$$

where D is distance and T is threshold.

Next the distances of the remaining points from C_1 and C_2 are calculated. At the next step, the minimum of these two distances is saved along with the cluster involved in obtaining the minimum value. The maximum of this list of minima is then obtained and compared with threshold 1. If it is less than threshold 1, the point is included in the cluster to which it is closest and the original cluster center is modified to be the mean of itself and the new member. Otherwise, a new cluster center is defined.

Assume that a center C_3 is formed, that C_3 is the vector whose distance from C_1 or C_2 was the maximum of the minimum distances and that its distance exceeded threshold 1. A second threshold is now computed:

$$(52) \quad T_2 = 0.5 \frac{D_{C_1, C_2, C_3}}{3}$$

where D is distance, where $C_1 \ldots C_N$ is the $0.5\, N(N-1)$ distances between cluster centers and where T is threshold. For example, the distance algorithm being used is distance (C_1, C_2, C_3) or the sum of $d(C_1, C_2)$, $d(C_1, C_3)$ and $d(C_2, C_3) \cdot d(u,v)$.

The procedure is continued until no new cluster centers are formed. It can be seen that the selection of the threshold is critical to the determination of the number of clusters and their relative density. A low value yields many clusters varying from a single point to a cluster with a high density of points. A high value leads to a lesser number of clusters with relatively low average point density. This problem is similar to the estimation of interval size for calculating probability density curves.

The generated cluster topology can be used to aid in selecting the type of algorithm, the number of classes to consider and so forth. Cluster analysis is particularly useful for the production of synthetic data.

Distance Measures

Before implementing certain pattern recognition routines, a distance measure must be defined. Distances are used to determine the degree of similarity between vectors or patterns.

The nature of the pattern space is an important consideration with respect to selecting a particular distance measure. Computational efficiency is also another important factor. Some of the more popular measures are euclidean distance:

$$(53) \quad D = \sqrt{\sum_{i=1}^{q} (U_i - V_i)^2}$$

where q = dimension of the space, U_i is a component of the vector U and V_i is a component of the vector V.

If r is even, the minkowski distance r is:

$$(54) \quad D = \left[\sum_{i=1}^{q} (U_i - V_i)^r \right]^{\frac{1}{r}}$$

and the manhattan distance is:

$$(55) \quad D = \sum_{i=1}^{q} |U_i - V_i|$$

and the square distance is:

$$(56) \quad D = \max_{i=1,q} \{ |U_i - V_i| \}$$

and the octagonal distance is:

$$(57) \quad D = \sum_{i=1,q} |U_i - V_i| + \sqrt{q} \max_{i=1,\ldots,q} |U_i - V_i|$$

Fuzzy Logic

Fuzzy logic is a term used to denote a form of sequential decision making. The process is sequential if a definite decision may based on a limited amount of information or call for more information.

Features are ranked according to some measure of their discriminating power. Feature 1 is the first feature because it has the smallest overlap or fuzzy area in the sense of probability density function curves. Definite decisions can be made on either side of the overlap interval. The data falling in the fuzzy region could possibly represent 10 percent of the values that occur. Therefore 90 percent of the occurring population could be classified at this first step. If feature 1 has values in the fuzzy area, more information would be needed to make a decision. Feature 2 would now be considered for more information. Decisions are made on the nonfuzzy areas of feature 2.

The decision at this stage may account for 70 percent of possible feature 2 values. In that case, 70 percent of the original 10 percent undecided is now classified. Using the two features allows classification (Fig. 31).

Linear Discriminants

A class of functions widely used in decision algorithm development is composed of linear discriminants. These are weighted linear combinations of feature values. The general form is shown below:

$$(58) \quad y = w_0 + w_1 x_1 + w_2 x_2 + \ldots + w_N x_N$$

or:

$$(59) \quad D = w^t x + w_0$$

FIGURE 31. Sorting algorithm for bond quality assessment.

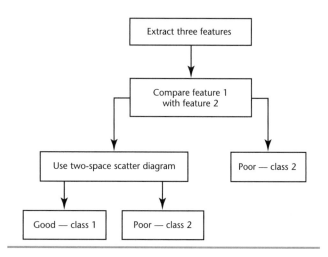

where w is the weighting coefficient, w_0 is the scalar weighting factor and x is the feature vector. Decisions are based on whether or not the value y exceeds a given threshold. The goal of linear discriminant analysis is to establish a criterion and a way to determine the weights that separate the data into a desired class structure.

The fisher linear discriminant is a popular function. One of the major problems encountered in pattern recognition is the vastness of the feature space. Procedures that are analytically and computationally manageable in low dimensional space become impractical in higher dimensional space. An ideal space is the one-dimensional space represented by a straight line. The advantage of a fisher linear discriminant is that it projects all of the data from an N-dimensional space onto the best line for separating the data. Once the data have been projected onto the line, a threshold value may be selected that divides the data into two classes. Thus the fisher linear discriminant is ideally suited to a two-class problem.

The simplest way to project an N-dimensional space onto a line is by forming a dot product:

$$(60) \quad [w_1, w_2, \ldots, w_N] \cdot \begin{bmatrix} x_1 \\ x_2 \\ \vdots \\ x_N \end{bmatrix} =$$

$$\sum_{i=1}^{N} w_i x_i = y$$

This also may be written as:

$$(61) \quad y = w^t x$$

Consider a set of K samples (vectors) divided into two classes, C_1 and C_2 with N_1 samples and N_2 samples where ($K = N_1 + N_2$). If the samples fall into two intermingling clusters, the result desired is that the clusters be shrunk and their means well separated. Another way of expressing this is to say that the difference of projected means is to be maximized and the scatter within each cluster is to be minimized. Figure 32a shows an arbitrary projection; Fig. 32b shows the projection using the fisher algorithm. Note the increased separation between the projected means and reduced scatter.

Minimum Distance Classifier

The minimum distance classifier is a mathematical algorithm that compares a test feature vector with average or prototype class vectors by way of a distance measure. Finally, a classification is made to the prototype closest to the test vector.

In minimum distance classifying, X is typically a feature vector with n components and P_i is a prototype vector from class i. A feature vector is generally representative of a particular class of vectors.

Prototype vectors are models — good representatives of a particular group or class of vectors. As an example, feature vectors may be obtained from ultrasonic signals coming from class 1, class 2, class 3 and so on. The class 1 vectors are grouped, the class 2 vectors are grouped and so forth. Each grouping may have a

FIGURE 32. Two-space plots showing fisher linear discriminant concept: (a) arbitrary projection; (b) fisher determined projection.

(a)

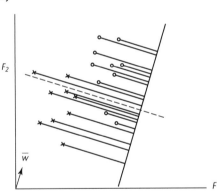

(b)

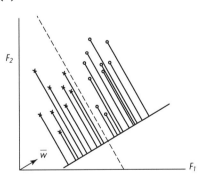

Legend
F_1 = fisher feature class 1
F_2 = fisher feature class 2
$\overline{w}$ = average weight

characteristic vector — a good estimation of what to expect from that class. The vector may be decided by testing or by a predetermined rule. The rule may use the mean vector, the median vector and so on.

A measure of similarity is needed for comparison between unknown vectors X and prototype vectors P_i. The euclidean distance between X and P_i is given by:

$$(62) \quad |X - P_i|^2 = X \cdot X - 2 \cdot X \cdot P_i + P_i \cdot P_i$$
$$= X \cdot X - 2 \cdot \left(X \cdot P_i - \frac{1}{2} P_i \cdot P_i \right)$$

The distance $|X - P_i|^2$ is a minimum when the term $(X \cdot P_i - 0.5\, P_i \cdot P_i)$ is a maximum. For the two-class case:

$$(63) \quad G(x) = G_1(x) - G_2(x)$$
$$= w^t x + w_0$$

with:

$$(64) \quad w^t = w_1^t - w_2^t$$

and:

$$(65) \quad w_0 = w_{01} - w_{02}$$

The decision rule is now simply that, if $G(x) > 0$, then x is in class 1 and that, if $G(x) \leq 0$, then x is in class 2. The concept can be extended to an in-class problem. The final form of $G(x)$ is characteristic of a class of functions known as *linear discriminant functions*. The fisher discriminant discussed above is also of this form. Discriminants may be differentiated by the manner in which the weights w^t and w_0 are determined.

Multiclass Problems

Multidiscriminant Analysis

Many times, problems arise where there are more than two classes. One way to solve these problems is by dichotomy: define class 1 as one particular set and class 2 as the collection of the $N - 1$ remaining classes, if there are N classes. After finding the discriminant that separates classes 1 and 2, class 2 is divided into two classes, class 1′ and class 2′, with class 2′ containing $N - 2$ sets. This process requires $N - 1$ discriminants for N classes. It should be a division that yields the highest index of performance. Errors at the first level of dichotomy are propagated into the lower levels, yet aside from this deficiency, this technique is often used when the initial levels have performance indices near 100 percent.

An alternative approach called *multiple discriminant analysis* is also possible. This technique projects from an N-dimensional space to a $(C - 1)$-dimensional space, where C is the number of classes and N is the dimension of the feature vectors involved. Other possibilities certainly exist.

Polynomial Discriminants

There are two techniques for the generation of nonlinear or polynomial discriminant functions. Both techniques involve the generation of pseudofeatures or features that are combinations of each other. The typical approach is to form the following combinations given two features f_i and f_j: $f_i \cdot f_j$ and f_j^2. This formulation results in a discriminant of the form:

$$(66) \quad d_{ij} = w_0 + w_1 f_i + w_2 f_j + w_3 f_{ij}$$
$$+ \ w_4 f_i^2 + w_5 f_j^2$$

One technique for determining the weight w_k is to generate the $0.5\ N(N - 1)$ data points. The $0.5\ N(N - 1)$ discriminants d_{ij} are then calculated using the fisher technique. Of these discriminants, those that perform the best are studied further whereas the others are discarded. The discriminants d_{ij} that were saved can be treated as features. Assume d_{12} and d_{23} were kept, then the discriminant d_{123} can be formed as:

$$(67) \quad d_{123} = w_0 + w_1 d_{12} + w_2 d_{23}$$
$$+ \ w_3 d_{12} \cdot d_{23} + w_4 d_{12}^2 + w_5 d_{23}^2$$

This is a fourth degree multinomial in x_1, x_2 and x_3.

Rather than using a fisher algorithm (maximizing the between-class scatter to within class scatter ratio), a least mean square criterion may also be used. Many additional procedures are being developed and are detailed in the literature on pattern recognition, expert systems, artificial intelligence and neural networks.[53-61]

Feature Mapping

The goal of a feature mapping technique or a decision technique is to go beyond the direct acoustical imaging modalities using amplitude in traditional B-scan or C-scan work. For a more physically based approach, tomographic arrival time and phase information may also be used. Such an approach uses feature mapping or feature imaging to outline feature changes, anomalies in materials or overall material characteristics.

The motivation behind the development of the feature mapping technique is that each anomaly or material interacts with an ultrasonic wave mode in a special way and this information can be extracted from the ultrasonic response through a detailed analysis of the signal. This analysis often produces a image useful for further analysis. It may also provide a final decision on material type and a decision image consisting of the decision rule as a function of several features. The exact amplitude, arrival time and phase information may not always be essential during anomaly identification in feature mapping. All of the items associated with pattern recognition and feature definition can be used in a feature map system.[62]

Neural Networks

As mentioned earlier, one tool used for pattern recognition, classification and decision uses an artificial neural network. This technique tries to mimic the decision mechanism associated with the human brain. It is composed of a large number of highly interconnected processing units — neurons. A biological neuron may have 10 000 different inputs and may send its output to several other neurons. Artificial neural networks try to mimic this capability but in a much simplified settings. For a particular neuron i, a collection of input data x_i are fed into it after being multiplied by weight function w_{ij}. The sum (Eq. 68), together with an optional bias value b_i yields v_i (Eq. 69) and is evaluated by an activation function h_i that decides on the output y_i:

$$(68) \quad u_i = \sum_{j=1}^{N} w_{ij} x_j$$

$$(69) \quad v_i = b_i + u_i = b_i + \sum_{j=1}^{N} w_{ij} x_j$$
$$= \sum_{j=0}^{N} w_{ij} x_j$$

$$(70) \quad y_i = h(v_i)$$

The neural network can be arranged with various level of topological complexity. An example of a multilayered network with one hidden layer can be seen in Fig. 33.[63] The network operates in two modes.

1. First, in the learning mode, the neural network is configured to perform its task by using a learning process. Adjusting the synapses, the connections between the neurons, changes the influence of one neuron on another. In a supervised network, the synapses are updated during the training to minimize the square mean error function, implying that the difference between the desired output and the obtained output should be reduced to a value that satisfies the determinate error threshold.[64] Thus, the network is trained to associate known outputs with input patterns.

2. Later, the network operates in the usage mode. It identifies the input pattern and tries to output the associated output pattern. If the input pattern is not identical to one of the taught inputs, the network gives an output that corresponds to the least different taught input. The ability to learn by example and generalize the learned information is the main attraction of the artificial neural network.

Spectral Analysis

Spectral analysis comprises a family of techniques that have been used to characterize discontinuities and to answer questions about material properties including surface roughness, strength, fracture toughness, velocity dispersion and bond quality. Spectra are measured for a range of frequencies. Because the sensor is in a fixed position, spectral analysis is not favored for discontinuity location or sizing. Spectral analysis is discussed in more detail elsewhere.[1,65-67]

Closing

There has been rapid development of the signal processing and data analysis techniques used in nondestructive testing. The primary purpose of these techniques is to enhance significant features of received signals and to facilitate the acquisition and evaluation of large data bases.

The driving forces behind the continuing development of data analysis are (1) the increasing need for automation and (2) the need to evaluate new materials and joining techniques. Developments result from the increased sophistication of digital computers and software packages. Emphasis on discontinuity detection and characterization in the twentieth century has shifted toward materials microstructure characterization and bond testing in the twenty-first.

FIGURE 33. Schematic of multilayer feed forward error back propagation artificial neural network. Parameters are given as input x_i to the neural network and as output z_k (discontinuity depth is computed continuously), where $[y_j = \sum w_1(i,j)x_i]$ and the sigmoidal function effects $f(x) = 1/(1+e^{-x})$.[63]

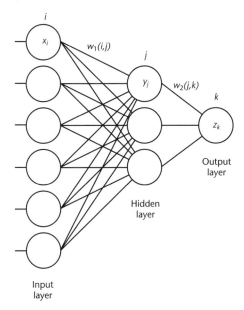

Legend
i,j,k = serial integers
w = weight function
x = input value
y = intermediate
z = output value

References

1. Adler, L., A. Jungman, P.B. Nagy and J.L. Rose. Section 6, "Waveform and Data Analysis Techniques." *Nondestructive Testing Handbook,* second edition: Vol. 7, *Ultrasonic Testing.* Columbus, OH: American Society for Nondestructive Testing (1991): p 131-185.
2. Benjamin, R. "Modulation." *Resolution and Signal Processing in Radar, Sonar and Related Systems.* Elmsford, NY: Pergamon (1966).
3. Luthi, B.P. *Signals, Systems and Communication.* New York, NY: Wiley (1967).
4. Simpson, R.S. and R.C. Houts. *Fundamentals of Analog and Digital Communication Systems.* Boston, MA: Allyn and Bacon (1971).
5. Goodyear, C.C. *Signals and Information.* London, United Kingdom: Butterworth (1971).
6. Roden, M.S. *Analog and Digital Communication Systems,* fourth edition. New York, NY: Pergamon (1996).
7. Lynn, P.A. *An Introduction to the Analysis and Processing of Signals.* London, United Kingdom: Macmillan (1973).
8. Srinath, M.D. and P.K. Rajasekaran. *An Introduction to Statistical Signal Processing with Applications.* New York, NY: Wiley (1979).
9. Urkowitz, H. *Signal Theory and Random Process.* Dedham, MA: Artech House (1983).
10. Orfanidis, S.J. *Optimum Signal Processing: An Introduction,* second edition. New York, NY: MacMillan (1988).
11. Bracewell, R.N. *The Fourier Transformation and Its Applications,* third edition. New York, NY: McGraw Hill (1999).
12. Love, A.E.H. *The Mathematical Theory of Elasticity,* fourth edition. New York, NY: Dover (1944).
13. Strutt, J.W. [Lord Rayleigh]. *The Theory of Sound.* Vols. 1 and 2. New York, NY: Dover (1877, 1965).
14. Schoch, A. "Schallreflexion, Schallbreihung und Schallbengung." *Ergebnisse der Exakten Naturwissenschaften.* Vol. 23. Berlin, Germany: Springer (1950).
15. Achenbach, J.D. *Wave Propagation in Elastic Solids.* Amsterdam, Netherlands: Elsevier Science Publishers (1984, 1999).
16. Morse, P.M. and K.U. Ingard. *Theoretical Acoustics.* Princeton, NJ: Princeton University Press (1968, 1986).
17. Fitting, D. and L. Adler. *Ultrasonic Spectral Analysis for Nondestructive Evaluation.* New York, NY: Springer (1981).
18. De Billy, M., L. Adler and G. Quentin. "Measurements of Backscattered Leaky Lamb Waves in Plates." *Journal of the Acoustical Society of America.* Vol. 75. Melville, NY: American Institute of Physics, for the Acoustical Society of America (1968): p 998.
19. De Billy, M., J. Doucet and G. Quentin. "Angular Dependence of the Backscattered Intensity of Acoustic Waves from Rough Surfaces." *Ultrasonics International.* Guilford, United Kingdom: IPC Science and Technology Press (1975): p 218.
20. Fink, M., F. Cancre, C. Soufflet and D. Beudon. "Attenuation Estimation and Speckle Reduction with Random Phase Transducers." *Proceedings of the Ultrasonics Symposium.* New York, NY: Institute of Electrical and Electronics Engineers (1987): p 951.
21. De Billy, M., F. Cohen-Tenoudji, A. Jungman and G. Quentin. "The Possibility of Assigning a Signature to Rough Surfaces Using Ultrasonic Backscattering Diagrams." *Transactions on Sonics and Ultrasonics.* SU-23(5). New York, NY: Institute of Electrical and Electronics Engineers (1976): p 356.
22. Saiie, J. and N.M. Bilgutay. "Quantitative Grain Size Evaluation Using Ultrasonic Backscattered Echoes." *Journal of the Acoustical Society of America.* Vol. 80. Melville, NY: American Institute of Physics, for the Acoustical Society of America (1986): p 1816.
23. Goebbels, K. "Structure Analysis by Scattered Ultrasonic Radiation." *Research Techniques in Nondestructive Testing.* Vol. 4. New York, NY: Academic Press (1980): p 87.
24. Doyle, P.A. and C.M. Scala. "Crack Depth Measurement by Ultrasonics." *Ultrasonics.* Vol. 16. Guilford, United Kingdom: IPC Science and Technology Press (1978): p 164.

25. Adler, L., J.H. Rose and C. Mobley. "Ultrasonic Method to Determine Gas Porosity in Aluminum Alloy Castings: Theory and Experiment." *Journal of Applied Physics*. Vol. 59. New York, NY: American Institute of Physics (1986): p 336.

26. Hsu, D.K. and S.M. Nair. "Evaluation of Porosity in Graphite-Epoxy Composite by Frequency Dependence of Ultrasonic Attenuation." *Review of Progress in Quantitative Nondestructive Evaluation* [San Diego, CA, August 1986]. Vol. 6B. New York, NY: Plenum (1987): p 1185.

27. Nagy, P.B., A. Jungman and L. Adler. "Measurements of Backscattered Leaky Lamb Waves in Composite Plates." *Materials Evaluation*. Vol. 46, No. 1. Columbus, OH: American Society for Nondestructive Testing (January 1988): p 97-100.

28. Engleson, M. *Spectrum Analyzer Measurements: Theory and Practice*. Beaverton, OR: Tektronix (1971).

29. Cooley, J.W., P.A.W. Lewis and P.D. Welch. "The Fast Fourier Transform and Its Applications." *Transactions*. E-12(1). New York, NY: Institute of Electrical and Electronics Engineers (1969): p 27.

30. Burgess, J.C. "On Digital Spectrum Analysis of Periodic Signals." *Journal of the Acoustical Society of America*. Vol. 58. Melville, NY: American Institute of Physics, for the Acoustical Society of America (1975): p 556.

31. Ramirez, R.W. *The FFT: Fundamentals and Concepts*. Part 070-1756-00. Beaverton, OR: Tektronix (1975).

32. Simpson, W.A. "A Fourier Model for Ultrasonic Frequency Analysis." *Materials Evaluation*. Vol. 34, No. 12. Columbus, OH: American Society for Nondestructive Testing (1976): p 261-264, 274.

33. Simpson, W.A. "Time-Frequency Domain Formulation of Ultrasonic Frequency Analysis." *Journal of the Acoustical Society of America*. Vol. 56. Melville, NY: American Institute of Physics, for the Acoustical Society of America (1976): p 1776.

34. Bogert, B.P., M.J.R. Healy and J.W. Tukey. *The Frequency Analysis of Time Series for Echoes: Cepstrum Pseudo-Autocovariance, Cross-Cepstrum and Sample Cracking, Time Series Analysis*. New York, NY: Wiley (1963).

35. Leow, M.H., R. Shankar and A.N. Mucciardi. "Experiments with Echo Detection in the Presence of Noise Using the Power Cepstrum and a Modification." *Proceedings of the International Conference on Acoustical Speech and Signal Processing*. New York, NY: Institute of Electrical and Electronics Engineers (1977).

36. Morgan, L.L. "The Spectroscopic Determination of Surface Topography Using Acoustic Surface Waves." *Acustica*. Vol. 30. Stuttgart, Germany: S. Hirzel (1976): p 222.

37. Niethammer, M., L.J. Jacobs, and J. Qu. "Application of STFT Techniques to Interpret Ultrasonic Signals." *Review of Progress in Quantitative Nondestructive Evaluation* [Montréal, Canada, July 1999]. Vol 19A. Melville, NY: American Institute of Physics (2000): p 703-708.

38. Daubechies, I. *Ten Lectures on Wavelets (CBMS-NSF Regional Conference Series in Applied Mathematics)*. Philadelphia, PA: Society for Industrial and Applied Mathematics (1992).

39. Chui, C.K. *An Introduction to Wavelets*. San Diego, CA: Academic Press (1992).

40. Murthy, R., N.M. Bilgutay and O.K. Kaya. "Detection of Ultrasonic Anomaly Signals Using Wavelet Decomposition." *Materials Evaluation*. Vol. 55, No. 11. Columbus, OH: American Society for Nondestructive Testing (November 1997): p 1274-1279.

41. McNamara, J. and F. Lanza di Scalea. "Improvements in Noncontact Ultrasonic Testing of Rails by the Discrete Wavelet Transform." *Materials Evaluation*. Vol. 62, No. 3. Columbus, OH: American Society for Nondestructive Testing (March 2004): p 365-372.

42. Han, J.-B., J.-C. Cheng, T.-H. Wang and Y. Bertholet. "Mode Analyses of Laser-Generated Transient Ultrasonic Lamb Waveforms in a Composite Plate by Wavelet Transform." *Materials Evaluation*. Vol. 57, No. 8. Columbus, OH: American Society for Nondestructive Testing (August 1999): p 837-840.

43. Duda, R.O., P.E. Hart and D.G. Stork. *Pattern Classification*, second edition. New York, NY: Wiley (2000).

44. Agrawala, A.K. *Machine Recognition of Patterns*. New York, NY: Wiley (1977).

45. Gericke, O.R. "Determination of the Geometry of Hidden Defects by Ultrasonic Pulse Analysis Testing." *Journal of the Acoustical Society of America*. Vol 35. New York, NY: Acoustical Society of America (1963): p 364.

46. Whaley, H.L. and L. Adler. "Flaw Characterization by Ultrasonic Frequency Analysis." *Materials Evaluation*. Vol. 29, No. 8. Columbus, OH: American Society for Nondestructive Testing (August 1971): p 182-188.

47. Rose, J.L., J.B. Nestleroth and Y.H. Jeong. "Component Identification Using Ultrasonic Signature Analysis." *Materials Evaluation*. Vol. 41, No. 3. Columbus, OH: American Society for Nondestructive Testing (March 1983): p 315-318.

48. Rose, J.L. "A 23 Flaw Sorting Study in Ultrasonics and Pattern Recognition." *Materials Evaluation*. Vol. 35, No. 7. Columbus, OH: American Society for Nondestructive Testing (July 1977): p 87-92.

49. Rose, J.L. and G.P. Singh. "A Pattern Recognition Reflector Classification Study in the Ultrasonic Inspection of Stainless Steel Pipe Welds." *Non-Destructive Testing*. Vol. 21, No. 6. Northampton, United Kingdom: British Institute of Non-Destructive Inspection (November 1979).

50. Mucciardi, A.N, R. Shankar, J. Cleveland, W.E. Lawrie and H.L. Reeves. *Adaptive Nonlinear Signal Processing for Characterization of Ultrasonic NDE Waveforms, Task 1: Inference of Flat-Bottom Hole Size.* AFML-TR-75-24. Wright-Patterson Air Force Base, OH: Air Force Wright Military Laboratories (January 1975).

51. Nilsson, N.J. *The Mathematical Foundations of Learning Machines.* San Mateo, CA: Morgan Kaufmann (1990).

52. Avioli, M.J., Y.H. Jeong and J.L. Rose. "Utility of a Probability Density Function Curve and F-Maps in Composite Material Inspection." *Experimental Mechanics.* Vol. 22, No. 4. Bethel, CT: Society for Experimental Mechanics (April 1982).

53. Rose, J.L. "Elements of a Feature Based Ultrasonic Inspection System." *Materials Evaluation*. Vol. 42, No. 2. Columbus, OH: American Society for Nondestructive Testing (February 1984): p 210-218.

54. Invernizzi, M. "Prospect of Artificial Intelligence in Nondestructive Testing." *Proceedings of the Seventh International Conference on NDE in the Nuclear Industry.* Materials Park, OH: ASM International (1985).

55. *Visual Communications and Image Processing.* SPIE Proceedings. Bellingham, WA: International Society for Optical Engineering (1998).

56. Fing, P.K., F.A. Iddings and M.A. Overbu. "Analysis of Knowledge Used for a Structured Selection Problem." *Proceedings of the Fall Joint Computer Conference.* New York, NY: Institute of Electrical and Electronics Engineers (1987).

57. *Proceedings of the International Symposium on Pattern Recognition and Acoustical Imaging.* SPIE Proceedings. Bellingham, WA: International Society for Optical Engineering (1987).

58. Avioli, M.J. "NDE Benefits from Artificial Intelligence." *EPRI Journal.* Vol. 13, No. 3. Palo Alto, CA: Electric Power Research Institute (1988).

59. Nugen, S.M., K.E. Christensen, L.S. Koo and L.W. Schmerr. "Flex — An Expert System for Flaw Classification and Sizing." *Review of Progress in Quantitative Nondestructive Evaluation* [Williamsburg, VA, June 1987]. Vol. 7A. New York, NY: Plenum (1988): p 445.

60. Baker, A.R. and C.G. Windsor. "The Classification of Defects from Ultrasonic Data Using Neural Networks: The Hopfield Method." *NDT International.* Vol. 22, No. 2. Guildford, United Kingdom: Butterworth Publishers (April 1989): p 97-105.

61. Ogi, T., M. Notake, Y. Yabe and M. Kitahara. "A Neural Network Applied to Crack Type Recognition." *Review of Progress in Quantitative Nondestructive Evaluation* [Brunswick, ME, July 1989]. Vol. 9A. New York, NY: Plenum (1990): p 689-696.

62. Rose, J.L., J.B. Nestleroth and K. Balasubramanian. "Utility of Feature Mapping in Ultrasonic Non-Destructive Evaluation." *Ultrasonics.* Vol. 26. Guildford, United Kingdom: Butterworth Publishers (1988): p 124.

63. Rao, B.P.C., B. Raj, T. Jayakumar and P. Kalyanasundaram. "Using Artificial Neural Networks to Quantify Discontinuities in Eddy Current Testing." *Materials Evaluation*. Vol. 60, No. 1. Columbus, OH: American Society for Nondestructive Testing (January 2002): p 84-88.

64. Haykin, S. *Neural Networks: A Comprehensive Foundation,* second edition. New York, NY: McMillan (1998).

65. Gericke, O.R. "Ultrasonic Spectroscopy." *Research Techniques in Nondestructive Testing.* Vol. 1. New York, NY: Academic Press (1970): p 31-61.

66. Scott, W.R. and P.F. Gordon. "Ultrasonic Spectrum Analysis for Nondestructive Testing of Layered Composite Materials." *Journal of the Acoustical Society of America.* Vol. 62, No. 1. Melville, NY: American Institute of Physics, for the Acoustical Society of America (1977): p 108-116.

67. Papadakis, E. "Ultrasonic Velocity and Attenuation: Measurement Methods with Scientific and Industrial Applications." *Physical Acoustics.* Vol. 12. New York, NY: Academic Press (1976): p 277-374.

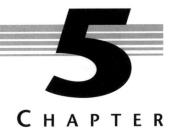

CHAPTER

Instrumentation for Ultrasonic Testing

Matthew J. Golis, Advanced Quality Concepts, Columbus, Ohio (Parts 2 and 4)

Robert E. Green, Jr., Johns Hopkins University, Baltimore, Maryland (Part 1)

PART 1. Scanning Approaches

Classification of Equipment[1]

Equipment selected for ultrasonic testing of solid materials typically falls into one of three categories, based on the parameter measured: (1) amplitude of reflected energy only, (2) amplitude and transit time of reflected energy and (3) loading of the transducer by the test object.

Other arbitrary subdivisions are possible. In some techniques, the effects combine.

Amplitude Systems

Transmission systems using only amplitude information depend on the principle that specific material characteristics of a test object produce significant changes in the intensity of an ultrasonic beam passing through it. The entire thickness of the object can be tested with this technique.

Structurally, the equipment must consist only of an ultrasound source, receiver, test object and suitable couplant (Fig. 1). Typically, however, a scanning mechanism, a gate and a recording or alarm device are needed because the ultrasonic beam area is likely to be much smaller than the test object cross section.

The discontinuity detectability of such a system depends principally on (1) the ratio of discontinuity area to beam size and (2) the separation between discontinuity and the transducers.

In addition to these limitations, other problems may arise from this system configuration, including spurious signals from multiple-path reflections, amplitude variations caused by minor geometry changes, undesirable resonances of test object or couplant and direct electrical cross talk between transducers. If contact coupling is used, pressure effects are large. If immersion is used, standing waves can sometimes occur when waves interfere after reflection. To minimize such variables, the electric signal applied to the transducer is often pulsed. In this way, resonances are averaged out and standing waves are reduced.

Amplitude and Transit Time Systems

The most versatile techniques for ultrasonic testing of solid materials use two parameters simultaneously: (1) the amplitude of signals obtained from internal discontinuities and (2) the time or phase shift required for the beam to travel between specific surfaces and these discontinuities.

These techniques are used in radar and depth sounding equipment, although the problems relating to interpretation, resolution and frequency range are different. A short electric pulse is generated and applied to the electrodes of the transducer. This pulse produces a short train of elastic waves coupled into the test object. Timing circuits then measure the intervals between the transmittal of the initial pulse and the reception of signals from within the test object.

This cycle is repeated (at rates varying from 60 Hz to 10 kHz) at regular periods so that a continuous indication is obtained. The pulse repetition rate on a pulse echo system is adjusted so that reverberations within the test object decay completely between pulses.

Several types of instrumentation are possible, depending principally on the means of timing and indicating. Many applications can also be used, depending on the number and style of transducers, the frequency range covered and the means for coupling or scanning. In addition, numerous variations and combinations of circuit components can be incorporated into the equipment. The breakdown of basic equipment types in Table 1 relates primarily to the means of presenting discontinuity data.

TABLE 1. Types of ultrasonic system displays.

Display Type	Indication
A-scan	discontinuity depth and amplitude of signal
B-scan	discontinuity depth and distribution in cross sectional view
C-scan	discontinuity distribution in plan view
Gated system	determined by technique; used for marker, facsimile or chart recorder

A-Scan Equipment

Most ultrasonic test systems use a basic A-scan presentation. The horizontal baseline on the display indicates elapsed time (from left to right) and the vertical deflection shows signal amplitudes. For a given ultrasonic velocity in the test object, the sweep can be calibrated directly in terms of distance or depth. Conversely, when the through-wall dimensions of the test object are known, the sweep time can be used to determine ultrasonic velocities from which elastic moduli can be calculated. The signal amplitudes represent the intensities of transmitted or reflected beams. These may be related to discontinuity size, test object attenuation, beam spread and other factors.

Several test techniques can be used, including through-transmission or reflection, single-transducer or double-transducer systems and contact or immersion coupling. Other possibilities include angle beam and surface wave techniques using single or dual transducers and various combinations of techniques. In the United States, single transducer operation is used for most reflection testing applications.

A-Scan Sensitivity

In industrial testing, the sensitivity of commercial A-scan instruments is typically adequate for detecting the smallest discontinuities of concern (including cracks, inclusions and

FIGURE 1. Types of through-transmission testing systems: (a) continuous frequency; (b) modulated frequency; (c) swept frequency; (d) pulsed; (e) gated.

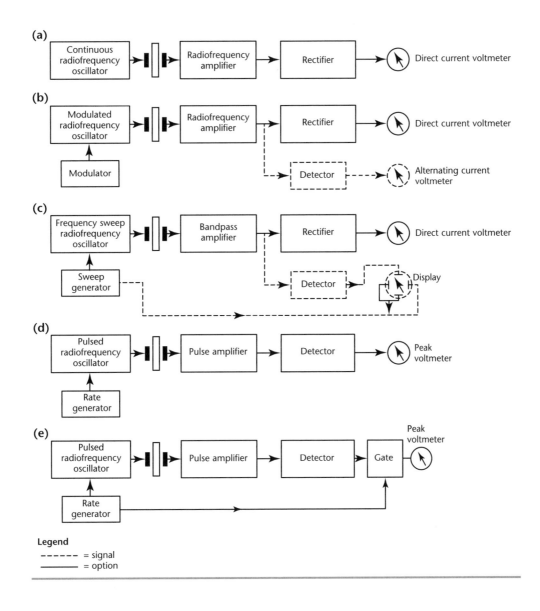

porosity), although other limitations such as the detail of the resolution may exist.

Reasonable amplifier linearity is desirable for calibration and discontinuity comparison. Reading accuracies of one part in twenty are adequate because most discrepancies are due to other variables such as coupling and alignment. Precision markers of high sweep linearity are ordinarily not required for discontinuity detection, although one or the other may be necessary for accurate thickness or velocity measurements. In some cases, precision markers are provided as system accessories.

Among the alternative configurations for ultrasonic circuit components are those listed in Table 2.

Special instrumentation needed for some testing applications may include the following: (1) provision for dual-transducer operation, (2) interference elimination circuitry, (3) compensation for long transducer cables, (4) stabilization for extreme line voltage changes, (5) exponential calibrator for attenuation measurements, (6) exceptional portability for field use, (7) remote indicators, (8) frequency range extended above 100 MHz, (9) high resolution and (10) computer interface and on-board digital memory.

B-Scan Presentation

When the shape of large discontinuities or their distribution within a test object cross section is of interest, the B-scan display is the most useful. In addition to the basic components of the A-scan unit, provision must be made for these additional B-scan functions: (1) intensity modulation or brightening of the pixel in proportion to the amplitude of the discontinuity signal, (2) deflection of the display trace in synchronism with the motion of the transducer along the test object and (3) retention of the display image by a long persistence phosphor.

B-Scan Equipment

Often a B-scan display is used with A-scan testing or as an attachment to standard A-scan equipment. Therefore, the system design criteria depend on A-scan equipment and the testing application.

TABLE 2. Alternative circuit components for ultrasonic test systems.

Characteristic	Options
Synchronizer	
pulse repetition rate	fixed, adjustable with fixed range, stepped with sweep range, variable (50 to 1000 Hz)
locking signal	line voltage (or harmonic), internal
Pulser	
wave shape	impulse, spike, gated sine wave, damped wave train
type	tunable, impedance matched, variable amplitude
circuit	thyratron, pulsed oscillator
Amplifier	
Type	tuned radio frequency, wide band
Response	linear, sharp cutoff, logarithmic
Sensitivity	time variable gain or constant
Controls	gain, input attenuation, reject, variable band width
Signal Display	
Type	radio frequency wave train, video
Source	radio frequency output, rectified (envelope), differentiated video
Sweep	
Type	logarithmic, high linearity, conventional
Delay	adjustable, automatic, none
Expansion	fixed, adjustable, related to sweep
Marker	
Type	fixed scale on display, precision electronic, adjustable square wave, movable step mark
Source	crystal oscillator, adjustable multivibrator, precision integrator
Display	superimposed on signals, alternate sweep, separate trace, intensity modulated
Signal Gate	
Type	amplitude proportional
Output	direct current level, modulated, rectangular wave, pulse stretched
System	
Frequency range	single; continuous tuning; low (50 to 200 kHz), intermediate (0.2 to 5 MHz), high (5 to 25 MHz)

Where high speed scanning is required, the longer persistence of the B-scan display may be an advantage to the operator.

Discontinuity Detectability

The effectiveness of the B-scan in showing discontinuity detail depends on the relationship of discontinuity size, beam area and wavelength. Optimum results are obtained with larger discontinuities, smaller transducers and higher frequencies. For other conditions, beam sharpening techniques such as focusing and electronic contrast enhancement may be needed.

C-Scan Presentation

By synchronizing the position of the display spot with the transducer scanning motion along two coordinates, a plan view of the test object can be developed similar to the common plan position indicator (PPI) radar display.

In addition to the circuitry required for a B-scan, provision must be made for eliminating unwanted signals such as the initial pulse, interface echo or back reflection, which obscure internal discontinuity signals. An electronic gate is used to render the display circuits sensitive only for the short intervals of sweep time when signals from the desired depth range occur.

In certain cases, hybrid systems present some data about discontinuity size and location with a sacrifice in discontinuity shape and position detail.

Gated Systems

In general, gating is needed for all automatic C-scan systems that alarm, mark, record, chart or otherwise replace visual interpretation. Such gating circuits may be built into the discontinuity detector or supplied as separate attachments.

Commercial recording attachments typically provide at least two gates, one to indicate the presence of discontinuities in the test object and the second to show a decrease in back reflection. Some units provide additional discontinuity gates so that two or more alarm levels can be set or so that different depth increments can be tested.

If the cross section of the test object varies during the scanning cycle in an automatic test, the gating periods must be simultaneously adjusted. In addition, other functions such as sensitivity, transducer angle and recorder speed may have to be controlled.

PART 2. Basic Send/Receive Instrumentation

Basic Instrument[2]

The basic electronic instrument used in pulsed ultrasonic testing contains a source of voltage spikes (to activate the sound source — that is, the pulser) and a display mechanism that permits interpretation of received ultrasonic acoustic impulses. Figure 2 shows a block diagram of the basic unit. The display can be as simple as a digital meter for a thickness gage or a multidimensional representation of signals over an extended area of interest.

The timer circuitry triggers the pulser (activates the transducer) and the sweep generator forces the electron beam within the display to move horizontally across the screen. Other special circuits triggered as needed include markers, sweep delays, gates, distance amplitude correction and other support circuits. Pulse signals from the receiver transducer are amplified to a level compatible with the display.

The term *pulse* is used in two contexts in ultrasonic testing. The electronic system sends an exciting electrical pulse to the transducer being used to emit the ultrasonic wave. This electrical pulse is usually a unidirectional spike with a fast rise time. The resulting acoustic wave packet emitted by the transducer is the ultrasonic pulse with both a positive and negative excursion. It is characterized by a predominant central frequency at the transducer's natural thickness resonance.

The received signals are often processed to enhance interpretation with filters (that limit spurious background noise and smooth the appearance of the pulses), rectifiers (that change the oscillatory radio frequency signals to unidirectional video spikes) and clipping circuits (that reject low level background signals). The final signals are passed on to the vertical displacement circuits of the display unit and produce the time delayed echo signals interpreted by the operator. This type of display is commonly referred to as an A-scan (signal amplitude displayed as a function of time).

Most functions are within the control of the operator, and their collective settings are the setup of the instrument. Table 3 lists the variables under the control of the operator and their impact on the validity of an ultrasonic test. If desired, a particular portion of the trace may be gated and the signal within the gate sent to some external device, an alarm or recording device that registers the presence or absence of echo signals being sought.

Characteristics of the initial ultrasonic, radio frequency pulse (shape and frequency content) are carried forward throughout the system, to the test object, back to the transducer, the receiver (amplifier), the gate and the display. In essence, the information content of the initial electrical pulse is modified by each of these items. It is the result of this collective signal processing that appears on the screen. The initial pulse may range from 100 to 500 V and have a very short rise time.

In some systems, the initial pulse may represent a portion of a sinusoidal oscillation, tuned to correspond to the natural frequency of the transducer. The sinusoidal driving pulses are needed to help penetrate highly attenuative materials such as rubber and concrete.

Signals from the receiving transducer (usually in the millivolt range) may be too small to be directly sent to the display unit. Both linear and logarithmic amplifiers are used to raise signal levels needed to drive the display. These amplifiers, located in the receiver sections of A-scan units, must be able to produce output signals linearly related to the input signals and which supply signal

FIGURE 2. Basic pulse echo system for ultrasonic testing.[2]

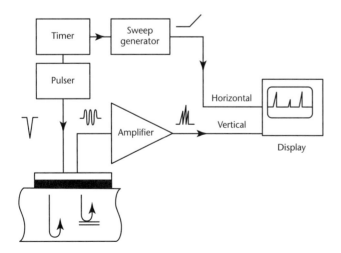

processing intended to assist the operator in interpreting the displayed signals.

Amplifiers may raise incoming signals to a maximum level, followed by precision attenuators that decrease the signal strength to levels that can be positioned on the screen face — capable of changing amplification ratios in direct response to the gain control.

Discrete attenuators (which have a logarithmic response) are currently used because of their ease of precise construction and simple means for altering signal levels beyond the viewing range of the screen. Their extensive use has made decibel notation a part of the standard terminology used in describing changes in signal levels, such as changes in receiver gain and material attenuation.

The ratio of two pulse amplitudes (A_2 and A_1) and their equivalence can be expressed in decibel notation (N_{dB}):

$$(1) \qquad N_{dB} = 20 \log_{10} \frac{A_2}{A_1}$$

Inversion of this equation results in the useful expression:

$$(2) \qquad \frac{A_2}{A_1} = 10^{\frac{N}{20}}$$

where a change of 20 dB, $N = 20$, makes:

$$(3) \qquad 10^{\frac{N}{20}} = 10^1 = 10$$

Thus 20 dB is equivalent to a ratio of ten to one. Signals may be displayed as radio frequency waveforms, replicating the acoustic wave as detected by the receiving transducer, or as video waveforms, (half-wave or full-wave rectified), used to double the effective viewing range of the screen (bottom to top rather than centerline to top and to bottom) but suppressing the phase information found only in radio frequency presentations.

To enhance the ability to accurately identify and assess the nature of the received ultrasonic pulses, particularly when there exists an excessive amount of background signals, various means of signal processing are used. Both tuned receivers (narrow band instruments) and low pass filters have been used to selectively suppress frequencies of the signal spectrum that do not contain useful information from the test material.

Linear systems, such as the ultrasonic instrument's receiver section (as well as each of the elements of the overall system), are characterized by the manner in which they affect incoming signals. A common approach is to start with the frequency content of the incoming signal (from the receiving transducer) and to describe how that spectrum of frequencies is altered as a result of passing through the system element.

When both useful target information (which may be predominantly contained in a narrow band of frequencies generated by the sending transducer) and background noise (which may be distributed randomly over a broad spectrum of frequencies) are present in the signal entering the receiver, selective passing of the frequencies of interest emphasizes the signals of interest while suppressing others that interfere with interpretation of the display.

When an ultrasonic instrument is described as being broad band, that means a very wide array of frequencies can be processed through the instrument with a minimum of alteration — that is,

TABLE 3. Effects of instrument controls.

Instrument Control	Comments on Signal Response
Pulser	
Pulse length (damping)	if short, improves depth resolution; If long, improves penetration
Repetition rate	if high, brightens images but may cause wrap-around ghost signals
Receiver	
Frequency response	wide band — faithful reproduction of signal, higher background noise
Frequency response	narrow band — higher sensitivity, smoothed signals, requires matched (tuned) system
Gain	if high, improves sensitivity, higher background noise
Display	
Sweep — material adjust	calibration critical for depth information
Sweep — delay	permits spreading of echo pulses for detailed analysis
Reject	suppresses low level noise, alters opponent vertical linearity
Smoothing	suppresses detailed pulse structure
Output (Alarm, Record) Gates	
Time window (delay, width)	selects portion of display for analysis; gate may distort pulses
Threshold	sets automatic output sensitivity
Polarity	permits positive and negative images, allows triggering on both increasing and decreasing pulses

the signal observed on the screen is an amplified representation of the electrical signal measured at the receiving transducer. Thus both useful signals and background noise are present, and the ratio of signal to noise may be bad. The shape and amplitudes of the signals, however, tend to be an accurate representation of the received response from the transducer.

A narrow band instrument, on the other hand, suppresses incoming frequencies above or below the pass frequency band. With the high frequency noise suppressed, the gain of the instrument can be increased, leading to an improved sensitivity. However, the shape and relative amplitudes of pulse frequency components are often altered.

Instrument Types[3]

Typical ultrasonic test instruments provide basic functions, including the generation of an elastic wave, the reception of ultrasonic signals, signal conditioning and processing, discontinuity signal gating and signal presentation. Depending on the intended application, ultrasonic instruments may incorporate other functions, including multiple-channel capability, additional signal gates, filters, computer interfaces and compensation for signal loss as a function of distance traveled and attenuation. The ultrasonic testing instrument has evolved into several distinct categories: manual instruments (typically portable send/receive units), customized systems (programmed for specific industrial applications) and special purpose systems (typically for the laboratory).

Basic Instruments

A distinction is made between basic, manual (portable) and laboratory instruments because their internal designs and external interfaces are considerably different. Portable instruments are generally self-contained in terms of their internal functions. Laboratory instruments often require peripheral components not normally found in nondestructive testing production environments: signal sources and processors, displays, desk top computers and other components.

Portable and industrial production instruments are calibrated differently than laboratory instruments. For example, the vertical and horizontal axes of portable instruments are generally calibrated in relative units with respect to known distances and reflector sizes. Furthermore, portable instruments are intentionally designed to allow adjustments and calibration by a human operator at the job site. Laboratory instruments are typically calibrated in absolute units (volts and microseconds).

A general purpose instrument designed for research laboratory applications has functions similar to a basic portable instrument but with different operator interfaces. The external and internal differences between manual and laboratory instruments reflect different user requirements. Basic, portable instruments are configured to satisfy the practical needs of an inspector whose test assignments may vary daily. Laboratory instruments are intended primarily for use by material research engineers and scientists who require ultrasonic frequency data in terms of highly reproducible engineering units. Industrial production systems are generally intended for special purpose, factory floor installations operated under computer control.

Industrial Production Systems

Industrial production systems are often modular and offer multiple-channel capabilities. Such systems can be easily optimized for a particular production environment through plug-in modules and changes in computer control software.

To accommodate different test requirements, modular systems typically use a general purpose enclosure internally compatible with a broad range of special function, plug-in modules. Each module is designed to perform a specific function. This approach offers the user the flexibility of designing a custom instrumentation package. As the requirements change, new modules can be added to the system at incremental cost. Maintenance of modular systems is facilitated by this approach. The initial cost of a basic modular system may be higher than that of a portable system.

Special Purpose (Laboratory) Systems

The category of special purpose systems includes all instruments designed to perform a specific ultrasonic test that cannot, for cost or performance reasons, be carried out with a portable, laboratory or modular system. This category includes bond testers, velocity determination instruments, high powered drivers for air coupled and special purpose electromagnetic acoustic transducers, scanners, imaging equipment and acoustic microscopes. The cost of installing a special purpose system can vary widely. Thickness gages are generally less expensive than portable ultrasonic instruments whereas acoustic microscopes can be much more expensive than modular systems.

Low frequency (less than 100 MHz) acoustic microscope systems are suited for ultrasonic tests of complex aerospace structures and electronic packages. High power laboratory instruments can be used with unconventional ultrasonic transducers, including air coupled and electromagnetic acoustic transducers. Using front panel controls, it is possible to reconfigure this instrument to generate a variety of pulse shapes, including spike, square wave and tone burst pulses.

Below, the principles of ultrasonic test instruments and auxiliary equipment are explained by using the operation of a portable instrument as an example. The special features of laboratory and modular industrial production instruments are explained and some basic modes of data presentation are discussed.

Portable Instruments[3]

Portable ultrasonic instruments are battery operated and principally used as discontinuity detectors. Some such instruments are designed for handheld operation and offer a limited range of functions. Other instruments are suitable for most remote or laboratory production applications and for procedure development. Such instruments are generally larger and heavier than handheld discontinuity detectors but offer many additional functions.

Basic portable instruments are most often operated in the pulse echo mode (described elsewhere in this volume) by using the same ultrasonic transducer for generating and receiving the ultrasonic signals. This mode of operation was first demonstrated by Firestone around 1940.[4] However, portable instruments may also be operated in a pitch catch or through-transmission mode, using separate transducers for generating and receiving ultrasonic signals.

Instrument Functions

Portable test systems typically offer a minimum range of basic functions: (1) pulse echo and pitch catch modes, (2) spike or square wave pulse generation, (3) adjustment of pulse amplitude and harmonic content, (4) selection of test frequencies, typically 1 to 50 MHz, (5) coarse and fine receiver amplifier gain adjustment, (6) signal gating, (7) signal detection and filtering, (8) accept/reject threshold setting and alarm and (9) display of received ultrasonic signals.

These functions typically satisfy most contact ultrasonic test requirements. However, additional functions are needed in applications such as contact tests of thick sections and immersion tests. Some of these additional functions are available in portable instruments but are usually standard in laboratory and production systems.

If properly configured, a portable instrument can be used in immersion testing in the pulse echo and through-transmission modes. It can also be used to test many thick section materials and structures. In addition, when used with data logging and scanning, the instrument offers B-scan and C-scan presentations. Other useful functions include interface triggering of gate and display, distance amplitude correction and simultaneous display of both video and radiofrequency signals.

Although nearly all portable instruments are compatible with piezoelectric ceramic transducers in the 1 to 50 MHz frequency region, they may not operate properly with special transducers. In particular, most piezoelectric polymer and low frequency (typically 0.5 MHz and lower) piezoelectric ceramic transducers will not operate properly if the equipment is not designed for these materials and frequencies.[5]

It is not generally recommended that portable instruments be used to drive unconventional transducers, including air coupled transducers and electromagnetic acoustic transducers. However, specialized high power drivers[6] and low noise preamplifiers are available for such transducers.[7]

Operation

Low cost, portable instruments are intended primarily for discontinuity detection and thickness gaging. The instrument provides a video display of the ultrasonic signals. Figure 3 illustrates the main functions of the instrument and shows representative internal and displayed waveforms.

Internally, the basic instrument is a display whose horizontal deflection (sweep) voltages are synchronized with the transmitted ultrasonic pulses. Two modes of operation are possible: pulse echo and pitch catch. The pulser excites an ultrasonic transducer with a high voltage spike or square wave pulse and has controls for adjustment of the amplitude (energy) and shape (harmonic content) of the transmitted ultrasonic pulses. The system's receiver processes ultrasonic signals returned from the test object (Fig. 4). Only the most elementary controls are provided for adjusting the

FIGURE 3. Block diagram of portable ultrasonic instrument (see also Fig. 4).

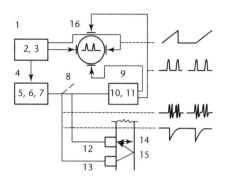

Legend
1. Timing section
2. Pulse repetition frequency
3. Sweep rate
4. Pulser
5. Pulse amplitude
6. Pulse frequency
7. Damping
8. Transmit/receive switch
9. Receiver
10. Gain
11. Frequency
12. Receiver
13. Transmitter
14. Pulse echo
15. Pitch catch
16. Display

frequency domain (filtering) and time domain (gain) parameters of the received signals. In addition, such a basic instrument has front panel controls for adjusting the sweep rate, usually calibrated in units of length or velocity. The sweep rates are made adjustable because ultrasonic propagation velocities vary with the test material. A signal gate, enabling the operator to set an alarm level, is provided as a standard function.

Timing and Synchronization

The operation of a basic instrument is timed and synchronized by the so-called *timing section*, which controls the system's pulse repetition frequency. The timing section also generates the internal sweep rate signals which determine the separation between the received ultrasonic signals on the instrument's display.

The pulse repetition frequency timing signals are fed directly to a pulser that drives the ultrasonic transducer through a manually selectable diplexer. Diplexers are also known as *transmit/receive switches*.

Following a propagation delay corresponding to the ultrasonic time of flight between the transducer and an internal reflector, the back scattered ultrasonic signals are received by the same transducer. These signals are then detected by the receiver preamplifier.

FIGURE 4. Principal functions of portable instrument's receiver and their effect on the received ultrasonic signals.

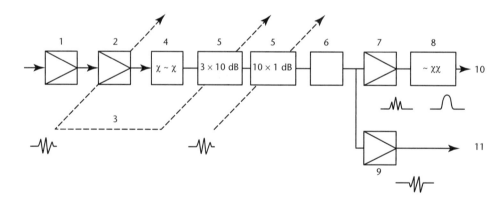

Legend
1. Preamplifier
2. First radiofrequency amplifier (gain block)
3. Gain adjust
4. Filters
5. Attenuators
6. Second radiofrequency amplifier
7. Video detector
8. Low pass filters
9. Buffer amplifier
10. Video out
11. Radiofrequency out

However, before the received signals can be processed and displayed, additional signal processing steps are needed. Processed signals are displayed for evaluation by inspectors or automatic detectors. It is assumed that the travel time is long enough to keep signals of different transmitter pulses from overlapping.

Receiver Gain Adjustment

After preamplification to help establish the best electrical signal-to-noise ratio, the amplitudes of the received signals on the display can be adjusted using a combination of fixed and variable attenuators. The overall gain of the amplifier can be selected by switching in two or three 20 dB gain circuits. Generally, this selection can be accomplished using controls at the front panel of the instrument. Receiver gains might be adjusted also through an external controller.

After amplification, band pass filtering and video detection (rectification and low pass filtering), the signals are amplified again by the video amplifier. This amplification is often followed by an adjustable low pass filter and the output of the filter is then applied to the vertical axis of the display, as function of time (horizontal axis of the display). The final detected and filtered signal is called the *video display* or *A-scan*. In some designs, it is possible to display radiofrequency waveforms directly.

Sweep, Signal Filtering and Display

The horizontal axis of the display device is driven by the sweep signals generated in the system's timing section. Generally, the start of each sweep signal is delayed with respect to the transmitter pulse or by an interface trigger. This delay is used to offset the start of the display to some convenient interface echo.

The amplitude of the displayed signals are determined principally by the receiver gain and frequency filter settings. They can also be affected by the low pass filter in the detector circuit. In addition, the setting of the transmitter pulse amplitude and pulse damping controls can affect the amplitude and the appearance of the displayed ultrasonic signals.

Signal Gating and Threshold Selection

Among the essential functions of a basic instrument are the signal gate and the alarm threshold controls. These functions enable the operator to isolate a specific portion of the received signal train and to compare its peak amplitude with a preset threshold level.

The signal gate delay, width parameters and alarm threshold level typically can be selected from the front panel. To ensure reliable results, receiver gain levels and the alarm threshold level within the gate interval should be adjusted before the test using an appropriate ultrasonic reference standard and an instrument calibration procedure.

Pulse Repetition Frequency

Battery powered discontinuity detectors can be operated at relatively high pulse repetition frequencies (500 Hz and higher) to ensure a bright display. Thickness gages can achieve even higher pulse repetition frequencies. However, high pulse repetition frequencies use more power and so make the instrument less portable. High pulse repetition frequencies can cause interference of ultrasonic signals generated by different transmitter pulses, in turn producing undesirable fluctuations in signal amplitude. Interference must be avoided because of its detrimental effect on test reliabilities.

In many advanced instruments, fast digital sampling, storage techniques and advanced display technologies increase display brightness while reducing power consumption. In these designs, pulse repetition frequencies can be as low as 40 Hz. Lower frequencies could result in perceptible flicker and make real time scanning inadvisable because of wide intervals between adjacent pulses.

Pulse Amplitude and Shape Control

Most portable ultrasonic instruments use relatively simple pulse circuitry. In the twentieth century, spike pulser designs were common. In the twenty-first century, many designs incorporate square wave pulsers.

If the instrument uses a spike pulser, then the operator may be able to modify the pulse amplitude by adjusting the energy of the pulse. Pulse energy is adjusted by selecting the value of the energy storage capacitor. In addition, an adjustment of the damping resistor value may be made to minimize transducer ringing.

If the instrument uses a square wave pulser, the operator is generally required to adjust pulse width individually for each transducer to exactly match the frequency characteristics. In addition, the value of the damping resistor should be adjusted to match the impedance characteristics. To protect the transducers from the effects of voltage overdrive, pulser voltages seldom exceed 400 V.

Avoidance of Receiver Saturation

Most ultrasonic testing procedures require the operator to adjust the gain of the input amplifier and attenuator to ensure that none of the components in the receiver amplifier chain are in saturation. Typically, the maximum displayed signal level is adjusted to the saturation value, about 80 percent of the full display. Such an adjustment can be made using front panel controls. The overall gain of a typical receiver may be adjustable over a range of 100 dB in discrete steps of 1, 2, 6 and 10 dB.

Signal Gate and Alarm Level Settings

The gain adjustment and signal gate functions are important because they can be used to control accept/reject thresholds. If the amplitude of the signal in a discontinuity gate exceeds a preestablished threshold, then the discontinuity alarm feature is activated. The discontinuity alarm is usually built-in and can be audible or visual.

Operation in Pitch Catch or Through-Transmission Modes

If the diplexer or transmit/receive switch is set in the open position, then it is possible to operate in the pitch catch or through-transmission modes. In this configuration, separate transducers are used to generate and receive the ultrasonic signals.

General Purpose Ultrasonic Test Equipment[3]

Portable ultrasonic systems intended for the field and laboratory can incorporate more functions than basic instruments, including distance amplitude correction, interface triggering, display of radiofrequency waveforms, multiple signal gates, interfaces to external control and others.

Distance Amplitude Correction

Distance amplitude correction helps control the gain of the instrument receiver section as a function of sweep time. This function is often used in contact testing of thick sectioned materials where signal attenuation as a function of depth can be severe. Distance amplitude correction allows signals reflected from similar discontinuities at different depths to be evaluated concurrently.

Interface Triggering

The interface triggering function is typically needed when the transducer separation from the front surface of the test object cannot be precisely controlled, as in immersion testing. This situation often occurs in pulse echo, water immersion testing of thin, flexible laminates. If the time delay of the signal gate is synchronized with the initial pulse, variations in distance between the transducer and the front surface cause the position of the gate to vary as well. In effect, on the basis of elapsed time, the gate position has remained constant, but the position of the test object has shifted from the original setup. This is highly undesirable because many potential discontinuities may be missed.

To ensure that the ultrasonic signals returned from the interior of the laminate always arrive within the signal gate, the beginning of each signal gate and display sweep waveform can be synchronized to the signal reflected from the front face of the laminate. This procedure is called *interface triggering.*

Interface triggering permits automatic tracking of the signal gate with respect to a selected portion of the ultrasonic sweep. When using interface triggering, the relative positions of the signals on the display remain unchanged as the transducer separation from the test object is varied (Fig. 5).

In practice, the signal gate and the sweep delays can be synchronized to other ultrasonic signals when a blocking gate is part of the equipment. Signals are disregarded at the blocking gate. Examples of such signals include those from the back faces of thick laminates, thick metal sections and other thick test objects.

In traditional instrument designs, the interface triggering function is realized using analog circuits. However, by using analog-to-digital converters, interface triggering also can be accomplished with digital signal processing techniques.[8]

Digital signal processing is generally superior to the traditional analog techniques, particularly in terms of near surface resolution. This capability is particularly important in the study of impact damage in polymer composites.

To isolate and process characteristic features of radiofrequency waveforms is increasingly important in discontinuity evaluation and material characterization. It is now widely recognized that radiofrequency waveforms can contain significant material information. Processing of radiofrequency waveforms is of particular interest in the study of polymer composite materials.[9] However, to fully exploit the information in a radiofrequency waveform, digital signal processing must be used.

Modular Ultrasonic Instruments[3]

Instruments in ultrasonic testing research are designed to be used with other high performance instrumentation in the laboratory: display screens, desktop computers, data logging equipment and other components. Equipment intended for production testing and procedure development is typically self-contained. By contrast, laboratory instruments can delegate many functions to other more efficient laboratory systems. This trend is reflected in the designs of many ultrasonic instruments that can be interfaced with other laboratory instruments by high speed computer interfaces.

Multiple Channels

A waveform digitizer, of 100 MHz for example, can be designed to allow custom integration of laboratory instruments by using an industry standard architecture bus. In combination with an ultrasonic transducer that interfaces with the same bus, the digitizer can form the nucleus of a flexible system for ultrasonic testing research.

Multiple-channel capabilities can be achieved by adding more pulser/receiver and digitizer boards. The instrument also can be adapted to different measurement needs by changing the control and signal processing software of the host computer. The data display functions are provided by the computer and its output devices.

Digital signal processing offers many advantages over analog techniques. Most importantly, digital processing allows expansion of the dynamic range of the ultrasonic signals. Digital instruments with high dynamic range are more easily calibrated and can acquire and record more data than analog instruments. Furthermore, setup information, including pulser/receiver and transducer parameters, can be stored in the headers of data files. This feature may facilitate comparison and standardization of results obtained with different instruments or at different times.

Modularity

Modules are used to configure an ultrasonic instrument for a specialized application: a multiple-channel preamplifier, a high energy pulser, a receiver module and a gate. The modules are integrated with a proprietary electrical back plane design that can accommodate both analog and digital signals. The operation of the instrument is controlled by a dedicated module that interprets digital control signals generated by an external computer. Generally, modules designed by one manufacturer are not compatible with instruments designed by other manufacturers.

Conceptually, the functions offered by modular instruments are similar to those of general purpose ultrasonic systems. However, modular instruments can be configured for concurrent, multiple-channel operation with the parameters of each channel optimized to perform a specific ultrasonic test. Thus,

FIGURE 5. Interface triggering function for automatic tracking of ultrasonic signal gate: (a) test configuration; (b) initial pulse triggering for transducer 1; (c) interface triggering for transducer 1; (d) initial pulse triggering for transducer 2; (e) interface triggering for transducer 2.

(a)

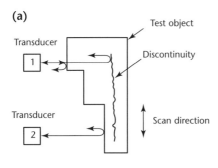

(b)

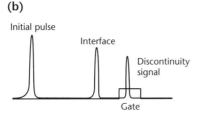

(c)

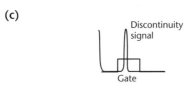

(d)

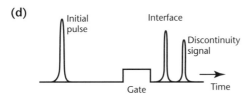

(e)

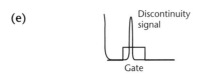

one channel can be configured for pulse echo testing while another channel is configured for pitch catch testing. In many designs, the setup parameters can be dynamically modified under computer control. This feature of modular instruments facilitates testing of complex structures.

Part 3. Special Purpose Ultrasonic Equipment[3]

Special purpose ultrasonic instruments have typically been developed to satisfy specific requirements of a particular industry segment. Examples of such instruments include thickness gages, acoustic microscopes, bond testers and others. With the exception of thickness gages, special purpose instruments account for a relatively small percentage of the ultrasonic test equipment market. The market is dominated by discontinuity detection equipment.

Thickness Gages

Thickness gages are widely used by the petrochemical, aerospace and other industries.[10] Because they serve a single purpose, thickness gages feature few panel controls. Typically, thickness gages can only operate with special transducers supplied with the instrument by the manufacturer. Contemporary thickness gages are highly integrated and very small.

Figure 6 shows a functional block diagram for a thickness gage. Basically, this gage is a pulse echo discontinuity detector using special pulse circuits and broad band, highly damped transducers to achieve high spatial resolutions.

Thickness gages use pulsers that excite specially designed transducers with waveforms whose rise times are generally shorter than 10 ns. They also use broad band receivers and special signal processing circuits for low amplitude, repetitive signals. The display is typically a digital readout. Sometimes, a supplemental amplitude is also displayed.

The time interval between the initial pulse and back surface echoes represents the travel time of the ultrasonic signal through the test object (Figs. 7 to 9). Test object thickness, a direct function of the back surface echo travel time and material ultrasonic velocity, can then be determined. To obtain correct readings, the operator must calibrate the instrument with appropriate procedures.

Special transducers are needed to operate in direct contact mode. Such transducers use thin plates made of special wear resistant materials. Contact transducers are coupled directly to the material using a film of liquid. This procedure and the resulting test signals are shown in Fig. 8.

When the transducer incorporates a delay line to separate the initial pulse from the material interface (delay line mode), a separate interface signal occurs. Figure 7 shows interface and back surface

FIGURE 7. Interface and back surface echoes from thick test object: (a) test setup; (b) display.

(a)

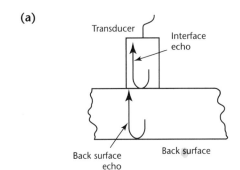

(b)

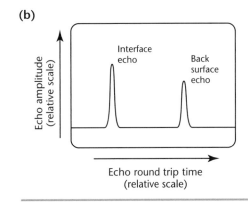

FIGURE 6. Function diagram of ultrasonic thickness gage.

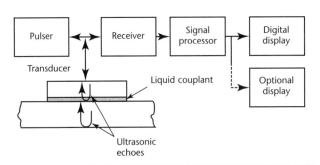

echoes from a test object. The back surface echoes are typically smaller than interface echoes because of material attenuation.

During contact gaging, material thickness is determined by measuring the time interval between the interface echo from the back surface echo. The thickness gage accomplishes this automatically through built-in signal processing circuits. Generally, echoes cannot be seen by the operator because most instruments use digital readout and do not have analog signal displays.

because acoustic microscopes form images through interference of at least two different ultrasonic signals.[13] However, many microscope designs also incorporate functions originally developed for traditional discontinuity detection applications, including interface gating and generation of C-scan presentations.

Currently, low frequency acoustic microscopes are mainly used for aerospace and microelectronic packaging applications. High frequency microscopes (1 GHz and higher) are mainly used to inspect surfaces of semiconductor devices.

Acoustic Microscopes

The principle of a mechanically scanned acoustic microscope was demonstrated in 1973.[11] The frequencies of early acoustic microscopes were in excess of 1 GHz, too high for most nondestructive test applications. Since then, significant developments have resulted in lower operating frequencies, between 5 and 100 MHz. These developments have made scanning acoustic microscopy accessible to the nondestructive testing community.[12] Consequently, acoustic microscopy has converged with more traditional nondestructive test equipment.

The design of receivers used in acoustic microscopy differs from designs used in conventional discontinuity detection

Continuous Wave Technique

Theory[14]

If a thin, low loss transducer is coupled to a test object and its effective impedance is measured by a high frequency impedance bridge or Q meter, sharp resonances in the impedance are observed whenever the frequency is such that an integral number of half wavelengths fits in the test object's thickness dimension.[15] If the frequency is near the resonant frequency of the

FIGURE 9. Delay line test using a buffer; buffer delay time is also called the water path for immersion transducers.

(a)

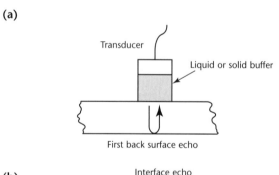

(b)

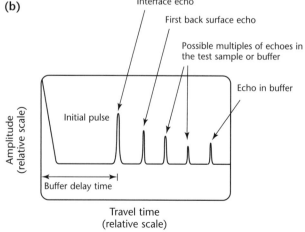

FIGURE 8. Contact test using thin film of liquid couplant: (a) test setup; (b) display.

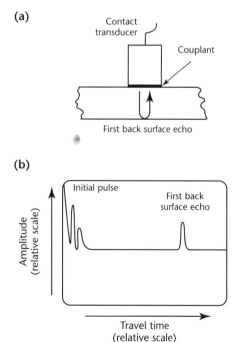

transducer and the couplant is thin, the velocity of sound in the test object is:

$$(4) \quad V = 2T\Delta f \left(1 + \frac{m}{M}\right)$$

where M is the total mass of the test object, m is the total mass of the transducer, T is thickness (meter) and Δf is the difference in frequency between two adjacent resonances (hertz).

The sharpness of the resonances and the accuracy of measuring Δf depends critically on the damping in both the test object and the transducer. Both damping factors must be small.

Continuous wave phase comparison techniques can be used to measure the phase and group velocities in dispersive materials by slowly sweeping the frequency over a wide range and recording the frequencies where the input and output signals are in and out of phase. The disadvantage of the continuous wave technique is its inability to discriminate between reflections, mode conversions or other interfering signals. This limitation may be overcome by pulsing the signal so that extraneous signals are separated in time from the main signal.[16]

Bond Testers

Most discontinuity detectors use pulses to excite the ultrasonic transducers. Bond testers use continuous wave excitation.[17] Bond testers are principally intended for laminates that cannot be adequately tested using conventional discontinuity detection equipment. For example, bond testers can be used for single-sided contact testing of aerospace honeycomb structures.

Continuous wave bond testers operate by setting up a 50 to 500 kHz standing wave within the test object. In principle, such instruments are sensitive to changes in the acoustic impedance of the laminate at preselected test frequencies.[18] The results, in the form of complex impedance values, are displayed on the display unit using a polar presentation appropriate for continuous wave measurements.

The major limitation of continuous wave bond testers arises from their insensitivity to delaminations near the free surfaces of the test objects. However, such discontinuities can generally be detected using other techniques.

Operation in Large Testing Systems

Many ultrasonic instruments, particularly modular industrial production systems,

are used as components of large, automated quality control systems (Fig. 10). In such environments, the ultrasonic instruments must function reliably near motion control mechanisms and other industrial equipment.

To ensure reliable operation, extreme care must be taken not to degrade the quality of the ultrasonic signals and to prevent noise.[19] In particular, transducers should not be mounted on scanning devices requiring long cable lengths. If cables must be long, then specially designed remote pulser preamplifier modules should be used. Such devices are generally small enough to allow positioning close to the transducer, minimizing the undesirable effects of excessive cable lengths.

FIGURE 10. Large automated quality control system containing modular ultrasonic test component.

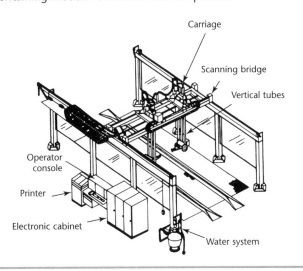

PART 4. Calibration[2]

Measuring System Performance

Ultrasonic test calibration is the practice of adjusting the gain, sweep and range and of assessing the impact that other parameters of the instrument and the test configuration may have on the reliable interpretation of ultrasonic signal echoes. Gain settings are normally established by adjusting the vertical height of an echo signal, as seen on the display, to a predetermined level. The level may be required by specification and based on echo responses from specific standard reflectors in material similar to that which will be tested. Sweep distance of the display is established in terms of equivalent sound path, where the sound path is the distance in the material to be tested from the sound entry point to the reflector.

It is important to establish these parameters. Gain is established so that comparisons of the reference level can be made to an echo of interest to decide whether the echo is of any consequence and, if so, then to aid in the determination of the size of the reflector. Sweep distance is established so that the location of the reflector can be determined. (Amplitude is subject to large, uncontrolled errors and its use in sizing a reflector must be cautious.)

Horizontal linearity is a measure of the uniformity of the sweep speed of the instrument. The instrument must be within the linear dynamic ranges of the sweep amplifiers and associated circuitry for electron beam position to be directly proportional to the time elapsed from the start of the sweep. It may be checked using multiple back echoes from a flat plate of a convenient thickness — say, 25 mm (1 in.). With the sweep set to display multiple back echoes, the spacing between pulses should be equal. The instrument should be recalibrated if the sweep linearity is not within the specified tolerance. Vertical linearity implies that the height of the pulse displayed on the A-scan is directly proportional to the acoustic pulse received by the transducer. For example, if the echo increases by 50 percent, the indicated amplitude on the display should also change by 50 percent. This variable may be checked by establishing an echo signal on the screen, by changing the vertical amplifier gain in set increments and by measuring the corresponding changes in A-scan response. An alternate check uses a pair of echoes with amplitudes in the ratio of two to one. Changes in gain should not affect the ratio, regardless of the amplifier's settings. When electronic distance amplitude correction is used in an ultrasonic system, the vertical amplifier's displayed output is purposefully made to be nonlinear. The nature of the nonlinearity is adjusted to compensate for the estimated or measured variation in the material's and system's aggregate decay in signal strength as a function of distance (travel time) from the sending transducer.

Reference Reflectors

Reflector types commonly used for establishing system performance and sensitivity include spheres, flat bottom holes, notches, side drilled holes and other designs. Table 4 summarizes these reflectors and their advantages and limitations.

Spherical reflectors are used most often in immersion testing for assessing

TABLE 4. Reference reflectors in ultrasonic testing.

Type	Characteristics	Uses
Solid sphere	omnidirectional reflector	transducer sound field assessment
Notches	flat, corner reflector	simulation of near surface cracks
Flat bottom hole	disk reflector	reference gain
Side drilled hole	cylindrical reflector	calibration for distance amplitude correction
Special	custom reflectivity	simulation of natural discontinuity conditions

transducer sound fields as shown in Fig. 11. Spheres provide excellent repeatability because of their omnidirectional sound wave response. The effective reflectance from a sphere is much smaller than that received from a flat reflector of the same diameter due to its spherical directivity pattern. Most of the reflected energy does not return to the search unit. Spheres of any material can be used; however, steel ball bearings are the norm because they are reasonably priced, are very precise in size and surface finish and are available in many sizes.

Flat reflectors are used as calibration standards in both immersion and contact testing. They are usually drilled, flat bottom holes of the desired diameters and depths. All flat reflectors have the inherent weakness that they require careful alignment of the axis of the sound beam to the reflector. Deviations of little more than about 50 mrad (a few degrees) will lead to significantly reduced echoes and become unacceptable for calibration. However, for discontinuities of cross section less than the beam width and with a perpendicular alignment, the signal amplitude is proportional to the area of the reflector. Generally, if a discontinuity echo amplitude is equal to the amplitude of the calibration reflector, it is assumed that the discontinuity is at least as large as the calibration reflector.

Notches are frequently used to assess the detectability of surface breaking discontinuities such as cracks, as well as for instrument calibration. Notches of several shapes are used and can either be of a rectangular or V cross section. Notches may be made with milling cutters (end mills), circular saws or straight saws. End mill or electric discharge machined notches may be made with highly variable length and depth dimensions. Circular saw cuts are limited in length and depth by the saw diameter and the configuration of the device holding the saw. Although the circular saw makes it more difficult to achieve a desired ratio of length to depth, these notches are used frequently because of their resemblance to fatigue cracks — for example, shape and surface finish. Notches may be produced perpendicular to the surface or at other angles as dictated by the test configuration. On piping, they may be on the inside surface or outside surface and are aligned either in the longitudinal or transverse directions.

Side drilled holes are placed in calibration blocks so that the axis of the hole is parallel to the entry surface. The sound beam impinges on the hole, normal to its major axis. Such a reflector provides very repeatable calibrations, may be placed at any desired distance from the entry surface and may be used for both longitudinal waves and a multitude of transverse wave angles. It is essential that the hole surface be smooth, so reaming to the final diameter is often the final step in preparing such holes.

Used in sets with differing distances from the surface and different diameters, side drilled holes are frequently used for developing distance amplitude correction curves and for setting overall sensitivity of transverse wave testing schemes. After the sweep distance is set, signals from each reflector are maximized (by maneuvering the search unit) and the results are recorded on the screen using erasable markers or stored in a digital format. The peak signals from each reflector are then connected by a smooth line. This line is called the *distance amplitude correction* (DAC) curve.

FIGURE 11. Spherical reflector for calibration of ultrasonic test system.

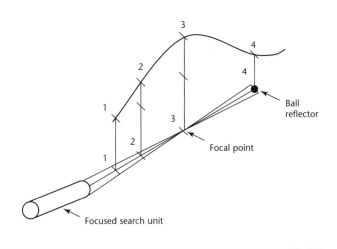

Calibration Blocks

The setting of basic instrument controls is expedited by several standard sets of blocks containing precision reflectors arranged to feature a specific characteristic of test systems (Table 5). For example, area amplitude blocks contain flat bottom holes of differing diameters, all at the same distance from the sound entry surface (Fig. 12). The block material is normally similar to that of the test material. In the distance and area amplitude blocks, a hole is placed in a separate cylinder, 50 mm (2 in.) in diameter. Other blocks, intended for the same purpose of establishing the correlation of signal amplitude with the area of the reflector, may contain a number of holes in the same block, usually a plate. Hole sizes increase in sixty-fourths of an inch and are

TABLE 5. Parameters checked with various calibration blocks.

Characteristic	Block Designation						
	IIW	DSC	ASME (SDH)	SC	DA	AA	AWS (RC)
Sweep Range	T, L	T, L	T, L	—	L	L	—
Sensitivity	T, L	T, L	T, L	T	L	L	—
Exit point	T	T	—	—	—	—	—
Exit angle	T	T	—	T	—	—	—
Distance Amplitude Correction	—	—	T, L	—	L	L	—
Depth Resolution	L	—	—	—	L, n	—	T
Curvature Compensation	—	—	T, c	—	—	—	—

Legend

AA = area amplitude block (flat bottom holes)
ASME = American Society of Mechanical Engineers (side drilled holes)
AWS (RC) = American Welding Society, resolution calibration (side drilled holes)
c = set of curved blocks
DA = distance amplitude block (flat bottom holes)
DSC = distance and sensitivity calibration (slots, side drilled holes, reference geometries)
IIW = International Institute of Welding (slots, side drilled holes, reference geometries)
L = longitudinal wave
n = near surface only
SC = sensitivity calibration
T = transverse wave

FIGURE 12. Flat bottom hole blocks for ultrasonic calibration: (a) set of 19 steel blocks; (b) diagram.

(a)

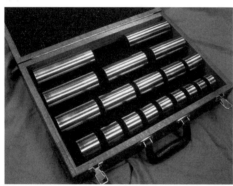

(b)

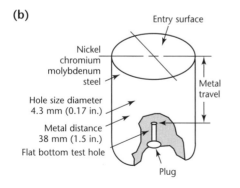

Entry surface

Nickel chromium molybdenum steel

Hole size diameter 4.3 mm (0.17 in.)

Metal distance 38 mm (1.5 in.)

Flat bottom test hole

Metal travel

Plug

designated by that value. For example, a 1.59 mm (4/64 = 0.062 in.) hole is a number 4 hole. Area amplitude blocks are used to establish the response curve of area to amplitude and the sensitivity of the ultrasonic test system. Maximum signals are obtained from each of the holes of interest, and the signal amplitude is recorded. These values may be compared to echoes from the same metal path and reflector sizes estimated for the test item. Figure 12b diagrams a cross section of a block composed of Unified Numbering System G43400 nickel chromium molybdenum steel, with a number 5 flat bottom hole measuring 2.98 mm (5/64 = 0.078 in.) and a travel distance of 38 m (1.5 in.).

Distance amplitude blocks differ from area amplitude blocks in that a single diameter, flat bottom hole is placed at incrementally increasing depths from very near the entry surface to a desired maximum depth. Sets of blocks are available in different materials and with diameters ranging from number 1 to number 16 and larger. Distance amplitude blocks are used to establish the distance amplitude response characteristic of the ultrasonic system in the test material; the measured response includes the effects of attenuation due to beam spread and scattering and/or absorption. With this curve established, the operator can compensate for the effects of attenuation with distance. Distance amplitude blocks are useful in setting instrument sensitivity (gain) and if present the electronic distance amplitude correction circuits.

There are numerous blocks commercially available for calibrating ultrasonic test instruments for sweep distance (sound path), sensitivity (gain) and depth resolution. Included in this group are various angle beam blocks, the ASME (American Society of Mechanical Engineers) basic calibration block and the IIW (International Institute of Welding) calibration block (Fig. 13). Some blocks are specified by standards.[20-29]

Other special blocks are often required in response to specification and code requirements based on the construction of the blocks, using materials of the same nature as those to be inspected. Included are the ASME weld inspection blocks — such as the side drilled hole for angle beam calibration, curved blocks for simulation of piping or nozzles and nozzle dropouts (circular blanks cut from vessel plates) for custom nuclear inservice inspection applications. It is possible to fabricate reflectors that can directly behave as cracks and generate actual cracks, particularly intergranular stress corrosion cracks. Table 5 summarizes many of these blocks and their intended uses.

FIGURE 13. Ultrasonic calibration blocks: (a) angle beam calibration block; (b) ASME basic calibration block; (c) International Institute of Welding calibration block. (1 degree = 17 milliradian. 1 inch = 25.4 millimeter.)

(a)

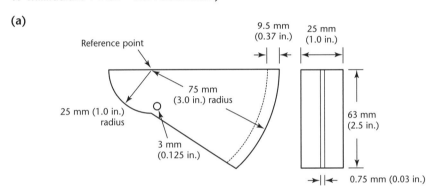

(b)

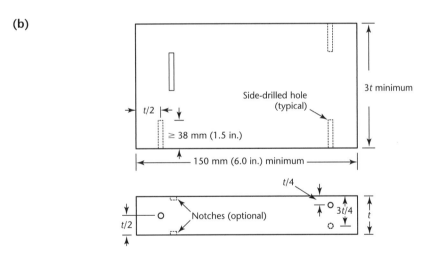

(c)

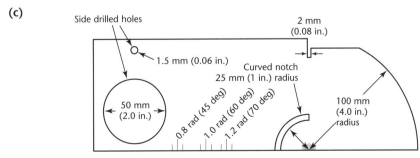

One of the best known calibration blocks is the IIW block, used primarily for measuring the refracted angle of angle beam search units, setting the metal path and establishing the sensitivity for weld inspection. To measure the refracted angle, the sound beam exit point is determined on the 100 mm (4 in.) radius. The angle is then determined by maximizing the signal from the large side drilled hole and reading the exit point position on the engraved scale.

Various reflectors are provided in modified IIW blocks to provide the capability to set the sweep distance. These include grooves and notches at various locations to yield echoes at precisely known distances. The block may also be used for setting distances for normal (straight beam) search units using the 25 mm (1 in.) thickness of the block. Distance resolution may also be checked on the notches adjacent to the 100 mm (4 in.) radius surface. Because different manufacturers provide variations in the configuration of the block, other specific uses may be devised.

The distance calibration block is specifically designed for setting up the sweep distance for both normal and angle beam testing for longitudinal, transverse or surface waves. For straight beam calibration, the search unit is placed on the 25 or 50 mm (1.0 or 2.0 in.) thick portion and the sweep distance adjusted. For angle beam calibration, the search unit is placed on the flat surface at the center of the cylindrical surfaces. Beam direction is in a plane normal to the cylinder axis. When the beam is directed in such a manner, echoes should occur at intervals of 25, 50 or 75 mm (1, 2 or 3 in.). With a surface wave search unit at the centerline, a surface wave may be calibrated for distance by observing the echoes from the 25 and 50 mm (1 and 2 in.) radii and adjusting the controls accordingly.

A miniature multipurpose block is 25 mm (1 in.) thick and has a 1.5 mm (0.06 in.) diameter, side drilled hole for sensitivity settings and angle determinations. For straight beam calibration, the block provides back reflection and multipliers of 25 mm (1 in.). For angle beams, the search unit is placed on the flat surface with the beam is directed toward either curved surface. If toward the 25 mm (1 in.) radius, echoes will be received at 25 mm (1 in.), 100 mm (4 in.) and 175 mm (7 in.) intervals. If toward the 50 mm (2 in.) radius, the intervals will be 50 (2 in.), 125 mm (5 in.) and 200 mm (8 in.). Refracted angles are measured by locating the exit point using either of the curved surfaces. The response from the side drilled hole is maximized and the angle read from the engraved

scales. Single point (zone) sensitivity can be established by maximizing the signal from the side drilled hole. Distance amplitude correction curves can be developed for any number of test part thicknesses using a side drilled hole block. By placing the angle beam transducer on surfaces which change the sound path distance, a series of peaked responses can be recorded and plotted on the display in the form of a distance amplitude correction curve over the range of distances of interest to inspection.

A more suitable, but expensive, approach to the testing of complex parts involves sacrificial samples into which are placed wave reflectors such as flat bottom holes, side drilled holes and notches.

Reference blocks based on imbedded natural reflectors such as cracks by diffusion bonding, although useful for establishing a baseline for self-teaching adaptive learning, are difficult to duplicate and cannot correlate with naturally occurring discontinuities. Of concern is the inability to duplicate test samples on a production basis; once destructive correlations are carried out, remaking the same configuration is questionable. Even when such reflectors can be duplicated to some extent, the natural variability of discontinuities found in nature still tends to make this approach to reference standards highly questionable. In all cases, the block materials used for calibration purposes must be similar to the test materials to which the techniques will be applied. The concept of transfer functions has been used with limited success in most critical calibration settings.

References

1. Green, R.E., Jr. Section 1, "Introduction to Ultrasonic Testing." *Nondestructive Testing Handbook,* second edition: Vol. 7, *Ultrasonic Testing.* Columbus, OH: American Society for Nondestructive Testing (1991): p 1-21.
2. Golis, M.J. *ASNT Level III Study Guide: Ultrasonic Method,* second edition. Columbus, OH: American Society for Nondestructive Testing (1992; fourth printing, corrected, 2006).
3. Fortunko, C.M. Section 5, "Ultrasonic Testing Equipment." *Nondestructive Testing Handbook,* second edition: Vol. 7, *Ultrasonic Testing.* Columbus, OH: American Society for Nondestructive Testing (1991): p 101-129.
4. Firestone, F.A. United States Patent 2 280 226, *Flaw Detecting Device and Measuring Instrument* (April 1942).
5. Silk, M.G. *Ultrasonic Transducers for Nondestructive Testing.* Bristol, United Kingdom: Adam Hilger (1984): p 4-20.
6. Rivera, O. and F.V. Vitale. "Airborne Ultrasonic Scanning." *Materials Evaluation.* Vol. 46, No. 4. Columbus, OH: American Society for Nondestructive Testing (April 1988): p 614-615.
7. Fortunko, C.M., J.O. Strycek and W.A. Grandia. "Nondestructive Testing of Thick Aerospace Honeycomb Structures Using Through-Transmitted Ultrasonic Guided Waves." *Review of Progress in Quantitative Nondestructive Evaluation* [La Jolla, CA, July-August 1988]. Vol. 8B. New York, NY: Plenum (1989): p 1643-1650.
8. Moran, T.J. and C.F. Buynak. "Correlation of Ultrasonic Imaging and Destructive Analyses of Low Energy Impact Events." *Review of Progress in Quantitative Nondestructive Evaluation* [La Jolla, CA, July-August 1988]. Vol. 8B. New York, NY: Plenum (1989): p 1627-1634.
9. Hughes, M.S., D.K. Hsu, S.J. Wormley, J.M. Mann, C.M. Fortunko and D.O. Thompson. "Comparison of Attenuation and Phase Velocity Measurements Made Using Unipolar and Bipolar Pulses." *Review of Progress in Quantitative Nondestructive Evaluation* [La Jolla, CA, July-August 1988]. Vol. 8A. New York, NY: Plenum (1989): p 1111-1118.
10. Lynnworth, L.C. *Ultrasonic Measurements for Process Control.* New York, NY: Academic Press (1989): p 55-58.
11. Lemons, R.A. and C.F. Quate. "Acoustic Microscope — Scanning Version." *Applied Physics Letter.* New York, NY: American Institute of Physics (1974): p 163-164.
12. Burton, N.J. "NDT Applications of Scanning Acoustic Microscopy." *IEE Proceedings.* Vol. 134, Part A, No. 3. United Kingdom: Institution of Electrical Engineers (1987): p 283-289.
13. Meeks, S.V., D. Peter, D. Horne, K. Young and V. Novotny. "Microscopic Imaging of Residual Stress Using a Scanning Phase-Measuring Acoustic Microscope." *Applied Physics Letters.* Vol. 55, No. 18. Melville, NY: American Institute of Physics (1989): p 1835-1837.
14. Alers, G. Section 11, "Methods for Velocity and Attenuation Measurement." *Nondestructive Testing Handbook,* second edition: Vol. 7, *Ultrasonic Testing.* Columbus, OH: American Society for Nondestructive Testing (1991): p 365-381.
15. Bolef, D.I. and M. Menes. "Measurement of Elastic Constants of RbBr, RbI, CsBr and CsI by an Ultrasonic CW Resonance Technique." *Journal of Applied Physics.* Vol. 31, No. 2. Melville, NY: American Institute of Physics (1960): p 1010.
16. *Nondestructive Testing Handbook,* second edition: Vol. 7, *Ultrasonic Testing.* Columbus, OH: American Society for Nondestructive Testing (1991): p 173.
17. Botsco, R.J. and R.T. Anderson. "Ultrasonic Impedance-Plane Analysis of Aerospace Laminates." *Adhesives Age.* Vol. 27, No. 7. Atlanta, GA: William Zmyndak Communication Channels (June 1984): p 22-25.
18. Highmore, P. and J. Szilard. "Resonance Methods." *Ultrasonic Testing: Nonconventional Testing Techniques.* New York, NY: Wiley (1982): p 263-296.
19. Ott, H.W. *Noise Reduction Techniques in Electronic Systems,* second edition. New York, NY: Wiley Interscience (1976): p 253-254.

Bibliography

Hagemaier, D.[J.] Section 13, "Ultrasonic Reference Standards and Control of Tests." *Nondestructive Testing Handbook,* second edition: Vol. 7, *Ultrasonic Testing.* Columbus, OH: American Society for Nondestructive Testing (1991): p 433-482.

Herman, P., Jr. "Manufacturing NDT Reference Standards." *The NDT Technician.* Vol. 4, No. 3. Columbus, OH: American Society for Nondestructive Testing (July 2005): p 1-3, 5.

Houf, J.[W.] "Practical Contact Ultrasonics — Angle Beam Calibration Using a Basic Calibration Block." *The NDT Technician.* Vol. 3, No. 4. Columbus, OH: American Society for Nondestructive Testing (October 2004): p 4-6, 9.

Houf, J.[W.] "Practical Contact Ultrasonics — Equipment Maintenance." *The NDT Technician.* Vol. 4, No. 3. Columbus, OH: American Society for Nondestructive Testing (July 2005): p 4-5.

Houf, J.[W.] "Practical Contact Ultrasonics — IIW Based Angle Beam Calibration." *The NDT Technician.* Vol. 3, No. 3. Columbus, OH: American Society for Nondestructive Testing (July 2004): p 4-6.

Makarwich, L.B. "Benefits and Limitations of Ultrasonic Testing Multiplexers." *The NDT Technician.* Vol. 4, No. 1. Columbus, OH: American Society for Nondestructive Testing (January 2005): p 1-3, 11.

Posakony, G.J. "Influence of the Pulser Parameters on the Ultrasonic Spectrum." *Materials Evaluation.* Vol. 43, No. 4. Columbus, OH: American Society for Nondestructive Testing (1985): p 413-419

Standards

ASTM E 127, *Standard Practice for Fabricating and Checking Aluminum Alloy Ultrasonic Standard Reference Blocks.* West Conshohocken, PA: ASTM International.

ASTM E 164, *Standard Practice for Ultrasonic Contact Examination of Weldments.* West Conshohocken, PA: ASTM International.

ASTM E 317, *Standard Practice for Evaluating Performance Characteristics of Ultrasonic Pulse-Echo Examination Instruments and Systems without the Use of Electronic Measurement Instruments.* West Conshohocken, PA: ASTM International.

ASTM E 428, *Standard Practice for Fabrication and Control of Steel Reference Blocks Used in Ultrasonic Examination.* West Conshohocken, PA: ASTM International.

ASTM E 1158, *Standard Guide for Material Selection and Fabrication of Reference Blocks for the Pulsed Longitudinal Wave Ultrasonic Examination of Metal and Metal Alloy Production Material.* West Conshohocken, PA: ASTM International.

ASTM E 1324, *Standard Guide for Measuring Some Electronic Characteristics of Ultrasonic Examination Instruments.* West Conshohocken, PA: ASTM International.

EN 12223, *Non-Destructive Testing — Ultrasonic Examination — Specification for Calibration Block No. 1.* Brussels, Belgium: European Committee for Standardization.

EN 12668, *Non-Destructive Testing — Characterization and Verification of Ultrasonic Examination Equipment.* Brussels, Belgium: European Committee for Standardization.

EN 27963, *Welds in Steel — Calibration Block No. 2 for Ultrasonic Examination of Welds.* Brussels, Belgium: European Committee for Standardization.

ISO 7963, *Welds in Steel — Calibration Block No. 2 for Ultrasonic Examination of Welds.* Geneva, Switzerland: International Organization for Standardization.

ISO 12715, *Ultrasonic Non-Destructive Testing — Reference Blocks and Test Procedures for the Characterization of Contact Search Unit Beam Profiles.* Geneva, Switzerland: International Organization for Standardization.

ISO 18175, *Non-Destructive Testing — Evaluating Performance Characteristics of Ultrasonic Pulse-Echo Testing Systems without the Use of Electronic Measurement Instruments.* Geneva, Switzerland: International Organization for Standardization.

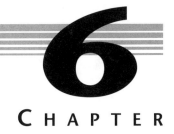

6

C H A P T E R

Ultrasonic Pulse Echo Contact Techniques

Francis H. Chang, Fort Worth, Texas (Parts 1 to 3)

Donald J. Hagemaier, Huntington Beach, California (Part 2)

Michael Moles, Olympus NDT Canada, Toronto, Ontario, Canada (Part 6)

G.P. Singh, Karta Technology, San Antonio, Texas (Parts 5 to 7)

Part 1. Straight Beam Pulse Echo Tests[1,2]

Introduction

In contact pulse echo ultrasonic testing, the transducer touches the test surface, sometimes with an intervening film of couplant. Although a single transducer typically is used as transmitter and receiver of the ultrasound, dual-element transducers are also used. The presence and location of a reflecting discontinuity is indicated by the echo signal amplitude and the time at which the echo signal arrives at the transducer.

The major advantage of the pulse echo contact technique is its adaptability to large and irregularly shaped objects. The test object does not need to be placed in a water tank, as in the immersion technique, or in a large fixture, as in the water jet technique. The contact technique can be used directly on a large stationary object or on confined areas of a complex structure.

The pulse echo contact technique offers high sensitivity to small discontinuities and permits accurate determinations of discontinuity depth beneath the entry surface. In many cases, pulse echo tests also permit determination of the size and orientation of internal discontinuities, particularly laminar discontinuities oriented perpendicular to the path of the incident ultrasonic beam. With rough surfaced discontinuities or nearly spherical small discontinuities (such as porosities in organic composites), the ultrasonic beam is often scattered and the echo signals are low in magnitude. In such cases, it is possible to recognize the presence of the discontinuity by the loss of the echo from the back surface of the test object if this surface is nearly parallel to the test object's front surface.

The instrumentation for the pulse echo technique can be quite simple. A single transducer, a pulser/receiver unit and a screen display are sufficient for tests without permanent records. If permanent records are required, there must also be equipment for indicating the amplitude of the signal and the transducer position on the test object.

The major disadvantage of the pulse echo contact technique is reduced near surface resolution caused by ringdown interference. This is caused by the direct contact of the transducer face and the test object and the presence of a large excitation pulse. This can be somewhat offset by introducing a solid delay line at the end of the transducer or by placing a partitioning column of liquid couplant between the transducer face and the test object.

Instrumentation for Straight Beam Tests

To meet mobility requirements of contact testing, smaller portable ultrasonic test systems often are preferred over larger, more sophisticated units. In a typical system, the dynamic gain range required for the pulser/receiver depends on the required penetration, usually a minimum of 20 dB.

Because the pulse echo contact technique is often performed in the field, the operation of the pulser/receiver should be as simple as possible — recent developments in pulser/receiver technology have produced digital control of gain, sweep delay and gate setting. Some test objects such as stainless steel welds need more sophisticated equipment.

Transducers for Straight Beam Tests

In the majority of cases, a single-element contact transducer is used in the pulse echo mode. A wear plate is placed on the face of the transducer to reduce damage from contact with test object surfaces. A wear plate with an acoustic impedance midway between that of the element and the test material optimizes the contact.

To improve the near surface resolution of the test, a delay line can be attached to the face of the transducer to separate the excitation pulse from the incident surface response and to better match the acoustic impedance of the test material. The length of the delay line should be such that the multiple reflections from the delay line fall well outside the back surface reflection. Many commercial contact transducers are designed with interchangeable delay lines. It is important to place a thin layer of gel between the transducer face and the delay line for good coupling.

The disadvantage of using a delay line is that its attendant attenuation and impedance mismatch (with metals) can diminish the penetration power of the ultrasound. Sometimes a dual-element transducer can be used instead of a single-element transducer with delay line. Separate elements for transmitting and receiving transducers are arranged side by side to eliminate interface signal interference. Multiple transducers or phased arrays arranged in a paint brush fashion are also used so that a wider path can be covered in a single scan.

Displaying Pulse Echo Test Results

Most pulse echo contact testing is performed visually using a pulser/receiver display in the A-scan mode as the only means of data presentation. Pulse echo contact systems that analyze test results and output the real time C-scan on a graphic display are discussed separately below.

Straight Beam Test Procedures

For accessible surfaces of a test object, pulse echo contact techniques are straightforward. As shown in Fig. 1 for a direct contact transducer, ultrasound enters the test object and is reflected off its back surface. On the screen display, the interface or front surface signal coincides with the initial pulse. The back surface reflection signal occurs later, corresponding to the thickness of the test object. If a discontinuity is encountered, its reflected signal occurs before the back surface signal. A gate can be set between the front and back surface signals to monitor responses from the material during scanning. Any gate signal with an amplitude exceeding a preset level can set off an audible alarm or transmit a computer message.

For a transducer with a delay line, the interface signal or front surface signal is separated from the initial pulse. The near surface resolution can be improved by this separation. It is important to set the length of the delay line so that multiple reflections from the delay line do not fall within the gate.

For test objects thinner than the path length of the ultrasound, the beam spread of the sound pattern may create interference from the side walls. If the longitudinal waves strike the side walls, transverse waves are generated in addition to longitudinal waves from the straight beam. The screen then displays spurious signals occurring after the back surface reflection signal. Such signals generally do not present problems in interpretation because they occur after the back surface reflection (see Fig. 2).

Other gating techniques can be used to interrogate or emphasize certain depth ranges in the test object. Some pulser/receiver units have the ability to use multiple gates. Gates and variable gain controls may be used concurrently to focus on certain depth ranges.

Signal processing techniques can be used for waveform analysis in

FIGURE 1. Ultrasonic test displays for two composites: (a) direct contact transducer; (b) transducer with delay line.

(a)

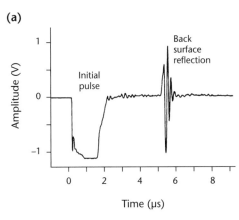

(b)

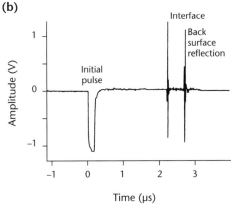

FIGURE 2. Ultrasonic beam spread in 44 mm (1.75 in.) diameter aluminum rod tested laterally.

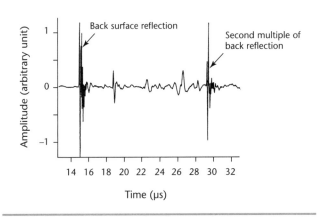

computerized contact test systems. The advantage of signal processing over conventional peak detection and gating techniques is better discontinuity resolution and discrimination. Signal processing is especially useful for achieving a high level of near-surface resolution. For example, a conventional pulser/receiver contact testing unit might have a minimum near-surface resolution of 0.38 mm (0.015 in.) in graphite epoxy composites.

Applications of Straight Beam Contact Tests

Manual Scanning

The pulse echo contact technique is most often applied manually or with scanning. The technique is rarely used for initial large area tests. Its primary use is for outlining or mapping discontinuity areas. In a manual scan, the technician places the transducer on the test object and watches the screen for discontinuity indications.

Whenever the inspector finds an indication, the corresponding spot on the test object surface is marked with a grease pencil or an indelible marker. The transducer is moved around the surrounding area and the periphery of the discontinuity is outlined by monitoring where the signal drops below a preset level. Sometimes discontinuity areas are traced on a transparent overlay and kept as a permanent record of the test.

Screen Indications of Discontinuities

A traditional straight beam ultrasonic contact test display is shown in Fig. 1. The horizontal displacement indicates the time delay between successive ultrasonic signals. The first vertical indication, reading from left to right, corresponds to the initial pulse of electrical energy applied to the transducer. In contact tests, this event occurs at a time just preceding the entry of the sound energy into the front surface of the test object, after leaving the transducer and passing through the face plate and liquid couplant. In the A-scan display, this signal is sometimes wrongly considered to represent the position of the front or entry surface of the test material.

A broadening of this pulse may be noted as the transducer is placed in contact with the test object. The horizontal axis of the A-scan signal display can be defined as (1) the time delay following the initial pulse or (2) the distance from the test object entry

surface. The latter interpretation is valid only when the sound pulse velocity is constant within the test material, so that the round trip sound pulse transit time is proportional to the depth from which the sound pulse is reflected. The assumption is generally valid for most uniform, nonporous, elastic test materials (metals, ceramics or glasses). Thermal gradients, heterogeneous regions and other effects can invalidate this assumption.

Initial Pulse

Widening of the initial pulse indication can result from transducer ringing (inadequate damping), lengthening of the excitation pulse, thick couplant layers or rough entry surfaces on the test object.

Such prolonged initial pulse indications can obscure or hide reflection signals from discontinuities or interfaces that lie close to the entry surface. This so-called *dead zone* is the distance from the test surface to the nearest depth at which discontinuities can be reliably detected. The extent of a dead zone can be reduced (1) by selecting a higher pulse frequency or (2) by selecting a minimal pulse length, thereby reducing the pulsing time on the instrument. In addition, another transducer may be selected with dual-element construction, a more efficient piezoelectric element or more effective damping. If pulse length is too long for the application, the material may be scanned from the reverse side to cover the obscured areas.

Discontinuity Signals

The second vertical indication in Fig. 3 represents an echo signal from a discontinuity in the test material. Its amplitude is lower than that of the front surface signal. The discontinuity reflects only a portion of the incident sound pulse

FIGURE 3. Typical ultrasonic test display showing interface signal, discontinuity indication and back surface reflection.

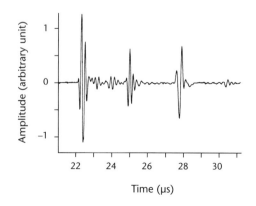

when the sound beam diameter is greater than the reflecting cross-sectional area of the discontinuity.

Many discontinuities are not flat or perpendicular to the incident sound beam and serve to scatter the ultrasonic energy so that it does not return to the transducer. Such discontinuities might be indicated by reduced echo signal levels. The amplifier type and its gain setting also have strong effects on the relative amplitude of discontinuity echo signals. Time varying signal amplifier gain controls are typically limited to the far field of the ultrasonic transducer.

Back Surface Reflections

The third vertical indication (on the right of Fig. 3) corresponds to the strong echo returned from the rear surface of the test material when (1) this surface is perpendicular to the sound beam and (2) the material transmits ultrasound with little attenuation. This back surface signal could be reduced in amplitude or could disappear completely if the intervening discontinuity is large enough in area to intercept most of the beam from the transducer. Loss of back surface indications without loss of coupling is an immediate warning that the sound beam from the transducer has been interrupted by a large discontinuity in the test object or has been scattered by rough or angled discontinuities.

The loss of back surface reflected signals can also occur in highly attenuative media. In this case, it may be necessary to reduce the test frequency to decrease the attenuation. Only when clear back surface signals are displayed can it be ensured that the ultrasonic beam intensity is adequate for producing detectable discontinuity signals. Because lower test frequencies decrease the detectability of small discontinuities, higher amplifier gains may be required to ensure detection of small discontinuities.

Only a small portion of the initial pulse energy is returned to the transducer at the end of its first round trip through the test material. As each echo returns to the front surface, only a small fraction of its energy passes through the material surface and the couplant to the transducer. The sound pulse energy remaining within the test material continues to bounce back and forth between the parallel front and back surfaces until the sound has dissipated within the test material.

While the decaying sound beam continues to reflect back and forth within the test object, the search unit continues to receive weakening signals when each echo reaches the entry surface under the transducer. A number of these multiple

back reflections and internal discontinuity signals may be observed on the screen by extending the time scale (Fig. 4). Because the signal multiples become more complex, it is often preferable to adjust the time sweep of the tube to display only one or two round trip periods.

Discontinuity Discrimination

The most commonly used technique of automated discontinuity discrimination is known as the *amplitude gating technique*. In this technique, a monitoring gate is set by electronically selecting a period of time in the horizontal time sweep of the pulser/receiver. The gate is typically set between the front and back surface reflection signals or in the specific area of interest and any signal appearing in the gate above a predetermined level triggers a discontinuity indication device.

Discontinuities between the front and back surfaces reflect sound energy back to the transducer within the time period set by the gate. The orientation and geometrical shape of the discontinuity, with respect to the test object surface and the transducer orientation, are important factors in determining the intensity of the ultrasound reflected back to the receiving transducer.

Figure 5 shows the ultrasonic signals reflected from a series of geometric shapes embedded in a plastic casing. A planar discontinuity parallel to the front surface is a good reflector, redirecting energy back to the receiving transducer (Figs. 5a and 5b). A spherical discontinuity scatters ultrasound and reflects only a small amount of the impinging energy at the apex closest to the test object surface (Fig. 5d). A planar discontinuity perpendicular to the test object surface presents a small area to the beam,

FIGURE 4. Multiple ultrasonic reflections in 7 mm (0.27 in.) aluminum block.

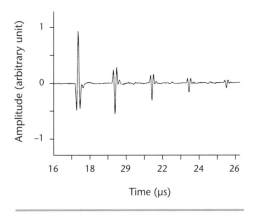

reflecting a small amount of the incident energy back to the receiver (Fig. 5c).

To detect clusters of small spherical discontinuities such as porosity in composites, a second gate may be set to monitor the amplitude of the back surface

echo. In the case of many small discontinuities (or any discontinuity that diverts the reflected signal away from the receiving transducer), the ultrasound reaching the back surface is less than normal and the signal amplitude is diminished. With a continuous automated recording procedure, this back surface amplitude technique can be used only in homogeneous material when the ultrasonic test system provides a second gate or digitized waveform analysis.

Discontinuities Detected with Straight Beam Technique

Discontinuities commonly seen in composites are delaminations, voids, porosities and ply gaps (Fig. 6). Inclusions in composites are difficult to detect because their composition is sometimes close to the acoustic impedance of the composite and insufficient energy is reflected from the discontinuity interfaces. Figure 7 shows signals reflected from a reference standard with implanted inclusions of polyethylene and polyester films.

In metals, common discontinuities are voids, foreign inclusions, cracks and other anomalies. As discussed in the preceding subsection, the signals reflected from these discontinuities depend on the shape and orientation of the principal reflecting surfaces. Few fatigue cracks are oriented with reflective surfaces parallel to the entry surface of the test object. For this reason, an angle beam ultrasonic contact technique is generally used to detect fatigue cracks.

Sizing Discontinuities[1,3]

When discontinuity sizes are larger than the diameter of the ultrasonic transducer, the outline of the discontinuity can be obtained by marking positions where the discontinuity signals drop by a preset amount, such as 50 percent. With an appropriate transducer diameter and test frequency, the contact pulse echo ultrasonic technique provides a reliable means for sizing discontinuities approximately.

In manual scanning, the outline is made by marking the location of the center of the transducer on the test object. In computerized pulse echo contact scanning, an algorithm can be written into the data analysis program to mark and refine the outline of the discontinuities.

If the size of a discontinuity is smaller than the diameter of the transducer, a

FIGURE 5. Straight beam ultrasonic reflections: (a) from right disk head on, (b) from hexagonal disk head on; (c) from side of right disk; (d) from sphere.

(a)

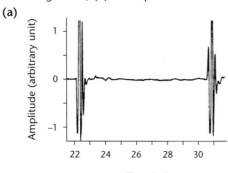

(b)

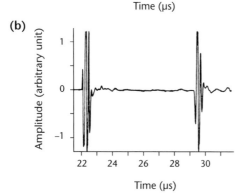

(c)

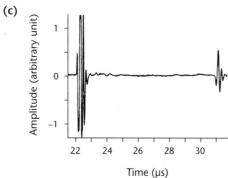

(d)

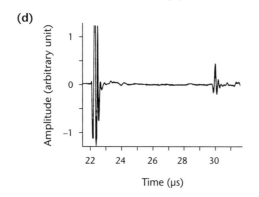

reference standard containing known discontinuity sizes is necessary for calibration. A common reference standard configuration has flat bottom holes of graduated sizes machined into assorted metals. Testing specifications of many metallic materials are often classified in terms of the diameter of these flat bottom holes. Distance amplitude correction devices are used to standardize the reflected signals from different depths in the material.

In the United States, it has been common to measure the amplitudes of discontinuity echoes in terms of their signal height on a video screen. In the twentieth century, such measurements were typically expressed in inches or as a

percentage of the maximum or full screen height or a percentage of the height of a fixed datum. The reproducibility of all these techniques depends on the type of ultrasonic instrument and the linearity of the amplifier response, the display and the gated output of automated equipment. Elaborate checks have been devised to test linearity[4] but there are simple techniques as well.[5,6]

A calibrated attenuator can reduce the size of the displayed signal independently of amplifier linearity, overcoming the problem of comparison. When a discontinuity signal is detected, the attenuator is used to adjust the A-scan signal height to a fixed level so that the discontinuity echo amplitude can be expressed unambiguously and repeatedly in decibels above or below the fixed level.

If the equipment has been set up so that a standard target also gives an echo to this level, then discontinuity echoes can all be referred back to the standard as so many decibels above or below it.

FIGURE 6. Typical ultrasonic test signals from six-ply fabric composite: (a) well bonded material front and back surface reflections; (b) porosities; (c) delamination at five-ply depth.

(a)

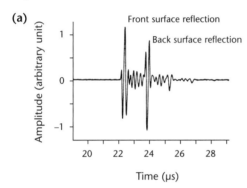

(b)

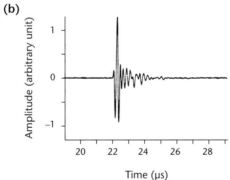

(c)

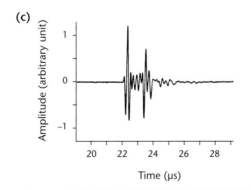

FIGURE 7. Ultrasonic test signals from 50-ply composite: (a) polyethylene inclusion; (b) polyester film inclusion.

(a)

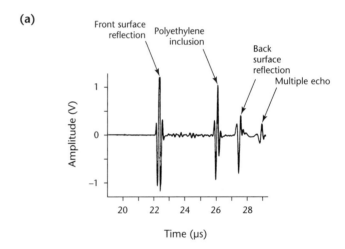

(b)

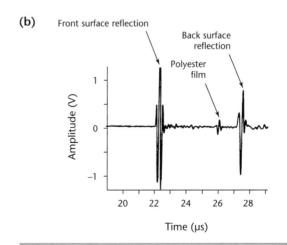

Because it is a unit of comparison or a relative measure, the decibel scale has a floating zero that can be chosen to correspond to the echo from a convenient standard target.

If the ultrasonic equipment includes an internally connected attenuator calibrated in decibels, a reflector of a single size may be used as a reference standard to evaluate the product to different quality levels. The instrument may be standardized using 2.0 mm (5/64 in.) flat bottom holes at different metal travels. Corrections for other size reflectors are established by adding or subtracting (Table 1).

Factors Determining Discontinuity Echo Signals[3]

The height of an echo depends on the size (reflecting area) of the discontinuity, its depth, shape, orientation and the nature of the test object surfaces (roughness, contour and acoustic impedance). For discontinuities covering a large area or for laminations in sheet, amplitude is not used and these factors are not significant — the size can be found by tracing the outline of the discontinuity with the transducer, noting where the signal amplitude drops by 6 dB, that is, by half.

When the discontinuity is smaller than the diameter of the sound beam, the size may be deduced from the height of the echo, provided the following essential conditions are fulfilled: (1) the plane of the discontinuity must be parallel with the sound entry surface, (2) surface roughness is less than 5 µm (0.0002 in.), (3) the reflectivity is 100 percent and (4) the discontinuity distance from the sound entry surface is in the far field and there is no edge interference.

Attempts have been made to reduce the number of reference blocks to determine discontinuity size. The situation is complex because the amplitude of the test signal varies with the position of the near and far field in the test object. The point of maximum response along the sound beam axis can be loosely described as the end of the near field zone. In Europe, it is called the

N point. In the United States, the term $Y_0(\text{max})$ is used (Fig. 8).

The position of this maximum sensitivity point in the ultrasonic beam is determined by the diameter of the transducer; its effective operating frequency and the velocity of sound in the test medium.

Distance Gain Size Diagram[3,6,7]

Attempts have been made to quantify the flat reflector system without actually using reference blocks. The distance gain size diagram allows discontinuity size estimations based on observed echo heights and a series of simple calculations. The diagram is straightforward once the physical characteristics of beam shapes are appreciated, the basic concepts used in this technique include (1) a reduced range (distance of transducer to discontinuity expressed as a multiple of the near field distance), (2) a reduced size (discontinuity diameter expressed as a fraction of the transducer diameter) and (3) a comparison of the discontinuity echo amplitude with that from a specular reflector on the rear surface of a flat plate, for standardization purposes.

This technique greatly simplifies discontinuity size determination in terms of an ideal flat bottom target. Using an ultrasonic discontinuity detector and the distance gain size diagram applicable to the test transducers, the size of a discontinuity may be obtained.[7,8] There are a number of diagram variants to suit particular test objects. A typical distance gain size diagram for longitudinal wave testing is shown in Fig. 9. The distance to the discontinuity is expressed in units N of the near field, and relative size is based on the transducer diameter.

Reference standards are also made for composites to aid in sizing small voids

TABLE 1. Test hole correction factors.

Applicable Calibration Diameter		Signal Factor (dB)	Amplitude (percent)
mm	(in.)		
0.8	(2/64)	–16	16
1.2	(3/64)	–9	36
2.0	(5/64)	0	100
3.2	(8/64)	8	256

FIGURE 8. Typical on axis straight beam distance amplitude correction curve.

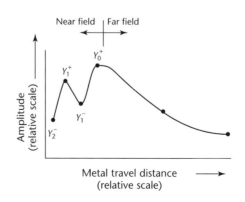

and delaminations. However, inclusions in composites are also a major concern, particularly because the detection of inclusions is more difficult than detection of delaminations. Composite reference standards are made using different materials as implants in a known matrix material. Such implant materials generally are synthetic fluorine resins or polyester films. Composite reference standards are more often used for setting of detection levels than for discontinuity sizing.

Mechanical Scanning[1]

Manual scanning is the most commonly used contact pulse echo ultrasonic testing technique. The disadvantage of manual scanning is that the only permanent record is an overlay with discontinuity locations traced from markings on the test object. In many cases, permanent C-scan records are needed to properly document the ultrasonic test procedure. To produce a C-scan recording, the location of the contact transducer during scanning must be known at all times. Encoding systems have been developed to provide the transducer location.

Mechanical Position Encoding

Mechanical encoding positioning can be obtained from a variety of commercial systems. The most common are encoding arms. They can be rectilinear sliders or pivot arms. The transducer is fixed to the arm and guided over the area of interest. The data typically are collected at a constant rate. If the sensor location is repeated, either the highest signal level or the newest signal level is recorded. If scanning is too fast or if areas are skipped, the data will be missing. Motorized mechanical scanners avoid this problem.

Mechanical scanners based on encoder wheels or mouse directed laser tracking are also possible. The devices are convenient but less accurate than mechanical arms because they can slip and lose location.

Array transducers can be used in scanning with encoding. Arrays in roller probes provide a mechanical scan of an area the width of the probe by the length of a roller scan. Array probes can also be slid on a surface, with an encoder to create a C-scan record.

Large mechanical devices are cumbersome when moving the transducer on the test object but are more adaptable to flat test areas. The main advantage of mechanical devices is that they provide more positive position information and are not subject to ambient disturbances.

Sonic Position Encoding

Sonic devices have been used for position encoding. Two point sensors are separated by a fixed distance, and a stylus emitting

FIGURE 9. Ultrasonic distance gain size diagram for longitudinal wave testing.

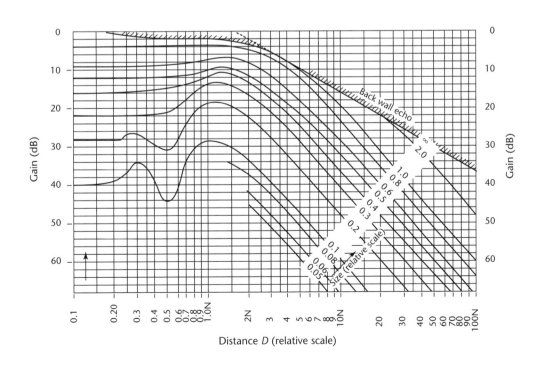

a low frequency signal is attached to the transducer so that the sound emitted by the stylus reaches the two-point sensors. The time of flight from the stylus to the two sensors is processed by computer. Together with the known fixed distance between the sensors, the location of the stylus (and the transducer) can be calculated by triangulation.

The main advantage of the sonic position encoding device is its portability and ease of operation. Sonic devices also can be used on contoured surfaces, so long as the stylus' sound can reach the point sensors. The main disadvantage of the sonic device is its susceptibility to sonic disturbances having the same frequency as the stylus and the sonic device's dependence on the accuracy of the stylus position. Some sonic sources are generated with a spark, which can be hazardous where fuel fumes are present.

Electromagnetic Position Encoding

Radio frequency position encoding is another approach for contact transducer encoding. A small sensor can be used that provides six axes of orientation. Resolution is similar to that of sonic techniques.

Selection of Ultrasonic Test Frequencies

Contact tests are generally limited to frequencies in the range from 0.1 to 10 MHz. The frequency most frequently used in tests of metallic materials is 2.25 MHz in the United States and 2 MHz elsewhere. Frequencies as low as 0.4 MHz are used for tests of coarse grained metals and alloys to reduce the scatter of the ultrasonic energy from grain boundaries which in turn reduces its penetrating ability.

With fine grained materials such as wrought aluminum alloys, frequencies of 5.0, 7.5 or 10 MHz can be used to provide improved resolution of small discontinuities. Composite materials are typically inspected at 2.25, 3.5 or 5 MHz. Transducers labeled as highly damped 25 MHz are also used to test advanced composites with improved near-surface resolution.

Effects of Ultrasonic Transducer Diameter

The diameter of the transducer face can have significant effects on ultrasonic test results. The distribution of sound intensities within the beam close to the face of the transducer is influenced by the face diameter D as well as by the selection of the test frequency f. In addition, the velocity of sound v in the medium adjacent to the face of the transducer influences the distance along the ultrasonic beam axis in front of the search unit within which nonuniform sound field intensity variations influence test signal characteristics.

In the near field, or fresnel field, the amplitudes of echo signals from discontinuities can vary widely and lead to misinterpretation of discontinuity size or location. Considerable caution should be exercised when interpreting test indications from the near field.

Transducer Near Field

The length of the near field zone is given by:

$$(1) \quad \ell = D^2 \frac{f}{4v} = \frac{D^2}{4\lambda}$$

where D is the diameter of the transducer (meter), f is the test frequency (hertz), v is the velocity of sound in the test material (meter per second) and λ is the wavelength of sound in the test medium (meter). The length of the near field zone should be routinely calculated to avoid interference with test procedures and signal interpretation.

Also significant in its influence on discontinuity signal amplitudes is the position of the discontinuity within the near field or far field of the transducer's ultrasonic beam. As might be expected, a specific loss in ultrasonic beam energy results from each unit of distance traveled by the beam. This rate of attenuation might be constant within a particular type of material. For example, it might be anticipated that the farther a discontinuity of specific size is from the front surface, the smaller is its reflection. Likewise, a lesser amount of reflected energy is received by the transducer and results in a smaller indication height on the oscilloscope. In practice, this is not always true.

If the height of the A-scan echo signal from a specific discontinuity is plotted as a function of the discontinuity's distance from the transducer, a curve such as that shown in Fig. 10 is obtained. Initially, the height of the A-scan signal becomes greater. This effect is characteristic when the discontinuity lies within the near field of the search unit. The maximum A-scan signal height is attained at a discontinuity depth determined by Eq. 1. The distance at which a given reflector produces this maximum A-scan signal indicates the limit of the near field under the specific test conditions and material.

Divergence of Ultrasonic Beams in Far Field

In the far field, coherent wave fronts tend to be spherical with increasing radii of curvature as distance increases. At positions well into the far field, wave fronts can approximate those of plane waves and ultrasonic beams diverge in this region. The intensity of the sound beam propagating from the transducer decreases with increasing distances into the far field according to an inverse square law.

The half angle of sound beam divergence in the far field is:

$$(2) \quad \sin \alpha = 1.22 \frac{\lambda}{D}$$

where D is the face diameter of the transducer (meter) and λ is the wavelength of ultrasound in the material (meter).

With most practical ultrasonic transducers, the beam divergence angle is small, typically under 170 mrad (10 deg). For this reason, Eq. 2 can be approximated by assuming the sine of the angle to be nearly equal to the angle itself:

$$(3) \quad \alpha = 1.22 \frac{v}{fD}$$

where D is the transducer face diameter (millimeter), f is frequency (megahertz), v is the velocity of sound in the test material (meter per second) and α is the ultrasonic beam half angle (radian).

For longitudinal waves in steel with a sound velocity of 5.84 km·s⁻¹, the divergence half-angle is about:

$$(4) \quad \alpha = \frac{7.11}{fD}$$

and, for longitudinal waves in steel with a sound velocity of 230 000 in.·s⁻¹, the divergence angle is about:

$$(5) \quad \alpha = \frac{0.28}{fD}$$

where D is the transducer face diameter and f is the frequency (megahertz).

For a transducer with a diameter of 25 mm (1 in.) and a low contact test frequency of 1 MHz, the product $f \cdot D = 1$. For this example, the divergence half angle in the far field in steel is about 250 mrad (16 deg). At a higher test frequency of 5 MHz, this angle is reduced to about 50 mrad (3 deg).

Under typical ultrasonic contact test conditions, the decrease in intensity because of geometrical beam spreading in the far field is usually relatively small, particularly where the total travel distance is limited. However, when the sound beam must travel long distances through a large forging, for example, the geometrical loss in beam intensity could contribute to a significant reduction in echo signal amplitudes.

Ultrasonic Beam Attenuation by Scattering

Much more important than beam divergence is the effect of ultrasonic beam scattering and incoherence resulting from the internal structures of metallic materials. In most cases, the primary cause of scattering is the coarse grain in many metals and alloys. Each grain boundary serves as a small reflector that sends out its own scattered and reflected signals. Large grain boundaries weaken the interrogating sound beam emitted by the transducer, in addition to attenuating echo signals returning from discontinuities deep in the test material. The overall effect is that of weakening significant signals and lowering the amplitude of the A-scan signal heights.

Coarse grain boundaries can return detectable echoes of their own. These appear as numerous vertical indications on the A-scan display (often called *grass*). Such nonrelevant signals can interfere

FIGURE 10. Typical resolution block calibration curve.

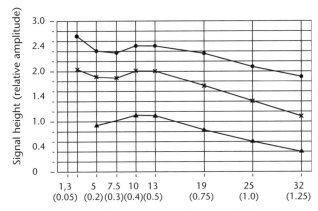

Distance from surface, mm (in.)

Legend
- • = 3.25 mm (0.13 in.) hole
- ✕ = 2 mm (0.08 in.) hole
- ▲ = 1 mm (0.04 in.) hole

with signals from significant discontinuities and may completely obscure important test results. In most cases, the only practical solution is to reduce the magnitude of grain boundary signals by switching to a lower frequency. This approach could also reduce the amplitude of signals from small discontinuities to the point that they might be missed during ultrasonic testing.

The heights of A-scan indications depend directly on the transmissibility of ultrasound in specific test materials. Such effects can be especially significant in tests of large steel castings or forgings (copper, nickel based alloys or austenitic stainless steels) whose grain size and ultrasonic scattering effects are much smaller. In aerospace aluminum structures, small discontinuities can be detected and located precisely with ease.

Effects of Mechanical and Thermal Processes

The microstructures and grain sizes of metals and alloys can be changed significantly by mechanical and thermal processes commonly used in primary mills and in subsequent manufacturing operations. It is essential for the ultrasonic test operator to know the actual condition of materials at the time of testing. Hot working and heat treatment of steels can produce radical changes in grain size and internal microstructure and these can in turn change ultrasonic test sensitivity and reliability. Forging and other hot working operations (at temperatures high in the austenitic range) involve plastic deformation and tend to refine grain size (that is, to reduce grains to smaller dimensions).

On the other hand, prolonged heating at the high temperatures used for forging can lead to grain size enlargement. When carbon steels are heated from ambient temperatures up through the critical ranges 720 to 880 °C (1333 to 1620 °F), grain refinement occurs as the steel is converted to its higher temperature microstructure. Such heating through the critical range occurs in processes such as normalizing, hardening or annealing of steels in heat treating operations.

In some cases, materials are coarse grained and transmit ultrasound poorly as cast or after fusion welding and can be difficult to test ultrasonically. After subsequent heat treating, mechanical working or reduction operations that refine their grain size, sound propagation improves, permitting precise discontinuity detection and location at considerable depths below the entry surface. It is for these reasons that some products are tested at particular stages of their

manufacture when ultrasonic transmissibility is improved.

Effects of Composite Structures

Compared to metals, composite materials generally have higher sound attenuation because of their heterogeneous nature. Thermosets and thermoplastics generally have about the same sound attenuation characteristics. Compared to unidirectional tapes, woven fabric composites have higher attenuation compared to unidirectional tapes.

Metal matrix composites have sound attenuation levels between those of metals and those of organic composites. Refractory composites such as carbon carbon have the highest sound attenuation level because of their high porosity. Testing refractory composites requires special care in frequency selection and signal interpretation.

Selection of Test Frequencies

Pulsed contact tests use frequencies from 25 kHz to 10 MHz (Table 2). Because of variations in metallic structure typically encountered during contact tests in industrial plants, it is often desirable to use the lowest frequency that locates specified minimum sizes and types of discontinuities with consistent results.

Proper selection of the test frequency requires experience with similar test materials, careful analysis or experimental tests. Tests with reference standards may be needed to check the reproducibility of

TABLE 2. Typical frequency ranges for conventional, straight beam, longitudinal, pulse echo, ultrasonic test applications.

Frequency Range	Applications
25 to 100 kHz	concrete, wood poles, rock and coarse grained nonmetallic materials
0.2 to 2.25 MHz	castings (gray iron, nodular iron)
	relatively coarse grained metal (copper, austenitic stainless steels, nickel alloys)
	plastics (solid rocket propellants)
	grains
0.4 to 5 MHz	castings (steel, aluminum, brass) and materials with refined grain size
1 to 2.25 MHz	welds (ferrous and nonferrous)
1 to 5 MHz	wrought metallic products (sheet, plate, bars, billets)
1 to 10 MHz	forgings (ferrous and nonferrous)
2.25 to 10 MHz	drawn and extruded ferrous and nonferrous products (bars, tubes, shapes)
	glass and ceramics

test procedures and the uniformity of response.

In fine grained steels, contact tests are usually made at 2.25 or 5.0 MHz, when the test is used to detect forging bursts, flaking, pipe and discontinuities of smaller size. A 10 MHz frequency is sometimes selected for detection of microscopic inclusions and segregations.

Large, medium carbon steel castings are generally tested at 1 to 5 MHz with ultrasonic beams penetrating 3 m (10 ft) or more. Small forgings are tested at 5 to 10 MHz and large forgings at 2.25 to 5 MHz. The central portion of forgings such as turbine rotors may have large grain sizes typical of the original cast shape, while the near-surface material may have received considerable grain refinement as a consequence of more extensive hot working during forging.

High carbon and high alloy steels may require the use of a lower test frequency (500 kHz to 1 MHz) if the ultrasonic beam is to penetrate over 1 m (3 ft). The frequency also depends on the degree of working or heat treatment of the material. Lower test frequencies are often used for cast iron, in which the flakelike graphite structure causes scattering of the ultrasonic beam and lowers its penetration, even at low frequencies.

In most metals and alloys, greater grain refinement from forging, rolling or heat treating produces a more homogeneous metallic structure so that a higher frequency can be used. Many brass alloy castings have a fine grain structure because of controlled cooling or heat treatment and may be tested at 2.25 MHz. Other castings of similar alloy may be difficult to test even at 500 kHz because of their extremely large grain size. Most wrought aluminum alloys have relatively fine grains and very good ultrasonic transmissibility. For these materials, test frequencies of 5, 7.5 or 10 MHz are preferred for high resolution of small discontinuities. Varying grain sizes may characterize cast and worked aluminum alloys, magnesium, titanium and other alloys, for which frequencies of 2.25 to 5 MHz might be used.

Austenitic stainless steel and high alloy castings used in nuclear power systems can often have grain sizes on the order of 2.5 mm (0.1 in.) or more. These may require combinations of low test frequencies, high pulse power levels or focused ultrasonic beams to compensate for the severe scattering and attenuation that occurs. As with most nondestructive tests, when performance or sensitivity is in doubt, results should be compared to reference standards with known, similar materials structures or similar ultrasonic transmissibility.

Selection of Test Frequency in Composites

Selection of test frequency for composite materials is generally based on penetrability. For thin composite laminates below 6.4 mm (0.25 in.), special transducers are required, operating at frequencies from 10 to 25 MHz to produce better discontinuity size discrimination and near surface resolution. To penetrate thicker laminates, test frequencies from 1 to 5 MHz may be used as a compromise between penetrability and resolution. For very thick laminates, frequencies below 1 MHz may be required to provide sufficient penetrability.

Selection of Test Frequency Based on Discontinuity Size

In addition to grain size, attenuation characteristics of the material and the size of the test object, it is important to consider also the minimum size and type of discontinuity that must be detected. At higher test frequencies, smaller discontinuities can be detected, if attenuation and scattering effects permit penetration and allow echo signals to return from all depths within the material. When test object size or grain size dictates lower test frequencies, the response to small discontinuities is reduced and they may not be easily detected.

In general, sensitivity to small discontinuities can best be determined using ultrasonic reference standards of the same material and grain characteristics as the test object. The amplitude of signals from a reference standard can be determined experimentally to estimate the size of the smallest discontinuity detected reliably at various depths.

It must always be recognized that flat bottom holes in reference standards are ideal sound reflectors, including those with large grain size and high ultrasonic attenuation. The shape, orientations and depth of discontinuities may alter the reflection path and reduce the possibility of detection. Rough, spherical or tilted discontinuities typically return to the transducer signals smaller than those from flat bottom holes whose faces lie perpendicular to the incident sound beam.

The echo signal from a rough tilted discontinuity in a large plate section is typically recognized as low in amplitude but broad at the base. It may shift position along the base line as the transducer is moved in the direction of the tilt. A reference standard's flat bottom holes with diameters smaller than the minimum size specified for the actual test must be clearly detected.

Lowering the test frequency may improve sound transmission within coarse grained materials by reducing the magnitude of signals from large grain boundaries. Different frequencies may alter the sensitivity of the test to small discontinuities. The need to suppress grain boundary scattering by lowering the test frequency involves a compromise with lower sensitivity to small discontinuities.

In critical cases, it may be necessary to use special techniques such as increasing the pulse power of the incident sound beam, selecting a transducer of lower damping or higher efficiency, selecting a smaller area search unit or devising means for focusing the sound beam to concentrate its energy at the location of the suspected small discontinuity. Alternative techniques include double transducer tests or through-transmission tests. Separate sending and receiving transducers may also be considered.

Effect of Discontinuity Orientation on Signal Amplitude

When a reflecting discontinuity is not oriented normal to the axis of the straight beam longitudinal wave transducer (and is not parallel to the front surface of the test object), the ultrasonic signal from it is significantly reduced in amplitude. This occurs because much of the reflected sound is directed at angles so that the maximum echo signal does not return to the transducer where it can be detected. If the sound beam could be directed perpendicularly to the face of a tilted, laminar discontinuity, it could provide the maximum signal from the discontinuity.

Theoretically, thin wedge shaped coupling blocks could angle the longitudinal wave to intercept discontinuities of known angles and to reflect maximum signals back to the transducer. In practice, however, when the angle is unknown and can vary widely, this costly and time consuming approach requires many tests with wedges graduated in small angles. With angle beam transverse wave tests, it is common practice to use transducers equipped with wedges. A choice of beam angles in the test material can be made by selecting a transducer with the desired wedge. Even with this procedure, it is usually not practical to make many tests with different angle beam transducers to explore each discontinuity.

Effect of Discontinuity Geometry on Echo Amplitude

In industrial test objects, discontinuity reflecting surfaces can vary widely. For example, a void may be almost spherical in a casting, fusion weldment or other metallic material that has received little or no mechanical working after solidification. During mechanical working such as forging or hot rolling and piercing, a gas hole or porosity in cast metal may flatten into a laminar discontinuity parallel to the rolling or metal flow direction. Because this direction is often parallel to the surface, as in a plate or sheet, it can offer a good sound reflecting surface perpendicular to the straight beam longitudinal wave in contact or immersion testing.

On the other hand, if refractory or brittle inclusions are associated with a discontinuity, the reflecting surface may conform to the shape of the inclusion, which could be rough or irregular. If a metallic inclusion is bonded into a metal matrix material, it may reflect only a small fraction of the incident sound beam, depending on the impedance mismatch at its surface. If such an inclusion breaks its bonds to the surrounding metal and produces a metal-to-air interface, the unbonded inclusion could be indicated by a strong reflection signal and may be easily detected.

Because of the factors that affect the height of an A-scan signal from a discontinuity, it is often difficult to determine the precise size of a discontinuity. Ultrasonic tests are more qualitative than quantitative in this respect. To a considerable degree, discontinuities that reflect the incident sound beam have characteristics like new sources of ultrasonic emission. The ratios of their dimensions to the sound beam wavelengths influence the patterns of the sound reflected and scattered from their surfaces, much like the beam patterns radiated from transducers.

Data Presentation

Contact tests can be used to produce all three forms of ultrasonic testing data: A-scan, B-scan or C-scan. The A-scan is a one-dimensional presentation of ultrasonic signal amplitude along the propagation path. If there is a discontinuity along the path, the occurrence of the ultrasonic signal in the time sweep of the test unit, in relation to the front and back surface reflections, indicates the depth of the discontinuity.

The amplitude of the signal reflected from the discontinuity can be a measure of the area of the reflector if the discontinuity is smaller than the beam.

A series of A-scan data obtained along a certain linear direction across the test object can be pieced together to form a B-scan. The horizontal axis of a B-scan represents the position of the transducer with respect to the test object. The vertical axis represents the time of flight or swept time in the A-scan. The time of flight for the front and back surface signals plotted in one direction forms a cross section of the test object. Any discontinuity cut by the cross section has its depth displayed on the B-scan. The B-scan therefore provides a picture of discontinuities in a plane parallel to the direction of wave propagation.

The C-scan provides a plan view of the position and size of discontinuities projected onto a plane normal to the direction of wave propagation. A C-scan may use either through-transmission or pulse echo techniques.

When the test object is scanned in a raster pattern, the signals reflected from discontinuities can be used to activate a plotter showing a top view of the test object with discontinuities indicated in place. Generally, C-scans are used to provide the location and size of a discontinuity. They are the most popular way to present data in ultrasonic testing.

Modern computerized ultrasonic contact systems can store all three forms of data simultaneously. The A-scan results are obtained by digitizing each ultrasonic signal waveform before storing it in memory. The waveforms are then analyzed by setting software gates and discrimination levels to apply accept/reject criteria. Time-of-flight information is gathered at the same time. Any of the three modes can be displayed after brief data processing.

If a computerized testing system is used, different signal processing programs can be used to enhance the discontinuity detecting capability of the system. Waveform averaging can be used to minimize electronic noise to improve front surface and back surface resolutions. Back surface reflection amplitude and discontinuity signal amplitude can be monitored simultaneously to improve detection reliability. Image enhancement can be used to improve discontinuity size and shape estimates.

The most significant contribution of computerization to contact ultrasonic testing is the ability to ensure coupling of the transducer to the test object surface. Maintaining coupling is the most difficult part of contact testing, especially with rough or contoured surfaces. Manual testing requires that the technician scrutinize the system display constantly to ensure coupling. Mechanical scanning with automatic discontinuity determination must have a provision to monitor the coupling efficiency to ensure the quality of the testing data.

Tests of Multilayered Structures and Composites

One of the major advantages of contact ultrasonic testing is the portability of the instruments. The technique can be applied to assembled structures that have adhesives as the joining medium between individual components. Testing the individual components and the adhesive bonds in the structures is often required.

The components or substrates in an adhesively bonded structure can be composite or metallic materials. They can be composite bonded to composite, composite bonded to metal or composite bonded to honeycomb core materials. It is essential to know in advance the thicknesses of the substrates for interpretation of signals appearing on the system display. The bondline thickness generally ranges from 100 to 300 nm (4×10^{-6} to 12×10^{-6} in.).

Tests of Adhesive Bonds

In an ultrasonic test of a typical adhesively bonded structure, time of flight corresponds to layer thicknesses. Identification of the return signals can be made by knowing the layer thicknesses and the sound velocity in the composite and in the metal. The bondline thickness is usually small compared to the substrates, so that the front and back surface reflections of the bondline are indistinguishable. Higher test frequencies can be used to resolve bond line thickness if the thickness and attenuation of the adherends are not too great.

Disbonds can be identified by monitoring the back surface reflection when the top and bottom layers do not have equal thickness. When a disbond exists at the bondline, elastic waves cannot get past the bondline. Multiple reflections from the top and bottom layers are of equal thickness and the back surface reflection cannot be distinguished from multiples of the top surface reflections.

A disbond condition is difficult to identify by viewing the reflected signal at the interface. A disbond at the interface may produce a larger reflected amplitude but the amplitude is also strongly influenced by the surface condition of the substrate at the disbonded area. At the bondline interface, the bondline thickness is usually so thin that the front and back surface reflections are indistinguishable. From the A-scan display, it is extremely difficult to tell whether the disbond exists at the front or back side.

If a computerized test system is used, signal processing techniques such as fourier transform can be used to determine the bondline thickness or to detect and locate disbonds. With the window of the fourier transform set in the neighborhood of the interface signal, a normal bond produces a dip in the power spectrum of the transform. When sound impinges at the metal/adhesive interface, it is going to an acoustically dense medium (metal) from a less dense medium (adhesive). When it emerges from the adhesive/metal interface, it is going from a less dense (adhesive) to a more dense medium (metal). The dip in the destructive interference indicates the bondline thickness. When the disbond occurs at the interface between the top layer and the adhesive layer, multiple reflections are seen in the A-scan display. The power spectrum from the fourier transform becomes a smooth curve with no interference. When the disbond occurs at the interface between the adhesive and the bottom layer, the power spectrum again shows interference. However, the reflective interface for the sound going from a more dense medium (adhesive) to a less dense medium (air) produces constructive interference contrary to the case of a good bond.

Under favorable conditions, discontinuities in the top and bottom substrates can be identified by extraneous signals appearing in the time periods between the top surface bond line and bottom surface bond line. If the top layer thickness is smaller than the bottom layer, the multiples of the interface signal are superimposed in the time period between the bond line and the bottom surface and could be misinterpreted as a discontinuity.

Part 2. Angle Beam Contact Testing[1]

Although the majority of contact testing is done with longitudinal waves propagating normal to the test surface, there are many instances when an angled beam is preferred. The predominant reason for angle beam testing is the detection of discontinuities with geometries and orientations other than parallel to the test surface. Planar cracks normal to the test object surface, voids with small reflective surfaces parallel to the test object surface and discontinuities in welds with uneven top surfaces are examples of situations that require angle beam techniques.

Verification of Transverse Wave Angle

Angled longitudinal waves, transverse waves or surface waves are generated in a test object by mounting the piezoelectric element at an angle in the contact transducer. The correct angle can be determined with Snell's law of refraction. Most of the commercial angle beam contact transducers are designed to produce transverse waves of 0.5, 0.8 and 1.0 rad (30, 45 and 60 deg) in steel. Some produce surface waves. For materials with different sound velocities, the angles of refraction can be calculated using Snell's law when standard transducers are used. The transducer angle can be verified using a calibration block like the one in Fig. 11a.[9]

The first step in angle beam calculation is to determine the transducer's beam exit point. The transducer is placed on the focal point of the calibration block and is moved back and forth until the monitor reaches maximum amplitude for the reflection from the large outside radius. The focal point on the block then corresponds with the beam exit point of the transducer.

The transducer is next placed on the other side of the block to obtain a reflection from the 50 mm (2 in.) diameter hole. The transducer again is moved back and forth until the reflection from the hole shows maximum amplitude on the monitor display. At this point, the angle of the sound beam matches the degrees stamped on the side of the calibration block.

The transducer sound beam exit point should always be checked first. If the exit point marking is not correct, then the angle cannot be measured accurately.

FIGURE 11. Calibration blocks: (a) International Institute of Welding (IIW), type 1; (b) transducer placement on IIW, type 1; (c) distance sensitivity calibration (DSC) block.

(a)

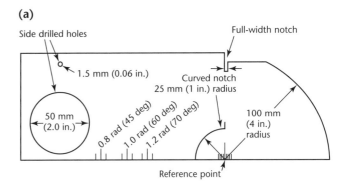

(b)

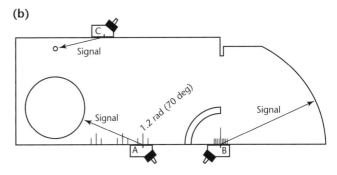

(c)

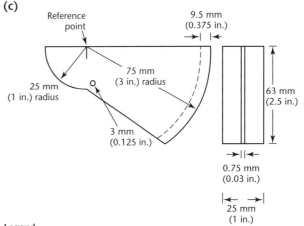

Legend
A. Wedge angle.
B. Distance calibration.
C. Sensitivity calibration.

Transverse wave transducer angle placement on an International Institute of Welding (IIW) block are shown in Fig. 11b. The miniature angle beam block, shown in Fig. 11c, can also be used to calibrate the transducer angle in far field work.

Ranging in Transverse Wave Tests

In angle beam testing with the beam directed away from the transducer, no back surface reflection appears on the monitor display. A reflected signal usually indicates a discontinuity. Ranging of the discontinuity is not as simple as in straight beam testing. In metals, a standard reference block such as the International Institute of Welding block can be used to calibrate the distance from the transducer to the discontinuity. In materials other than steel, a conversion must be made, taking into account the ratio of velocities in the material to the velocities in steel.

In range estimating, the beam spread of the angle beam should also be taken into account. The sound beam radiating from the transducer fans out or diverges.

FIGURE 12. Possible sound beam paths in angle beam testing: (a) crack at front surface; (b) crack at back surface; (c) crack in middle.

(a)

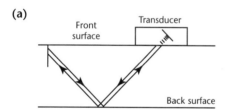

(b)

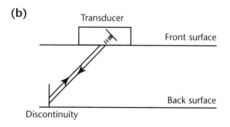

(c)

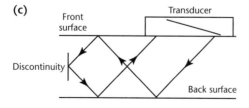

The exact location of the discontinuity represented by the reflected signal on the monitor display may be difficult to judge because of the beam spread. Another difficulty in discontinuity ranging lies in the uncertainty of where the discontinuity may be relative to the boundary surfaces. As in Fig. 12a, the sound beam undergoes four slanted trips to complete a round trip to a crack at or near the top surface. When the crack is near the bottom surface, the sound beam takes only two trips to make the round trip (Fig. 12b). In Fig. 12c, where the crack is located near the middle of the plate, the sound beam bounces off both the upper and lower surfaces and may return to the transducer if the plate is not too thick. Whenever possible, the plate should be tested from both sides to judge the crack location more accurately.

Ultrasonic Tests of Tubes

Angle beam testing of tubes uses transverse waves reflected repeatedly along the tube wall. Occasionally longitudinal waves are used but they suffer much from mode conversion. Figure 13 shows a sound beam bouncing off inner and outer walls of a tube during a typical ultrasonic test. Longitudinal cracks in the path of the sound beam reflect the sound and are indicated on the test system's monitor. To cover the entire area of the tube, the transducer or the tube must be rotated while either one moves in the longitudinal direction.

FIGURE 13. Sound beam bouncing off inner and outer walls in ultrasonic tube test.

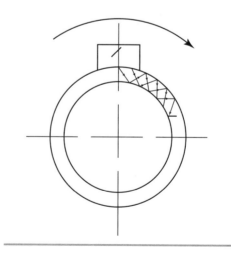

Weld Testing

The angle beam technique is extensively used for weld testing (see Fig. 14a). Typically, the weld is tested in using a full skip, using the two test directions provided by the angle beam test as shown in Figs. 14b and 14c. To help interpret the results of angle beam tests, a direct reading ultrasonic calculator may be developed (Fig. 15a). The horizontal scale across the top of the card represents the horizontal distance from the exit point of the transducer. Distance from the exit point and the center of the weld is laid out along this scale. The vertical scale represents distance in the thickness direction. Specimen thickness is indicated on this scale and the arc shows the angle of the sound beam.

As an example of using the calculator, assume a double-V weld with an opening of 0.5 rad (30 deg) in a 50 mm (2 in.) steel plate. The weld is to be tested using a 1 rad (60 deg) transverse wave transducer. A line is first drawn from the point of incidence at the upper left corner of the calculator through the 1 rad (60 deg) mark on the arc, extending to the 50 mm (2 in.) point representing the plate thickness.

Calibrate the horizontal sweep of the monitor to represent beam travel distance in the test material. The full skip distance of the sound beam is obtained by doubling the 86 mm (3.4 in.) intersecting point at the bottom of the plate and

marking the point at 175 mm (6.9 in.) on the upper plate surface. The 0.5 rad (30 deg) V weld is next drawn on transparent paper positioned over the monitor screen — here at a value of 140 mm (5.5 in.). The distance between the center of the transducer (exit point) and the center of the weldment is then measured, giving 116 mm (4.6 in.). The transparent paper is moved by the same distance. The position of the discontinuity is indicated and can be evaluated.

Pitch Catch Contact Testing

Angle beam contact testing can also be conducted using two transducers in a pitch catch mode. The transmitting transducer pitches a sound beam that skips in the plate and is caught by a receiving transducer (Fig. 16).

The distance between the two transducers can be calibrated to maximize the received signal amplitude. As shown in Fig. 16b, a planar discontinuity perpendicular to the plate surface in the path of the sound beam deflects the sound beam and prevents it from reaching the receiving transducer. Therefore, a loss of signal on the monitor indicates the presence of a discontinuity.

FIGURE 14. Ultrasonic angle beam weld tests: (a) wave path; (b) insonification near weld; (c) insonification farther from weld.

(a)

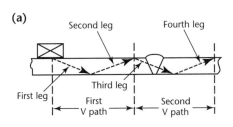

(b)

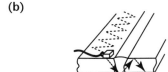

(c)

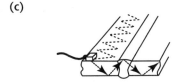

FIGURE 15. Direct reading ultrasonic discontinuity location calculator: (a) showing angles; (b) example showing beams. (1 radian = 60.3 degrees.)

(a)

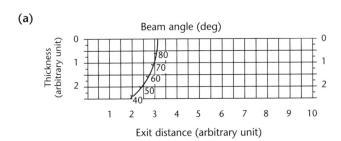

(b)

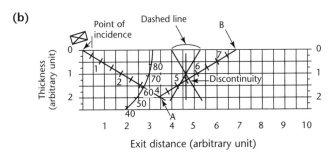

Surface Wave Testing Techniques

With a proper wedge angle, the sound beam entering the test object surface can reach a refracted angle of 1.5 rad (90 deg). The refracted waves in this case propagate along the surface of the test object and are referred to as *surface waves*. Surface waves are typically used in metals, with a travel distance up to 100 mm (4 in.).

Surface wave techniques are used to detect fatigue cracks along the surface of metallic components. The sensitivity of the technique is quite good on smooth surfaces. With proper instrumentation, a 1 mm (0.04 in.) crack length can be detected in aluminum and steel.

FIGURE 16. Pitch catch angle beam testing: (a) in sound material; (b) with discontinuity.

(a)

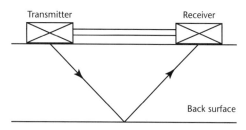

(b)

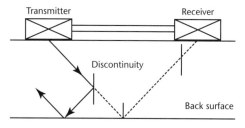

PART 3. Coupling Media for Contact Tests[1]

Transducer Shoes

Wedge Shaped Shoes

Wedge shaped shoes are used to refract an ultrasonic beam to angles off normal from the entry surface, particularly in metallic test objects. Introducing straight beams at an angle to the entry surface also causes mode conversions, in which surface waves propagate along the surface and transverse (shear) waves are propagated into the test object, in addition to the refracted straight beam.

In most contact tests, a wedge shaped shoe can reduce signal amplitude or eliminate the usual front surface echo signal. In almost all uses of a single search unit, the front surface echo is directed at an angle through the wedge so that some portion of it may not return to the transducer. In many dual-transducer techniques, the receiving unit is positioned to receive echo signals that do not return to the sending search unit.

Contoured Shoes for Curved Test Surfaces

When testing curved surfaces with contact techniques, flat faced transducers may be inappropriate because only a point (or at best, a line) of the transducer face can actually touch the curved entry surface. With slightly contoured surfaces, viscous couplants may help transmit ultrasonic waves from a larger portion of the transducer face into the test material, but this is imprecise and variations in signal amplitudes often occur. Also, excess couplant can increase transducer ringing. For these reasons, contoured shoes are preferred over flat faced transducers on curved test surfaces. In all cases, the effects of beam refraction are significant and must be considered.

As shown in Fig. 17, acrylic coupling shoes can be shaped to fit the flat surface of the transducer on one side and the curved surface of a test object on the other side. It is essential to use a good couplant at both of these interfaces because ultrasonic waves cannot be transmitted through an air gap. Petroleum jelly or heavier greases or oils can be used to provide good coupling between the face of the transducer and the coupling

shoe. Oil or another of the commonly used couplants may serve at the interface between the contoured surface of the coupling shoe and the test object. In most applications, the contoured shoe can be locked in place on the transducer after a layer of couplant has been applied to the interface. Both layers of couplant should be thin, uniform in thickness and completely free of voids or bubbles.

During contact tests with contoured shoes, care should be taken to protect the surface of the shoe. This is a secondary function of the couplant, to lubricate the shoe and protect it from damage by a rough test object surface.

Contoured shoes can help maintain contact perpendicular to a portion of the test object. However, it must be recognized that sound waves passing through the interface between the acrylic shoe and the test object may refract

FIGURE 17. Contoured testing shoes: (a) straight beam shoe; (b) angle beam contact shoe.

(a)

(b)

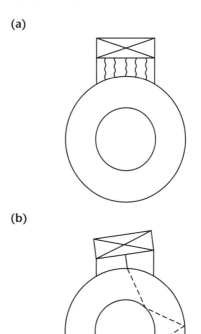

(Fig. 18). When a curved shoe is applied to a convex surface (a round bar or tube), the outer portions of the ultrasonic beam tend to diverge within the test material and so reduce the beam intensity. The test signal amplitude and the test sensitivity may also be reduced in the peripheral regions of the spreading sound beam. Focused immersion test techniques may be superior for these applications.

Couplant and Membranes

Solid or flexible membranes may be attached to a transducer for the purpose of directing the sound beam at angles off normal incidence or for cushioning the transducer from a rough or contoured test object surface. Membranes containing fluid couplant or solid, flexible materials are often used for ultrasonic tests. Such membranes must be coupled to the entry surface with a suitable liquid or semiliquid couplant layer.

When a flexible membrane covers the ceramic transducer element, it becomes the front face of the search unit. Some transducer cases are designed so that replaceable membrane covers can be installed when one is damaged. A suitable viscous fluid couplant fills the space between the face of the transducer and the membrane. All air bubbles must be excluded from this interface.

Oil, water or another liquid couplant must be applied between the membrane and the entry surface to avoid air interfaces and to enable transmission of

FIGURE 18. Beam spreading in convex test object caused by off-normal beam incidence on curved surface. Signal amplitudes are reduced and less clear than discrete reflections obtained with flat surfaced test objects.

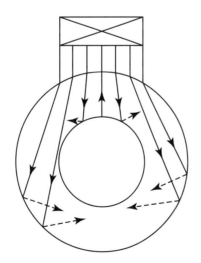

the ultrasound into the test object. In the 1950s, permeable plastic membranes were developed in the United States to couple and, in some applications, to match with the impedance of the porous heat shield structures. These membranes were liquid coupled to the transducer but dry coupled to the structure because of its porous nature.

Delay Lines

Plastic coupling blocks are often used between the face of the contact transducer and the front surface of the test object. Such blocks are also known as *delay lines, buffer rods* or *standoffs*. Their function is analogous to that of an equivalent water path distance in ultrasonic immersion tests. Much of the near field zone can be confined to the delay line. In addition, the ringing of the transducer falls off before the front surface echo returns from the test object. To some degree, this technique may enhance near-surface discontinuity resolution.

When a sonic delay line is used, it should be long enough so that multiple reflections do not appear in the A-scan signal trace ahead of the back surface reflection signal from the test object. Such multiple reflections can mask discontinuity signals from the test object.

High Temperature Applications

A special use of standoffs is made for testing high temperature materials, particularly metals. Some delay line configurations can be water cooled to prevent heat from reaching the transducer.

Cooled standoffs are also used in research, as when measuring the modulus of elasticity in metallic bars over a wide temperature range. In such applications, the test object is placed in a furnace so that temperature variations can be controlled. The standoff extends beyond the wall of the furnace and is cooled so that the transducer operates near normal temperatures.

Selection of Coupling Media

A contact ultrasonic test ordinarily cannot function without a suitable couplant to transmit ultrasound between the transducer and the test material. A couplant may be liquid, semiliquid or paste that (1) provides positive acoustic coupling for reliable testing (consistent back surface echo amplitude), (2) wets both the surface of the test object and the face of the transducer, excluding air between them, (3) can be easily applied, (4) does not run off the surface too quickly, (5) provides adequate lubrication for easy movement of the transducer over the test object surface, (6) is homogeneous and free from solid particles or bubbles, (7) does not freeze or evaporate under test conditions, (8) is easily removed or evaporates after testing is complete and (9) is free of contaminants (such as from lead or sulfur) and is not corrosive, toxic, flammable or otherwise hazardous or polluting.

Another critical characteristic for a couplant is that its acoustic impedance is between that of the transducer face and that of the test material or is identical to that of the test material.

For rough or porous test surfaces, soft rubber sheets are sometimes effective as coupling materials.

Selection of Couplants

It is critical to select the proper couplant for specific ultrasonic testing applications.

Water as Couplant

Water is widely used as a couplant for ultrasonic tests. Wetting agents or detergents are sometimes added to ensure good surface wetting and to eliminate air films.

However, water's viscosity is so low that it will not stay on some test surfaces long enough to complete the ultrasonic test procedures. For example, water cannot be used as a couplant on vertical or angled surfaces unless it is continuously replenished with a hose and pump setup or with a water coupled dolly transducer system. Water is not suitable for tests of absorbent materials or those that react to it adversely.

Water Based Gelatin Couplants

Water based gelatin is most widely used on test objects made of advanced composites. Such materials absorb water and as a result experience critical property degradation. Because of its higher viscosity, a gel can also serve as a filler for rough composite surfaces. Such gels are water soluble and can be easily cleaned after testing is completed.

Oil and Grease Couplants

For contact ultrasonic tests, various grades of oil are used more frequently than water mainly because they stay on the test surface longer. Oils containing wetting agents, as in many commercial motor oils, are most desirable for test applications.

Heavier oils and greases are used as couplants on hot surfaces, on vertical surfaces and to fill in irregularities on very rough test surfaces. These heavier grades are retained on the test surface much longer than lighter grades.

Glycerin Based Couplants

Glycerin is often used as a contact test couplant because it adheres to surfaces more effectively than water or light oil and because it is a better acoustic impedance match for transducers and test objects.

On forged component surfaces, higher amplitude echo signals are obtained with glycerin than with water. In many experimental situations, propylene glycol serves as a convenient liquid couplant. In some cases, a small amount of wetting agent helps the glycerin adhere to the surface.

Resins and Special Purpose Commercial Products

Hair grooms, cellulose gums (gravy thickeners) and petroleum jelly have found applications as sonic couplants in special circumstances because of their adherence to vertical, overhead or rough surfaces and because of their availability and economy.

Unusual materials such as chewing gum have been used as couplants in emergencies.[10] High viscosity resins and honey are useful in transverse wave contact tests at normal incidence.

Pressure Coupling

Pressure coupling has been used to dry couple longitudinal and transverse waves at normal incidence to test objects at temperatures well above 1000 °C (1800 °F). Pressure coupling has also been used with contact tests at oblique incidence at cryogenic temperatures.

Nuclear Component and Transverse Wave Couplants

Couplants on nuclear components are required to meet stringent specifications to ensure that tested components do not corrode.

Couplants for vertically polarized transverse waves at oblique incidence can be the same as for longitudinal waves.

Operator Techniques to Ensure Good Coupling

Operator technique can be a significant factor in successful coupling for contact tests. Before applying couplants, test materials should be wiped clean and free from grit, metal chips or liquids. Touching the surface with the fingers and sliding them about can ensure that no wedges or burred edges of metal prevent good, flat contact.

For general testing, a surface finish of 250 root mean square or better is required. For higher sensitivity and reliability, smoother surfaces are needed. Waviness exceeding 1.5 mm (0.06 in.) over a 50 mm (2 in.) span is unacceptable.

Ringing Technique

A technique of ringing the transducer to the couplant coated surface (similar to the placing of precision gage blocks in intimate contact) is often used. The operator places the transducer gently on the test surface, then rotates it or moves it back and forth while watching the test signal indication responses. The procedure is complete when maximum amplitude signals are consistent.

Constant pressure on the transducer during this movement helps to expel air bubbles and to make the thickness of the couplant film more uniform.

Test Object Surface Preparation

Liquid couplants are used successfully on test surfaces created by swing grinding, rolling, forging, sand blasting and other elaborate surface preparations. Smaller A-scan signals are received from internal discontinuities when testing through the grooved, milled surface of a steel block. This effect is frequency dependent and can be severe at certain test frequencies. Proper choice of couplant helps to minimize this effect.

The type of couplant used in contact testing of forged surfaces can affect detection of discontinuities. Forged and shot blasted surfaces can reduce the amplitude of discontinuity signals when surface roughness exceeds 6.5 mm (250×10^{-6} in.). However, no significant reduction in echo signal amplitude is observed with surface finishes less than 5 μm (200×10^{-6} in.).

Rough machined test objects sometimes produce spurious echo signals between the front surface and back surface indications in A-scan presentations. Such signals typically disappear if the rough surface can be smoothed with a hand grinder and fine grit abrasive. Rough surface effects can be severe when test objects are thin and the resolving power of the ultrasonic system is nearly half of the test object thickness.

PART 4. Imaging of Butt Weld Pulse Echo Tests[1]

To ensure the quality of welds, film radiography and ultrasonic testing are the two nondestructive techniques generally used. Film radiography is a repeatable technique that provides a permanent record of discontinuity location and size, with the following disadvantages: (1) a health hazard is posed to personnel near the test, (2) the technique is insensitive to thick sections, (3) discontinuity depth information is not provided and (4) access to both sides of the test object is required.

Conventional ultrasonic testing does not present a personnel hazard. It provides depth information and detects discontinuities that radiography could overlook. Conventional ultrasonic techniques have these potential disadvantages: (1) variance in test results because of variables controlled by the operator, (2) requirements for a high degree of operation subjectivity, (3) lack of a suitable means for producing a repeatable, permanent record and (4) low probability of repeated test results on small but rejectable discontinuities.

Ultrasonic imaging helps overcome these limitations and provides the advantages of both nondestructive techniques. For example, the automation of data acquisition and the recording of transducer location and test parameters provide a repeatable, permanent record. The text below discusses the application of ultrasonic imaging techniques for weld tests. Several examples of discontinuities commonly found in welded joints are presented, including lack of fusion, porosity and intergranular stress corrosion cracking.

Ultrasonic Imaging Procedures

To determine the acceptability of weld indications, two measurements are taken from ultrasonic signals: amplitude and time of flight. Figure 19 shows a video display of a typical ultrasonic signal (an A-scan). The display represents a plot of amplitude as a function of time. A gate is set to record signals in the region of interest while a threshold is set so that noise is not recorded.

Signals that occur in the gate and exceed the threshold trigger the measurement circuits to digitally record the time of flight and signal amplitude. These measurements can be done in hardware on analog signals or in software on digitized signals. Several imaging systems record the first signal in the gate while others record the peak signal. The resolution of the electronics determines the accuracy of the measurements.

Position is recorded with optical encoders or stepping motor pulses. Because stepping motors are prone to skip counts under certain loading conditions, optical encoders provide a more accurate measurement of transducer position. A scan grid is generated for recording the transducer position (see Fig. 20). Each cell in the grid (called a *grid spacing*) determines the spatial resolution of the scan. For each grid spacing, the transducer location, time of flight and amplitude information are recorded and images may then be generated in real time.

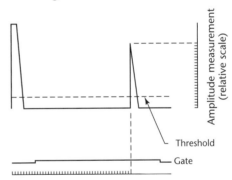

FIGURE 19. Measurement of amplitude and time-of-flight data.

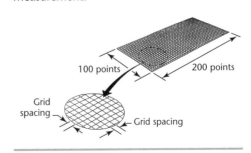

FIGURE 20. Scan grid for position measurement.

In addition to saving the scan data, most ultrasonic imaging systems record other information with each scan, including a list of test parameters that detail the test setup. These parameters include administrative information, scanner setup, calibration data and the ultrasonic equipment settings. This information serves as the basis for generating repeatable scans.

Contact Weld Tests

Test Frequency

The majority of weld tests are done with angle beam transducers. The test angle is selected to obtain the optimum signal from the expected indications. Most weld testing is done with frequencies between 2 and 5 MHz. There are special cases for testing outside the typical frequency range: thick, coarse grained materials require lower test frequencies (0.5 to 2 MHz) whereas thin, fine grained materials can tolerate higher frequencies (5 to 15 MHz).

When choosing test frequencies, several considerations should be noted: high frequencies provide better resolution and sensitivity whereas low frequencies offer better propagation.

Transducer Positioning

Weld discontinuities with specific orientations can be detected at specific transducer positions relative to the weld (Fig. 21). The sound path of the transducer is divided into zones that correspond to multiples of the test object thickness. The sound path between the transducer and the back surface is the first position and is commonly referred to as a *half-skip* or *half*-V *test*. The sound path from the back surface to the top surface is second and is called a *full-skip* or *full*-V *test*.

Data are collected from the first position when the transducer is closest to the weld; second position data are collected when the transducer is farther from the weld (Fig. 22). In applications where the scan is limited by weld configuration or transducer access, data are collected from a third position. At this point, the sound beam has diverged significantly and small discontinuities are more difficult to resolve.

Two transducers can also operate in tandem, one transmitting the ultrasonic signal and the second receiving the reflected signals. The configuration lends itself to detection of discontinuities poorly oriented for single transducer applications.

Ultrasonic Images of Welds

The images in Figs. 23 to 25 are from tests conducted with an angle beam transducer

FIGURE 22. Scan area for weld tests.

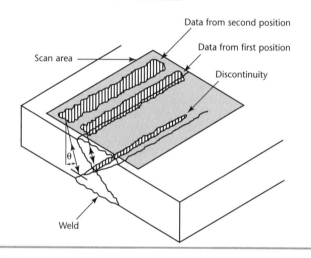

FIGURE 21. Weld testing with pulse echo contact transducer.

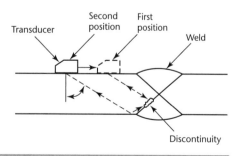

FIGURE 23. Ultrasonic image of lack of fusion.

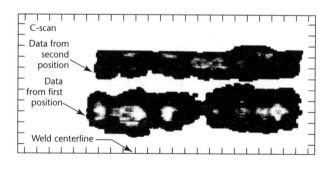

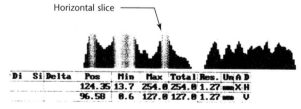

in pulse echo mode. Tests were made on three welded objects containing lack of fusion, porosity and intergranular stress corrosion cracking.

The first test object is a high yield strength carbon steel plate having a double-V butt weld containing lack of fusion. The scan shown in Fig. 22 was made with a 5 MHz transducer aimed toward the weld. Data were collected from the first and second positions by setting the ultrasonic gate to register signals over the appropriate skip distances. Normally, the gate is set to record data from a single position. To compensate for signal loss from beam divergence and attenuation, time controlled gain was applied to the received signal.

To show an ultrasonic image from lack of fusion, a C-scan displays a map of the ultrasonic signal amplitude. Data from the second position are shown at the top of the image. As the transducer is moved toward the weld centerline, data from the first position come into view. High signal amplitudes are shaded light and low signal amplitudes are darker. The white area surrounding the indications corresponds to data that did not exceed the trigger threshold. In angle beam tests, signals are returned only from echoes that reflect back to the transducer — if no signals are present, no data are recorded.

The slice at the bottom of the display represents a horizontal cross section of amplitude through the cursor on the C-scan display. During analysis, viewing thresholds can be set to various amplitude levels and the indications appropriately sized for acceptance or rejection according to the test criteria.

The second test object has the same weld geometry and material composition as the first but contains porosity in the weld (Fig. 24). Porosity is typified by low amplitude signals clustered together, as the image shows. The horizontal slice at the bottom of the display shows similar indications.

The third test object is an austenitic stainless steel pipe weld containing intergranular stress corrosion cracking. The weld has a single-V full penetration butt configuration (Fig. 25a). Intergranular stress corrosion cracks propagate in a branching manner along the grain boundaries of the material. The cracking occurs in the heat affected zone of a weld when the microstructure is sufficiently sensitized and exposed to critical conditions of stress and strain in a corrosive environment. Typically, such cracking is next to the counterbore, so the toe of the weld and signals can be difficult to differentiate.

Figure 25c shows an ultrasonic time-of-flight map of intergranular stress corrosion cracking — thick sections are shaded light and thin sections are darker.

FIGURE 25. Intergranular stress corrosion cracking: (a) cross section of butt weld; (b) example setup of tube weld; (c) image with points keyed to Fig. 25b.

(a)
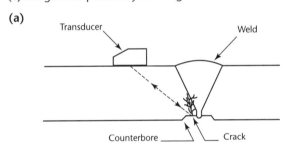

(b)
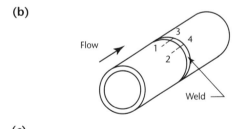

(c)
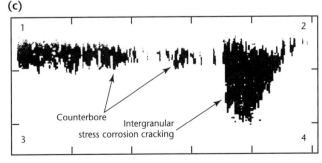

FIGURE 24. Ultrasonic image of porosity.

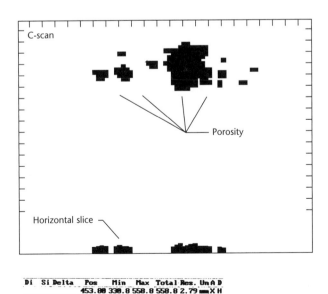

Di	Si	Delta	Pos	Min	Max	Total	Res.	UnA D
			453.88	338.8	558.8	558.8	2.79	X H
47.44	1.4		252.8	279.4	2.79			V

The horizontal indication at the top is caused by signals from the counterbore and has a thickness near the nominal thickness of the pipe. The darker indication is from intergranular stress corrosion cracking and is easily distinguished from the counterbore.

Ultrasonic imaging of weldments is a practical technique giving accurate volumetric information about discontinuities in welds. Because the area is well defined, the test can be performed by automated scanning processes. Images can be archived and retrieved for comparison as additional data are collected. The technique lends itself to periodic monitoring for assessing weld integrity. With this knowledge of discontinuity shape, size and location, the critical nature of the discontinuity can be determined.

PART 5. Multiple-Transducer Ultrasonic Techniques[11]

Introduction to Multiple-Transducer Tests

Ultrasonic techniques for nondestructive testing have two purposes: (1) the detection and characterization of discontinuities in materials and (2) the evaluation of material properties. A single ultrasonic transducer used for pulse echo tests can have several limitations for certain kinds of applications: (1) poor signal-to-noise ratios in highly attenuative materials, (2) limited discontinuity indication and characterization capabilities, (3) inability to detect all discontinuities because of component geometry and (4) a generally slow test procedure.

The use of multiple transducers provides improvements in all of these areas. However, because of many beam entry points, they are generally more susceptible to poor couplant or rough surfaces than single-transducer systems. Multiple-transducer systems may be configured in three primary categories (Fig. 26).

In the first category, the transducers are physically separated. The geometry of the test object and the locations of the transducers influence the detection and characterization of discontinuities. This category includes through-transmission and various pitch catch setups. Most of these techniques use only two transducers. However, transducers can be arranged as multiple pairs of a particular two-transducer technique to increase the speed of testing. Transmission and reception are then controlled by a multiplexer.

In the second category, the transducers are close to each other and depend on complex electronics for timing of transmission and reception. The various phased array configurations make up this category. Because the ultrasonic beam can be steered and focused, discontinuity detection and characterization are excellent with these techniques and real time imaging is practical.

In the third category, a single transducer is moved over the test object surface and individual A-scans are stored and then combined using sophisticated computer algorithms to form an image. Ultrasonic synthetic aperture focusing techniques are in this category. These techniques are excellent for discontinuity detection and characterization but are slow. They need multiple scans and processing.

FIGURE 26. Different types of multiple transducer configurations.

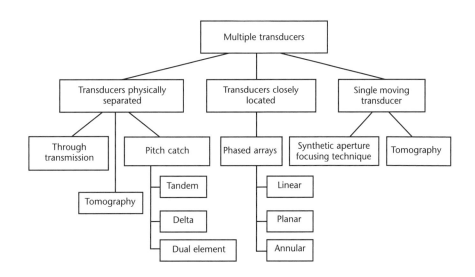

Tests with Separated Transducers

Through-Transmission Configurations

The normal through-transmission configuration uses two ultrasonic transducers located on opposite sides of a test object. One transducer acts as an ultrasound transmitter and the other transducer is lined up to passively receive the ultrasound. The transducers can be in contact with the material, immersed in liquid couplant or connected to the test object using water column transducers or squirters to transmit the sound to the material surfaces.

However, the through-transmission technique does have several limitations in that it is unable to distinguish between voids and delaminations because the attenuation characteristics of the two discontinuities are identical. Also, a discontinuity's location in the thickness of the material cannot be determined with through-transmission tests. If the thickness is known, the ultrasonic signal's time of arrival can be used to calculate the velocity and this can then be used to characterize the acoustic impedance of the material. Changes in the acoustic impedance represent changes in the composition of the test material. Through-transmission can be used for thickness measurements by recording the time of flight for the ultrasonic beam in a material whose acoustic impedance is known. Computer control technology enables ultrasonic instrumentation to use the most beneficial features of both through-transmission and pulse echo simultaneously. This feature avoids the limitations by letting the ultrasonic signal be received from both transducers at the same time.

Pitch Catch Tests

The pitch catch technique is an ultrasonic test with transmitting and receiving transducers where the path of the ultrasonic beam is not straight but is reflected one or more times before reaching the receiver. The transducers may be on the same surface of the test object with the sound beam bouncing off reflecting surfaces. When the component geometry does not allow a reflection between sender and receiver, the transducers may be located on different surfaces. The transducers must be precisely aligned, usually connected by a fixture or holder.

Direct Pitch Catch. There are several widely used pitch catch techniques for discontinuity detection and characterization. However, the pitching and catching of the ultrasonic beam can be broadly divided into two categories: direct and indirect. In direct pitch catch, the receiver is placed where the reflected ultrasonic beam is expected if there is no discontinuity. Objects free of discontinuities produce a good reflection and a discontinuity is detected when the beam is obscured and no reflection is received.

This technique is less prone to errors caused by discontinuity orientation, facets or roughness but it may cause errors because of the transparency of areas within a discontinuity or the ultrasonic diffraction at the edges of discontinuities. Full testing of a component is possible by continuously recording the transmitted signal but large numbers of spurious indications may occur because of beam angle and material properties.[4]

Figure 27 shows an in-service testing procedure for shrink fitted turbine disks using a direct pitch catch technique for the detection of stress corrosion cracking. Because of the geometry, the centers of the disks cannot be tested with a single transducer and the pulse echo technique. The pitch catch technique allows access to the centers of the disks.[5]

Indirect Pitch Catch Tests. With indirect pitch catch tests, the receiver is placed where the ultrasonic beam is expected to be if reflected by a discontinuity (Fig. 28).[12] This technique has speed advantages but may miss some discontinuities because of their orientation.

A digital imaging system based on a specialized indirect pitch catch technique

FIGURE 27. Pitch catch technique for testing turbine disks.[14]

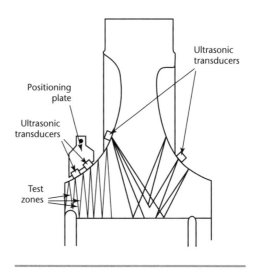

has been developed as shown in Fig. 29.[6] A transducer transmits a normal incidence longitudinal wave above the discontinuity and an image is formed from the scattered waves and is received at the rayleigh wave array transducer.

Experiments with this configuration produced images having three distinct waves along with other less distinct features. Figure 30 shows the origins of the three detected waves, each from a different area of the discontinuity.[6] The first to be detected is a transverse wave from the crack tip as it travels diagonally toward the coupling strip. The second is a rayleigh wave scattered by the crack opening. The third is a rayleigh wave that scatters at the crack tip and then propagates down the length of the crack and the surface of the test object. Using Eqs. 6 to 8, the depth of the crack h can be calculated:

$$(6) \quad \Delta t_1 = \frac{h}{V_L} + \frac{h}{V_R} + \frac{\sqrt{Z^2 + h^2}}{V_T}$$

$$(7) \quad \Delta t_2 = \frac{h}{V_R} - \frac{h}{V_L}$$

$$(8) \quad \Delta t_3 = \frac{h + Z}{V_R} + \frac{\sqrt{Z^2 + h^2}}{V_T}$$

Where V_L is the velocity (meter per second) of longitudinal waves in the test object, V_R is the velocity of rayleigh waves in the test object and V_T is the velocity of transverse waves in the test object.

Time-of-Flight Diffraction Tests

A well known variation of the pitch catch technique is the time-of-flight diffraction technique.[4,13-15] Ultrasonic waves from a transmitting transducer are diffracted from the tips of a crack as well as transmitted along the scanning surface and reflected from the back wall. The diffraction technique is therefore a hybrid of the direct and indirect pitch catch tests. The diffractions are separated in space so their reception by the receiving transducer

FIGURE 28. Setup for indirect pitch catch test.[13]

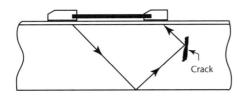

FIGURE 30. Diagram of three waves scattered by discontinuity: (a) test setup (b) transverse wave from crack tip, rayleigh wave from crack opening and a rayleigh wave from crack tip.[6]

(a)

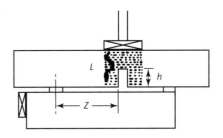

FIGURE 29. Indirect pitch catch technique for discontinuity imaging.[6]

(b)

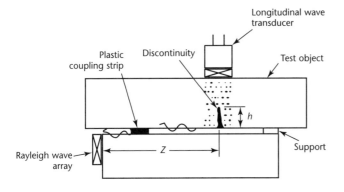

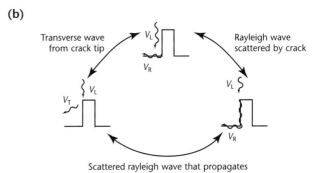

Legend
h = crack depth
Z = rayleigh wave travel

Legend
h = crack depth
L = longitudinal wave travel
Z = rayleigh wave travel
V_L = the velocity of longitudinal waves in test object (meter per second)
V_T = the velocity of transverse waves in test object (meter per second)
V_R = the velocity of rayleigh waves in test object (meter per second)

is separated by time. This difference in time can be used to locate and size the crack.

Time-of-flight diffraction is used in nondestructive tests of piping and pressure vessels because of its advantages over a pulse echo technique: its speed, objectivity, repeatability and its insensitivity to weld surface conditions and discontinuity orientation.[16] Time-of-flight diffraction techniques are typically used for sizing after the discontinuity is detected with another ultrasonic technique — diffraction techniques accurately determine the length and depth of surface breaking and submerged cracks. The technique has also been used on nonplanar discontinuities.[17] The applicability of the technique may be limited because the lower crack tip may not always diffract enough energy to be detected; however, the continuing improvements in developing ray based models and evolving applications with phased array systems continue to make the technique highly useful for sizing and locating discontinuities.

Tandem Transducer Tests

The tandem transducer technique is a common pitch catch test that uses two transducers close together on the same material surface, sometimes connected together, one acting as a transmitter of an inclined ultrasonic wave and the other acting as a passive receiver.[18] This technique is used for discontinuity detection and materials characterization.

The path of the ultrasound has three distinct segments caused by two reflections of the ultrasonic beam. The amplitude signal and time-of-flight data interpretation are based on knowledge of this geometry. Received signals that fall outside of a statistical confidence limit indicate a discontinuity. Discontinuity roughness, orientation and specular reflection from facets affect this technique's ability to detect and size discontinuities.[19]

Several transducers could be lined up to receive the transmitted signal, assisting determination of the optimum depth of discontinuity detection. The direct tandem technique has been used to test abrasive wheels composed of silicon carbide for radial cracks with a dry couplant.[20] Because of the orientation of the discontinuities, the through-transmission technique did not work. For these tests, the ultrasonic energy propagates through the silicon carbide and is reflected off the mounting hole at the wheel's center. The system is calibrated with a reference standard to get the maximum amplitude of the reflected signal. Radial cracks were found to reduce

the amplitude appreciably and the amount of the reduction can be used as a measure of crack dimensions. Sometimes the signal undergoes multiple reflections, causing a shift in the signal pattern.

The tandem technique can be used to characterize discontinuities, differentiating between voids and cracks when the transmitting transducer also receives the reflected signal. If the discontinuity is a void, then it probably has a spherical shape (Fig. 31a) — the transmitter receives a signal of amplitude A_1 and the receiver receives a signal of amplitude A_2. Because of reflection and attenuation:

$$(9) \quad \frac{A_1}{A_2} \gg 1$$

If the discontinuity is planar (Fig. 31b), then the transmitting transducer receives reflections such that:

$$(10) \quad \frac{A_1}{A_2} \ll 1$$

However, the potential orientations of planar discontinuities must be taken into consideration.

The tandem technique also has been adapted for the characterization of composites to compute the stress wave factor.[13,21-24] The stress wave factor may be defined:[22]

$$(11) \quad \epsilon = grn$$

FIGURE 31. Ultrasonic test setup for characterizing (a) spherical discontinuities where $A_1 \div A_2 \gg 1$; (b) planar discontinuities where $A_1 \div A_2 \ll 1$.

(a)

(b)

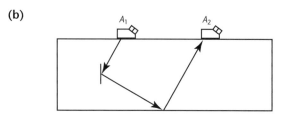

Legend
A_1 = transmitting transducer
A_2 = receiving transducer

where g is the accumulation time after which the counter is reset (microsecond), n is the number of oscillations exceeding a threshold in the output waveform and r is the transmitter repetition rate. The stress wave factor depends on the input signal characteristics, transducer characteristics, system gain, reset time, distance between transducers and other system dependent factors. When these factors are kept constant, the stress wave factor indicates the ability of a material to transmit ultrasound.

In one application, the stress wave factor was redefined as the summation of the amplitudes of the oscillations on the output signal trace.[13] The stress wave factor can be used as an indicator of residual tensile strength in the composites.

A technique developed on the tandem concept can be used to characterize a material with mild anisotropy.[16] Anisotropy changes the skip distance as a function of the angle (Fig. 32). The deviation of this function from a constant value could be used as a measure of a material's anisotropy.

Bond strength between adhesively bonded materials may also be determined with the tandem technique.[25] In this configuration, two broad band, mildly focused transducers are mounted on a holder that allows them to move. Longitudinal waves emitted by the transmitter are mode converted into a transverse wave focused on the interface between the two bonded objects. Signal processing algorithms performed on the received signal yield a diagnosis of the adhesive interface condition.[25]

FIGURE 32. Setup for measuring material anisotropy.[16]

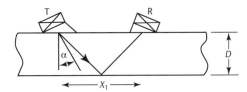

Legend
D = test object thickness
R = receiving ultrasonic transducer with location in neighborhood of maximum response point
T = sensing transducer with incident angle steering capability calibrated on a reference standard
X_1 = skip distance measured as function of incident angle which differs from actual angle of energy propagation
α = incident angle

Delta Testing

The delta technique is an indirect pitch catch test developed for weld discontinuities.[17] The transmitting transducer is not in contact with the test surface but is inclined at an angle that typically produces refracted transverse waves in the test object at an angle of 1 rad (60 deg). When this ultrasonic beam encounters a discontinuity, it is scattered.

A receiving transducer positioned normal to the test object surface detects the scattered waves. Figure 33 shows how the sound energy is partitioned when the incident transverse wave strikes a crack.[18] Some of the transverse waves are reflected, some are mode converted into longitudinal waves and the rest are simply reradiated. This reradiation may be caused by edge waves according to Huygen's principle or may be the result of mode converted rayleigh waves that propagate along the length of the discontinuity. When these rayleigh waves reach the edge of the discontinuity, they are mode converted to transverse waves. Because of these three different effects, a wide ultrasonic beam is created. This creation is known as the *delta effect*.

The delta technique has two advantages over the pulse echo technique: (1) the receiving transducer detects a signal only when there is a discontinuity and (2) the width of the redirected ultrasonic beam increases the probability that randomly oriented discontinuities will be detected. The delta technique has a better signal-to-noise ratio and better back wall resolution.[18] If a discontinuity is located near the back wall, there is no echo off the back wall to interfere with the discontinuity signal.

However, there is little correlation between discontinuity size or the depth of the discontinuity and the amplitude of the signal received. Therefore, the delta technique is excellent for detecting discontinuities but is limited in its ability to locate the depth of the discontinuity and to size it. Discontinuities have been sized by monitoring the discontinuity

FIGURE 33. Energy partition at smooth crack during delta test.[18]

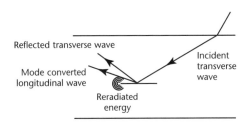

Reflected transverse wave

Mode converted longitudinal wave

Incident transverse wave

Reradiated energy

signal as the transmitting transducer is scanned across the test object.[26]

An example of a process optimization of the parameters using the delta technique for inspection of electron beam welds in titanium aircraft parts has been demonstrated.[27]

Dual-Element Transducers

Dual-Element Design

A dual-element transducer consists of two transducers (a transmitter of longitudinal waves and a receiver) mounted on delay lines side by side and separated by an acoustic barrier.[14] The electronics of the two transducers are separated so that the receiver can start detecting echoes before the transmitter ends transmission (Figs. 34 and 35). The two transducers are pitched at an angle to the vertical plane dividing them, called the *roof angle* or *squint angle*, usually around 150 mrad (8 deg). This angle causes the longitudinal wave beams of the two transducers to overlap, creating a pseudofocusing effect in the focal zone and increasing the ratio of signal to noise. For this reason, the dual-element transducer performs well for detecting discontinuities in highly attenuative materials like concrete and stainless steel weld metal.

In a dual-element transducer and its sensitivity diagram, sensitivity can be high at short focal distances, so different transducers with various roof angles are used for detection at different distances. As with a single transducer, the basic test measurement is the time between the transmission and the reception of an echo.

The path of the ultrasound is shaped like a V: from the transmitting transducer to the reflecting surface and then to the receiving transducer. This path introduces an error that may be large for short

distances but microprocessor controls correct such errors. The transmitting transducer's ultrasonic beam can be of normal incidence to the test surface (for thickness measurements) or it can be an angle beam (to detect surface and near surface discontinuities).

Dual-element transducers were designed to overcome problems encountered by a single transducer when measuring very thin materials or when detecting near surface discontinuities. When a piezoelectric crystal is excited, it vibrates and generates an elastic wave. The crystal vibration has a finite duration or ringing time. During this time, the crystal cannot act as a receiver for the reflected echo and the receiver amplifier may be saturated by the transmitted pulse. This is called the *dead zone* and may extend several millimeters into the test object for a low frequency transducer.

In an application where the discontinuities are farther, the dead zone is not a problem. For locating and characterizing anomalies near the surface, ringing time is critical. Also, if the test surface is rough it may produce long ringing interface echoes. A dual-element transducer overcomes these disadvantages because the receiver can receive the reflected signal even before the transmitter has ceased transmitting.

Dual-Element Applications

A major application of the dual-element measurement of piping and pressure vessels. In many such applications, the test object material is coarse grained, highly attenuative and has suffered from

FIGURE 35. Ultrasonic beam profile for dual-element transducer.

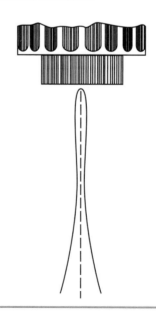

FIGURE 34. Schematic of dual-element, delay line transducer.[30]

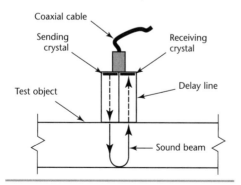

corrosion in the form of pinhole failures. It is desirable that the ultrasonic beam be focused and of minimal diameter because of the geometry of the discontinuity (small, rounded, reflecting surface).

A single transducer using the pulse echo technique is inadequate under such conditions, mainly because of its low signal-to-noise ratio and the lack of focusing ability. The dual-element transducer provides a good beam profile for these applications (Figs. 34 and 35) and has the additional advantage of near-surface detection of pinhole corrosion.[29] The beam angle is normal to the surface of the test material and, depending on the thickness, thickness accuracies of 0.01 mm (0.0004 in.) are possible.[30]

Another major application of dual-element tests is detecting discontinuities in regions of cladding and austenitic welds.[26,31,32] Short pulses, heavily damped transducers and a broad band receiver system enhance resolution and may increase the ratio of signal to noise. Depending on the anticipated orientation and type of discontinuity, the beam angle can be oblique or normal to the material surface.

Another dual-element technique for discontinuity detection, characterizing and sizing of welds uses creeping waves. In steel, for example, the transducers emit and detect several different waves: longitudinal creeping surface waves, longitudinal bulk waves and two types of transverse waves. The wedge of the transducer is designed to have a high angle of incidence for the creeping wave or head wave, which also emits an indirect transverse wave. There is also a longitudinal wave beam between 1.1 and 1.3 rad (65 and 80 deg). A direct transverse wave is emitted between 0.5 and 0.6 rad (30 and 35 deg). The transverse waves are mode converted on the opposite surface back into longitudinal waves and creeping waves. Surface breaking cracks can be detected on inside and outside surfaces.

Other Two-Transducer Systems

Other specialized techniques have been developed using two transducers for industrial nondestructive testing and medical imaging.

Two transducers have been used as a means of constructing a C-scan of the thickness variations in ceramic and composite materials.[14] The system locates the test material in an immersion tank between two transducers. Each transducer uses the pulse echo effect to measure the

distance between itself and the material through the water. The two distances are added together and the distance between the two transducers is known, so the thickness of the material can be accurately measured.

A technique called *multibeam satellite pulse observation technique* has been developed for identifying and sizing near-surface cracks in cladded reactor pressure vessels. The system's two transducers (Fig. 36) transmit 1 rad (60 deg) longitudinal waves and 0.7 rad (40 deg) transverse waves.[19] These two signals produce a doublet, a pair of associated signals that travel across the screen of the test system display. By interpreting the separation between these two signals, the size of a crack can be estimated (larger separation indicates a longer crack).

Tests with Closely Positioned Transducers

Multiple-Transducer Systems

Many ultrasonic testing systems use more than two transducers, either as transmitters or receivers or both. These systems use multiplexers to enhance speed of testing and reduce electronics. A computer typically controls the firing of the transducers.

For test of welds, for example, a multiple-transducer system has been developed based on the time-of-flight diffraction technique.[33] Using multiple transmitters and receivers controlled by a computer, the test is designed for automated detection and sizing of cracks in welds. The multiple-transducer system is designed so that each transducer

FIGURE 36. Bimodal transducers in multiple-beam satellite pulse observation technique.[19]

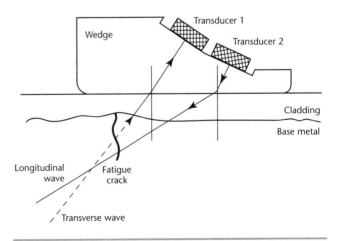

transmits at an angle that differs from any other transducer in the array. These angles lie between 0.7 and 1.3 rad (45 and 80 deg). Figure 37 shows the weld coverage from a system with eight transmitters and eight receivers.[33] The transducers transmit one at a time and the computer collects A-scans of the received signal from the corresponding receiver. The A-scans are used to construct a B-scan image and from comparison of B-scans from different transducer pairs, discontinuities are detected and sized.

A technique called *travel time mode conversion* has been developed for the detection and characterization of fatigue cracks in steel plates.[34] Figure 38 shows the multiple-transducer configuration used for a surface breaking crack. The transducers are positioned by scanning the tip and root of the crack. Each transducer acts as both a transmitter and receiver so that the crack is completely covered by each ultrasonic beam and each transducer receives the scattered waves. The sizing of the crack is accomplished by comparing the relative time-of-flight information on the reflected, diffracted and mode converted ultrasonic waves.

A different type of multiple-transducer configuration uses long and intermediate wavelength inverse scattering with a pitch catch technique.[35,36] The test data are then used for three-dimensional discontinuity reconstruction.

From a combination of transmitting and receiving transducers, multiple waveforms from different angles are recorded. The signals from the transducers must intersect at the discontinuity for different angles of incidence if the pitch catch (or pulse echo, when the transmitter is also the receiver) is to be effective. A measurement model is used to correct the backscatter waveforms for attenuation, diffraction and interface losses to produce waveforms that only represent the backscatter. A one-dimensional born approximation is applied to each waveform to obtain a size parameter for the discontinuity from each of the angles.

These parameters and the viewing angles are then used in a regression analysis to construct an ellipsoid that best fits the data. Because low and intermediate frequencies are used, discontinuities of some depth can be characterized. This technique can also provide material property data, such as the normalized stress intensity factor for cracks. An arbitrarily oriented discontinuity may not be completely reconstructed but this may be compensated for by increasing the aperture of the multiple-view transducer.

Another multiple-transducer system has been developed for the detection of small discontinuities near the surface in castings.[37] The system was designed to overcome problems with the dead zone, surface roughness, scattering echo and other impediments. Figure 39 shows the construction of the three transducers: the outer two are transmitters of transverse waves and the central transducer acts as a receiver of mode converted longitudinal waves. This combination helps overcome any decrease of signal-to-noise ratio caused by increased attenuation of

FIGURE 37. Design of multiple-transducer system to cover volume of weld.[33]

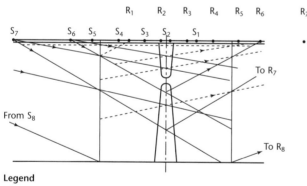

Legend
R = receiving transducer
S = sending transducer

FIGURE 38. Multiple-transducer configuration for detecting surface breaking cracks in steel.[34]

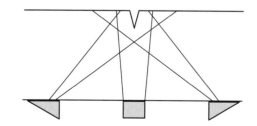

FIGURE 39. Construction of multiple-transducer configuration for tests of castings.[37]

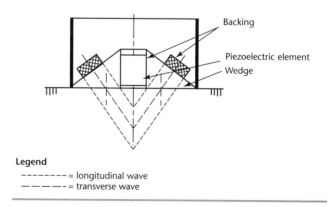

Legend
------- = longitudinal wave
— — — — = transverse wave

longitudinal waves reacting with graphite in the casting. The transducer is designed to act in different modes as shown in Fig. 40.

Figure 41 is the distance amplitude characteristic curve for this multiple transducer, showing maximum sensitivity between 6 and 7 mm (0.23 and 0.28 in.) below the surface. Experimental results demonstrated that the transducer could detect discontinuities of 0.5 mm (0.02 in.) diameter at depths up to 5 mm (0.2 in.).[37]

Research on improving ultrasonic measurements with multiple transducers through newer signal processing approaches has continued. An optimal approach to estimating the material reflection sequence for a linear signal generation model using maximum *a posteriori* estimation was performed.[38]

Experimental data and simulation experiments were performed to verify the correctness of the multiple-transducer model and the estimation scheme.

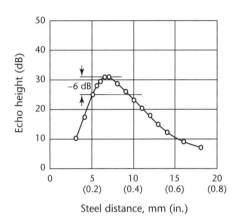

FIGURE 41. Distance amplitude characteristic curve of multiple transducer, transmitting wave at 5 MHz and receiving longitudinal wave.[37]

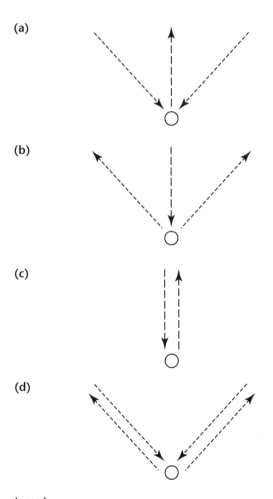

FIGURE 40. Combination patterns of transmitting and receiving for multiple transducer configuration: (a) two to one; (b) one to two; (c) one to one; (d) two to two .[37]

(a)

(b)

(c)

(d)

Legend
- - - - - - - = longitudinal wave
— — — — - = transverse wave

Part 6. Phased Arrays

Arrays are arrangements of transducer elements that offer capabilities greater than single- or multiple-transducer systems for the determination of shape, size and orientation of discontinuities.[29,39] There are three major types of arrays: linear, planar (or mosaic) and annular. In a phased array, a prescribed phase shift is controlled electronically and provided to each of the transducers for ultrasonic transmission. Phased arrays provide significant control over the shape and direction of the transmitted ultrasonic beam, thereby fulfilling two requirements for sophisticated nondestructive testing applications: dynamic focusing and real time scanning.

Transducers with a flat face project a beam pattern like the one shown in Fig. 42a — constant in the near field and uniformly conical in the far field.[40] Lateral resolution in the near field is limited by the diameter of the transducer. In the far field, the beam widens so that the lateral resolution of the transducer decreases. Decreasing the diameter of the transducer decreases the transition distance and increases the angle of divergence. To counter these effects, the frequency may be increased but this decreases the wavelength which, in turn, increases attenuation.

To create a smaller ultrasonic beam within the near field, the transducer can be focused by curving the transducer element or by attaching a lens to a flat transducer. A lens can cause reverberations within the piezoelectric material, so curving the transducer is preferable. The focusing ability of a transducer is described by radius of curvature and the beam width can be reduced either by increasing the diameter of the transducer or by increasing the frequency (Figs. 42b and 42c). The amount of focusing affects the depth of beam penetration: the stronger the focusing, the shallower the focal zone. Therefore, the focused transducer is limited in possible depth and lateral resolution. These transducer focal abilities cannot be changed because they are characteristics of design and construction.

In an array transducer system, timing of the transducer's firing can be controlled — the transmitted ultrasound from all the elements of the array combine to form an overall wave front, providing dynamic focusing. This wave front can be well controlled (shaped) by firing the outermost elements first and then firing the elements toward the interior of the transducer. Figure 43 is a representation of a linear phased array transducer and demonstrates the principle of using

FIGURE 42. Beam patterns for typical commercial fixed focus transducers: (a) long focus at 3.5 MHz; (b) medium focus at 3.5 MHz; (c) medium focus at 5 MHz.[40]

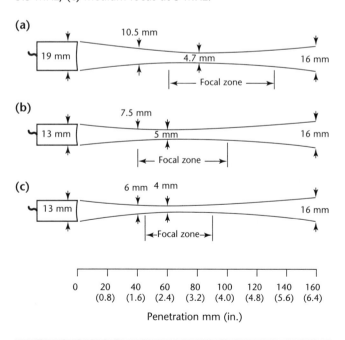

FIGURE 43. Time delays for focusing of phased linear array.[41]

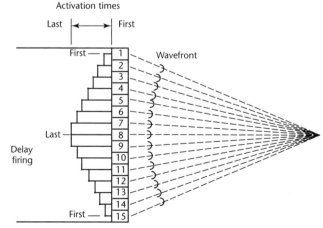

multiple small wave fronts to create a focused overall wave front.[41]

Figure 44 is the layout of an annular array transducer.[40] An annular array can be thought of as a cylindrical transducer that has been sliced into concentric rings or annuli, each forming a separate transducer. The time of transmission and reception of these annuli are controlled by electronics, thereby controlling the shape and the focal point of the overall wave front, always on the axis of the transducer. Reflections produced by objects closer to the transducer arrive sooner than those farther away. By changing the receiver delay lines, the focus can be changed during signal reception to concentrate on different depths along the axis.

A second advantage offered by phased array transducer systems is ultrasonic beam steering, a crucial feature in real time ultrasonic imaging. In real time imaging, fast moving structures can be imaged and evaluated and the procedure can be automated to eliminate diagnostic variability caused by differing technician skill levels.[41] Figure 45 shows three ways in which a scan can be performed for real time imaging: a sector scan, a linear scan and a linear scan with sector scans at the boundaries of the linear scan.[42]

High speed multiplexing can achieve effects similar to those of phased arrays (Fig. 46).[42] For linear scanning, a single transducer is quickly moved back and forth over the test object. A sequential linear array accomplishes the linear scan by transmitting from each of the array elements (or small groups of elements) one at a time and receiving the reflection with the same element (or group of elements) to form one line of a B-scan (Fig. 47a).[40] By moving down the array, an image is produced with the number of lines equal to the number of array elements and the field of view equal to the length of the array.

A mechanical sector scan is accomplished by encasing the transducer assembly in a fluid filled holder with an acoustically transparent window.[41] The assembly can be (1) a stationary transducer that directs its beam onto an oscillating mirror and through the window, (2) a disk that oscillates about its diameter or (3) a number of transducers mounted on a rotating wheel, with each transducer transmitting as it reaches the window. A phased linear array or planar array performs a sector scan by sequencing the transmission and reception of transducers to steer the ultrasonic beam (Fig. 47b). The planar array provides steering in three dimensions.

Phased arrays are widely used in medical ultrasonic imaging but had limited use in nondestructive testing in the twentieth century, mainly because of

FIGURE 45. Single-pass scanning technique: (a) single sector scan; (b) linear scan; (c) combination of linear and sector scan.[42]

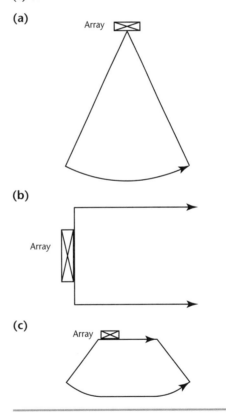

FIGURE 44. Layout of annular array transducer and its associated electronics.[40]

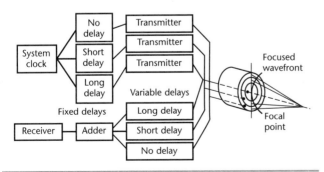

FIGURE 46. Types of real time scanning instrumentation.[42]

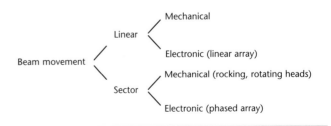

the complexity and cost of the systems. One application uses a steered, focused ultrasonic beam for tests of tubes.[43] An experimental array of 24 transducers was developed in a ring that fit over the tube and had four consecutive elements transmitting sequentially as a group, similar to the sequential linear array.

When using a sector scan for testing materials, the ultrasonic beam is steered over a wide sector from a fixed position. Compound scanning (scanning the same general area from different positions) offers several benefits: high redundancy, exact determination of discontinuity location and high detectability when using high intensity beams, especially for crack tip detection.[29]

For discontinuity characterization, there are two approaches to take with compound scanning.

1. In discontinuity reconstruction by scanning with a beam width as narrow as possible. The results from all the positions are superimposed to produce a cross sectional B-scan presentation of the discontinuity.
2. In discontinuity classification by scanning with a beam large compared with discontinuity size. Figure 48 shows how the maximum echoes from each transducer position can be combined to form a compound scan amplitude locus curve.

Contact Modes Phased Arrays

Phased arrays can operate in three basic contact modes: manual, semiautomated and automated. Like other types of ultrasonic testing, phased arrays can also operate in immersion. The following discussion describes the three contact modes and how they are applied.[87]

Manual Contact Phased Arrays

Normally, a portable phased array unit is used. These compact units have much of the capability of larger units and typically have 128 channels. Manual phased arrays operate in a similar manner to conventional discontinuity detectors but use a sector scan displayed on the screen. This allows real time imaging with true depth positioning.

Discontinuities can be imaged in spectral color at true depth. The displayed waveform corresponds to the angled line

FIGURE 47. Linear array: (a) simple linear scan; (b) sector scan (phased linear array).[40]

(a)

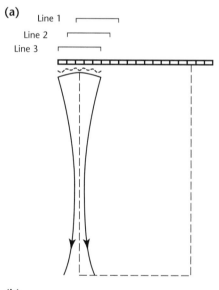

(b)

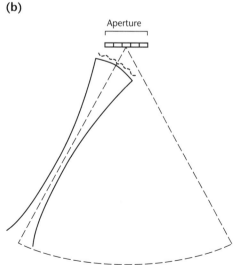

FIGURE 48. Generation of compound scan amplitude locus curve: (a) maximum echo amplitude; (b) beam profiles and transducer locations.[29]

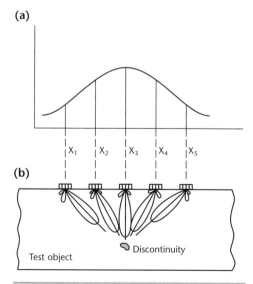

on the electronic scan and the gate corresponds to the two corresponding lines in the S-scan. Cursors are also available for discontinuity sizing.

With manual phased array tests, the operator calibrates and couples in the usual contact manner but typically watches the electronic scan while scanning for early detection and characterizing of discontinuities. This gives improved probability of detection and faster testing rates. For welds, a transverse wave is used; the operator can increase scanning speed by using the electronic scan. For other applications, such as shaft inspections, a longitudinal wave electronic scan may be more appropriate.

Because no encoder is used, it is not possible to generate a C-scan, However, screen shots can be saved — a major advantage of manual phased arrays. Saving images reduces subjectivity, gives better reporting and more repeatable rescanning. Focused beams significantly improve the ratio of signal to noise (and hence the probability of detection).

Semiautomated Contact Phased Arrays

Semiautomated tests are similar to manual tests with one major difference; the scans are encoded and all the data are stored. The simplest semiautomated system is an array with an encoder attached but handheld scanners and belt scanners are also used for some applications (Fig. 49).

The operator calibrates in the usual manner; coupling is either with commercial gels/oils or pumped water, depending on the application, requirements and test speeds. The operator pushes the probe by hand, whether using just an encoder or a handheld scanner.

Semiautomated tests are typically used for weld inspection, corrosion mapping

FIGURE 49. Typical semiautomated handscanner for piping test.

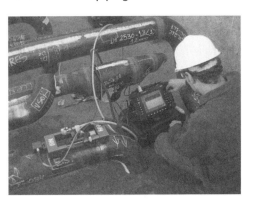

and other applications where full data storage and display is required. With these inspections, the results can be displayed as corrosion maps, A-scans, B-scans, C-scans, D-scans (or top, side and end views) as shown in Fig. 50 or as required.

FIGURE 50. Phased array test of weld, showing indications: (a) top view; (b) side view; (c) end view; (d) waveform.

(a)

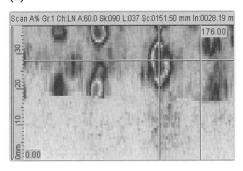

(b)

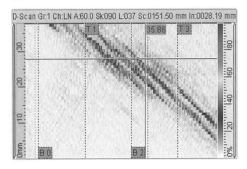

(c)

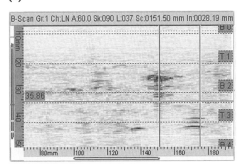

(d)

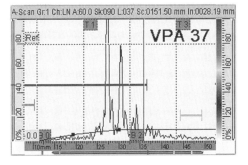

Semiautomated scans permit a high degree of reliability and reproducibility, with minimal cost and maintenance.

Automated Contact Phased Arrays

Fully automated test systems are totally mechanized; the operator controls the scanner from a computer, and all data are collected automatically. With phased arrays, fully automated test systems are normally single-axis systems because the second axis is performed by electronic scanning, discussed elsewhere in this volume. Typically, fully automated phased array systems are high end products with significantly better capability than semiautomated systems. For example, scanning speed is typically at mechanical speeds of 100 mm·s⁻¹ or faster. The ultrasonic test performed may be complex, the data collection rate may be high and the arrays may be bigger.

Calibration is made to the code or specifications, which may be specifically tailored to the application and equipment. The couplant is typically pumped, and is probably water unless otherwise required. Some form of coupling check is often required, for example, a through transmission for welds or a normal beam signal. Generally, the large array wedges run smoothly and give less coupling problems than an equivalent multiple-probe system.

At high scanning speeds, the plastic wedges wear quickly, especially on carbon steel. Standard practice is to use wear pins (often tungsten carbide), positioned with a specified maximum allowed gap to ensure good water flow.

Linear Phased Arrays

Linear phased arrays are an excellent means of implementing a real time ultrasonic imaging system. They allow beam steering and focusing, signal processing during image formation and a potential for parallel processing to increase data rates.

Beam Steering

Beam steering is based on the principles of geometric optics.[44,45] Figure 51 shows a representative linear array with eight elements, where D_A is the total lateral dimension or aperture, L_A is the elevation dimension, d_A is the interelement spacing and W_A is the size of the elements.

Steering can be performed in the lateral dimension for both transmitting and receiving at the azimuthal angle θ. The lateral dimension D_A can be between 13 and 25 mm (0.5 and 1.0 in.), with 16 to 64 elements.

Studies show that the best number of elements to have in an array aperture between 20 and 30.[46] Less than twenty decreases the resolution and more than thirty has little effect on improving the lateral and axial resolution. The same research also concludes that both the lateral and axial resolution are inversely proportional to the aperture.

A linear array is typically constructed by cutting through a single piezoelectric ceramic to isolate the individual elements (a technique called *slotting*) or by electroding the surface and leaving the plate intact. The latter type of array is called *monolithic*.[47-49] The lateral dimension of the array is always larger than its elevation dimension $D_A > L_A$) but the individual element is always smaller than its elevation dimension ($L_A > W_A$), so that each element can be approximated as a line source.

Beam Focusing

As described above, a linear array can produce an ultrasonic wave front at any azimuth by timing the sequence of array element transmissions so that the maximum acoustic intensity of all the elements creates a line perpendicular to the direction of overall propagation. The timing of the sequence dictates the direction of the wave front. For a steering angle *r*, each of the array elements must be delayed:[44]

FIGURE 51. Design of multiple element linear array.[44]

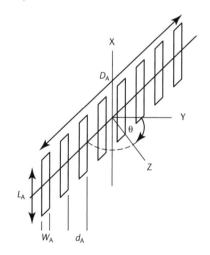

Legend
d_A = element separation
D_A = aperture depth
L_A = aperture length
W_A = element width
X,Y,Z = dimensional axes
θ = steering angle

$$(12) \quad t_n = n\frac{d_A}{c} \sin\theta + t_0$$

where c is the velocity of ultrasound in the test material, where $n = 0, \pm 1, \pm 2 \ldots$ with respect to the center element for the individual elements from the center of the array outward and where t_0 is a constant large enough to avoid negative delays.

A spherical timing relationship can produce focusing within a certain range of the ultrasonic beam. Focal points are limited by the transition range Z_{TR} of the array and may be approximated:[44]

$$(13) \quad Z_{TR} = \frac{d_A^2}{4\lambda_0}$$

where λ_0 is the wavelength corresponding to the center frequency of the transmitted acoustic burst. For an ultrasonic beam focused at range F with a direction of θ, the delay times for the individual elements are:[44]

$$(14) \quad t_n = \frac{F}{c}\left[1 - \sqrt{1 + \left(\frac{nd}{F}\right)^2 - 2\frac{nd}{F}\sin\theta}\right] + t_0$$

This focusing is restricted to the region around the focal point, a region known as the *depth of field*. The depth of field is inversely proportional to the square of the array aperture at a given focal distance.

The depth of field of a strongly focused system can be improved during reception using dynamic focusing. The receive focus of the array is rapidly changed to track the range of reflections synchronously. Multiple foci are possible by focusing the receiver on a point close to the transducer. After those reflections are received, the focus is moved by increasing the delay times to receive more reflections.

Linear Array Field Patterns

A real time scan is composed of a complete transmission and reception in multiple azimuthal directions. A phased array could be steered in any azimuthal direction but practical considerations limit steering to ±0.8 rad (±45 deg) from the center element, depending on the element size and frequency.[44,45] A far field pattern for a phased array transmitting straight ahead has a main lobe with some small grating lobes, each lobe having a width of $\lambda \cdot (D_A)^{-1}$. The grating lobes occur at angular spacings of $\lambda \cdot (d_A)^{-1}$.

As the far field pattern of a linear phased array beam is steered to greater angles, the amplitude of the main beam decreases and one of the adjacent grating lobes increases in amplitude. For good imaging, only the reflections from targets in the path of the main lobe should be received.

Grating lobes reduce the range for imaging and in some cases create multiple images. The amplitudes of grating lobes can be reduced by using the nyquist sampling criterion, where the array element spacing is half the wavelength or less.[50] This small spacing translates into more transducers for the array and increases the angle between the main lobe and the grating lobes. Also, using short pulses reduces the relative amplitude of the grating lobes.[44]

Limitations of Phased Arrays

Linear phased arrays have a number of limitations. For example, the response of transducer arrays is not ideal. This occurs because of the coupling of the thickness mode and radial mode vibrations, which leads to a decrease in the thickness mode resonant frequency. It has been shown that a width-to-thickness ratio of 0.65 provides the optimum transducer sensitivity.[51]

In addition, there are limitations to the uniform angular response of the array elements, due in part to coupling of energy to adjacent elements through the transducer faceplate and interelement material.[52] Another problem is caused by the fact that the time delays that control the sequencing of transmission and reception are discreet, which results in a quantized approximation of the smooth, continuous curves needed for ideal focusing and steering. The jagged curve produces error grating lobes in the image, especially at high steering angles. The best way to reduce this effect is to decrease the time delay increments.[53-56]

Phased Linear Array Design

The design of a phased linear array considers many critical factors, including (1) the number of elements (especially with regard to focusing), (2) whether the transducer is in contact with test material or immersed in a liquid, (3) whether the electrical excitation is burst or pulsed and (4) control of signal transmission and reception.

The electronics of the phased linear array are crucial to its operation. The problem with focusing the received reflections is to provide signal delays so that the echoes arriving at different times are made coincident when they are summed.[56-59] One approach to this is multiplexing each array element onto a fast analog-to-digital converter and storing the results in memory. The data are taken out of memory with the appropriate delay, then summed. The delays are related to the geometry of the targets: (1) the reflections from the different ranges arrive at increasingly higher rates after transmission and (2) the curvature of the received wave front varies inversely with the time delay after transmission.

Also, targets produce a linear time delay in their echoes at the receiver aperture. In one representative system, charged coupled devices are used as analog delay lines, each array element sending its output signal through two delay lines controlled by independent clocks. Clock 1 is linear across the array and produces the steered beam; clock 2 has a parabolic curvature. The variation of the frequency of clock 2 has a parabolic curvature. This variation of clock 2 controls the summation of the different curved wave fronts produced by the different ranges, so reception can be focused. Combining the received reflections can also be implemented in software if all of the signals are stored. An alternative technique uses a pipelined sampled delay focusing technique that eliminates memory addressing and some hardware.[58]

The elements of the linear array do not have to be equidistant. For example, in one phased linear array the elements are spaced according to a sine distribution:[29,38]

$$(15) \quad x_i = \frac{D_A}{n}\left[i - p\left(\frac{\pi}{ni}\right)\right]$$

where i is the number of that element in relation to the array center, n is the total number of elements and p is a positive number smaller than $n \cdot (2\pi)^{-1}$. This distribution concentrates elements in the center and thins them out toward the ends — the directivity diagram has a main lobe surrounded on both sides by regions of high angular damping.

Before 1990, almost all phased array imaging systems had been developed for medical applications. A monolithic phased array (Fig. 52) has used both longitudinal and transverse waves appropriate for nondestructive testing.[47-49]

A sequential linear array with 32 contacting transducers has been developed for tests of aluminum.[60] The array uses longitudinal waves with a center frequency of 3 MHz. A second array was designed to use transverse waves at half the wavelength of the longitudinal wave. Another technique, called *interlaced scanning*, uses a linear array for the helical scanning of cylindrical objects for discontinuities, especially longitudinal cracks.[61] Because of the geometry of the testing problem, a phased linear array is not needed, just a linear array with each transducer transmitting and receiving.

Phased Planar Arrays

A phased planar (or matrix) array is basically an extension of the two-dimensional phased linear array into the third dimension. This extension produces the planar array's major advantage — the ability to steer the ultrasonic beam — but this comes at a high cost: a considerable increase in the complexity of electronics to control the sequencing of individual transducers. For this reason, phased planar arrays have had limited use in nondestructive testing. The theory for controlling the phased planar array is similar to that of phased linear arrays and is based on the timing of the array element's firing.

Charge coupled devices have been used as delay lines in a square $N \times N$ transducer array that requires the use of $N + 1$ delay line modules.[59] Each row is thought of (in the X direction) as a linear array connected to a delay line that controls the Y direction steering. The phase delays for any single element add linearly, therefore the X and Y direction delay lines produce independent phase effects. Phased planar arrays are described mathematically elsewhere.[62-68]

During reception, the focus is shifted to each zone by using switchable delay elements, creating an expanding aperture.[63] Design approaches include the application of different spatial sampling patterns for sparse array transducer design[62] and both experiments and simulations for designing phased array transducers.[63-66] Newer techniques in transducer design also include the miniaturization of the transducer arrays, which not only improves the

FIGURE 52. Monolithic phased linear array for nondestructive testing.[49]

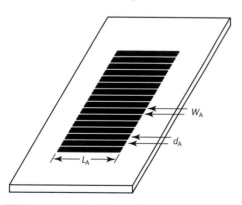

characteristics of the arrays but also expands the range of applications.[67,68]

Phased Annular Arrays

Annular arrays cannot be steered but their focusing abilities along the central axis can be considerably enhanced. Focusing is enhanced by time delays in the path of the reflections detected by the array elements and then summing those results. As described earlier, dynamic focusing during reception of the ultrasonic reflections is achieved by varying the time delays. In transmission mode, the ultrasonic beam may not be dynamically focused because it originates from only one annulus. However, the focal length along the axial direction can be varied by changing the delays between the sequential excitation of the annuli, the outermost to the center.

Annular Array Design

The primary factors for the design of an annular array are the size and number of array elements and the frequency of transmission. The primary factors influencing the use of an annular array are the calculation of the focal depth and the time delays. Much of the theory for the design and use of annular arrays is based on the theories of geometric optics. The characteristics of sound propagation, however, do not closely follow those of light. Specifically, parallel light rays do not focus whereas parallel sound beams emanating from a flat source focus at $D^2_A \cdot (4\lambda)^{-1}$.

If this difference is ignored, then the sound beam's focal length is shorter than expected. In the discussion of annular array theory that follows, this consideration should be kept in mind and strict experimentation should be performed to verify any results predicted by the theory.

Phased annular arrays were first discussed in the mid 1950s as a means of extending the depth of field of strongly focused apertures while maintaining adequate lateral resolution.[69] However, it was not until the 1970s that the technique was perfected for practical applications.

In one developmental system, a device was designed with a single annulus that was not a phased annular array but a segmented configuration that allowed different subelements to transmit and receive (see Fig. 53).[59,70] All elements were capable of transmitting and receiving but the reception could not be dynamically focused. To reduce side lobe effects, two pulses were used, with the transmitting segments shifted one segment over between the pulses. Then the reflected pulses were combined.

Early designs of phased annular arrays had flat faces and focusing only with the receive mode. The transmit mode was typically only a weakly insonifying pulse. To determine the beam pattern characteristics of the annular array, the beam profiles of the transducers are measured during transmission. According to the reciprocity principle, the sensitivity of a transducer acting as a receiver is identical to its beam pattern distribution when transmitting.[71]

A seven-element phased annular array has been designed with the capability of dynamic focusing using separate transmitters and receivers in each element.[72] The lack of dynamic control during the transmit phase of scanning has been circumvented by different researchers by transmitting with the center element only, by conical or line focusing of the entire aperture or by using switched zone focusing (described below).[73] Otherwise, the image is limited to a predetermined depth of focus.[72]

A flat faced 12-element array (one element per annulus) has been developed with an expanding aperture. In this system, four central annuli are always active. The outer eight are inactive for short focal distances and active for longer distances, to effect dynamic focusing.

FIGURE 53. Transmitting and receiving segments for first and second pulses of segmented transducer array.[70]

(a)

(b)

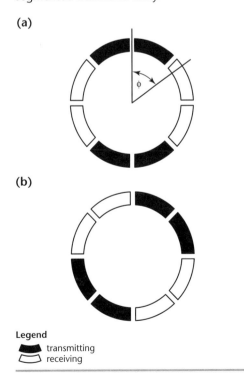

Legend

transmitting
receiving

The f number is a characterization of the focusing ability of a transducer and is the ratio of the focal length to the aperture diameter. The beam width and therefore the lateral resolution in the focal plane have a linear relationship with the f number when the f number is greater than 2.[74] The design allows for larger elements, lower time delays and lower refocusing rates.

A time delay is needed for an annulus of radius r located away from the central element of the array:[74]

$$(16) \quad t = \frac{\sqrt{r^2 + z^2} - z}{c}$$

where c is the acoustic velocity through the material (millimeter per microsecond) and z is the axial distance of the reflection source (millimeter).

The largest time delay is at the minimum focal distance for any active element. The key to dynamic focusing is refocusing the array on receive as the phase shifts occur across the elements of the array. For a frequency f_0 with a phase shift of 0.5 π, the maximum refocusing rate t_S must be designed for:[74]

$$(17) \quad t_S = \frac{f_0 r^2}{z^2}$$

This design assumes that the plane of observation is in the far field and the annular elements are treated as infinitely thin.

It has been shown that superior focusing, lower side lobe levels and simplified electronics can be achieved by using concave annuli.[73,75] To focus a concave annular array with a radius of curvature R_c at a depth of field d_f, the time delay t_j between the jth element of radius a_j and the central element is approximated:[75]

$$(18) \quad t_j \approx a_j^2 \frac{\left(\dfrac{1}{R} - \dfrac{1}{d_f} \right)}{2c}$$

This expression is a good approximation for all depths of field where the outer annulus radius a_N satisfies $[a_N \cdot (d_f)^{-1}]^2 \ll 1$. R_c is chosen to minimize the maximum time delays:[75]

$$(19) \quad \frac{1}{R} = \frac{1}{2}\left(\frac{1}{d_{f1}} - \frac{1}{d_{f2}} \right)$$

where d_{f1} is the shortest focal depth used and d_{f2} is the longest focal depth used.

Switched zone focusing has been proposed as an alternative to the faster dynamic focusing because of the improved lateral resolution, lower side lobe effects and simpler electronics.[73] A separate ultrasonic pulse is transmitted for each zone, so it takes several pulses for each A-scan. A means has been developed for choosing zones according to the depth of field. To determine the depth of field, the axial pressure distribution about the Z axis is based on H.T. O'Neil's theory of focusing radiators:[73,76]

$$(20) \quad p(z) = \frac{\rho v_0 f_0 \pi a^2}{z} \left(\frac{\sin \dfrac{\Delta\phi(z)}{2}}{\dfrac{\Delta\phi(z)}{2}} \right)$$

where a is radius of beam at point z (millimeter), f_0 is the center frequency (hertz), v_0 is the amplitude of the particle velocity at the source, $\Delta\phi(z)$ is the phase shift along the Z axis and ρ is the density of the medium (gram per cubic millimeter).

Figure 54 shows a typical pulse echo distribution about the area of focus.

Depth of field also may be defined as the depth over which the axial response multiplied by z^2 remains over 50 percent of its value at the focus:[73]

$$(21) \quad D_f = 7.1 \lambda \left(N_f \right)^2$$

where D_f is the depth of field (meter) and N_f is the f number.

This definition can be used to define the transition distances between the

FIGURE 54. Typical pulse echo distribution for focused array, showing depth of field.[73]

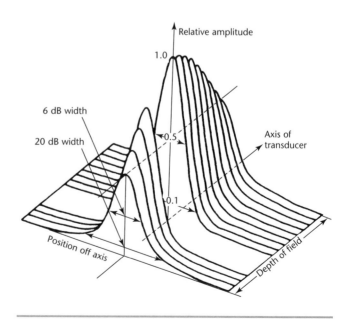

different focal zones. With different focal zones, both the transmit and receive modes can be strongly focused. To choose the number of focal zones N_z for an array, Eq. 22 may be used:[73]

$$(22) \quad N_z = \frac{z_{max} - z_{min}}{D_{f\,av}}$$

where $D_{f\,av}$ is the depth of field with the average f number, and:[73]

$$(23) \quad N_{f\,av} = \frac{z_{min} + z_{max}}{4a}$$

where a is the radius of the beam at the focal point of interest. Despite the success of this design, dynamic focusing remains the primary technique for implementing a phased annular array.

The design of a phased annular array requires several difficult compromises. Elements of equal width proportional to the f number of the system have been used for expanding the aperture system.[74] Each element of the array should have the same area so that they have similar electrical impedance properties and identical phase shifts across each element for any axial position. However, elements of equal area cause lateral modes of vibration leading to pulse degradation.[77]

The frequency is usually chosen according to the attenuation characteristics of the test material.[78] However, a higher frequency is desired because it optimizes the lateral resolution and the depth of field is proportional to the frequency.[73] According to mode coupling theory, the ratio of width to thickness should be at least 2. This provides a sufficient separation between the thickness and lateral modes of vibration of the piezoelectric crystals.[79]

The equivalent source resistance of an array element in receive mode, and therefore its maximum attainable signal-to-noise ratio, is inversely proportional to the square root of the element area. Element area should be maximized but must be weighed against overall transducer size and the number of elements. Studies with concave annular arrays have tried to approximate a focused solid-to-solid aperture. This approximation is affected by the number, the width and the spacing of the annuli and affects how closely an array matches the theory.[74]

The annular array's ultrasonic beam can be shaped but, to achieve uniform wide and narrow beams, many elements are required, increasing the complexity and cost of the electronic control hardware and initiating the need for compromise.[78]

A concave design with the highest frequency possible and the largest aperture was chosen for a handheld transducer design.[77] To choose the number of elements for the array, an acceptable level of beam degradation was sought by diagramming the lateral point response for transducers with different numbers of elements using a simulation program.[75] The number of elements has little effect on the –6 dB resolution of the transducer but significant influence on the side lobe levels.

The gaps between elements should be minimized to achieve maximum sensitivity and to lower the sensitivity of side lobes. To determine the width of each annulus, it is necessary to test the phase shift. The phase shift across a focused aperture, with respect to a given focal point, is determined from the difference between the longest and shortest distances from the aperture to that point. The phase shift for each focal zone must not exceed a certain value, say 0.5 π. The phase shift affects the maximum width of an element with respect to any point in the focal zone. The maximum phase shift occurs at the minimum focal distance:[74]

$$(24) \quad w \approx \frac{\lambda z_{min}}{4r}$$

This is the common geometry for a flat annular array. The phase shift across a concave array is related to the difference between these two distances from the aperture to the point of interest. For a depth of field d_f, the phase shift is given:[75]

$$(25) \quad w = \frac{\pi a^2}{\lambda} \left(\frac{1}{d_f} - \frac{1}{R} \right)$$

Annular Array Applications

Applications for annular arrays include medical imaging, pulsed doppler volume flow meters and tests of turbine disks.[80,81] An annular array was chosen to reduce the number of individual transducers needed to test the turbine disk. The array is segmented into quarters with randomly spaced but equal area elements (Fig. 55). Each segment has its own channel and the elements are randomly spaced to reduce the effects of grating lobes.

Another annular array has been designed for nondestructive testing with the capability of three-dimensional steering by heavily segmenting the rings.[82] The divided ring array has 48 segments on two rings (Fig. 56). It can be steered in the range of ±0.8 rad (±45 deg) by longitudinal wave excitation and ±0.5 to ±1.2 rad (±30 to ±70 deg) by transverse wave excitation. The system performs better than a phased linear array for discontinuity reconstruction.

Applications of Phased Array Systems

Applications of phased array systems for inspection and health monitoring take advantage of improvements in transducer design and signal processing capabilities.[83] Examples include monitoring for cracks in industrial plant facilities at high temperatures[84,85] and the development of piezoelectric wafer active sensors which can be embedded into thin walled structures and scan the structure for cracks using lamb waves.[86,87]

Commercial phased array systems have user friendly software that performs all calculations. For example, the operator can program a 0.8 rad (45 deg) transverse

wave focused at 50 mm (2 in.), and the instrument will calculate the time delays and focus.

Pressure Vessel Inspections

The ultrasonic test patterns can be complex, as can the geometry.[88] For example, pressure vessels normally require tests in compliance with the *ASME Boiler Code,* having two separate transverse wave angles.[89] Good practice would also include time-of-flight diffraction, all of which can be performed in a single linear scan with phased arrays. Figure 57 shows a typical pressure vessel test using a delivery system that follows a magnetic strip.

Results are often displayed as merged data displays, with multiple views such as top, side and end views plus time-of-flight diffraction (Fig. 58). The software often has special features for data analysis, including linked the cursors,

FIGURE 55. Diagram of segmented annular array with random spacing and 1.5 rad (90 deg) segmentation.[80]

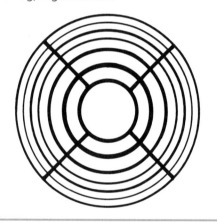

FIGURE 56. Optimized arrangement of divided ring array.[82]

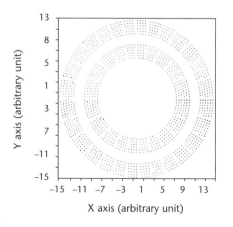

FIGURE 57. Magnetic wheel tracker performing contact phased array weld test.

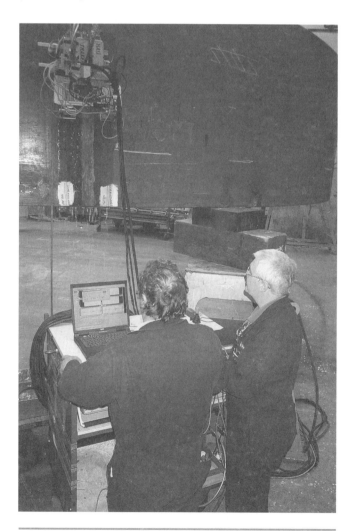

three-dimensional cursors, overlays and full data storage.

Tailored Weld Inspections

Phased arrays are well suited for tests customized for a specific component or weld profile and for the expected discontinuities. A standard for customized weld tests is for automated ultrasonic testing of pipelines, which uses the zone discrimination technique.[89,90] Here, the weld is divided into zones, and each zone is inspected using a well focused, correctly angled beam. This type of test is easily performed using phased arrays and the setups can be automated.

Welding bands are used for delivery systems. Scanning speed is high, 100 mm·s^{-1} (240 in.·min^{-1}), so a 0.9 m (36 in.) pipe is scanned in under 60 s. Depending on the configuration, up to 20 MB of data are collected each minute and are saved to two separate storage locations. The data are displayed in real time so the operator can make rapid accept/reject decisions.

As with pressure vessels, the coupling is pumped water (or methanol water mix in cold countries). Wedges are mounted with wear pins, and coupling checks are performed. This approach has been used for millions of welds.

Pipe Mills

Pipe mills are extensive users of contact ultrasonic testing, usually continuously with many different pipe diameters and wall thicknesses. Phased arrays have significant setup advantages over conventional systems, allowing fast configuration of several oblique discontinuity detection setups by simply downloading focal laws.[91] No mechanical adjustments are needed, and better coverage is obtained. Figure 59 shows a photograph of a full-body inspection system, which uses contact phased arrays to inspect for longitudinal, transversal and up to six different oblique discontinuities, measuring ±0.21, ±0.38, ±0.79, ±1.17 and ±1.36 rad (±12, ±22, ±45, ±67 and ±78 deg). Different water wedges hold each array group; each water wedge is usually optimized for detection of one or two discontinuity types.

FIGURE 59. Phased array technique for full-body test of rotating pipe.

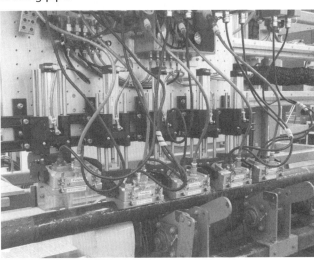

FIGURE 58. Phased array test of weld: (a) top view and side view; (b) end view and waveform.

(a)

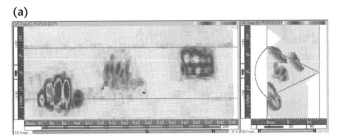

(b)

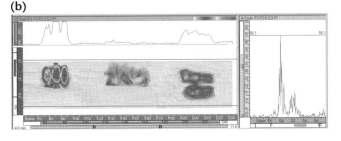

PART 7. Moving Transducers[11]

Ultrasonic Tomography

Computed tomographic imaging is the reconstruction by computer of a tomographic plane or slice of a test object. Such imaging is achieved using several different types of energy, including ultrasound, electrons, alpha particles, lasers and radar. By definition, a tomograph of an object is a two-dimensional visualization of a very thin cross section through the object. The Greek word τομοσ, *tomos,* means "slice." A cross section of an object can be at any location and orientation. In ultrasonic transmission tomography, the image of the cross section is a two-dimensional reconstruction of many one-dimensional A-scans taken from many directions.

This cross sectional technique eliminates the superposition of features that occurs when a three-dimensional object is displayed in a two-dimensional imaging format. The superposition, sometimes called *structural noise,* makes discontinuity detection and characterization more difficult because reflective objects from outside the plane of interest are included. Tomographic imaging is much more highly detailed. In addition, computers that reconstruct the image also provide access to image enhancement algorithms.

Tomography can be divided into two types with different applications: reflective and transmission tomography. Reflective ultrasonic tomography is used to locate and size discontinuities, erosion and corrosion of metals and can be used to characterize voids and inclusions. Transmission ultrasonic tomography can be used for determining differentiations in material density, composition or residual stress. Both sides of the test object must be accessible and the lateral resolution is limited by the lateral resolution of the transmitting and receiving transducers.

Reflection Tomography

Ultrasonic reflection tomography is an outgrowth of the transmission technique and is designed for providing quantitative images displaying a specific acoustic parameter of the test material. The size and location of the detected discontinuity or material interface can be closely estimated by the amplitude and time of flight of the reflected signal. The gross shape of the discontinuity or material interface can be estimated by successive scans around the boundary of the discontinuity.

However, because most ultrasonic energy is scattered in the forward direction, the receiving transducer must have high sensitivity and electronics are required to measure backscattered signals at high signal-to-noise ratios. A technique based on time of flight has been developed for the reconstruction of the image from backscattered ultrasound when a fan beam is used.

Ultrasonic tomography requires more computer hardware and software than conventional ultrasonic techniques. The hardware has three basic components: (1) data acquisition, (2) data storage and processing and (3) image display of the processed data. A data acquisition system consists of the transducer (single or phased array) in an immersion tank and can be either normal to the material surface or at an oblique angle.

During scanning the transducer is moved across the plane of the test object. This movement can be with about 0.15 rad (several degrees) of freedom to follow the contour of irregularly shaped components. The storage and processing system stores the raw scanned data and then performs calculations on the data to produce the cross sectional image. The image may be a two-dimensional plot constructed by comparing many adjacent cross sections. Software is required to perform this processing. Because of the number of scans required, a tomographic image takes longer to construct than a conventional ultrasonic image.

Synthetic Aperture Focusing

Ultrasonic synthetic aperture focusing is a computer enhanced imaging technique for the detection and characterization of discontinuities. It takes advantage of the nonlinear phase shift of a reflection as a discontinuity is linearly scanned. Improved lateral resolution and a higher signal-to-noise ratio are achieved by using this phase shift, mathematically simulating the focusing of an ultrasonic lens that is focused on every point in a test object.

Synthetic aperture focusing requires a computer. Processing many signals for a single final image has a great advantage: the system assists in signal interpretation and displays a visually understandable image. The synthetic aperture focusing technique can produce unambiguous images of discontinuities, especially those with irregular refractive surfaces, and can eliminate the blurring caused by complex angular scattering at discontinuities. These effects are averaged out by the processing of the technique.

In conventional ultrasonic testing, the resolution depends on the size of the aperture, the area over which data can be collected from a single point and is limited by the physical size of the transducer. Synthetic aperture focusing simulates an aperture larger than those that can be realistically used with a small aperture transducer. The focus of the transducer is assumed to be a point of constant phase at the interface of couplant to material, where all the sound waves pass before diverging in a cone.

The angle of the cone is determined by the diameter of the transducer and the focal length. The width of the cone at a given depth corresponds to the aperture that can be synthesized. The path length and travel time to any reflector located beneath the focal point is calculated from the corresponding ray path. The path length corresponds to the phase shift seen in the signal for the transducer position. The signals from the adjacent positions in the synthesized aperture are shifted by the phase and then added to the signal. The final images are usually three-dimensional maps of the discontinuities and the area surrounding the discontinuities.

Because the synthetic aperture focusing technique is based primarily on the processing of stored data, different algorithms can be applied to the data. A conventional, large aperture transducer has a limited depth of field, a drawback that can be circumvented by simultaneous, multiple-depth focusing algorithms. Multiple-depth focusing lets the scanning be much more flexible because the final image shows discontinuities at various depths for a component with a relatively complex shape.

The raw data are A-scans stored as the broadband transducer is scanned over the surface of the test object. A curve is made of the peak amplitudes caused by the reflection from the discontinuity for each aperture element. The size of this curved path is determined by the width of the ultrasonic beam. The curvature and apex of the curve depend on the depth of the discontinuity, the ultrasonic velocity in

the test material and the coupling medium. This collection of A-scans then must be processed to create a single image.

Processing of Synthetic Aperture Data

The processing of the data begins by choosing A-scans processed as a unit to construct the synthetic aperture (the synthetic aperture can be considered a synthetic transducer, the S transducer). The number of A-scans is determined by the spacing between scans. The beam width at the depth of field, usually composed of an odd number of scans, is used to facilitate the processing described below. The increase in resolution and signal-to-noise ratio in synthetic aperture focusing is degraded if scans are included that do not contain the target discontinuity.

The basic process includes giving each aperture element signal a time shift that is the inverse of the time shifts resulting from the geometry, the ultrasonic velocity in the test material and in the immersion couplant. The signals then are summed point by point along the length of the center aperture element and divided by the number of signals summed.

For synthetic aperture focusing to work, the target discontinuity must be in the near field of the S transducer. To achieve one-wavelength lateral resolution, the transducer must be focused at a depth about equal to its diameter. However, as the target discontinuity is scanned by aperture elements further away from the discontinuity, the ultrasonic beam intensity decreases. When the S transducer is created during processing, this phenomenon effectively apodizes the S transducer aperture, smoothing the near field fluctuations and improving the image.

The data processing can be either analog or digital but the digital has advantages, such as ease of manipulation. More than one sample may be taken at each aperture element and these signals can be averaged. If the electronic amplifiers in the system have zero mean gaussian noise, then this signal averaging increases the signal-to-noise ratio by the square root of the number of sums.

The averaging increases the amplitude accuracy by giving a better estimate of the exact level of the signal relative to the quantization steps in the analog-to-digital converter. One concern to note is the accuracy of the time shift that must be incorporated during processing. Quantization errors in calculating this time shift cause phase errors in the image. The suggested limit on this phase shift is 0.44 rad (26 deg).

The final image can be displayed as a two-dimensional line isometric plot, an isometric projection of contour plots, a two-dimensional gray scale image or a color coded isometric projection.

Linear Synthetic Aperture Focusing

The synthetic aperture focusing technique can be performed in two-dimensions, producing a linear scan. This so-called *linear synthetic aperture focusing technique* produces a discontinuity distribution in a plane perpendicular to the surface (a B-scan) that shows the discontinuity size and position.

Another variation uses linear synthetic aperture focusing and ultrasonic holography. The two-dimensional holography results in a C-scan image of the discontinuities and the linear synthetic aperture focusing results in a B-scan. Combining these two scans gives a top view and a cross sectional view of the discontinuity distribution. This decreases the computation time compared to that required for synthetic aperture focusing.

Errors can be introduced in processing if there are deviations in the test surface. Researchers have worked to compensate for scanning on deviating surfaces by using enhanced processing algorithms. A ray is traced from the focal point of the transducer to the desired range of the target discontinuity.

If the lateral position of the ray is close enough to the desired position, then the ultrasonic path and the time delay to the target discontinuity is calculated. Otherwise, the ray angle is changed and traced again. Some A-scans do not contain the discontinuity because of the sloping of the surface.

Conclusion

There are many techniques for using more than one ultrasonic transducer. These techniques have generally arisen in response to specific testing problems that could not be solved with the use of one transducer. This process has led to the development of through-transmission, various pitch catch and other techniques whose applications are controlled by the geometry and acoustic characteristics of the test material.

Another area that has influenced the application of sophisticated ultrasonic tests is medical imaging. Through extensive medical research, techniques requiring large investments in electronics and other equipment have been successfully developed (various array configurations and tomography are examples). This development allows use of such techniques and their adaptations for ultrasonic testing of materials.

A third factor that has influenced the development of ultrasonic testing is the proliferation of high speed computers. Their availability has enabled the practical use of calculation intensive procedures such as synthetic aperture focusing and ultrasonic tomography.

References

1. Chang, F.H. and G.A. Andrew. Section 7, "Ultrasonic Pulse Echo Contact Techniques." *Nondestructive Testing Handbook,* second edition: Vol. 7, *Ultrasonic Testing.* Columbus, OH: American Society for Nondestructive Testing (1991): p 187-217.
2. Bar-Cohen, Y., A.S. Birks and F.H. Chang. Section 11, "Ultrasonic Pulse Echo Techniques." *Nondestructive Testing Handbook,* second edition: Vol. 10, *Nondestructive Testing Overview.* Columbus, OH: American Society for Nondestructive Testing (1996): p 379-424.
3. Hagemaier, D.J. Section 13, "Ultrasonic Reference Standards and Control of Tests." *Nondestructive Testing Handbook,* second edition: Vol. 7, *Ultrasonic Testing.* Columbus, OH: American Society for Nondestructive Testing (1991): p 433-482.
4. Rogerson, A. and A. Murgatroyd. "Defect Characterization Using Ultrasonics Techniques." *Research Techniques in Nondestructive Testing.* Vol. 4. New York, NY: Academic Press (1982): p 451-507.
5. Jestrich, H.A. and J. Ewald. "Ultrasonic In-Service Inspection of Shrunk-On Turbine Disks." *Sixth International Conference on NDE in the Nuclear Industry.* Materials Park, OH: ASM International (1983): p 675-679.
6. Peterson, D.K., S.D. Bennet and G.S. Kino. "Real-Time Digital Imaging." *Proceedings of the Ultrasonics Symposium.* Vol. 1. New York, NY: Institute of Electrical and Electronics Engineers (1981).
7. Krautkrämer, J. and H. Krautkrämer. *Ultrasonic Testing of Materials,* fourth edition. Berlin, Federal Republic of Germany: Springer-Verlag (1990): p 204-205.
8. Krautkrämer, J. and H. Krautkrämer. *Pocket-Book on Ultrasonic Testing of Materials.* Stamford, CT: Krautkramer (1963).
9. Houf, J.[W.] "Practical Contact Ultrasonics — Equipment Maintenance." *NDT Technician.* Vol. 4, No. 3. Columbus, OH: American Society for Nondestructive Testing (July 2005): p 4-5.
10. Brunk, J.A. "Chewing Gum and Other Useful Testing Accessories." *NDT Technician.* Vol. 4, No. 3. Columbus, OH: American Society for Nondestructive Testing (July 2005): p 6.
11. Singh, G.P. and J.W. Davies. Section 9, "Multiple Transducer Ultrasonic Techniques." *Nondestructive Testing Handbook,* second edition: Vol. 7, *Ultrasonic Testing.* Columbus, OH: American Society for Nondestructive Testing (1991): p 267-309.
12. Whittle, M.J. "The Reliability of NDT or PWR: The CEGB Case at the UK Public Inquiry." *Sixth International Conference on NDE in the Nuclear Industry.* Materials Park, OH: ASM International (1983): p 9-18.
13. Williams, J.H. and N.R. Lampert. "Ultrasonic Evaluation of Impact-Damaged Graphite Fiber Composite." *Materials Evaluation.* Vol. 38, No. 12. Columbus, OH: American Society for Nondestructive Testing (December 1980): p 68-72.
14. Gruber, J.J., J.M. Smith and R.H. Brockelman. "Ultrasonic Velocity C-Scans for Ceramic and Composite Material Characterization." *Materials Evaluation.* Vol. 46, No. 1. Columbus, OH: American Society for Nondestructive Testing (January 1988): p 90-96.
15. Charlesworth, J.P. and J.A.G. Temple. *Engineering Applications of Ultrasonic Time-of-Flight Diffraction.* Chichester, United Kingdom: Wiley (1989).
16. Rose, J.L. and A. Tverdokhlebov. "Ultrasonic Testing for Metals with Mild Anisotropy." *British Journal of Non-Destructive Testing.* Vol. 31, No. 2. Northampton, United Kingdom: British Institute of Non-Destructive Testing (February 1989): p 71-76.
17. Posakony, G.J. Report TR66-24, *The Delta Technique.* Boulder, CO: Automation Industries (1966).
18. Granville, R.K. and J.L. Taylor. "The Improvement in Signal-to-Noise Ratio during the Ultrasonic Testing of Titanium Alloys." *British Journal of Non-Destructive Testing.* Vol. 28, No. 4. Northampton, United Kingdom: British Institute of Non-Destructive Testing (July 1986): p 228-231.

19. Gruber, G.J. and G.J. Hendrix. "Sizing of Near Surface Fatigue Cracks in Cladded Reactor Pressure Vessels Using Satellite Pulses." *Sixth International Conference on NDE in the Nuclear Industry.* Materials Park, OH: ASM International (1983): p 83-95.

20. Thavisimuthu, M., P. Palanichamy, C.V. Subramanian, D.K. Bhattacharya and B. Raj. "Evaluation of Abrasive Wheels by an Ultrasonic Dry Couplant Technique." *British Journal of Non-Destructive Testing.* Vol. 31, No. 7. Northampton, United Kingdom: British Institute of Non-Destructive Testing (July 1989): p 388-390.

21. Bernard, L. "Time-of-Flight Diffraction Technology for Ultrasonic Inspection of Piping and Pressure Retaining Components." *Materials Evaluation.* Vol. 45, No. 5. Columbus, OH: American Society for Nondestructive Testing (May 1987): p 506-507.

22. Vary, A. and K.J. Bowles. TM-78813, *Ultrasonic Evaluation of the Strength of Unidirectional Graphite-Polyimide Composites.* Cleveland, OH: NASA Lewis Research Center (February 1978).

23. Dos Reis, H.L.M. and D.M. McFarland. "On the Acousto-Ultrasonic Non-Destructive Evaluation of Wire Rope Using the Stress Wave Factor Technique." *British Journal of Non-Destructive Testing.* Vol. 28, No. 3. Northampton, United Kingdom: British Institute of Non-Destructive Testing (May 1986): p 155-156.

24. Dos Reis, H.L.M., L.A. Bergman and J.H. Bucksbee. "Adhesive Bond Strength Quality Assurance Using the Acousto-Ultrasonic Technique." *British Journal of Non-Destructive Testing.* Vol. 28, No. 6. Northampton, United Kingdom: British Institute of Non-Destructive Testing (November 1986): p 357-358.

25. Pilarski, A. and J.L. Rose. "Ultrasonic Oblique Incidence for Improved Sensitivity in Interface Weakness Determination." *NDT International.* Vol. 24, No. 4. Guildford, Surrey, United Kingdom: Butterworth Scientific (August 1988): p 241-246.

26. Wüstenberg, H., A. Erhard and G. Engl. "Improved Ultrasonic Flaw Detection and Analysis Techniques for Inservice Inspection of Pressure Vessels." *Periodic Inspection of Pressurized Components* [London, United Kingdom, May 1979]. London, United Kingdom: Mechanical Engineering Publications, for the Institution of Mechanical Engineers (1979).

27. Matikas, T.E. "Optimization of the Delta Technique and Application to the Evaluation of Electron-Beam Welded Titanium Aircraft Parts." *Nondestructive Testing and Evaluation.* Vol. 18, No. 1. Abingdon, United Kingdom: Taylor and Francis (2002): p 21-35.

28. "Corrosion Gaging with Dual Element Transducers." *NDT Applications.* No. 18. Waltham, MA: Panametrics (September 1988).

29. Gebhardt, W., F. Bonitz and H. Woll. "Defect Reconstruction and Classification by Phased Arrays." *Materials Evaluation.* Vol. 40, No. 1. Columbus, OH: American Society for Nondestructive Testing (January 1982): p 90-95.

30. Houf, J.[W.] and [W.A.] Svekric. "Practical Contact Ultrasonics — Straight Beam Testing." *NDT Technician.* Vol. 3, No. 1. Columbus, OH: American Society for Nondestructive Testing (January 2004): p 4-6.

31. Wüstenberg, H. and E. Mundry. "Limiting Influences in the Reliability of Ultrasonic In-Service Inspection Methods." *Periodic Inspection of Pressurized Component: A Conference* [London, United Kingdom, June 1974]. London, United Kingdom: Mechanical Engineering Publications, for the Institution of Mechanical Engineers (1975).

32. Neumann, E., M. Romer, T. Just, E. Nabel, K. Matthies and E. Mundry. "Development and Improvement of Ultrasonic Testing Techniques for Austenitic Nuclear Components." *International Conference on Nondestructive Evaluation in the Nuclear Industry* [Salt Lake City, UT, February 1978]. Materials Park, OH: ASM International (1978).

33. Curtis, G.J. and B.M. Hawker. "Automated Time-of-Flight Studies of the Defect Detection Trial Plates 1 and 2." *British Journal of Non-Destructive Testing.* Vol. 25, No. 5. Northampton, United Kingdom: British Institute of Non-Destructive Testing (September 1983): p 240-248.

34. Bond, L.J. and M. Punjani. "New Multitransducer Techniques for Crack Characterization." *Review of Progress in Quantitative Nondestructive Evaluation* [Santa Cruz, CA, August 1983]. Vol. 3A. New York, NY: Plenum (1984): p 297-307.

35. Thompson, D.O., S.J. Wormley and D.K. Hsu. "Apparatus and Technique for Reconstruction of Flaws Using Model-Based Elastic Wave Inverse Ultrasonic Scattering." *Review of Scientific Instruments.* Vol. 57, No. 12. Woodbury, NY: American Institute of Physics (December 1986): p 3089-3098.

36. Hsu, D.K., D.O. Thompson and S.J. Wormley. "Reliability of Reconstruction of Arbitarily Oriented Flaws Using Multiview Transducers." *Transaction on Ultrasonics, Ferroelectrics and Frequency Control.* Vol. UFFC-34, No. 5. New York, NY: Institute of Electrical and Electronics Engineers (September 1987): p 508-514.

37. Onozawa, M., A. Katamine, Y. Ishi and G. Ohira. "Ultrasonic Testing for Near Surface Flaws in Castings." *British Journal of Non-Destructive Testing.* Vol. 31, No. 11. Northampton, United Kingdom: British Institute of Non-Destructive Testing (November 1989): p 611-615.

38. Olofsson, T. and T. Stepinski. "Maximum a Posteriori Deconvolution of Ultrasonic Signals Using Multiple Transducers." *Journal of the Acoustical Society of America.* Vol. 107, No. 6. Melville, NY: American Institute of Physics, for the Acoustical Society of America (2000): p 3276-3288.

39. Gebhardt, W., H.P. Schwartz, F. Bonitz and H. Woll. "Application of Phased Arrays in Basic and In-Service Inspection." *Sixth International Conference on NDE in the Nuclear Industry.* Materials Park, OH: ASM International (1983): p 717-723.

40. Carpenter, D.A. "Ultrasonic Transducers." *New Techniques and Instrumentation in Ultrasonography.* New York, NY: Churchill Livingstone Publishing (1980).

41. Leo, F.P. "Real-Time Ultrasound Technology." *Ultrasound Annual.* New York, NY: Raven Press (1983): p 47-65.

42. Taylor, K.J.W. "Real-Time Instrumentation, Automated Imaging, Pulse Doppler Devices." *Manual of Ultrasoundography.* New York, NY: Churchill Livingstone (1980).

43. Whittington, K.R. and B.D. Cox. "Electronic Steering and Focussing of Ultrasonic Beams in Tube Inspection." *Ultrasonics.* Saint Louis, MO: Elsevier (January 1969): p 20-25.

44. Von Ramm, O.T. and S.W. Smith. "Beam Steering with Linear Arrays." *Transactions on Biomedical Engineering.* Vol. BME-30, No. 8. New York, NY: Institute of Electrical and Electronics Engineers (August 1983): p 438-452.

45. Macovski, A. "Ultrasonic Imaging Using Arrays." *Proceedings of the IEEE.* Vol. 67, No. 4. New York, NY: Institute of Electrical and Electronics Engineers (April 1979): p 484-495.

46. Hosseini, S., S.O. Harrold and J.M. Reeves. "Resolution Studies on an Electronically Focused Ultrasonic Array." *British Journal of Non-Destructive Testing.* Vol. 27, No. 4. Northampton, United Kingdom: British Institute of Non-Destructive Testing (July 1985): p 234-238.

47. McNab, A. and I. Stumpf. "Monolithic Phased Array for the Transmission of Ultrasound in NDT Ultrasonics." *Ultrasonics.* Vol. 24. Saint Louis, MO: Elsevier (May 1986): p 148-155.

48. Campbell, M.A. and A. McNab. "A Novel Instrument for the Control of the Phased Array for NDE." *Proceedings on the Ultrasonics Symposium.* New York, NY: Institute of Electrical and Electronics Engineers (1985): p 994-997.

49. McNab, A. and M.A. Campbell. "Ultrasonic Phased Arrays for Nondestructive Testing." *NDT International.* Vol. 20, No. 5. Guildford, Surrey, United Kingdom: Butterworth Scientific (December 1987): p 333-337.

50. Steinberg, B.D. *Principles of Aperture and Array System Design.* New York, NY: Wiley (1976).

51. Sato, J., M. Kawabuchi and A. Fukumoto. "Dependence of the Electrochemical Coupling Coefficient on the Width to Thickness Ratio of Plank Shaped Piezoelectric Transducers Used for Electronically Scanned Ultrasound Diagnostic System." *Journal of the Acoustical Society of America.* Vol. 66, No. 6. Melville, NY: American Institute of Physics, for the Acoustical Society of America (1979): p 1609-1611.

52. Kino, G.S. and C.S. Desilets. "Design of Slotted Transducer Arrays with Matched Backings." *Ultrasonic Imaging.* New York, NY: Academic Press (1979): p 189-209.

53. Wooh, S. and Y. Shi. "Influence of Phased Array Size on Beam Steering Behavior." *Ultrasonics.* Vol. 36. *Ultrasonics.* Saint Louis, MO: Elsevier (1998): p 737-749.

54. Deutsch, W.A.K., A. Cheng and J.D. Achenbach. "Self Focusing of Raleigh Waves and Lamb Waves with a Linear Phased Array." *Research in Nondestructive Evaluation.* Vol. 9, No. 2. Columbus, OH: American Society for Nondestructive Testing (1997): p 81-95.

55. Azar, L., Y. Shi, and S.-C. Wooh. "Beam Focusing Behavior of Linear Phased Arrays." *NDT&E International.* Vol. 33. Kidlington, United Kingdom: Elsevier (2000): p 189-198.

56. Walker, J.T. and J.D. Meindl. "A Digitally Controlled CCD Dynamically Focussed Phased Array." *Proceedings of the Ultrasonics Symposium.* New York, NY: Institute of Electrical and Electronics Engineers (1975): p 80-83.

57. Hosseini, S., S.O. Harrold and J.M. Reeves. "Computer Controlled Focused Ultrasonic Transmitting Array." *Transactions on Sonics and Ultrasonics.* Vol. SU-31, No. 4. New York, NY: Institute of Electrical and Electronics Engineers (July 1984): p 432-435.

58. Song, T.K. and S.B. Park. "A New Digital Phased Array System for Dynamic Focusing and Steering with Reduced Sampling Rate." *Ultrasonic Imaging.* Vol. 12. New York, NY: Academic Press (1990): p 1-16.

59. Beaver, W.L. "A Method of Three-Dimensional Electronic Focusing and Beam Steering Using Electronic Delay Lines." *Proceedings of the Ultrasonics Symposium.* New York, NY: Institute of Electrical and Electronics Engineers (1975): p 88-90.

60. Baer, R.L., A.R. Selfridge, B.T. Khuri-Yakub, G.S. Kino and J. Souquot. "Contacting Transducers and Transducer Arrays for NDE." *Proceedings of the Ultrasonics Symposium.* New York, NY: Institute of Electrical and Electronics Engineers (1981): p 969-973.

61. Beck, K.H. "Ultrasonic Transducer Array Configuration for Interlaced Scanning." *Materials Evaluation.* Vol. 46, No. 6. Columbus, OH: American Society for Nondestructive Testing (May 1988): p 771-778.

62. Hassler, Honig and D. Schwarz. "Ultrasound B-Scanner with Multi-Line Array." *Ultrasonic Imaging.* Vol. 4. New York, NY: Academic Press (1982): p 32-43.

63. Nikolov, S. and J.A. Jensen. "Application of Different Spatial Sampling Patterns for Sparse Array Transducer Design." *Ultrasonics International* [Copenhagen, Denmark, 1999]. *Ultrasonics.* Vol. 37. Saint Louis, MO: Elsevier (February 2000): p 667-671.

64. Mahaut, S., O. Roy, C. Beroni and B. Rotter. "Development of Phased Array Techniques to Improve Characterization of Defect Located in a Component of Complex Geometry." *Ultrasonics.* Vol. 40. Saint Louis, MO: Elsevier (2002): p 165-169.

65. Mahaut, S., C. Gondard, M. El Amrani, P. Benoist and G. Cattiaux. "Ultrasonic Defect Characterization with a Dynamic Adaptive Focusing System." *Ultrasonics.* Vol. 34. Saint Louis, MO: Elsevier (1996): p 121-124.

66. Mahaut, S., S. Chatillon, E. Kerbrat, J. Porre, P. Calmon and O. Roy. "New Features for Phased Array Techniques Inspections: Simulation and Experiments." *16th WCNDT 2004 — World Conference on NDT: CD-ROM Proceedings* [Montréal, Canada, August-September 2004]. Hamilton, Ontario, Canada: Canadian Institute for NDE (2004).

67. Jain, A., D.W. Greve and I.J. Oppenheim. "A MEMS Ultrasonic Transducer for Monitoring of Steel Structures." *Smart Structures and Materials* [San Diego, CA, March 2002]. SPIE Conference Proceedings, Vol. 4696. Bellingham, WA: International Society for Optical Engineering (2002): p 31-37.

68. Jain, A., D.W. Greve and I.J. Oppenheim. "A MEMS Transducer for Ultrasonic Flaw Detection." *18th International Symposium on Automation and Robotics in Construction* [Washington, DC, September 2002]. Göteborg, Sweden: International Association for Automation and Robotics in Construction (2002).

69. Reid, J.M. and J.J. Wild. "Current Developments in Ultrasound Equipment for Medical Diagnosis." *Proceedings of the National Electronics Council.* Vol. 12. London, United Kingdom: Institution of Engineering and Technology (1956): p 44-58.

70. Burckhardt, C.B., P.A. Grandchamp and H. Hoffmann. "Focusing Ultrasound over a Large Depth with an Annular Transducer — An Alternative Method." *Transactions on Sonics and Ultrasonics.* Vol. SU-22, No. 1. New York, NY: Institute of Electrical and Electronics Engineers (January 1975): p 11-15.

71. Wells, P.N.T. *Physical Principles of Ultrasonic Diagnosis.* London, United Kingdom: Academic Press (1969).

72. Bernardi, R.B., P.J. Peluso, R.J. O'Connell, S. Kellogg and C. Shih. "A Dynamically Focused Annular Array." *Proceedings of the Ultrasonics Symposium.* New York, NY: Institute of Electrical and Electronics Engineers (1976): p 157-159.

73. Arditi, M., W.B. Taylor, F.S. Foster and J.W. Hunt. "An Annular Array System for High Resolution Breast Echography." *Ultrasonic Imaging.* No. 4. New York, NY: Academic Press (1982): p 1-31.

74. Dietz, D.R., S.I. Parks and M. Linzer. "Expanding-Aperture Annular Array." *Ultrasonic Imaging*. Vol. 1, No. 1. New York, NY: Academic Press (1979): p 56-73.
75. Arditi, M., F.S. Foster and J.W. Hunt. "Transient Fields of Concave Annular Arrays." *Ultrasonic Imaging*. No. 3. New York, NY: Academic Press (1981): p 37-61.
76. O'Neil, H.T. "Theory of Focusing Radiators." *Journal of the Acoustical Society of America*. Vol. 21, No. 5. Melville, NY: American Institute of Physics, for the Acoustical Society of America (1949): p 516-526.
77. Foster, F.S., J.D. Larson, M.K. Mason, T.S. Shoup, G. Nelson and H. Yoshida. "Development of a 12 Element Annual Array Transducer for Realtime Ultrasound Imaging." *Ultrasound in Medicine and Biology*. Vol. 15, No. 7. New York, NY: Pergamon (1989): p 649-659.
78. Melton, H.E., Jr. *Electronic Focal Scanning for Improved Resolution in Ultrasound Imaging*. Dissertation. Durham, NC: Duke University (1972).
79. Evans, J.M., R. Skidmore, N.P. Luckman and P.N.T. Wells. "A New Approach to the Noninvasive Measurement of Cardiac Output Using an Annular Array Doppler Technique: Part 1, Theoretical Considerations and Ultrasonic Field." *Ultrasound in Medicine and Biology*. Vol. 15, No. 3. New York, NY: Pergamon Press (1989): p 169-178.
80. Light, G.L., T.A. Mueller, T.L. Allen and E.A. Bloom. "Initial Evaluation of Annual Array Technology for Use in Turbine Disc Inspection." *Nondestructive Evaluation Program Progress*. NP-3347-SR.77. Palo Alto, CA: Electric Power Research Institute (March 1984).
81. Singh, G.P., G.A. Lamping, G.M. Light, M.J. Kolar and S.N. Lui. "Nondestructive Examination of Low-Pressure Steam Turbine Rotors." *Sixth International Conference on NDE in the Nuclear Industry*. Materials Park, OH: ASM International (1983): p 739-749.
82. Schwarz, H.P. "Development of a Divided-Ring Array for Three-Dimensional Beam Steering in Ultrasonic Nondestructive Testing: Theoretical and Experimental Results of a Prototype." *Materials Evaluation*. Vol. 45, No. 8. Columbus, OH: American Society for Nondestructive Testing (August 1987): p 951-957.
83. Granillo, J. and M.[D.C.] Moles. "Portable Phased Array Applications." Materials Evaluation. Vol. 63, No. 4. Columbus, OH: American Society for Nondestructive Testing (April 2005): p 394-404.
84. Kirk, K.J., A. McNab, A. Cochran, I. Hall and G. Hayward. "Ultrasonic Arrays for Monitoring Cracks in an Industrial Plant at High Temperatures." *IEEE Transactions on Ultrasonics, Ferroelectrics and Frequency Control*. Vol. 46. New York, NY: Institute of Electrical and Electronics Engineers (1999) p 311-319.
85. McNab, A., K.J. Kirk and A. Cochran. "Ultrasonic Transducers for High Temperature Applications." *IEE Proceedings — Science, Measurement and Technology*. Vol. 145, No. 5. London, United Kingdom: Institution of Engineering and Technology (September 1998): p 229-236.
86. Giurgiutiu, V. and J. Bao. "Embedded-Ultrasonics Structural Radar for Nondestructive Evaluation of Thin Wall Structures." *Proceedings of the 2004 ASME International Mechanical Engineering Congress and Exposition* [New Orleans, LA, November 2000]. New York, NY: ASME International (2004): p 1-8.
87. Giurgiutiu, V. Paper 17, "Lamb Wave Generation with Piezoelectric Wafer Active Sensors for Structural Health Monitoring." SPIE Conference Proceedings, Vol. 5056, *Smart Structures and Integrated Systems* [San Diego, CA, March 2003]. Bellingham, WA: International Society for Optical Engineering (2003).
88. Davis, J.M. and M.[D.C.] Moles. Resolving Capabilities of Phased Array Sectorial Scans (S-Scans) on Diffracted Tip Signals. *Insight*. Vol. 48, No. 4. Northampton, United Kingdom: British Institute of Non-Destructive Testing (April 2006): p 233-239.
89. *Introduction to Phased Array Ultrasonic Technology Applications*. Québec, Canada: R/D Tech (2004).
90. ASTM E 1961, *Standard Practice for Mechanized Ultrasonic Examination of Girth Welds Using Zonal Discrimination with Focused Search Units*. West Conshohocken, PA: ASTM International (2003).
91. Moles M.[D.C.], S. Labbé and J. Zhang. "Improved Focusing for Thick-Wall Pipeline Girth Welds Using Phased Arrays." *Insight*. Vol. 47, No. 12. Northampton, United Kingdom: British Institute of Non-Destructive Testing (December 2005): p 769-776.
92. *ASME Boiler and Pressure Vessel Code*. New York, NY: ASME International.

Bibliography

Contact Techniques

Houf, J.[W.] "Practical Contact Ultrasonics — Angle Beam Calibration Using a Basic Calibration Block." *NDT Technician*. Vol. 3, No. 4. Columbus, OH: American Society for Nondestructive Testing (October 2004): p 4-6, 9.

Houf, J.[W.] "Practical Contact Ultrasonics — Angle Beam Scan Patterns and Defect Location." *NDT Technician*. Vol. 4, No. 1. Columbus, OH: American Society for Nondestructive Testing (January 2005): p 4-6.

Houf, J.[W.] "Practical Contact Ultrasonics — Angle Beam Testing." *NDT Technician*. Vol. 3, No. 2. Columbus, OH: American Society for Nondestructive Testing (April 2004): p 5-6, 8-9.

Houf, J.[W.] "Practical Contact Ultrasonics — Defining Terms and Principles." *NDT Technician*. Vol. 2, No. 4. Columbus, OH: American Society for Nondestructive Testing (October 2003): p 5-7.

Houf, J.[W.] "Practical Contact Ultrasonics — Defect Characterizations and False Indications." *NDT Technician*. Vol. 4, No. 2. Columbus, OH: American Society for Nondestructive Testing (April 2005): p 3-5.

Houf, J.[W.] "Practical Contact Ultrasonics — IIW Based Angle Beam Calibration." *NDT Technician*. Vol. 3, No. 3. Columbus, OH: American Society for Nondestructive Testing (July 2004): p 4-6.

Synthetic Aperture Focusing

Kovalev, A.V., V.N. Kozlov, A.A. Samokrutov, V.G. Shevaldykin and N.N. Yakovlev. "Pulse Echo in Concrete Monitoring: Interference and Spectral Selection." *NDT&E International*. Vol. 30, No. 4. Amsterdam, Netherlands: Elsevier Science (August 1997): p 264.

Krause M., F. Mielentz, B. Milman, W. Muller, V. Schmitz and H. Wiggenhauser. "Ultrasonic Imaging of Concrete Members Using an Array System." *NDT&E International*. Vol. 34, No. 6. Amsterdam, Netherlands: Elsevier Science (September 2001): p 403-408.

Levesque, D., A. Blouin, C. Neron and J.-P. Monchalin. "Performance of Laser-Ultrasonic F-SAFT Imaging." *Ultrasonics*. Vol. 40, No. 10. Saint Louis, MO: Elsevier (December 2002): p 1057-1063.

Marklein, R., K. Mayer, R. Hannemann, T. Krylow, K. Balasubramanian, K.J. Langenberg and V. Schmitz. "Linear and Nonlinear Inversion Algorithms Applied in Nondestructive Evaluation." *Inverse Problems*. Vol. 18, No. 6. London, United Kingdom: Institute of Physics (2002): p 1733-1759.

Martinez, O., M. Parrilla, M.A.G. Izquierdo and L.G. Ullate. "Application of Digital Signal Processing Techniques to Synthetic Aperture Focusing Technique Images." *Sensors and Actuators A: Physical*. Vol. 76, No. 1. Amsterdam, Netherlands: Elsevier Science (August 1999): p 448-456.

Osetrov, A.V. "Non-Linear Algorithms Based on SAFT Ideas for Reconstruction of Flaws." *Ultrasonics*. Vol. 38, No. 1. Saint Louis, MO: Elsevier (March 2000): p 739-744.

Schmitz, V., K.J. Langenberg, W. Kappes and M. Kroning. "Inspection Procedure Assessment Using Modelling Capabilities." *Nuclear Engineering and Design*. Vol. 157, No. 1. Amsterdam, Netherlands: Elsevier Science (July 1995): p 245-255.

Schmitz, V., S. Chakhlov and W. Muller. "Experiences with Synthetic Aperture Focusing Technique in the Field." *Ultrasonics*. Vol. 38, No. 1. Saint Louis, MO: Elsevier (March 2000): p 731-738.

Sicard, R., J. Goyette and D. Zellouf. "A SAFT Algorithm for Lamb Wave Imaging of Isotropic Plate-Like Structures." *Ultrasonics*. Vol. 39, No. 7. Saint Louis, MO: Elsevier (April 2002): p 487-494.

Spies, M. and W. Jager. "Synthetic Aperture Focusing for Defect Reconstruction in Anisotropic Media." *Ultrasonics*. Vol. 41, No. 2. Saint Louis, MO: Elsevier (March 2003): p 125-131.

Tao, L., X.R. Ma, H. Tian and Z.X. Guo. "Phase Superposition Processing for Ultrasonic Imaging." *Journal of Sound and Vibration*. Vol. 193, No. 5. Amsterdam, Netherlands: Elsevier Science (June 1996): p 1015-1021.

Ylitalo, J. "A Fast Ultrasonic Synthetic Aperture Imaging Method: Application to NDT." *Ultrasonics*. Vol. 34, No. 2. Saint Louis, MO: Elsevier (June 1996): p 331-333.

Ylitalo, J. "On the Signal-to-Noise Ratio of a Synthetic Aperture Ultrasound Imaging Method." *European Journal of Ultrasound*. Vol. 3, No. 3. Amsterdam, Netherlands: Elsevier Science (July 1996): p 277-281.

Ultrasonic Tomography

Brown, G.J. and D. Reilly. "Ultrasonic Tomographic Imaging of Solid Objects in Air Using an Array of Fan-Shaped-Beam Electrostatic Transducers." *Ultrasonics.* Vol. 34, No. 2. Saint Louis, MO: Elsevier (June 1996): p 111-115.

Chow, T.M., D.A. Hutchins and J.T. Mottram. "Simultaneous Acoustic Emission and Ultrasonic Tomographic Imaging in Anisotropic Polymer Composite Material." *NDT&E International.* Vol. 30, No. 2. Amsterdam, Netherlands: Elsevier Science (April 1997): p 112-112.

Hoyle B.S., X. Jia, F.J.W. Podd, H.I. Schlaberg, H.S. Tan, M. Wang, R.M. West, R.A. Williams and T.A. York. "Design and Application of a Multi-Modal Process Tomography System." *Measurement Science and Technology.* Vol. 12, No. 8. London, United Kingdom: Institute of Physics (September 2001): p 1157-1165.

Koshovyy, V., E. Kryvin, A. Muraviov and I. Romanyshyn. "Special Features of the Ultrasonic Tomography of Thick-Sheet Products." *Russian Journal of Nondestructive Testing.* Vol. 40, No. 7. Wilmington, DE: Pleiades Publishing, for MAIK Nauka Interperiodica, Moscow, Russia (July 2004): p 431-441.

Mahaut, S., C. Gondard, M. El Amrani, P. Benoist and G. Cattiaux. "Ultrasonic Defect Characterization with a Dynamic Adaptive Focusing System." *Ultrasonics.* Vol., No. 2. Saint Louis, MO: Elsevier (June 1996): p 121-124.

Martin, J., K.J. Broughton, A. Giannopolous, M.S.A. Hardy and M.C. Forde. "Ultrasonic Tomography of Grouted Duct Post-Tensioned Reinforced Concrete Bridge Beams." *NDT&E International.* Vol. 34, No. 2. Amsterdam, Netherlands: Elsevier Science March 2001): p 107-113.

Rathore, S.K., P. Munshi and N.N. Kishore. "A New Tomographic Reconstruction Method for Anisotropic Materials." *Nondestructive Testing and Evaluation.* Vol. 18, Nos. 3-4. Philadelphia, PA: Taylor and Francis (July 2003): p 171-182.

Schlaberg, H.I., M. Yang and B.S. Hoyle. "Ultrasound Reflection Tomography for Industrial Processes." *Ultrasonics.* Vol. 36, No. 1. Saint Louis, MO: Elsevier (February 1998): p 297-303.

Schlaberg, H.I., M. Yang, B.S. Hoyle, M.S. Beck and C. Lenn. "Wide-Angle Transducers for Real-Time Ultrasonic Process Tomography Imaging Applications." *Ultrasonics.* Vol. 35, No. 3. Saint Louis, MO: Elsevier (May 1997): p 213-221.

Socco, L., L. Sambuelli, R. Martinis, E. Comino and G. Nicolotti. "Feasibility of Ultrasonic Tomography for Nondestructive Testing of Decay on Living Trees." *Research in Nondestructive Evaluation.* Vol. 15, No. 1. Columbus, OH: American Society for Nondestructive Testing (January-March 2004): p 31-54.

Ultrasonic Scanning

Yoseph Bar-Cohen, Jet Propulsion Laboratory, Pasadena, California (Parts 1 to 9)

Byron B. Brenden, Battelle Pacific Northwest Laboratories, Richland, Washington (Part 10)

Govinder P. Singh, Karta Technology, Incorporated, San Antonio, Texas (Part 2)

PART 1. Ultrasonic Coupling[1]

An ultrasonic wave, propagating from a transducer to a test object, crosses several interfaces with different acoustic impedances (the product of density and acoustic velocity) before being detected by the receiving transducer. If the receiving transducer is the same as the source, the configuration is called pulse echo, whereas if the receiving transducer is a different transducer, then the configuration is known as *through transmission*. In either case, the mismatch of the acoustic impedances causes an energy loss from reflections, which can be very high if air is present in the wave path.

To improve the energy transfer from the transducer to the test object, two coupling techniques are used: contact and immersion. The difference between these two techniques is related primarily to the length, or depth, of the couplant medium between the transducer and the test object.

Contact Coupling

With contact coupling, the transducer is pressed onto the test object surface to reduce the couplant thickness to a minimum. This thickness needs to be such that its resonance frequency is much higher than the transducer spectral response range.

$$(1) \quad d \ll \frac{V}{2f_{max}}$$

where d is the couplant thickness (millimeter), f_{max} is the transducer's maximum frequency measured at 6 dB below peak frequency (hertz) and V is the couplant's acoustic velocity (millimeters per second). The thickness d should be less than 0.25 λ (an antiresonance) or $d \leq V \cdot (4f)^{-1}$.

Immersion Coupling

Immersion coupling uses a long fluid delay line. The distance between the transducer and the test object is long enough to separate in the time domain the reflections from the test object front surface and the transducer's excitation signal. In addition, a separation is maintained between the test object's internal reflections and the repetitive reflections in the water path. This adjustment is necessary to avoid interference between the various reflections and to simplify the evaluation of the response.

Couplant path length is related to test object thickness for immersion coupling:

$$(2) \quad d_c > \frac{V_c}{V_{tm}} N d_{tm}$$

where d_c is couplant path length (millimeter), d_{tm} is test material thickness (millimeter), N is desirable number of repetitive reflections in the test material, V_c is acoustic velocity of the couplant (meter per second) and V_{tm} is acoustic velocity of the test material (meter per second).

Limitations of Immersion Coupling

As a rule in immersion coupling, the velocities ratio (couplant to test media) is about 1:6 for ceramics, 1:4 for metals and 1:2 for composites and plastics. A constraint over the path length of the coupling medium as expressed in Eq. 2 limits the practical usage of the immersion method to relatively thin sections. Because most aerospace structures meet this requirement, the immersion technique is very popular for testing aircraft components.

There are other limitations of the immersion technique.

1. Because of weight, immersion systems lack portability and are impractical in the field.
2. The hardware is complex and relatively expensive.
3. The technique is not recommended for test objects susceptible to corrosion.
4. Tests can be performed only on objects with a thickness below the limit of Eq. 2.

Advantages of Immersion Coupling

Immersion testing has significant flexibility. It is possible, for instance, to use immersion techniques in most contact coupling applications. The immersion technique also provides significant coupling uniformity and the simplicity of changing the insonification angle without changing the transducer. In addition, the transducer is not exposed to wear during use and immersion techniques are ideal for automated testing. The immersion technique provides good acoustic impedance matching to composite materials.

Water is the most common fluid used for immersion coupling, because of its availability and low cost. To inhibit chemical or biological aqueous reactions, various inhibitors can be added to water.

To prevent air bubbles from forming and accumulating on the surface of test objects, detergent additives are commonly mixed with the water. Such additives reduce the surface tension between the water and test object, making air bubbles less likely.

When the tank is filled or the water is moved (in scanning or filtering, for example), air tends to dissolve in the water and increase the attenuation. This attenuation increase can be as high as 6 dB and can be avoided by keeping water movement slow or by allowing the air to be outgassed before testing. The outgassing process can last from 15 to 60 min after filling the water tank. Generally, water is filtered before and during use to ensure that it does not contain particles that create false test indications.

Immersion scanning has seven primary advantages.

1. No special transducer adapters or shoes are required when changing the size or shape of the test object.
2. Simple continuous adjustment of the incidence angle of the sound beam is permitted. This capability is essential for contour following of complex shaped structures or when developing a test procedure.
3. The coupling liquid is continuously available.
4. Because intimate contact is not required, testing speed is significantly faster.
5. The immersion technique is not influenced so greatly as the contact technique by loss of coupling due to ovality of tubing, surface conditions or dimensional variations.
6. Total immersion in a water bath helps suppress surface waves that inordinately increase signals from minor outside surface discontinuities.
7. The water column provides a delay line that allows the very strong initial signal to pass through the amplifier before the weaker signals return to the instrument. This is particularly advantageous when testing small tube sizes and thin plates.

PART 2. Ultrasonic Test Techniques[1,2]

Ultrasonic test systems can be used with three forms of ultrasonic scanning: A-scan, B-scan and C-scan (Fig. 1). Each kind of scan provides a different set of information. Computer based test systems can display the results of all three scanning techniques.

A-Scan Technique

The ultrasonic A-scan presents one-dimensional data showing the response along the beam path at a specific location of the test object. Such scans can produce detailed information about discontinuities in the scanned material.

The depth of discontinuities is indicated by the time of flight as measured from the time base of the cathode ray tube. The size of

FIGURE 1. Comparison of scanning techniques: (a) lamination in plate; (b) A-scan of discontinuity; (c) B-scan of discontinuity; (d) plan view of C-scan (entire surface of plate must be scanned to produce plan view).

(a)

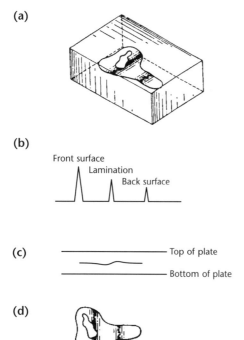

(b)

Front surface
Lamination
Back surface

(c)

Top of plate
Bottom of plate

(d)

discontinuities can be estimated from the amplitude of the reflected signal. The type of discontinuity can be determined by analysis of the amplitude and phase information. The A-scan technique is the most widely used and can be displayed on most standard ultrasonic instruments.

B-Scan Technique

With the ultrasonic B-scan, the test object is scanned along one axis to produce a presentation of its cross section. The location along the scanning path is shown on the X axis and time of flight values are shown along the Y axis. Because a cross section is produced, the B-scan is less practical for large volumes of material.

The B-scan is popular for medical diagnosis where cross sections are useful. In medical applications, the angular manipulation of the transducer is monitored to prevent image distortion and the display is adjusted to account for changes in the beam angle along the cross section of the examined area.

C-Scan Technique

The ultrasonic C-scan is applied to the test object in a raster pattern and presents a view of the discontinuity's area as seen from above. Discontinuity location and size data are available from changes in amplitude as a function of position.

Modern C-scan systems use computers to control the transducer position and to acquire, display, document and store the test results. The computer synchronously acquires the digitized position of the transducer and the associated value of a specific ultrasonic parameter. The position can be obtained by various means, including optical encoders or sonic digitizers.

In most cases, the parameters obtained include position, time of flight or the amplitude of reflection or transmission at a certain time range. These parameters are digitized with the aid of an analog-to-digital converter and stored in the memory of the computer for further processing.

C-scan systems can typically scan at speeds up to 500 mm·s⁻¹ (20 in.·s⁻¹) or higher. Speeds must be kept at a level that does not induce water turbulence, which introduces noise and degrades the reliability of the test.

Multiple transducers can be used in C-scan tests for through-transmission tests or phased array configurations. As an alternative to mechanical scanning, these phased array transducers perform synchronously and their scanning location is indicated by the cursor position on the computer display.

Ultrasonic C-scan systems are large in size and most are limited to on-site testing conditions. With the increasing availability of inexpensive computing capability, scanners for field applications have also been designed.

Through-Transmission Tests

The through-transmission technique uses two ultrasonic transducers located on opposite sides of a test object. One transducer acts as an ultrasound transmitter and the other transducer is passively receives the ultrasound. The transducers can be in contact with the material, or the test object can be immersed in liquid couplant. If this is not possible, water column transducers or squirters can be used to transmit the sound to the material surface (Fig. 2).[3]

Transducer Alignment

Because of the directivity pattern of the transducers, the two transducers must be exactly oriented so that the receiving transducer receives the maximum amount of sound energy. Otherwise, an incorrect measurement of velocity or signal amplitude is taken. The impedance and frequency characteristics of the two transducers must be exactly the same — the transducers must be calibrated to minimize signal modulation problems caused by instrumentation or the test setup. The angle of the ultrasonic beam can be normal to the test object surface (Fig. 3)[4] or at an oblique angle (Fig. 4)[5] but the receiver must be precisely aligned with the transmitter. Table 1 is a list of constraints for a normal incidence transducer and a typical test object, along with the ambiguities eliminated when these constraints are followed.

The through-transmission technique can be used for discontinuity detection,

FIGURE 3. Diagram for sending and receiving signals in through-transmission configuration.[3]

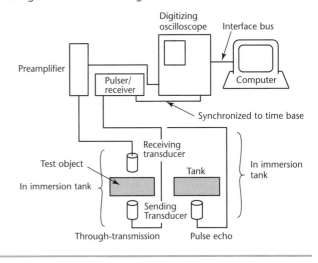

FIGURE 2. Through-transmission transducer configuration: (a) in immersion tank; (b) using water columns.[2]

(a)

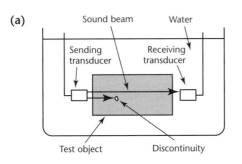

(b)

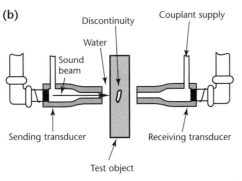

FIGURE 4. Through-transmission configuration with transducers at oblique angle.[4]

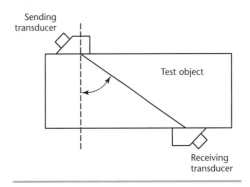

for material characterization and for thickness measurement, except in materials that are thick and highly attenuative. The usual test setup is to align the two transducers and move them simultaneously over the component. When a discontinuity or a change in a material's composition is encountered, the signal amplitude changes because the ultrasonic beam is reflected, scattered or obscured by the discontinuity.

However, the through-transmission technique cannot distinguish between voids and delaminations because the attenuation characteristics of the two discontinuities are identical. Also, a discontinuity's location in the thickness of the material cannot be determined using through-transmission tests.[6] If the thickness is known, the ultrasonic signal's time of arrival can be used to calculate the velocity, and its velocity can then be used to characterize the material's acoustic impedance. Changes in the acoustic impedance represent changes in the composition of the test material. Through-transmission can be used for thickness measurements by recording the time of flight for the ultrasonic beam in a material whose acoustic impedance is known.

TABLE 1. Ultrasonic wave attenuation in water as function of temperature.

Temperature		Attenuation	
°C	(°F)	10^{-15} Np·m^{-1}·Hz^{-2}	10^{-12} dB·m^{-1}·Hz^{-2}
0	(32)	56.9	0.494
5	(40)	44.1	0.383
10	(50)	36.1	0.313
15	(60)	29.6	0.257
20	(68)	25.3	0.219
30	(86)	19.1	0.165
40	(104)	14.6	0.127
50	(122)	12.0	0.104
60	(140)	10.2	0.089

PART 3. Immersion Coupling Devices[1]

The key to immersion coupling is the presence of a continuous fluid medium in the path between the transducer and the test object. This condition can be maintained by the various devices detailed below. While immersion of the transducer and the test object in a water tank is the most widely used form of immersion coupling, other forms are also finding widespread usage, particularly the water jet.

The cost of an ultrasonic test increases with the complexity of the coupling device. Therefore, choosing the device is a budgetary decision that must be weighed against the intention of the test procedure. Any of the coupling devices below can be used for automated testing.

Immersion Tanks

The technique of coupling a transducer to a test object by submerging both in a water tank has been in use for ultrasonic testing since the early 1940s. In the 1980s, the use of immersion tanks increased substantially with the development of automated scanning systems.

In a typical configuration, scanning systems are assembled on the immersion tanks and the transducer is moved sequentially in at least two normal directions, either manually or automatically, following a programmed scanning plan. A manipulator permits adjustment of the beam angles and remote control of the distance between the transducer and test object.

An immersion tank can be used to test many shapes, including plates, wires and contours. Computer controlled systems can follow complex shapes by changing the insonification angles to maintain a constant angle of incidence.

The immersion testing of stiff materials with a constant cross section (such as pipes and rods) can be simplified to avoid the high cost of large tanks.[4] These materials may be tested by passing them through a short tank with two windows that match the test object cross section (Fig. 5). To prevent water leakage, the windows have rubber seals in the gap between the test object and the window. After the test object is inserted through the windows, the water level in the tank is raised above the transducer and the ultrasonic test is performed.

Bubbler Devices

The device known as a *bubbler* contains a transducer and a captured water column. The test object is positioned below the water column opposite the transducer. The bubbler maintains a constant flow of water through the gap between the bubbler adapter (Fig. 6) and the test object. The transducer mounting unit is designed to provide the desired angle of incidence for the beam.

For continuous tests, it is preferable to couple the bubbler to the test object's bottom. With a weak water flow, this arrangement makes it easier to ensure that the area between the transducer and the test object is always filled with water. When the test object is placed below the bubbler, a strong water flow is required to expel air from the system. As shown in Fig. 6, water is fed to the bubbler cavity through a pipe nipple. If this is done at sufficient pressure, a water cushion is formed and the bubbler can slide over the test object without touching it.

FIGURE 5. Short immersion tank for scanning test objects with constant cross section.

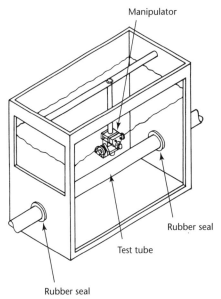

Manipulator

Rubber seal

Test tube

Rubber seal

The bubbler is used in a variety of field applications. As an example, one has been installed on a manual scanner to conduct a normal beam test of glass epoxy tubing.[5] The bottom section of the bubbler was machined to fit the outside diameter of the tube, and a fixture was designed to hold the bubbler and its angle steady while scanning.

Water Jet Devices

If enough pressure is available, a water jet can provide noncontact coupling of the transducer to a test object over a distance of 120 mm (4.75 in.) or more. Special hydrodynamic considerations are used in the design of the squirter to ensure a minimum of bubbles or turbulence. This capability is important for rapid automated testing where the manipulator might collide with an uneven surface or with a projection from the test object. Water jet coupling has an advantage over immersion when testing large structures. No large volume of water or tank is required: coupling is maintained by pressurizing a water column and draining the water after it strikes the test object. Examples of a water jet are shown in Fig. 7). Figure 7b is an automated manipulation system that can follow a contour.

Water jets are widely used in the aerospace industry, where many assemblies have a large volume of air in their internal structures. This air causes flotation capability and immersion is not practical. Furthermore, water can penetrate into such structures and induce corrosion.

A squirter produces many disturbing reflections at the contact point behind the front surface reflection, even when the water jet is smooth. These reflections can sometimes make the squirter coupling unsatisfactory for the pulse echo technique. Squirters are more commonly used with the through-transmission technique, where water jets are applied on both sides of the test object.

When using squirters with the pulse echo technique, the response is very sensitive to the angle of incidence. To ensure a sufficient signal-to-noise ratio, the water jet should be within 0.04 rad (2 deg) of normal to the surface. The surface needs to be smooth and free of scratches or wrinkles, a difficulty when testing composite laminates.

FIGURE 7. Water jet for ultrasonic tests: (a) schematic diagram; (b) automated system capable of contour following.

(a)

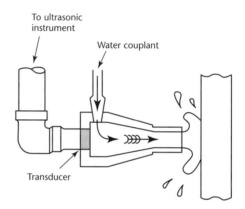

(b)

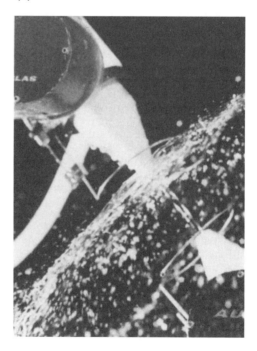

FIGURE 6. Cross section of bubbler device for immersion tests.

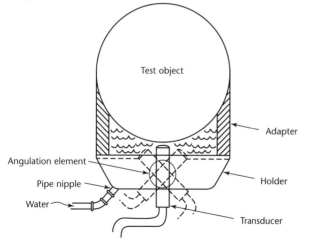

Wheel Transducers

Wheel transducers (Fig. 8) consist of a plastic tire filled with coupling fluid under pressure. During an ultrasonic test, the tire rolls over the test object and maintains a continuous coupling between it and the transducer. The transducer is attached solidly to the wheel's shaft and is positioned a few millimeters from the surface of the tire. The transducer can be manipulated to transmit at an angle that excites transverse waves in the test object. The angle between the plane of incidence and the rolling direction of the transducer can be adjusted to any rotation angle between 0 and 1.57 rad (0 and 90 deg).

Testing with the transducer wheel is performed by rolling the transducer with light pressure while scanning the test object manually or automatically. The tire creates reflections that need to be discriminated from the significant reflections of the test object.

Boot Attachment

The boot attachment uses a rubber or plastic enclosure to maintain a water path between the transducer and the test object (as in the wheel transducer).

A rubber cup is attached to the transducer assembly and the cup is filled with fluid (Fig. 9). Either a flat or a focused transducer can be used with the boot attachment and the angle of incidence can be controlled by the manipulator on which the transducer is mounted.

FIGURE 9. Boot attachment for water column capture.

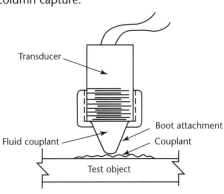

FIGURE 8. Wheel transducers: (a) straight ultrasonic beams; (b) angle beams.

(a)

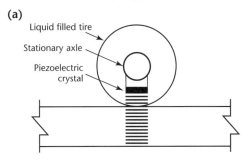

(b)

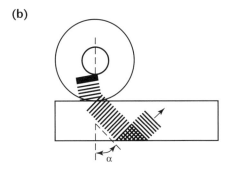

Part 4. Water Couplant Characteristics[1]

Frequency Downshift

Water as a coupling medium distorts transmitted signals at high frequencies, where the ultrasonic wave is significantly attenuated and the peak frequency of a broad band signal is downshifted. Neglecting losses due to diffraction, attenuation can be expressed as follows:

$$(3) \quad A = A_0 \exp\left(-\alpha f^n X\right)$$

where A is attenuated amplitude, A_0 is unattenuated amplitude, f is frequency (hertz), n is an exponent of the frequency dependence, X is propagation distance (meter) and α is a frequency dependent amplitude attenuation coefficient of the medium ($Np \cdot m^{-1} \cdot Hz^n$).

Note that the attenuation (decibels per meter) unites at a specific frequency: $dB \cdot m^{-1} = +8.6859 \, \alpha \, f^n$. The value of α for water is 2.4×10^{-14} $Np \cdot m^{-1} \cdot Hz^2$ and varies with water temperature and purity.

The following expression has been reported for the downshift of the frequency when $n = 2$:[5]

$$(4) \quad f_{peak} = \frac{f_0}{2\alpha X \nabla^2 + 1}$$

where f_0 is unattenuated peak frequency (hertz) and ∇ is $f_0 \times$ percent bandwidth $\div 236$.

The percent bandwidth (–6 dB) is from the unattenuated spectrum. The propagation distance X in Eq. 4 is for the signal's trip from the transducer to the target and back. The bandwidth refers to the width of the pulse echo spectrum under an impulse excitation. As an example, 5 percent downshift can be observed when a 25 MHz signal is reflected from a target 12.7 mm (0.5 in.) away from the transducer with a bandwidth of 50 percent.

When the downshift becomes too high, it is recommended to replace the water as a coupling medium with a high velocity, low attenuation solid medium. This medium serves as a bond between the transducer and the test object.

Wave Velocity in Water

The velocity of sound in water varies as a function of temperature. The equation relating the ultrasonic velocity of fresh water to its temperature is:

$$(5) \quad V_{fw} = 1410 + 4.21\,T - 0.037\,T^2$$

where T is the water temperature (celsius) and V_{fw} is fresh water ultrasonic velocity (meter per second).

Additional factors such as pressure and salinity contribute to an increase in ultrasonic velocity. These conditions play an important role when tests are in sea water. Under such conditions, the following correction factor needs to be added.

$$(6) \quad V_{sw} = V_{fw} + 1.1\,S - 1.8 \times 10^{-5}\,d$$

where d is the depth below the water surface (meter), S is salinity of water (parts per thousand) and V_{sw} is salt water ultrasonic velocity (meter per second).

It is common to use the term *standard water velocity*, to refer to 1.5 $km \cdot s^{-1}$. This value corresponds to sea water near the surface at a temperature of 15 °C (60 °F) and a salinity of 32 parts per thousand at a depth of 1 m (40 in.).[7]

Attenuation in Water

Ultrasonic attenuation in water changes as a function of temperature. Typical experimental values of attenuation versus temperature are listed in Table 1.[8] Attenuation in water also changes with pressure. Typical values of attenuation as a function of pressure are given in Table 2.

TABLE 2. Ultrasonic wave attenuation in water as function of pressure at 30 °C (86 °F).

Pressure		Attenuation	
MPa	(atm)	10^{-15} $Np \cdot m^{-1} \cdot Hz^{-2}$	10^{-12} $dB \cdot m^{-1} \cdot Hz^{-2}$
0	(0)	18.5	0.161
50	(500)	15.4	0.134
100	(1000)	12.7	0.110
150	(1500)	11.1	0.097
200	(2000)	9.9	0.086

PART 5. Pulse Echo Immersion Test Parameters[1]

Parameter Analysis

Pulse echo immersion test systems can use four parameters to detect and characterize discontinuities: (1) back surface reflection amplitude, (2) amplitude of extraneous reflections, (3) time-of-flight measurements and (4) spectral response.

A schematic view of a typical pulse echo response is shown in Fig. 10. Time gates, superimposed on an A-scan display, are used to examine the first three parameters. Windows are used in combination with a fast fourier transform to analyze the frequency domain response.

The analysis of a parameter can be done with analog hardware or a computer based digital system. Analog systems have high speed performance but also have predefined options that are relatively limited. If signals are digitized and analyzed by a microprocessor, a large variety of options become available. For real-time performance, hard coded firmware is used with a program that can acquire specific parameters. This approach provides high speed data acquisition but the test parameters are predefined and cannot be changed. Generally, such systems are similar in performance speed to the analog systems.

For high versatility, the desired parameters can be acquired and processed digitally. Digital instruments can digitize a full, single-shot A-scan signal at rates above 500 MHz. For frequencies up to the gigahertz range, sampling techniques are used. Such high frequency systems are more useful for surface wave devices. Various signal processing functions (filtering, windowing, transforming) can be used with such systems.

Computer based systems use image enhancement techniques to improve the detectability of discontinuities. Such systems can also characterize discontinuities in automatic systems by evaluating the received parameters. One suggestion is to combine C-scan imaging and discontinuity identification by using unique ultrasonic features that characterize the discontinuities.[9] The technique is called *feature mapping* and uses an array processor to examine signals in real time.

Generally, test results are presented on the computer monitor in colors (or in shades of gray scale) to provide high resolution. This technology is supported by developments in image processing and enhancement techniques from related fields such as X-ray tomography.

Back Surface Reflection Amplitude

Back surface reflection amplitude serves as a measure of the material attenuation and as a detector for anomalies that affect the energy of a traveling acoustic wave. This parameter is a fast indicator of discontinuities and is widely used to detect delaminations, porosity and microcracks.

Back surface reflection amplitude is an indirect indicator and can be sensitive to irrelevant sources. For example, geometry, surface roughness and variations in front and back surface conditions can cause changes in back surface reflection amplitude. Rejection of the test object on the basis of a change in this parameter can be done only after careful consideration because of the uncertainty in determining the source of the change.

The loss or absence of back surface reflection is evidence that the transmitted sound is being absorbed, refracted or reflected so that the energy does not return to the transducer. Loss of back surface reflection can result from many causes and does not serve as a quantitative measure of material properties. With the gain levels used in ultrasonic tests, at least several back

FIGURE 10. Schematic view of typical pulse echo test parameters.

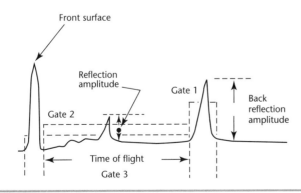

surface reflections are obtained in acceptable materials, particularly in metals.

Loss of back surface reflection may be determined by measuring the ratio of the number of back surface reflections in a reference material of thickness equivalent to the number of back surface reflections in the test material. The loss may also be evaluated by reducing the gain setting to give slightly less than a saturated (maximum undistorted) signal from the first back surface reflection in a reference material. The amplitude of this signal is then compared with the amplitude of the back surface reflection in the test object.

Amplitude of Extraneous Reflections

Discontinuities can be detected directly by examining their reflections from the bulk of the material. These reflections appear between the reflections from the front and the back surfaces (Fig. 10). Time gates are set in this region, and signals above a preset threshold indicate discontinuities. The reflection pattern can indicate the discontinuity. The reflection amplitude provides a measure of the discontinuity size.

Small Discontinuities

Individual discontinuities that are small compared to the effective beam diameter are evaluated by comparing their amplitude of reflection with the amplitude of reflection from a standard hole in a reference block. Extensive experience in the aerospace industry has shown this technique to have acceptable reliability.

Efforts have been made to develop quantitative techniques for determining the size of small discontinuities. Algorithms using born approximation[10] were developed but showed limited success because they require prior knowledge of several material and discontinuity parameters.

When using reference blocks to evaluate small discontinuities, the estimated discontinuity size is generally smaller than the actual discontinuity size. The surface of a test object and the surface of a discontinuity in a test object are usually not so flat and smooth as the surface of the reference block and the flat bottom hole in the reference block. In addition, the attenuation in the test object is commonly different than the one in the reference standard.

Large Discontinuities

Individual discontinuities larger than the effective beam diameter are also indicated by reflections between the front and back surfaces. However, the discontinuity size cannot be determined by comparing it with a reference block. The extent of the discontinuity can be obtained by moving the transducer along the surface of the test object and finding the points at which the discontinuity indication is still maintained.

The boundaries of the discontinuity are determined by marking the points where the reflection drops 6 dB below the amplitude of the reflection at the center of the discontinuity. As an alternative approach, a C-scan system can be used with its receiver gain or attenuation calibrated so that, when a reference standard is scanned, the exact size of discontinuities is displayed.

Time of Flight

Time-of-flight measurements typically are made between the test object's front surface and the next significant reflector. When this reflector is the object's back surface, there are no discontinuities. Pulse echo measurements of time of flight provide very good resolution. Test surface resolution of 0.5 mm (0.02 in.) and far surface resolution of 0.25 mm (0.01 in.) can be reliably obtained with a 5 MHz, highly damped transducer.

Time-of-flight measurements are made with the aid of a time gate that defines the boundaries of the time domain area of interest. To reduce the effect of ultrasonic noise, only signals above a preset threshold are measured. To avoid the pulse emitted by the transducer (called the *initial pulse* or *main bang signal*) and to synchronize the time gate with a specific material depth, it is common to trigger the system on the first significant signal that arrives at the receiver after the initial pulse.

When testing complex structures, the transducer's angle of incidence and its distance from the test object can change as a function of location. As a result, the reliability of the test is hampered. The capability of triggering the system with the first reflection overcomes the effect of water path length changes. This function is very useful for flat structures such as steps or slightly curved surfaces.

To maintain a constant angle of incidence, some computer based systems have the ability to follow contours. This is performed by software that contains information about the contour or by sensing devices that maintain perpendicularity of the beam to the test object front surface. The programmed technique is preferable for high scanning speeds, but it is time consuming to manually enter the test object's configuration into the computer before testing. Contour sensing devices are practical for tests of many objects with the same configuration.

Time-of-flight (depth) data as a function of position can be used to produce a three-dimensional display of discontinuities. Figure 11 shows a C-scan three-dimensional view of impact damage in a composite laminate. The distribution of delaminations as a function of depth is visible in the figure.

Frequency Domain Analysis

A transformation of broad band signal reflections to the frequency domain can reveal information that is difficult to identify in the time domain. Commercially available systems can produce fast fourier transforms at speeds very close to real time.

The spectral response allows visualization of features that are associated with discontinuity characteristics. Spectral analysis has been reported as a potential nondestructive testing tool for bonded structures[11] and composite materials.[12]

FIGURE 11. Computerized three-dimensional C-scan image of impact damage in composite laminate.

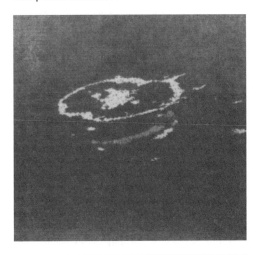

PART 6. Interpretation of Immersion Ultrasonic Test Indications[1]

Indications from Reference Standards

If a discontinuity's size is smaller than the ultrasonic beam diameter, then the size can be related to the response from known discontinuities in the A-scan. Figure 12a illustrates ultrasonic indications from reference blocks having 83 mm (3.25 in.) from the discontinuities to the surface and hole sizes from 0.04 to 3 mm (0.015 to 0.125 in.) in increments of 0.4 mm (0.015 in.). The same instrument setting was used for all test blocks.

Figure 12a shows that the 0.4 mm (0.015 in.) hole is barely discernible while the reflections from others are clearly indicated (increases with the size). Figure 12b shows B-scan presentations obtained with a constant gain setting for all eight reference blocks.

Indications from Small Discontinuities

The simplest type of discontinuity to detect has three basic characteristics: (1) relatively smooth surfaces, (2) effectively two dimensions but several wavelengths in width and (3) major dimensions parallel to the test surface so that the ultrasonic beam intersects the major dimension with normal incidence.

Small discontinuities form a significant part of the discontinuities encountered in ultrasonic tests of airframe components, particularly in wrought aluminum products. Foreign materials or porosity in the cast ingot are rolled, forged or extruded into wafer thin discontinuities during fabrication. Fabrication tends to orient the maximum dimensions of the discontinuity parallel to the surface.

The display in radio frequency form shows the front surface reflection, the echo from the discontinuity and the back surface reflection. The indication has the same amplitude as that obtained from a reference block with a 2.0 mm (0.075 in.) flat bottom hole.

Indications from Large Discontinuities

Discontinuities that are large compared with the ultrasonic beam size are generally easy to detect if their surfaces are reasonably smooth and parallel to the test surface. A large discontinuity in a die forging is illustrated in Fig. 13.

When using normal gain settings, the discontinuity indication saturates the display and the amplitude of the indication has little quantitative meaning. Typically, a strong loss of back surface reflection is observed because the discontinuity reflects nearly all the ultrasonic energy. The dimensions of the discontinuity may be determined from the distance the transducer can be moved while maintaining an indication.

Indications from Three-Dimensional Discontinuities

Discontinuities in materials that have been forged, rolled or extruded are essentially two-dimensional. Occasionally a three-dimensional discontinuity is encountered. Figure 14 shows a section from 56 × 75 mm (2.25 × 3 in.) rolled steel bar. In Fig. 15a, the indication is from a 2.0 mm (0.015 in.) flat bottom hole whose surface distance is equal to that of the discontinuity. The display on Fig. 15b is from the discontinuity in the test object. The first indication is from the front surface and the second indication is from the discontinuity (note that it saturates the display). No reflection is obtained from the back surface because sound is not transmitted through the discontinuity.

Testing from one surface does not indicate whether the discontinuity is a void as in Fig. 15c or whether it is a thin, laminar discontinuity with only two major dimensions. This can be ascertained by testing from two opposite surfaces. A test from the top surface of the object (Fig. 15b) indicates that the discontinuity is below the object surface about 60 percent of the thickness. Testing from the two opposite surfaces (not shown) indicates that the discontinuity has a

FIGURE 12. Ultrasonic indications from reference blocks with flat bottom holes; 0.4 to 3.2 mm (0.015 to 0.125 in.) in diameter, all reflecting surfaces at same distance: (a) A-scans; (b) B-scans.

(a)   (b)

0.4 mm
(0.015 in.)

0.8 mm
(0.03 in.)

1.2 mm
(0.045 in.)

1.6 mm
(0.06 in.)

25 Percent

2.0 mm
(0.075 in.)

2.4 mm
(0.1 in.)

2.8 mm
(0.11 in.)

3.2 mm
(0.125 in.)

thickness on the order of 20 percent of the thickness. The possibility of two discontinuities is eliminated by testing from all four sides. However, the likelihood of such an occurrence is considerably more remote than that of a single discontinuity of the type shown in Fig. 15.

Loss of Back Surface Reflection

Loss of back surface reflection is an important parameter that can be examined with many ultrasonic discontinuity detectors. Special care is required when interpreting or measuring loss of back surface reflection to ensure that geometrical considerations (such as roughness or taper) are not responsible for the reflection loss.

The process is simple to implement for test objects with relatively smooth surfaces and with nearly parallel front and back surfaces. Both large or small discontinuities can cause this loss of reflection since part or all of the energy is reflected from the discontinuity. The loss of back surface reflection is a very important parameter when there is no significant individual discontinuity. Among the causes for such a condition

FIGURE 13. Ultrasonic indication of discontinuity in aluminum alloy die forging: (a) A-scan indication; (b) cross section through discontinuity.

(a)

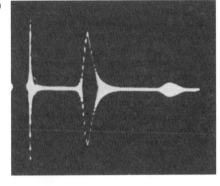

(b)

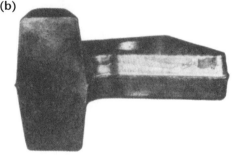

are (1) discontinuities with rough surfaces or orientations at steep angles to the surface, (2) large grain size, (3) a number of very small discontinuities (such as porosity) and (4) fine precipitate particles.

Figure 15) illustrates ultrasonic indications from an aluminum plate. The A-scan shown in Fig. 15a is from a 75 mm (3 in.) aluminum plate (cross sectioned in Fig. 15b). The A-scan in Fig. 15c is from a porous plate of the same material and thickness (Fig. 15d). The solid plate shows five repetitive reflections and the porous plate shows four reflections. Figure 15c shows no indication of discontinuities between the front and back reflections. Figure 15e is the same as Fig. 15c with a higher gain setting and an expanded time base scale. The high peaks in Fig. 15e are reflections from the front and back of the material.

Figures 15c and 15e show indications of excessive porosity or coarse grain — a loss of back surface reflection occurs at low gain with no occurrence of reflections. However, at high gain there is noise between the front and back reflections, indicating porous material. The photomicrograph of Fig. 16 reveals the size of this porosity.

FIGURE 15. Ultrasonic A-scan indications from aluminum plate: (a) multiple back reflections from solid aluminum plate; (b) cross section of solid plate; (c) multiple back reflections from porous plate with same gain setting as in Fig. 15a; (d) cross section of porous plate; (e) indication from porous plate with gain higher than Fig. 15a or 15c and expanded time base.

(a)

(b)

(c)

(d)

(e)

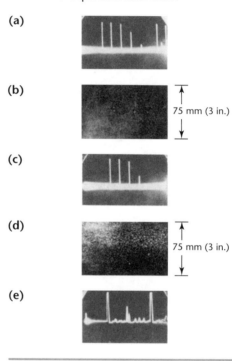

FIGURE 14. Ultrasonic scan of three-dimensional discontinuity: (a) A-scan indication from 2 mm (0.075 in.) reference block; (b) A-scan indication from discontinuity shown in Fig. 14c, using the same gain setting as in Fig. 14a; (c) discontinuity detected in rolled steel bar.

(a)

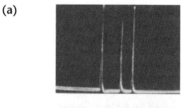

(b)

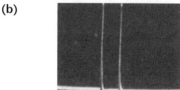

(c)

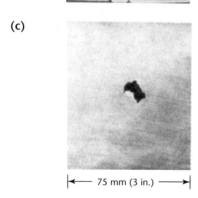

FIGURE 16. Photomicrograph of aluminum alloy containing porosity (94×).

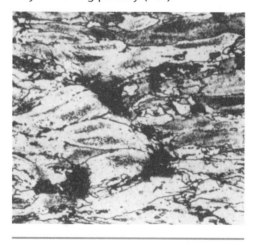

Metallurgical Factors in Indication Formation

Consideration of the metallurgical and fabrication history of materials is extremely valuable for interpreting of ultrasonic test indications.

In general, discontinuities in wrought products tend to be oriented in the direction of grain flow. The maximum dimension of the discontinuity is in the direction of maximum metal flow during fabrication. This generalization is not true for discontinuities that result from processes subsequent to forging, extrusion or rolling.

Plate and Extrusions

Grain direction (the direction the metal flows during working) is relatively simple to determine in a plate. Discontinuities are generally parallel to the plate surface and elongated in the direction that received the maximum amount of rolling, although there are variations to this generalization (Fig. 17).

Discontinuities in extrusions are nearly always elongated in the direction of extrusion (along the long axis of the extrusion). In the case of plate and extrusions, it is very important to note recurring discontinuity indications when scanning parallel to the direction of grain flow.

Such a situation can be seen in a cross section of an extrusion. Ultrasonic tests from the surface can indicate discontinuities equivalent to an indication from a 2.0 mm (0.08 in.) flat bottom hole in a reference block. The indications may occur along a 1.2 m (4 ft) length of the extrusion even if no continuous discontinuity is evident. Loss of back surface reflection occurs with the individual indications. An important clue that the discontinuity is large and continuous is if the discontinuities appear to be about the same distance below the surface and in a line coinciding with the grain. Extrusions are usually visible on the butt end of the extrusion. In this case, the discontinuity is extended across the complete length of the extrusion but was not evident on the ends, even after they were caustically etched.

Die Forging

Grain flow is a complex process in die forgings. Discontinuities are not necessarily oriented parallel to the surface or elongated in the long dimension of the test object. With the typically complicated geometry of forgings, these factors make detection and evaluation of discontinuities difficult.

In some instances where large, complex die forgings are being tested, it is possible to section a sample forging to determine grain flow in various parts of the test object. Results of such destructive procedures help determine the most likely orientation of discontinuities for subsequent ultrasonic test setups.

Test Indications Requiring Special Consideration

Contoured Surfaces

Reflections from fillets and concave surfaces may produce test indications between the front and back reflections and these can be confused with indications from discontinuities. Such spurious indications result from sound reflected back to the transducer at a time equivalent to the time of flight from a discontinuity at a given distance below the surface. It is sometimes difficult to

FIGURE 17. Discontinuities oriented in transverse direction in Unified Numbering System A97075, heat treatable, temper 6, wrought aluminum alloy rolled plate: (a) A-scan indication; (b) cross section of discontinuity.

(a)

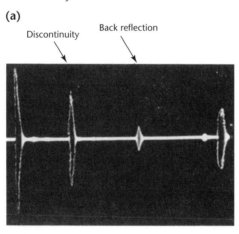

Discontinuity   Back reflection

(b)

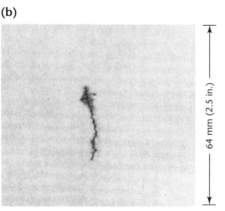

64 mm (2.5 in.)

distinguish between discontinuities and false indications from curved surfaces.

Frequently, if a false indication results from a contoured surface, the amplitude of the indication is related to the amplitude of the reflection from the front surface. In this case, the amplitude of the front surface echo diminishes as the false indication increases.

A false indication tends to be consistent as the transducer is moved along the contoured surface. A reflection from a discontinuity tends to be strongly localized. False indications from contoured surfaces are more likely to result in a broad based indication. Discontinuity indications are typically sharp spikes.

If false indications result from reflections around a contoured surface, it is sometimes possible to distinguish them by interrupting the ultrasonic beam between the transducer and the surface of the test object with a foreign object (a piece of sheet metal, for example). If the indication is a reflection from a curved surface, shielding a portion of the curved area may eliminate the false indication and allow the major portion of the beam to enter the test object.

Edge Effect

Irrelevant indications are sometimes produced near the edges of rectangular shapes. This type of indication is observed when the transducer is placed close to the test object's edge. This effect is the result of reflections from the edges, even though the ultrasound enters the top of the object and is not refracted by the corner.

One distinguishing characteristic of the edge effect is its consistency. There can be some variation in the distance below the surface (typically a fourth to a half of the test object thickness) but the location and characteristics of edge effect indications are consistent. As the transducer travels parallel to the edge of the test object, the indication remains relatively uniform in appearance and amplitude. In contrast to this, an indication from a discontinuity generally shows variation in amplitude because of roughness in the discontinuity's surface. In addition, discontinuities that give a continuous indication over several millimeters of transducer travel are generally of sufficient size to reduce back reflections.

Surface Conditions

Occasionally, test objects with smooth, shiny surfaces produce irrelevant or false indications. When testing plates with smooth finish surfaces, for example, consistent indications may exist beyond the front surface reflection. The indications remain relatively uniform in shape and magnitude when the transducer is moved around the edge. The false indication is caused by surface waves reflected from a nearby edge on the extremely smooth surface.

Such false indications can be eliminated by slightly disturbing the entry surface — coating with wax crayon or a thin film of petroleum jelly. One of the distinguishing characteristics of this false indication is its consistency. It is good practice to be suspicious of any indication that is unusually consistent in amplitude and appearance when the transducer is passing over the test object.

Location of Discontinuities

Because of the near zone effect and equipment recovery time, discontinuities very close to the test surface cannot always be detected at angles normal to the surface. However, indications of discontinuities are sometimes evident at a distance slightly less than that at which a definite individual peak is observed. The sound wave reflected from the discontinuity near the surface interferes with sound waves reflected from the front surface but the ultrasonic equipment is unable to resolve or separate the energy into two distinct signals.

A slight variation in the appearance of the front reflection does not necessarily indicate a front-surface discontinuity: a variation in the flatness or roughness of the test surface can also produce a variation in the indication. Roughness or flatness variations sufficient for causing fluctuations in a front surface indication can usually be detected by touch. When fluctuations of the front reflection cannot be attributed to surface condition, the possibility of a discontinuity near the surface should be investigated by testing from the opposite surface. Front surface discontinuities may also cause a loss of back surface reflection. To improve the detection of front surface discontinuities, double transducer techniques can be used.

Another technique to verify the presence of front surface discontinuities is the use of thin tungsten foil as a reflector. Because tungsten has a very high acoustic impedance (more than 10^8 kg·m^{-2}·s^{-1}), the reflection coefficient is very high. Such foil can be placed over a suspect area to obtain a reference reflection near the front surface reflection.

Discontinuities Oriented at Angle to Surface

Discontinuities oriented at an angle to the front surface may be difficult to detect and evaluate if care is not exercised.

Generally, it is desirable to scan first at a comparatively high gain level to detect discontinuities oriented at an angle to the test surface. It has been shown that a 2.0 mm (0.08 in.) diameter flat bottom hole oriented at 0.44 rad (25 deg) to the front surface is not discernible on the display if the transducer is parallel to the surface.[13] This test was conducted using a gain level giving a peak height 50 percent of the screen from a 2.0 mm (0.08 in.) flat bottom hole at normal incidence.

Ultrasonic waves obey Snell's law in a fashion similar to light. Therefore, it is necessary to manipulate the transducer when evaluating discontinuities oriented at an angle to the surface so that the sound beam strikes the plane of the discontinuity at right angles. Even though manipulation is accomplished, discontinuities oriented at angles to the surface result in indications with magnitudes slightly lower than those for discontinuities parallel to the surface. This difference is not large. Indication amplitude is a function of angle between the discontinuity and the front surface. The transducer can be manipulated to obtain maximum indication height.

In some instances, not only is the general plane of the discontinuity oriented at an angle to the surface but the surface of the discontinuity may also be irregular. The amplitude of the indication may not indicate a large discontinuity because most of the sound may be reflected to the transducer. Discontinuities of this type are generally large compared with the transducer size and evidence of the indication may persist as the transducer is moved over the test object.

Occasionally, discontinuities large compared to the transducer have a relatively smooth, flat surface but lie at an angle to the surface. Bursts in large forgings fit this category and tend to lie at 0.79 rad (45 deg) to the surface. Such discontinuities present a nearly continuous test indication. Because of the change in distance that the sound must travel, the indication moves along the base line of the display instrument as the transducer is moved.

Grain Size Discontinuities

In an ultrasonic test of Unified Numbering System G43400 nickel chrome molybdenum alloy steel at 5 MHz, an unusually high noise level was detected.[14] A study of this material showed very large grain size compared with ASTM grain size standards of 1 to 4 (Fig. 18a). The large grains found in the as-received condition resulted from (1) high temperature during hot working and (2) subsequent improper annealing.

Ultrasonic testing was performed on a similar sample again heat treated to attain grain refinement. The sample showed an absence of noise on the reference line, indicating that with proper heat treatment a finer grain size was obtained (Fig. 18c). Microscopic examination revealed a refined grain size of ASTM standards 6 to 8.

In another test performed on forgings of a nickel based alloy, a frequency of 5 MHz was used. One forging produced seven back reflections whereas another showed no back reflections with the same

FIGURE 18. Effect of grain size on ultrasonic indications from Unified Numbering System G43400 nickel chromium molybdenum alloy steel (both A-scans obtained with the same gain): (a) photomicrograph of large grain material; (b) ultrasonic A-scan indication for Fig. 18a; (c) photomicrograph of fine grain material; (d) ultrasonic A-scan indication for Fig. 18c.

(a)

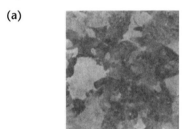

(b)

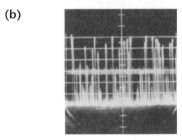

(c)

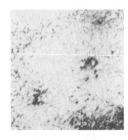

(d)

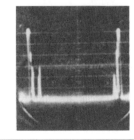

gain level, transducer and test frequency. Microscopic examination was made of these and other forgings to determine if any internal discontinuities were responsible for the ultrasonic pattern and to compare the grain size. The forgings with the unusually large grain size showed a loss of back reflections even though no internal discontinuity was present. Further investigations revealed that prolonged or improper forging temperature could cause the abnormally large grain size.

Interpretation of Indications from Rotor Wheels

The tests discussed below use as an example the straight beam immersion test of an aircraft component. Figure 19a illustrates the area tested ultrasonically in an aluminum compressor rotor wheel. The ultrasonic beam from the transducer is directed at an incidence angle of 0.09 rad (5 deg) at the surface periphery.

According to Snell's law, the angle of the refracted beam θ_1 is about four times

greater than θ_{in}, or about 0.35 rad (20 deg) to normal. A schematic description of the A-scan at this point is shown in Fig. 19b. The initial pulse (emitted by the transducer) is shown at the left and the reflection from the front surface is shown next. As the transducer moves in an axial direction, the refracted beam (position 1) is just cutting across the corner of the rabbit groove and producing an insignificant indication. The reflection from a far surface is shown at the right side.

Crack Indications

In Fig. 20a, the transducer has been moved farther right in an axial direction and the sound beam (position 2) is reflected from a crack. This produces an indication on the A-scan (Fig. 20b). The rabbit groove indication has disappeared because the ultrasonic beam has been repositioned. Because the ultrasonic pulse requires about 8 µs to make a round trip through 25 mm (1 in.) of aluminum, the time interval between the indication from the front surface and that from the crack is 2 ms. At the position shown in Fig. 20, the crack starts at about 6.5 mm (0.25 in.) below the surface.

As the transducer is moved axially, the refracted ultrasonic beam is reflected from the face of the crack at a depth of about

---

FIGURE 19. Ultrasonic testing of aluminum compressor rotor wheel at beam position 1: (a) beam hits corner of rabbit groove; (b) A-scan from position 1, showing indication from corner of rabbit groove.

(a)

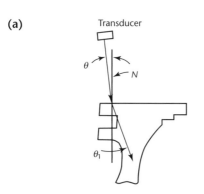

(b)

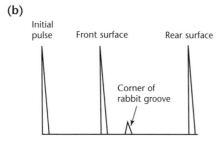

Legend
N = normal incidence
θ = angle of incidence
θ_1 = angle of propagation

FIGURE 20. Ultrasonic testing of aluminum compressor rotor wheel at beam position 2: (a) beam misses rabbit groove and strikes crack; (b) A-scan indication from position 2 shows crack reflection.

(a)

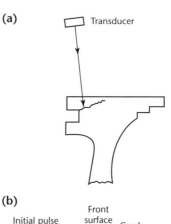

(b)

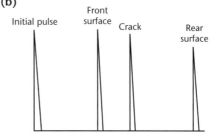

---

3 mm (0.125 in.) below the surface. The crack indication moves toward the front surface indication and the time interval between the two indications becomes about 1 μs. As the transducer moves, the crack indication seems to move toward the front surface reflection. This indicates that the crack is not parallel to the surface but instead is approaching the surface (the sound beam's angle of incidence has not changed with the change in the transducer's axial position).

Indications of Weld Cracks

A cross section of a welded turbine rotor is shown in Fig. 21. In this wheel, a rim of forged stainless steel is welded to a hub of forged ferritic material. Despite advanced welding techniques, cracks occasionally develop in the rim's heat affected zone. These occur often enough to require 100 percent testing.

The wheel cracks lie in a plane parallel to the face of the wheel and extend in a radial direction. Ultrasonic testing is the only means to detect cracks in this

FIGURE 21. Ultrasonic testing of welded turbine rotor: (a) beam position for crack in heat affected zone; (b) A-scan indication over sound material; (c) A-scan indication over crack, also showing loss of back reflection; (d) B-scan indication over crack.

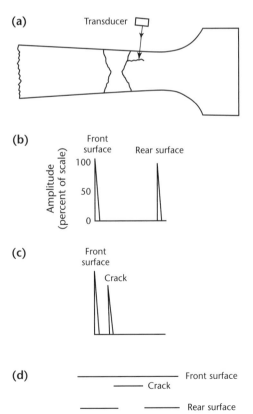

orientation. Figure 21a shows the direction of the ultrasonic waves and the position of the discontinuity in the cross section of the wheel.

During testing, the wheel is rotated on a turntable immersed in water. The A-scan display is shown in Fig. 21a for the condition in which the transducer is oriented over a solid metal path. Both the A-scan and B-scan presentations are shown (in Fig. 21) with the transducer over an area containing a crack. The discontinuity is large enough in this case to cause a reflection of high amplitude and a complete loss of back surface reflection (Fig. 21d).

The distance between front surface reflection and the reflection from the crack indicates the crack's depth below the surface. Care must be exercised when angulating the sound beam close to the interior interface of weld and rim material — the beam can be reflected off these faces and is rapidly attenuated. Consequently, this area is not always effectively tested by the ultrasonic method. Radiographic tests are also used for the weld area.

Indications of Metallic Inclusions and Segregations

Metallic inclusions in the same plane as cracks give similar indications in the heat affected zone. They are found most frequently in the rim and farther away from the weld area.

Ultrasonic testing is also used for solid forged turbine rotor wheels of certain stainless steel alloys fabricated without welding. The technique is used chiefly to detect sharp cracks from forging.

Forgings may also contain segregates that reflect ultrasonic beams. These indications cannot be distinguished from those caused by cracks. Metallurgists have determined that the mechanical properties of materials containing segregates meet normal service requirements for room temperature tensile and elevated temperature stress rupture properties. These segregates can cause indications with amplitudes of 15 to 90 percent of the front surface reflection (Fig. 21c). The more highly concentrated ones cause higher amplitude indications. These peaks can appear between the first and second multiples of the rear surface reflection.

Discontinuities in this stainless steel occur in either a loose or tightly bound condition. Fortunately, these discontinuities do not occur frequently. Although they do not adversely affect the mechanical properties, they cannot be accepted. If they should occur in a critical area like the serrations of the rotor wheel, they might propagate and cause catastrophic failure.

Indications of Forging Bursts

Figure 22 illustrates the cross section of a stainless steel rim of a turbine wheel containing forging bursts. These are irregularly shaped cavities caused by rupture of the material during forging. Forging bursts are rejectable, are likely to be clustered in groups and produce many A-scan indications of various amplitudes. The reflections from inclusions may also be of varying amplitude but are more likely to be widely scattered. By comparison, the indication from a crack is sometimes continuous for as much as one fourth the circumference of the rim, with complete loss of reflection from the far surface.

Indications of Small Inclusions

The rotor wheel rims are also ultrasonically tested for nonmetallic inclusions too small to be detected radiographically. These inclusions do not seriously affect the mechanical properties of the materials as do cracks and forging bursts.

The inclusions are often randomly located. If they are exposed on a machined surface such as a serration used for the insertion of a bucket, a costly rejection is the result. Rim acceptance

specifications do not permit any ultrasonic indications between front and rear surface reflections.

Indication from Surface Contour Blending

Surface conditions may cause false indications during ultrasonic tests. The safest way to avoid false indications is to have the surface prepared to completely avoid ultrasonic wave scattering. A common practice is to require that the surface of test objects have at least a 2 μm (8×10^{-5} in.) root mean square finish.

Surface treatment such as blending or grinding can produce misleading ultrasonic test results. Figure 23 shows the cross section of a turbine rotor where a slight depression has been made by a blending operation in the otherwise smooth surface. The depression has been exaggerated to illustrate the condition more clearly. In actual cases these depressions may be so slight that they cannot be seen under water and their presence can be verified only by touch.

Under certain conditions, such depressions can produce false indications as shown in the A-scan in Fig. 23b. If the sound waves enter the surface at the edge of the blended area, they can be scattered in such a way that part of the beam travels across the surface of the blend, reflects from the opposite edge and appears as a discontinuity indication. Because sound travels much slower in water than in metals, the amplitudes and position of false indications with respect to front and back surface reflections

FIGURE 22. Ultrasonic testing of stainless steel rotor wheel with forging bursts: (a) beam position on fillet area; (b) A-scan indications from forging bursts between front surface and rear surface.

(a)

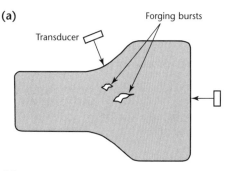

(b)

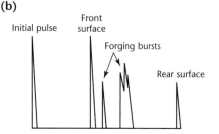

FIGURE 23. False indication from surface blending: (a) path of ultrasonic beam producing the false indication (dashed); (b) A-scan showing false indication between front surface and rear surface indications.

(a)

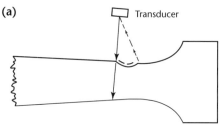

(b)

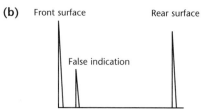

depend largely on the size, depth and contour of the blended area and the path length in the metallic test object.

A good practice is to machine the as-forged rotor wheel to a 2 μm (8×10^{-5} in.) root mean square finish with opposite faces parallel wherever possible so that the effects of varying shape and contour can be minimized. This is more necessary when testing materials that may contain inclusions, such as carbide bands whose reflections can be confused with those from serious discontinuities.

In these cases, the forging vendor (who also tests the wheels ultrasonically) is hired to prepare the test objects by machining. Enough stock is provided in the forging and after machining, before ultrasonic testing, so that the machine finish contours and tolerances can be maintained. This procedure is costly but pays for itself in greater reliability of ultrasonic testing for critical components. After preliminary machining and ultrasonic testing, the rotor wheels are heat treated before shipment from the forging vendor's plant.

Indications from Heat Treating Scale

Heat treating can produce a thin imperceptible scale or film on the surface of rotor wheels and this can in turn produce confusing ultrasonic test indications. Figure 24a shows the cross section of a machined turbine rotor wheel as obtained from a forging vendor.

The transducer is directed onto the surface of the rotor in an area containing a thin scale. The size of this scale has been exaggerated to illustrate the condition

more clearly. The indications from this surface condition are depicted on the A-scan in Fig. 24 and are generally characterized by an increased number of scattered signals next to the particular surface reflection.

Slight surface etching can remove the cause of these reflections. They are a concern because they can mask indications from an actual discontinuity.

FIGURE 24. False indications from heat treating scale: (a) path of ultrasonic beam entering scaled surface; (b) A-scan indications showing false indications between front surface and back surface indications

(a)

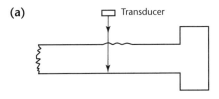

(b)

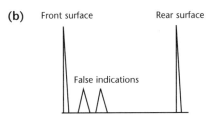

PART 7. Immersion Testing of Composite Materials[1]

Discontinuities in Composite Laminates

Composites are used in applications requiring materials with high ratios of stiffness to weight or of strength to weight. Composites possess a complex failure mechanism which causes difficulties in establishing design criteria and nondestructive test techniques.

Most composites are made of layers containing many fibers bonded with a matrix of different or equal composition. The layers are stacked at various fiber orientations, depending on design requirements. The resulting heterogeneous, anisotropic, layered characteristics hamper some nondestructive test techniques well established for homogeneous, isotropic materials.

In aerospace, three composite systems are commonly used: graphite epoxy (for critical structures), glass epoxy and plastic epoxy. The diameter of the fibers varies from 1 to 10 µm (4×10^{-5} to 4×10^{-4} in.) for graphite and 5 to 15 µm (0.0002 to 0.0006 in.) for glass. Several types of discontinuities are commonly induced during the manufacture and service life of a composite structure.

Causes of Composite Discontinuities

Composite systems have a tendency to nucleate porosity if the volatile components in the resin are not properly removed during cure. At curing, trapped air is pushed out along the fibers, typically along the fibers and between composite layers because of the high resin content in these regions. Once the curing composite passes the gel stage, it begins to harden and air is trapped in porosity or voids. In addition to porosity, improper cure can lead to a partial delamination of the composite plies.

Generally, delaminations result from hole drilling and impact damage. Delaminations can also be the result of stresses at the free edges of the composite, when the transverse tensile or shear strength is exceeded. During layup, foreign materials tend to be introduced, particularly the plastic carrier film and the release paper on which impregnated (uncured) composite plies are delivered.

Another foreign material that can be left in the composite is peel ply. Peel plies are used to prevent bonding of the laminate to the mold during cure and sometimes pieces of peel plies are introduced into the laminate bulk. Generally, the presence of such inclusions inhibit bonding between plies.

During layup, ply gap can occur in a laminate if the various impregnated composite tapes are not properly positioned and a gap is left between them. This gap is filled with a pocket of resin and causes a thickness reduction at its center.

Discontinuities such as delaminations, inclusions, porosity and ply gap can lead to property degradation not accounted for in design and ultimately can shorten the composite's service life.

Results of Composite Discontinuities

At less than 2 percent of volume, porosity provides *improved* fracture toughness. However, porosity also reduces compressive and interlaminar shear strength and compromises the fatigue life of the material. Porosity can produce an increase in the moisture equilibrium level and aggravates the thermal spike phenomenon. Both of these conditions lead to deterioration in the material's elastic properties.

Delaminations are a more severe discontinuity because they do not transfer interlaminar shear stresses. Under compressive loading, delamination can cause rapid and catastrophic buckling failure. The presence of a peel ply inside the laminate is harmful because of the low interlaminar shear it provides.

The effect of ply gaps depends on the stacking order and the discontinuity location. As an example, for [0, +45, 90, –45]$_{2S}$ laminate, a 2.5 µm (0.0001 in.) gap in the 0 rad (0 deg) layers reduces the tensile strength by 8 percent. The same size gap in the 1.57 rad (90 deg) layer reduces the strength by 17 percent.[15]

Ultrasonic Testing of Composite Laminates

Composites are usually tested for delamination using the straight beam immersion technique. Time of flight is measured to map the depth distribution of discontinuities. Loss of back surface reflection provides a profile of severity. Time of flight can be used to identify delaminations of less than 1 mm (0.04 in.) diameter in graphite epoxy laminates with ±0.2 mm (±0.008 in.) accuracy.[16]

Figure 25 shows A-scan images obtained from a 16-layer graphite epoxy composite bonded to an aluminum honeycomb through a protective layer of glass epoxy and adhesive bond. The ultrasonic test uses short duration pulses in the range of 100 ns.

Figure 26 shows time-of-flight C-scan imaging of delaminations that resulted from impact damage. Using the computer to conduct a three-dimensional rotation, the depth distribution of the delaminations is clearly identified as shown above (Fig. 11).

The examination of back surface reflection amplitude provides a measure of the attenuation and can reveal the presence of material changes and discontinuities. Typical discontinuities that affect attenuation are porosity, voids, impact damage and deviations in volume ratio of resin to fiber.

Many factors not related to material quality may also affect attenuation, so that attenuation changes serve as a discontinuity indicator only when a severe change is observed. Porosity, for example, is typically detected by its effect on attenuation. However, at low volume (below 3 percent), porosity can have about the same effect as surface roughness or geometrical variations.

Reflector Plate

In some thin structures, the ultrasonic beam attenuation may not be high enough for testing. When this occurs, it is common to use a reflector plate to detect small discontinuities. The reflector plate may be highly polished metal designed for the purpose. The bottom of the submersion tank may also be used.

The plate is used with the straight beam immersion technique and the test object is placed between the transducer and the plate. Tests are conducted by monitoring the changes in reflection amplitude from the front surface of the plate after passing twice through the test object.

Tests of Composite Tubing

Composite tubing is commonly manufactured by a filament winding process rather than by stacking layers to build a laminate. During the manufacture of composite tubing, several types of discontinuities can be induced and some of these may cause deterioration in performance. For such tubes, straight

FIGURE 25. Delamination detection in graphite epoxy (depth of discontinuities is indicated by time of flight): (a) trace without delamination; (b) trace with delamination.

(a)

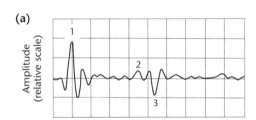

Travel time
(relative scale)

(b)

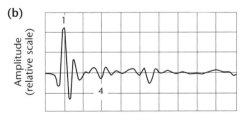

Travel time
(relative scale)

Legend
1. front surface reflection.
2. reflection from fiber/glass layer.
3. rear surface reflection from adhesive layer.
4. reflection from 1 mm (0.04 in.) delamination.

FIGURE 26. Computerized C-scan of impact damage in graphite-to-epoxy laminate.

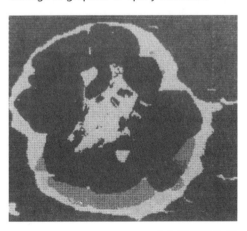

beam ultrasonic tests can be performed with water jet or bubbler instruments.[4]

Characteristic Responses of Tubing Discontinuities

The discontinuities below can be induced in a filament winding process. The characteristic responses when tested with straight beam ultrasonics are also detailed below. Each of these discontinuities has distinct characteristics that can be used with computer software to identify the discontinuity automatically (Table 3).

1. Concealed cut, or ply gap, is a discontinuity that produces a resin pocket. The mismatch of acoustic properties in the discontinuity area, as well as the presence of increased resin, cause a loss of back surface reflection as shown in Fig. 27.

2. Knot appears as a local increase in tube thickness. As the discontinuity is approached, an additional reflection splits off from the front reflection. The additional reflection advances gradually with respect to the front reflection and its amplitude grows steadily. In parallel, there is a decrease in the amplitudes of the other echoes. When the center of the discontinuity is reached, the reflection pattern acquires the appearance of a standard echo train, advanced in time and strongly attenuated. This behavior is shown in Fig. 28.

3. Lack of rovings appears in a helical configuration around the tube as a local decrease in tube thickness. When the transducer is near the discontinuity, a decrease of the echo train amplitude is observed and simultaneously the whole train is displaced from the main radio frequency pulse because of the increase in the time delay. Lack of rovings also involves shorter time of flight but with no significant effect on ultrasonic velocity. Whenever the severity of this discontinuity increases, the ultrasonic changes are more distinct. Reflection patterns from lack of rovings are shown in Fig. 29.

FIGURE 27. Ultrasonic A-scan indication of concealed cut: (a) 3 mm (0.1 in.) away from discontinuity center; (b) at discontinuity center.

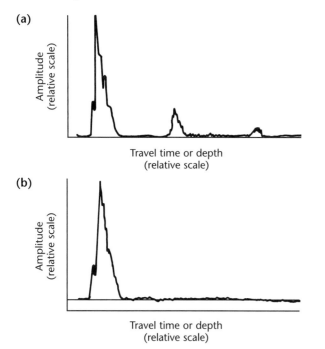

(a)

Amplitude (relative scale)

Travel time or depth (relative scale)

(b)

Amplitude (relative scale)

Travel time or depth (relative scale)

FIGURE 28. Ultrasonic A-scan indications of knot (dashed line indicates location of front surface reflection): (a) 10 mm (0.4 in.) from discontinuity center; (b) 4 mm (0.15 in.) from discontinuity center; (c) 2 mm (0.08 in.) from discontinuity center; (d) at discontinuity center.

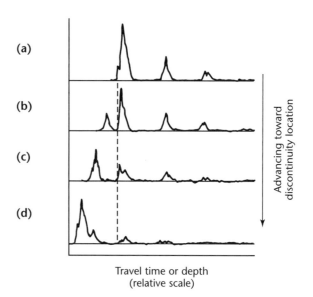

(a)

(b)

(c)

(d)

Advancing toward discontinuity location

Travel time or depth (relative scale)

4. Impact damage involves the appearance of local cracks and delaminations. When the transducer is near the discontinuity, additional reflections appear and the reflection from the inner diameter surface is decreased. This decrease reaches a maximum at the center of the damage and small reflections may also appear in the interval between the first and second reflections. The amplitude of the reflection from the outer tube surface is not changed at the discontinuity location and increased attenuation is measured. The reflection pattern of impact damage is shown in Fig. 30.

5. A resin starved layer has a nonlocalized nature, extending through a tube over a large area. This discontinuity causes the appearance of additional reflections originating at the surface of the starved layer. The time of flight between the discontinuity reflection and the front reflection depends on the depth of the resin starved layer. This discontinuity has some of the characteristics of delaminations in laminates (Fig. 31).

FIGURE 29. Ultrasonic A-scan indications of lack of rovings (dashed line indicates location of front surface reflection): (a) 10 mm (0.4 in.) from discontinuity center; (b) 4 mm (0.15 in.) from discontinuity center; (c) 2 mm (0.08 in.) from discontinuity center; (d) at discontinuity center.

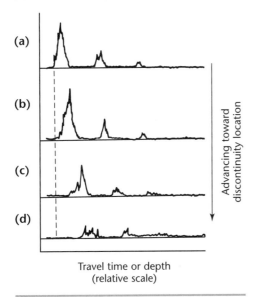

Travel time or depth
(relative scale)

FIGURE 30. Ultrasonic A-scan indications from impact damage: (a) 10 mm (0.4 in.) from discontinuity center; (b) 4 mm (0.15 in.) from discontinuity center; (c) 2 mm (0.08 in.) from discontinuity center; (d) at discontinuity center.

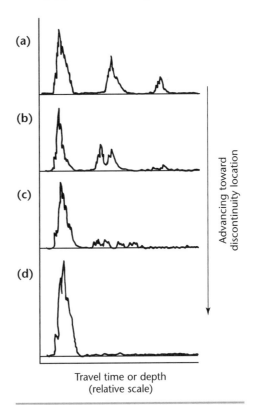

Travel time or depth
(relative scale)

FIGURE 31. Ultrasonic A-scan indications of resin starved layer: (a) reference pattern; (b) discontinuity characteristics.

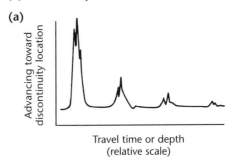

Travel time or depth
(relative scale)

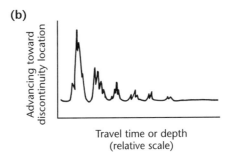

Travel time or depth
(relative scale)

TABLE 3. Characteristic parameters of various discontinuities in filament wound tubes.

Discontinuities	Additional Reflection	Increase of Attenuation	Shift of First Reflection	Change of Time of Flight[a]	Velocity Change	Changes near Discontinuity[b]
Concealed cut	—	yes	—	—	—	—
Knot	yes	yes	yes	yes	—	yes
Lack of rovings	—	yes	yes	yes	—	yes
Impact damage	yes	yes	—	—	—	yes
Resin starved layer	yes	—	—	yes	—	—
Flexible resin	—	yes	—	yes	yes	—
Low modulus fibers	—	—	—	yes	yes	—

a. Change in time of flight can indicate thickness variation without corresponding change in ultrasonic velocity.

b. Several discontinuities in one location can be detected ultrasonically before positioning of transducer at discontinuity location.

6. Flexible resin is a nonlocalized discontinuity caused by the wrong resin, an incorrect amount of hardener or unsatisfactory curing. Ultrasonic pulses are attenuated in flexible resin much more than in a properly hardened resin (17 dB in glass epoxy, for example). In addition, flexible resin is associated with some decrease in the ultrasonic velocity. The identification of this discontinuity requires that reference velocity and attenuation values be compared with those of the tubing being tested.

7. Low modulus fibers constitute another nonlocal discontinuity. It is caused by use of the wrong fibers in the composite. This discontinuity exhibits a decrease in ultrasonic velocity by as low as 10 percent of the original velocity. No significant attenuation change is observed.

These discontinuity types are listed in Table 3.

PART 8. Angle Beam Immersion Techniques[1]

Beam refraction occurs when the ultrasonic wave is not perpendicular to the test object surface. Immersion coupling provides the versatility of choosing any desired incidence angle. There are several reasons for performing angle beam tests: (1) to induce transverse waves, (2) to insonify at an angle that provides maximum reflection from discontinuities, (3) to avoid specular reflection from the test object's front surface, (4) to induce surface waves and (5) to induce lamb waves.

Principles of Angle Beam Tests

When an ultrasonic beam impinges on a surface at an incidence angle other than normal, the transmitted wave is refracted according to Snell's law. This phenomenon is used in the immersion ultrasonic test of tubular shapes. Because the angles of the sound beam are adjusted from 0.18 to 0.52 rad (10 to 30 deg), the refraction sends the beam around the tubular annulus.

Mode of Beam Propagation

The sound is propagated around a pipe wall in a saw tooth or zigzag pattern, and the mode of propagation is either transverse or longitudinal vibration. The saw tooth pattern is fairly sharp and a discontinuity can be detected only when its position coincides with the beam path.

Empirical data indicate that the sound is propagated around the thin wall of the small diameter tubing as a severely distorted longitudinal wave. As the boundaries of the material approach each other, they offer increased interference and the longitudinal velocity is appreciably reduced. This behavior indicates that the wave mode is modified.

With progressively thinner tube walls, the reflection nodes become less sharp. When the wall is very thin, the sound floods around the very narrow metal wall. These two concepts of the travel pattern are depicted in Fig. 32. Observations of thin walled tubing tests indicate that the sound wave phenomenon may be explained by comparison with the formation of lamb waves.

Scanning Systems

For disks, cylinders, tubes and various other shapes with axial symmetry, a turntable may be used in combination with the rectilinear bridge of C-scan ultrasonic systems. Turntable systems are provided with self-centering chucks or other handling devices to hold test objects in a properly aligned and secured position. Even though the rotation speeds can reach thirty revolutions per minute, the tendency to produce turbulence at such speeds enforces slower speeds.

When testing cylinders with a turntable, C-scan images can be produced on paper wrapped around a drum placed on a recorder. The drum height is at least equal to the test object's height and its

FIGURE 32. Propagation of sound in tube wall: (a) sawtooth pattern of distorted longitudinal wave; (b) sound flooding around thin walled tube.

(a)

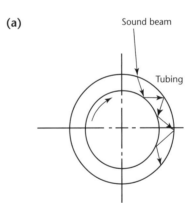

(b)

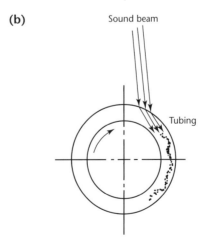

diameter is the same as (or a certain ratio of) the test object's. Ultrasonic C-scan imaging on a computer monitor is done by synchronizing the display cursor so that it simulates the location of the transducer.

Scope of Application

The immersion technique has been used successfully for critical tests of small diameter tubes down to 5 mm (0.2 in.) outside diameter by 0.6 mm (0.02 in.) wall and 6.5 mm (0.25 in.) outside diameter by 0.4 mm (0.02 in.) wall and pipe sizes of 280 mm (11 in.) outside diameters.

In general, this technique is designed to detect longitudinal discontinuities with an orientation along the tubular axis. Typical examples of longitudinal discontinuities are cracks, laps, seams, folds, incomplete weld penetration, severe intergranular corrosion, scratches, gouges and laminations.

The apparent size of the discontinuity is a function of two variables: (1) the reflecting area as determined by the cross section size of the discontinuity and its orientation relative to the sound beam and (2) changes in acoustic impedance related to a discontinuity.

The more nearly perpendicular the discontinuity is to the sound beam, the larger is the reflected signal. It is difficult to differentiate between short, deep discontinuities and long, shallow discontinuities having equal reflecting areas.

Limitations in Discontinuity Detection

A crack returns the maximum signal only if the plane of the longitudinal discontinuity contains a radius of the tubular shape. If this condition is not met, the discontinuity is detectable when the sound beam is propagated around the tube in one direction. However, this same discontinuity may not be detectable if the sound is propagated in the other direction. For this reason, all tubular objects should receive a double test to increase the probability of detection of nonradial discontinuities.

Discontinuities that offer little reflecting interface are difficult to detect by the angle beam technique. These include rounded grooves or gouges, pickling pits, small dimensional variations, small amounts of foreign metal, intergranular corrosion, pinholes (at normal test speeds) and internal metallurgical changes such as small variations in grain size. Experience shows that the angle beam technique should be used only for detection of longitudinal discontinuities.

Angle Beam Techniques and Procedures

Longitudinal cracks are the most common discontinuity in pipe and tubing. The simplest and most reproducible reference standard for such a crack is a very narrow longitudinal notch, equal in depth and length to a rejectable discontinuity. Such notches are machined on the inner and outer surfaces and on the same circumference of the reference standard. At best, this kind of standard is a go/no-go gage, used to determine the comparative size of discontinuities and to prove detectability of discontinuities on the inside surface of the pipe.

It is not easy to prepare a reference standard for small diameter tubing, mainly because of the difficulty of working on the inside surface of bores with diameters as small as 3 mm (0.1 in.). For this reason, a naturally occurring discontinuity is sometimes used as a reference standard for small diameter tubing.

Positioning of Transducer

For tests of tubular shapes, the transducer is aligned so that the sound beam produces a range of incident angles. These angles are optimized for the particular ratio of wall thickness to diameter and for the velocity of sound propagation peculiar to the test material.

Control of Sensitivity to Discontinuities

To interpret both inside and outside diameter discontinuities, a compromise must be made between the angular ranges sensitive to discontinuities in each location. This is achieved by careful adjustment of the angle range based on tests with a reference standard. The transducer is positioned to detect both inside and outside notches with comparable signal amplitude when the reference discontinuity signals are the same distance from the front surface signal.

This adjustment does not give the maximum signal from either discontinuity but it does present discontinuities in their relative size, regardless of their location in the tube or pipe wall. Discontinuities located on the inner surface are the most difficult to detect and it is necessary to demonstrate detectability.

Beam Collimation

When testing tubes that are smaller than the diameter of the transducer, only a short chord of the transducer is used. A collimator is used to confine the sound beam to the proper range of angles. As a result, the linear translation of the transducer per revolution is smaller and full coverage is time consuming.

If proper collimation is used, the effective width approaches the transducer diameter and the linear translation is limited only by the beam diameter. When dealing with larger pipe sizes, collimation may not be necessary — the radius of the pipe is large compared with that of the transducer and a natural collimation occurs. Limited success is encountered when using square or rectangular transducers to obviate collimation. Even with these transducers, proper collimation is essential for best sensitivity.

Gated Discontinuity Alarm

A reference standard is used as an aid in the initial alignment of the transducer relative to the test object. At the same time, instrument adjustments are made to ensure adequate identification of discontinuities with reflecting interfaces equivalent to the notches in the reference standard. As an aid to qualitative interpretation, a gated alarm can be used. If this circuit is adjusted properly with regard to time and sensitivity, only relevant signals actuate the alarm.

The short, diagonal signals on the B-scan pattern do not extend into the gated region and may be ignored because they indicate only of scratches or other insignificant discontinuities. The two diagonal signals that extend into the gate have sufficient amplitude to actuate the alarm and are causes for rejection. Attenuation correction increases the amplification as a function of the distance from the front surface signal. Its application can be helpful by amplifying relevant indications above nonrelevant signals.

Interpretation of Angle Beam Test Indications

Any determination of discontinuity size as a function of a reflected ultrasonic signal is simply a comparison with a known discontinuity in similar material. Inconsistencies may arise from this procedure if the detected discontinuity is not favorably oriented or if it is a nonradial discontinuity.

An estimation of relative discontinuity depth can be obtained from the magnitude of angular rotation through which a tube may turn and still present a detectable discontinuity signal. In general, shallow discontinuities are detectable through less than 1.05 rad (60 deg) of rotation. Signals from deeper

discontinuities may be detected for 1.57 rad (90 deg) or more. Some variation from this rule may occur when testing very small tubes with rejectable discontinuities at depths nearly equal to those of surface scratches.

Nonrelevant Indications

False and nonrelevant discontinuity signals make interpretation difficult but ultrasonic angle beam techniques eliminate the difficulty. Because the test object is rotating, discontinuities move with the same rotational speed, either increasing or decreasing the distance from the transducer or the time from the transducer. A signal that does not exhibit this characteristic time change may be ignored.

Sources of False Indications

Typical causes for false indications, particularly with tubular test objects, include dirt, grease or air bubbles on the inside or outside diameters. If these adhere to the surface, they move with the object and represent an acoustical mismatch leading to sonic reflection. In most instances, such false indications can be removed by cleaning. The inside of a tube should be purged to ensure that the bore is completely filled with water or air, an air-to-water interface being undesirable.

In general, nonrelevant signals originate from small scratches and discontinuities not serious enough to constitute rejectable discontinuities. Several dimensional variations in pipe (ovalness, eccentricity, outside diameter flats or inside diameter gouges) can produce characteristic ultrasonic indications that may or may not be relevant, depending on the test specification.

Crack Indications

Figure 33 illustrates the typical B-scan pattern from an outside diameter crack 0.3 mm (0.01 in.) deep in a 5.8 mm × 0.6 mm (0.2 in. × 0.02 in.) tube. The crack is comparatively short but still presents a readily detectable signal.

Figure 34 illustrates a typical large discontinuity detected by ultrasonics, along with the B-scan pattern obtained from a 0.7 mm (0.03 in.) deep crack in a 6.4 × 1.5 mm (0.25 × 0.06 in.) tube. This crack extends through 55 percent of the tube wall and is longer than the effective sound beam width. The larger B-scan indication is evident through 4.71 rad (270 deg) of rotation.

Among the smallest detectable discontinuities confirmed metallographically is a 38 μm (0.0015 in.)

deep by 1.6 mm (0.06 in.) long crack on the inside diameter of a 4.8 × 0.6 mm (0.20 × 0.02 in.) nickel base alloy tube. The B-scan indication may be identified readily but is much smaller and less brilliant than previous indications.

Figure 35a shows a seam detected with ultrasonic waves on the inside diameter of 19 mm (0.75 in.) schedule 40 pipe. Figure 35b is a typical B-scan pattern obtained from such a discontinuity.

FIGURE 33. Nickel base alloy tube measuring 5.8 × 0.6 mm (0.2 × 0.02 in.) with crack 0.3 mm (0.01 in.) deep: (a) 100× photomicrograph showing cross section of crack in tubing; (b) ultrasonic B-scan indication of crack.

(a)

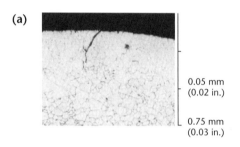

0.05 mm (0.02 in.)

0.75 mm (0.03 in.)

(b)

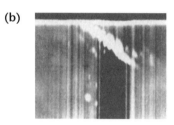

FIGURE 34. Tube measuring 6.4 × 1.5 mm (0.25 × 0.06 in.) with crack 0.7 mm (0.03 in.) deep: (a) 100× photomicrograph showing cross section of crack in tubing; (b) B-scan indication of crack.

(a)

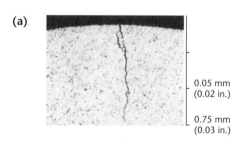

0.05 mm (0.02 in.)

0.75 mm (0.03 in.)

(b)

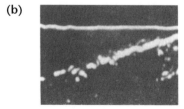

Specifications for Angle Beam Tests

Quality requirements depend on a component's service life and such considerations as the erosion environment, thermal gradients of stresses and mechanical loading, plus cyclic fluctuations in any of these variables. With these requirements in mind, it may be possible to determine the limits of acceptable discontinuities for particular applications.

In many instances, required quality levels may be obtainable from fabricators' stock items. If required quality is higher than normally available from vendors, two approaches may be followed.

1. Components may be specially manufactured and bought at a premium price.
2. Mill run stock is bought and tested at receiving to separate the required high quality materials.

Specified Characteristics

Typical specifications should be very specific and detailed, including statements about the following: outside and inside diameter surface finishes, minimum lengths, dimensional tolerances, the acceptability of certain fabrication techniques (sand blasting, heat treatment, polishing or grinding), in-plant test procedures and acceptable sizes of typical discontinuities.

FIGURE 35. Seam in 19 mm (0.75 in.) pipe: (a) 100× photomicrograph; (b) B-scan.

(a)

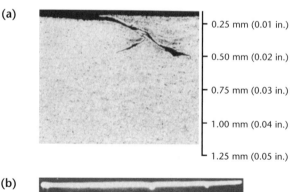

0.25 mm (0.01 in.)

0.50 mm (0.02 in.)

0.75 mm (0.03 in.)

1.00 mm (0.04 in.)

1.25 mm (0.05 in.)

(b)

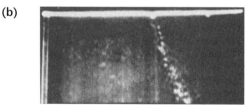

Angle Beam Tests for Misalignment

Angle beam techniques have been applied successfully to seamless tubing, welded and redrawn tubing, welded pipe, welded and rolled pipe and welded and swaged pipe. In general, welds that have been worked or reduced about 25 percent do not offer sufficient mismatch for an echo at the weld interface.

If there has been little or no work subsequent to the welding, a small reflection can occur at the weld interface. This is caused by variations in thickness of the initial metal strip. The resulting echo amplitude is not comparable with a physical misalignment of the parent metal faces at the weld point. Ultrasonic techniques offer an excellent gaging tool for measuring the degree of misalignment for the entire length of the pipe.

Ultrasonic Backscattering

When the limitation of front or far surface resolution is critical, avoiding specular reflection from the front and back test object surfaces can provide a substantial advantage. This approach has been effective for discontinuities in composites, for corrosion and for tests of aluminum laminate materials.[17] The technique is based on the fact that discontinuities (fibers, corrosion, microcracks, porosity) scatter waves backward when the incident wave is normal to their surface.

Angle Beam Testing of Composites

The test setup for composites is shown in Fig. 36. The angle of incidence α is measured with the Z axis (normal to the

plate) and β is the angle of the trajectory with the Y axis.

Figure 37 shows the scattering as a function of rotation angle at a constant angle of incidence for a unidirectional graphite epoxy laminate. Maximum scattering is observed when impinging on fibers at an angle normal to their axes. Surface roughness also contributes to the scattering angular spectrum but is relatively small in amplitude (about 1 dB compared to 8 dB from the fibers). This scattering effect can be eliminated by polishing the surface or by using a coating applied as a fluid over the surface and stripped away after testing.

If the transducer is placed in a plane normal to the fiber axis and the angle of incidence is changed, then the typical response has three maxima: (1) the specular reflection at 0 rad (0 deg), (2) the longitudinal critical angle and (3) the transverse critical angle (Fig. 38). Because maximum scattering is obtained at the

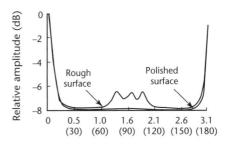

FIGURE 37. Backscattering as function of rotation angle for unidirectional graphite epoxy composite. Amplitude is relative to response at 0 rad (0 deg).

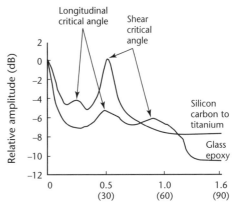

FIGURE 38. Backscattering from composites as function of incidence angle.

FIGURE 36. Setup for ultrasonic tests of backscattering from composites.

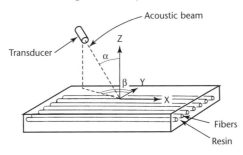

Legend
α = angle of incidence
β = angle between Y axis and the transmitter beam trajectory on the layer plane

critical angles, a high signal-to-noise ratio of backscattering can be obtained.

The excitation of maximum backscattering at angles of rotation normal to the fiber axis can be used to determine fiber orientations. The backscattering pattern for a $[0, \pm45, 90]_S$ laminate is shown in Fig. 39. The various fiber orientations are indicated through the backscattering peak at the appropriate angles. Using a polar scanner, the fiber orientations are made visible in Fig. 40.

FIGURE 39. Backscattering from quasiisotropic graphite epoxy laminate at 0.5 rad (30 deg) angle of incidence.

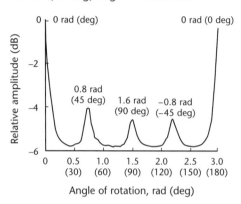

FIGURE 40. Polar backscattering C-scan of various laminates: (a) $[0]_8$; (b) $[0, 90]_{2S}$; (c) $[0, \pm45, 90]$.

(a)

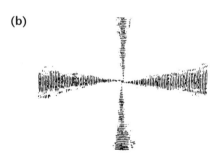

(b)

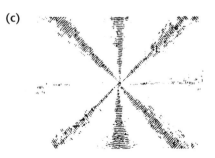

(c)

Backscattering is very sensitive to fiber alignment. This sensitivity provides the ability to make an image of a misalignment with the aid of a polar C-scan system. An example of this application is shown in Fig. 41 for graphite phenolic laminate.

Matrix cracks are common in composites and can serve as origin sites for delaminations. Matrix cracks extend through the thickness of the lamina (a *lamina* being a stack of layers of a given orientation within a laminate). In most cases, matrix cracks are more than an order of magnitude larger than the fiber diameter. For example, the thickness of a graphite ply is about 125 μm (0.005 in.) and the diameter of a fiber is about 5 μm (0.0002 in.).

The backscattering from transverse cracks is more than 30 dB higher than the scattering from the 1.57 rad (90 deg) fibers in a $[0, 90]_{2S}$ laminate. This fact allows the detection and imaging of transverse cracks using a C-scan system, discriminating the scattering amplitude of the cracks from the fibers.

Because fibers generate scattering only at specific angles, they produce a spatial window in the backscattering field. In this window, discontinuities of different scattering directions can be characterized.

As an example, porosity can be detected using such a window in the backscattering spectrum. Porosity tends to accumulate between various layers of the composite laminate. As randomly scattered spheres, porosity does not have a preferred orientation and generates backscattering of equal amplitude for all angles of rotation at a constant incidence angle. Ultrasonic tests for porosity can therefore be conducted with backscattering measurements at angles not normal to any fiber axis.

FIGURE 41. Fiber misalignment in graphite phenolic mold shown by backscattering C-scan imaging.

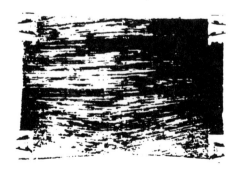

Angle Beam Tests of Metal Composite Laminates

Some common laminated materials are made of aluminum layers bonded with aramid epoxy layers. Cracking can occur in any of these layers. Ultrasonic backscattering techniques are useful for locating interlaminar cracks. The angle of rotation is set in a plane normal to the cracking direction and the angle of incidence is set in the range between the first and the second critical angles for aluminum. The sample test shows cracks at two different layers of aluminum in the laminate. The cracks extend from a hole drilled at the center of the plate and are normal to the direction of the cyclic tensile load.

Corrosion Detection

Corrosion exists in various forms and is typically expressed as a modification of an object's surface shape. A wave impinging on a corroded area is scattered with a relatively large component in the back direction. A typical ultrasonic test setup for corrosion is shown in Fig. 42.

To use the highest signal-to-noise ratio, a condition that allows maximum transmitted transverse waves needs to be determined. Theoretical curves of the reflected and transmitted coefficients for half-space aluminum, immersed in water and impinged by a longitudinal wave, are shown in Fig. 43. The maximum transverse wave transmission coefficient is obtained at a 0.28 rad (16 deg) angle of incidence.

This value has been verified experimentally[16] using a C-scan system and two angles of incidence, 0.28 and 0.35 rad (16 and 20 deg). An aluminum plate was exposed to a salt fog environment for 720 h and then tested with angle beams. Figure 44 shows the results and indicates the advantage of testing at 0.28 rad (16 deg). The corrosion detected in this experiment was not detectable with the straight beam ultrasonic technique.

FIGURE 44. Backscattering C-scan images from corroded aluminum plate:
(a) 280 mrad (16 deg) incidence angle;
(b) 350 mrad (20 deg) incidence angle.

(a)

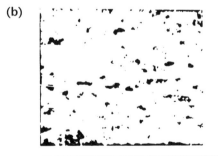

(b)

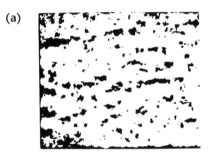

FIGURE 42. Detection of corrosion in multilayered structure by using ultrasonic backscattering.

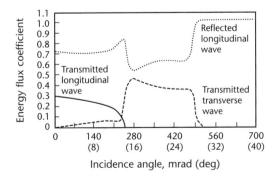

FIGURE 43. Reflection and transmission coefficients versus incident angle for water-to-aluminum interface.

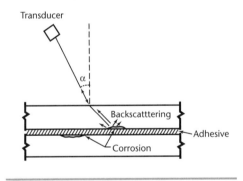

PART 9. Focused Beam Immersion Techniques[1]

Focused Transducers

Sound can be focused by lenses in a manner analogous to focusing light. The basic difference between the two is the ratio of the lens thickness to the wavelength. In optics, the lens thickness is 10^4 to 10^5 times the wavelength. In ultrasonics, the lens thickness is about 10 times the wavelength. As a result, sound waves with opposite phases are emitted from the surface of an acoustic lens in concentric rings several millimeters apart, interfering at the focal plane.

Acoustic lenses can improve testing reliability by reducing and controlling certain energy losses. They are usually an integral part of the transducer assembly. In most applications, the lens concentrates the energy into a long and narrow beam, increasing its intensity. Special sharp focused transducers can be made with a usable test range less than 6.4 mm (0.25 in.). Such a focused technique can resolve a 0.4 mm (0.015 in.) flat bottom hole located 1 mm (0.04 in.) beneath the surface of a steel block. These techniques are particularly useful for tests of thin materials, high resolution C-scan imaging and the determination of bond quality in sandwich structures.

Generally, focused transducers allow the highest possible resolving power with standard equipment because the front surface is not in the focal zone and the concentration of energy at the discontinuity makes its reflection very high, providing a ratio of up to ten thousand to one ($\leq$10 000:1) between the front surface and the discontinuity echo.

Using a cylindrical lens, an improvement in resolving power can be achieved to a lesser degree without decreasing the horizontal width of the beam. With this construction, a 75 mm (3 in.) wide beam can provide clear resolution of discontinuities from about 2.0 mm (0.08 in.) below the surface to a depth of 13 mm (0.5 in.). For standard ultrasonic equipment operating at 10 MHz, such transducers are produced for tests of thin airframe aluminum extrusions.

Focused beams reduce the effect of surface roughness and the effect of multiple minute discontinuities such as grain boundaries and porosity. In addition, these transducers produce plane wave behavior at the focal spot and are used in experimental studies.[18]

Focused techniques are more commonly used in immersion tests, where they are not exposed to wear or erosive conditions. Such transducers are also preferred for tests of curved surfaces. An ultrasonic beam encounters divergence at a curved surface when a flat transducer is used. A focused beam maintains a circular or cylindrical wave front and is not distorted by a curved surface (Fig. 45).

Ultrasonic Lenses

Ultrasonic beams are focused using three basic techniques: (1) a curved, ground piezoelectric material, (2) a plano concave lens cemented to a flat piezoelectric crystal and (3) a biconcave lens placed in front of the transducer. Curved transducers provide a well defined acoustic field with limited noise and energy losses. The need to fix a damper on the back of the crystal (to obtain broad band characteristics) makes curved crystals less practical. Instead, lenses are commonly glued to crystals.

Spherical lenses are used in most nondestructive test applications. When a line focus is needed, cylindrical transducers are used. In some special applications, an external lens is attached in front of a flat transducer to focus its beam and improve test sensitivity. Such lenses produce a certain amount of disturbance and absorption because of materials (such as vulcanized rubber) that contain fillers.

Lens Design Criteria[19]

Lenses can be made of solids or liquids. For most nondestructive test applications, the lens is a solid and the host or the conducting medium is fluid. Under these circumstances, the acoustic velocity is higher in the lens than in the host medium. This produces a converging lens that is concave (the reverse of optic lenses).

When designing an ultrasonic lens, there are several necessary considerations, including acoustic impedance, acoustic velocity, attenuation, fabrication and nonhazardous materials.

Matching acoustic impedances is required to minimize energy loss due to reflections from and within the lens:

(7) $\rho_1 V_1 = \rho_2 V_2$

where V is acoustic velocity (meter per second) and ρ is density. Index 1 values are for the water medium; index 2 values are for the lens medium.

A high index of refraction ($V_2 \cdot V_1^{-1}$) is required to allow a relatively small radius of curvature. The energy absorption and scattering must be as small as possible.

It is difficult to find materials that completely meet lens design requirements. Lenses undergo specific and, in some ways, unique fabrication processes, demanding particular material characteristics within limited tolerances. In addition, when a fluid lens is used, the fluid must not be harmful to personnel and must be inert to the materials it contacts. Materials that meet lens design criteria are listed elsewhere.[1]

The reflection coefficient for most host and lens combinations is significantly high unless a fluid or a lithium lens is used in a fluid host. Note that air has a very low acoustic impedance and cannot be present in any form in an ultrasonic focusing system.

Biconcave Lenses[20]

When a lens is immersed in front of a transducer, the lens must be concave on both surfaces to accommodate beam divergence from the transducer.

Plano-Concave Lenses

When an ultrasonic lens is glued directly to a transducer, then the near field is usually longer than the focal length of the lens and no clear focus can be produced.[20]

With the increase of the angle of aperture, the focus moves toward the lens and the focal area is widened. This reduces the concentration of energy and the accuracy of the focal position.

Focused Beam Profile and Intensity

The theory of focusing radiators are discussed in the literature.[21,22]

The main disadvantages of acoustic lenses are aberrations and the energy loss from reflections and attenuation. Most lenses are made from plastics for a low reflection coefficient, unfortunately plastics are highly attenuative. To reduce attenuation, ultrasonic applications use so-called *zone lenses*, the acoustic equivalent to fresnel lenses in optics.

In a zone lens, rings are scribed on a plate so that every second ring is in phase, generating constructive interference at a predetermined point. This point is dependent on the frequency and is regarded as the focal spot. The rings that are out of phase are covered to eliminate their contribution. Zone lenses have found very limited application in nondestructive testing.

Focal Distance

The focal distance of a transducer is measured experimentally by measuring the reflection from a small ball target. It is assumed that a spherical wave front is produced and the surface of the ball

---

FIGURE 45. Improvement obtained by using focused transducer on curved test surface: (a) distorted A-scan image obtained by flat transducer; (b) elimination of distortion with focused transducer.

(a)

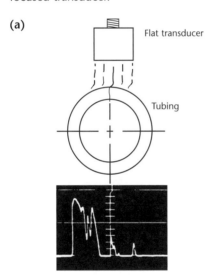

Flat transducer

Tubing

(b)

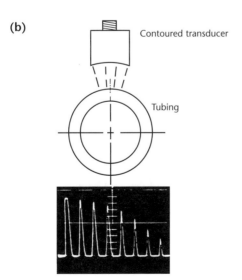

Contoured transducer

Tubing

behaves as an equal phase reflector. The focal point is inferred to be at the geometric center of the ball. When the ball diameter is larger than the diffraction limit, then it is common to add the radius of the ball to the water path. This path is measured by a pulse echo time of flight test. The transducer is moved back and forth with the sphere along its axis until maximum amplitude is measured.

The focal distance becomes shorter when the ultrasonic beam propagates from a fluid to a solid material. The reduction of the focal distance can be determined from a geometrical analysis of the position of the front surface of the material along the beam path (Fig. 46).

Because of the difference in velocities for metal and water, changes of the water path have a relatively small effect on the focal depth in the metal. The metal surface forms a second lens much more powerful than the acoustical lens itself. This effect pulls the focal spot very close to the metal surface, compared to the focal length of a transducer in water.

The second lens has three other important effects: it sharpens the beam, increases the sensitivity to objects in the focal zone and it makes the transducer act as a very directional and distance sensitive receiver. Large increases in sensitivity are produced by these complex interactions. This makes it possible to locate minute discontinuities and to study areas that produce very low amplitude reflections — for example, the bond between stainless steel and electroformed copper.

Pencil Shape Focus

In many ultrasonic applications, a long focused beam is required to test a large depth range. Two lens configurations produce such a focused beam.[23] The long axial test ranges are limited mainly by the rate at which signal amplitude falls off in the far field of the beam.

Acoustic Microscopy

An acoustic microscope uses acoustic waves and a set of one or more lenses to obtain information about the elastic microstructural properties of test objects. The finest detail resolvable by an acoustic microscope is determined by the diffraction limit of the system. Such microscopes are available commercially for tests of thin structures such as integrated circuits.[24] The acoustic microscope can also be used to study bond integrity, microstructure formation and material stress effects.

In scanning acoustic microscopes (SAM), a piezoelectric crystal is bonded to a sapphire or quartz substrate to which it transmits plane waves. At the back of the substrate is a spherical lens machined with a low reflection coating (Fig. 47). The lens produces a highly focused beam in water allowing the pair — transducer and lens — to operate as a focused transducer in a pulse echo mode. A shallow region close to the surface of the test material is examined.

The scanning procedure is similar to an ultrasonic C-scan and produces an image of the test area on the monitor. The contrast of the image is determined by the

FIGURE 47. Diagram of scanning acoustic microscope.

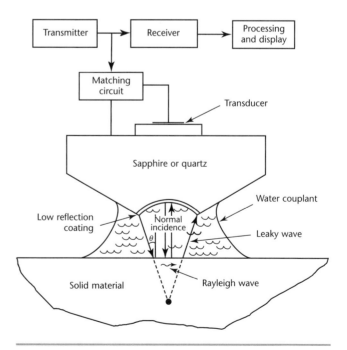

FIGURE 46. Ultrasonic focus effect in metals, demonstrating effect of second lens as result of immersion in water.

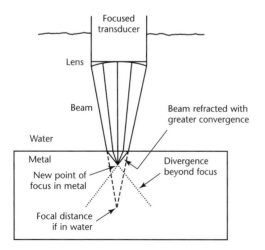

surface reflectivity of the test object and the phase of the reflected wave. Some of the rays from the lens are incident to the rayleigh angle on the surface, as determined by Snell's law:

$$(8) \qquad \sin \theta_r \ = \ \frac{V_w}{V_r}$$

where V_w is the acoustic wave velocity in water (meter per second) and V_r is the rayleigh or surface velocity of the test material (meter per second).

The rayleigh wave leaks energy into the couplant and this is transmitted by the lens to the transducer. Thus, the lens receives two components: specular reflection and the leaky rayleigh waves. The two components interfere, depending on the distance h between the surface and the focal point. The received amplitude $V(h)$ changes (1) as a function of h and (2) when scanning parallel to the surface and insonifying a material discontinuity. The interference associated with the leaky rayleigh waves provides the scanning acoustic microscope with high sensitivity to surface property changes.

A single lens can be used to produce a scanning acoustic microscope (SAM). An acoustic pulse is transmitted and examined by the SAM system, for reduced phase sensitivity. A microscope at low megahertz frequencies has been used in a detailed study of damage distribution in composites.[25]

Laminate Test Indications

Focused Beam Tests of Laminates

Focused beam techniques have proven valuable for testing multilayered structures composed of aluminum sheets bonded with layers of aramid. Such laminate structures tend to suffer from disbonding in various layers. Focused beams can be used to detect delaminations and to determine their depth.

With the aid of a pulse echo technique and a broad band high frequency focused transducer, images of delaminations at the various layers have been made.[17]

Focused Beam Bond Testing

When a reflected ultrasonic wave impinges on a bonded structure, its amplitude is reduced. This occurs because of a partial transmission of energy to the adhesive media rather than complete reflection by the interface of solid to air in the unbonded plate.

A focused transducer and a normal beam can detect relatively small unbonds

in both metals and composite assemblies.[26] The test object is scanned and its response is analyzed by comparison to a reference standard.

Summary of Pulse Echo Immersion Techniques

Ultrasonic techniques are implemented primarily in the pulse echo and through-transmission modes, with contact or immersion coupling. Pulse echo immersion is a coupling technique not commonly used in field applications because of the difficulty of maintaining the couplant. Several means are commercially available to overcome the limitations of immersion coupling, including wheels and boots.

Pulse echo techniques provide very detailed information about test objects. This capability is attributed to the various parameters that can be analyzed, including time of flight, amplitude of back surface reflection and amplitude of extraneous reflections.

Pulse echo immersion may be used with materials made of metal, plastic, composites and ceramics — the raw materials for most engineering structures. A wide variety of discontinuities can be detected and characterized with pulse echo techniques, where the location, depth, size and discontinuity type can be determined.

PART 10. Acoustical Holography[27]

Acoustical holography is a technique used to form an optical image of an ultrasonic field. Although not widely applied, it is useful in nondestructive testing because of its excellent lateral resolution, its ability to focus deep within the test volume and its speed of data collection.

Focused Piezoelectric Crystal

Two types of acoustical holography equipment have proven useful for nondestructive test applications. In one system, a hologram is formed by scanning a focused piezoelectric crystal over a plane. This technique has been used to map voids and inclusions in thick walled metal components.[28] The technique also has proven superior to conventional pulse echo techniques for sizing and determining the true geometry of discontinuities.[29]

The piezoelectric element is usually focused on the test surface and is used as the ultrasonic source and receiver. A complete scan provides a holographic record. Although versions before 1980 captured the hologram on photographic film, the practice since 1990 has been to make a digital record of the holographic data. These data can then be processed by computer to focus at any depth. This focusing capability makes possible the measurement of the size and shape of any object or discontinuity in the field of view. Holograms can be made using either longitudinal or transverse waves.

Measurement accuracy depends on the depth of the discontinuity, the size of the scan plane and the wavelength of the ultrasound in the test material. The uncertainty of lateral dimensional measurement ΔB is given by:

$$(9) \quad \Delta B = \frac{r}{2L}\lambda$$

where L is the width of the square scan plane (millimeter), r is discontinuity depth (millimeter) and λ is wavelength (millimeter) of ultrasound in the test material.

The depth at which the discontinuity lies is best obtained by time-of-flight techniques as used in conventional ultrasonic testing.

Liquid Surface Detector

The second type of acoustical holography equipment uses a liquid surface as an ultrasonic detector.[30]

Holographic images of ultrasonic fields produced by liquid surface detectors give realistic displays of relative ultrasonic intensity levels. A tone burst of ultrasound, 50 to 100 μs in duration, is generated by an object beam transducer. Ultrasound from the objective beam transducer propagates through the test material. Ultrasonic lenses act on the transmitted ultrasound to project an image of the test object on the liquid surface. A second beam of ultrasound, generated by the reference beam transducer, is mixed with the object beam at the liquid surface (detector) to form an interference pattern that shapes the liquid surface into a grating. The amplitude of the grating is proportional to the product of the object beam and the reference beam pressure amplitudes.

When the grating is illuminated by coherent infrared energy from a laser diode, some of the energy is diffracted. Where the grating amplitude is great, more infrared radiation is diffracted; where it is small, less infrared radiation is diffracted. A video system forms an image of the test object by using the light diffracted into the first order. Thus, the liquid surface, illuminated by a laser diode, converts an ultrasonic field pattern into an optical field pattern that can be read by a closed circuit video system.

Images formed in 100 μs are produced at video frame rates (60 images per second). The response time of the liquid surface allows the formation of up to 300 images per second. This characteristic of the liquid surface allows testing rates up to 20 m²·h⁻¹ (215 ft²·h⁻¹). At any instant, a 75 × 75 mm (3 × 3 in.) field in the test object is seen. Using 5 MHz ultrasound, the field displays 5625 resolvable picture elements instantaneously. Thus, test speed and resolution are the strong features of the system.

The system can be calibrated to measure the absolute attenuation of the object. Video pixel brightness is used as an indicator of attenuation.[31]

Liquid surface imaging systems have been very useful on the quality assurance programs of manufacturers of large graphite composite materials used in the aircraft industry where they have been proven to provide superior resolution of detail coupled with an inspection speed six times greater than that of conventional scanned technique systems.

References

1. Bar-Cohen, Y. Section 8, "Ultrasonic Pulse Echo Immersion Techniques." *Nondestructive Testing Handbook,* second edition: Vol. 7, *Ultrasonic Testing*. Columbus, OH: American Society for Nondestructive Testing (1991): p 219-266.
2. Singh, G.P. and J.W. Davies. Section 9, "Multiple Transducer Ultrasonic Techniques." *Nondestructive Testing Handbook,* second edition: Vol. 7, *Ultrasonic Testing*. Columbus, OH: American Society for Nondestructive Testing (1991): p 267-309.
3. Kulkarni, S.B. "NDT Catches Up with Composite Technology." *Machine Design*. Cleveland, OH: Penton (April 1983): p 38-45.
4. Krautkrämer, J. and H. Krautkrämer. *Ultrasonic Testing of Materials,* fourth edition. New York, NY: Springer (1990).
5. Bar-Cohen, Y., E. Harnik, M. Meron and R. Davidson. "Ultrasonic Nondestructive Evaluation Method for the Detection and Identification of Defects in Filament Wound Glass Fiber-Reinforced Plastic Tubes." *Materials Evaluation*. Vol. 37, No. 8. Columbus, OH: American Society for Nondestructive Testing (July 1979): p 51-55.
6. Ophir, J. and P. Jaeger. "Spectral Shifts of Ultrasonic Propagation through Media with Nonlinear Dispersive Attenuation." *Ultrasonic Imaging*. Vol. 4. New York, NY: Academic Press (1982): p 282-289.
7. Kinsler, L.E, A.R. Frey, A.B. Coppens and J.V. Sanders. *Fundamentals of Acoustics,* fourth edition. New York, NY: Wiley (1999).
8. Herzfeld, K. and T. Litovitz. *Absorption and Dispersion of Ultrasonic Waves*. New York, NY: Academic Press (1959).
9. Rose, J. "Elements of Feature-Based Ultrasonic Inspection System." *Materials Evaluation*. Vol. 42, No. 2. Columbus, OH: American Society for Nondestructive Testing (February 1984): p 210-226.
10. Gubernatis, J. "Elastic Wave Scattering Methods: Assessments and Suggestions." *Review of Progress in Quantitative Nondestructive Evaluation* [Williamsburg, VA, June 1985]. Vol. 5A. New York, NY: Plenum (1986): p 21-23.
11. Chang, F.H., P.L. Flynn, D.E. Gordon and J.R. Bell. "Principles and Application of Ultrasonic Spectroscopy in NDE of Adhesive Bonds." *IEEE Transactions on Sonics and Ultrasonics*. Vol. SU-23, No. 5. New York, NY: Institute of Electrical and Electronics Engineers (October 1976): p 334-338.
12. Gericke, O. and B. Monagle. "Detection of Delaminations by Ultrasonic Spectroscopy." *Transactions on Sonics and Ultrasonics*. Vol. SU-23, No. 5. New York, NY: Institute of Electrical and Electronics Engineers (1976): p 339-345.
13. Kleint, R. "Relationship between Defect Orientation and Ultrasonic Indications." *Nondestructive Testing*. Vol. 15, No. 1. Columbus, OH: American Society for Nondestructive Testing (January-February 1957): p 30-34.
14. *Investigation of Metallurgical Sample of 4340 Steel*. Report No. 330, Seattle, WA: Boeing (1955).
15. Bar-Cohen, Y. "NDE of Fiber Reinforced Composite Materials — A Review." *Materials Evaluation*. Vol. 44, No. 4. Columbus, OH: American Society for Nondestructive Testing (April 1986): p 446-454.
16. Bar-Cohen, Y., U. Arnon and M. Meron. "Defect Detection and Characterization in Composite Sandwich Structures by Ultrasonics." *SAMPE Journal*. Vol. 14, No. 1. Covina, CA: Society for the Advancement of Material and Process Engineering (1978): p 4-9.
17. Bar-Cohen, Y. "Nondestructive Characterization of Defects Using Ultrasonic Backscattering Measurements." *Ultrasonics International 87* [London, United Kingdom, July 1987]. Surrey, United Kingdom: Butterworth (July 1987): p 345-352.
18. Born, M. and E. Wolf. *Principles of Optics*. Oxford, United Kingdom: Pergamon (1970).
19. Lees, S. "Useful Criteria in Describing the Field Pattern of Focusing Transducers." *Ultrasonics*. Vol. 16, No. 5. Surrey, United Kingdom: Butterworth (1978): p 219-436.

20. Tarnoczy, T. "Sound Focusing Lenses and Waveguides." *Ultrasonics.* Vol. 3. Amsterdam, Netherlands: Elsevier (July-September 1965): p 115-127.

21. Madsen, E., M. Goodsitt and J. Zagzebski. "Continuous Waves Generated by Focusing Radiators." *Journal of the Acoustical Society of America.* Vol. 70, No. 5. Melville, NY: American Institute of Physics, for the Acoustical Society of America (1981): p 1508-1517.

22. O'Neil, H. "Theory of Focusing Radiators." *Journal of the Acoustical Society of America.* Vol. 21, No. 5. Melville, NY: American Institute of Physics, for the Acoustical Society of America (1949): p 516-526.

23. Turner, J. Report No. 313, *Development of Novel Focused Ultrasonic Transducers for NDT.* Cambridge, United Kingdom: The Welding Institute (1986).

24. Lemons, P. and C. Quate. "Acoustic Microscope." *Physical Acoustics: Principles and Methods.* Vol. 14. New York, NY: Academic Press (1979): p 1-92.

25. Khuri-Yakub, B.T., P. Reinholdtsen and J.L. Arnaud. "Nondestructive Evaluation of Composite Materials Using Acoustic Microscopy." *Review of Progress in Quantitative Nondestructive Evaluation* [Williamsburg, VA, June 1985]. Vol. 5B. New York, NY: Plenum (1985): p 1093-1098.

26. Hagemaier, D. and R. Fassbender. "Nondestructive Testing of Adhesive Bonded Structures." *SAMPE Quarterly.* Vol. 9. Covina, CA: Society for the Advancement of Material and Process Engineering (July 1978): p 36-58.

27. Brenden, B.B. "Acoustical Holography." *Nondestructive Testing Handbook,* second edition: Vol. 7, *Ultrasonic Testing.* Columbus, OH: American Society for Nondestructive Testing (1991): p 794-796.

28. Brenden, B.B. and H.D. Collins. "Acoustical Holography with Scanned Hologram Systems." *Holographic Nondestructive Testing.* New York, NY: Academic Press (1974): p 405-428.

29. Holt, A.E. and W.E. Lawrie. "Ultrasonic Characterization of Defects." *Acoustical Holography.* Vol. 7. New York, NY: Plenum (1977): p 599-609.

30. Sokolov, S. United States Patent 2 164 125, *Means for Indicating Flaws in Materials* (1937).

31. Hildebrand, B.P. and B.B. Brenden. *An Introduction to Acoustical Holography.* New York, NY: Plenum (1972).

CHAPTER

Ultrasonic Characterization of Material Properties[1]

Alex Vary, North Olmsted, Ohio

PART 1. Fundamentals of Material Property Characterization

To different degrees, elastic moduli, material microstructure, morphological conditions and associated mechanical properties can be characterized by ultrasonic testing. Elastic moduli are determined by speed measurements. Material microstructure can be characterized by speed and attenuation measurements. Ultrasonic assessments of mechanical properties (strength or toughness) are indirect and depend on either theoretical inferences or empirical correlations. Four categories of ultrasonic materials characterization are shown in Table 1: (1) measurements that determine elastic constants such as tensile, shear and bulk moduli, (2) microstructural and morphological factors such as grain size and distribution, grain aspect ratio and texture, (3) diffuse discontinuity populations such as microporosity or microcracking and (4) mechanical properties such as strength, hardness and toughness. Mechanical properties are extrinsic and depend on elastic properties and material microstructure and morphology. The directly measured

quantities are ultrasonic speed and attenuation.

Rationale for Using Ultrasonic Techniques

The usual objective in nondestructive testing is to detect and characterize a variety of discrete hidden discontinuities that can impair the integrity and reduce the service life of a structure. Such discontinuities include cracks in metals, delaminations in composites and inclusions in ceramics. Although a structure may be free of distinct identifiable discontinuities, it may still be susceptible to failure because of inadequate or degraded mechanical properties. This can arise from faulty material processing, over aging, degradation under aggressive service environments or from the other factors listed in Table 2. Because of poor microstructure and morphology, a solid may lack strength, toughness or may exhibit degraded resistance to impact,

TABLE 1. Ultrasonic materials characterization categories dependent on physical and geometric constraints given in Table 3.

Elastic Constants[a]	Microstructure and Morphology[b]	Diffuse Discontinuity[b]	Mechanical Properties[c]
Tensile modulus	Mean grain size	Microcracking	Tensile strength
Shear modulus	Grain size distribution	Crazing	Shear strength
Flexural modulus	Grain aspect ratio	Microporosity	Interlaminar strength
Bulk modulus	Texture	Inclusions	Yield strength
Young's modulus	Anisotropy	Aggregates	Ductility
Poisson's ratio	Density variations	Precipitates	Hardness
Lamé constant	Dispersoid variations	Fiber breakage	Fracture toughness
	Whisker/fiber bunching and maldistribution	Segregations	Fatigue resistance
		Porosity	Impact resistance
		Shock damage	
		Impact damage	
		Fatigue damage	
		Creep damage	
		Fiber/matrix interface voids	

a. Well established speed relations and dynamic resonance relations for simple shapes and laboratory samples. Both are comparative when applied to complex geometries.
b. Indirect; based on scatter attenuation and speed dispersion models and theories.
c. Indirect; comparative and based primarily on empirical correlations with speed and attenuation characteristics governed by microstructural and morphological factors.

fatigue or fracture. For these reasons, it is important to have nondestructive methods for characterizing local or global anomalies in microstructure or morphology and their associated mechanical property deficiencies.[2-5]

The best approach to reliability assurance combines nondestructive characterization of discontinuities with characterization of material environments in which the discontinuities reside. Assessments of structural integrity and service life can be improved by providing more complete information for fracture analysis and life prediction. This approach is needed to assess the structural reliability and residual life of components made of advanced materials in systems that demand efficient performance under extreme operating conditions.[6]

Relation to Materials Research

In materials research, the term *materials characterization* is conventionally understood to involve some form of destructive testing. However, nondestructive techniques should be used in materials research before and during destructive testing. This is especially the case for complex materials such as advanced polymeric, metallic and ceramic matrix composites. Application of ultrasonic and other nondestructive methods enhances materials characterization, understanding of failure mechanisms and explanation of behavior.

TABLE 2. Causes of material failure that can be characterized and assessed by ultrasonic nondestructive testing.

Processing Faults	Service Degradation
Texture and anisotropy	Altered microstructure
Wrong phase composition	Corrosion or chemical attack
Inclusions, agglomerates	Excessive deformation
Embrittling impurities	Excessive residual stress
Wrong grain structure	Overheating, decomposition
Faulty heat treatment	Fatigue or creep damage
Faulty case hardening	Decarburization
Faulty surface treatment	Stress corrosion
Incomplete polymerization	Radiation damage
Wrong fiber fraction	Gas embrittlement
High microvoid content	Moisture damage, absorption
Fiber bunching, segregation	Matrix softening, crazing
Fiber or ply misalignments	Impact or shock damage

Relation to Fracture Analysis

Nondestructive testing is frequently based on the need to detect critical discontinuities with dimensions specified by fracture analysis. Fracture analysis and the prediction of safe service life, in turn, depend on the assumption of an accurate set of mechanical properties. Fracture analysis presupposes discontinuity growth in materials with *known* moduli, ultimate strength, fracture toughness and fatigue and creep properties. Nondestructive methods that verify and characterize these properties can be used to validate fracture analyses and life predictions. Fracture analysis and analytical life prediction methods should be supplemented by ultrasonics and other nondestructive test techniques that can verify properties, structural integrity and reliability.[7]

Relation to Structural Materials

A survey of ultrasonic technology is presented below to indicate potential applications for nondestructive characterization of mechanical properties in structural materials. Ultrasonic techniques are covered that can be used to monitor extrinsic properties (tensile, shear and yield strengths, fracture toughness, hardness and ductility), elastic moduli and underlying microstructural and morphological factors.

The emphasis is on nondestructive testing of structural materials that arise in applications where high strength and toughness, low weight and high durability are required under aggressive service conditions, such as high temperature power and propulsion systems. The materials can include structural ceramics, metallics and their composite forms, such as particulate and whisker toughened ceramics and such as metallic, intermetallic and ceramic fiber reinforced composites. The usual applications are directed toward the evaluation of bulk properties in engineering solids with extensions to surfaces, substrates, bonded interfaces and protective coatings.

PART 2. Material Characterization Methods

There are a variety of mechanical wave techniques suitable for nondestructive materials characterization, including sonic and dynamic vibration methods. Acoustic emission testing is also included here because of its ability to reveal crucial material variables. Pulse echo, through-transmission and other ultrasonic interrogation techniques are discussed, along with signal analysis.

Although methods for global property evaluation are described, the emphasis is on methods that deal with smaller volumes within components at a given time. These methods include acoustic microscopy and analytical ultrasonics for quantitative characterization of materials down to the microstructural level. In materials research, such methods are used to monitor and characterize material response and microstructural behavior.

Sonic and Dynamic Vibration Techniques

Sonic Analysis

Sonic tests are among the oldest forms of nondestructive testing. They typically involve striking (coin tapping) an object to determine if it rings true.[8] In some types of instrumented sonic testing, the signals are inaudible and must be acquired electronically.

Sonic analysis tests are nondestructive if strain amplitudes are quite small and leave the material unaltered. They may be applied to simple laboratory specimens and also to structural components having complex shapes. Automated signature analysis is used to infer the integrity and internal condition of a range of structural components.[9]

Dynamic Resonance

Dynamic resonance testing assesses physical and mechanical properties of certain materials by evaluating the resonant vibration frequency.[10] If excited properly, most solids exhibit sonic resonances, typically in the frequency range below 20 kHz. Elastic moduli can be calculated if the dimensions, density and resonant frequency are known.

There are direct empirical relations between tensile moduli and resonant frequencies of structural components. It is possible to quickly confirm mechanical properties of a test object by comparing it with a known reference standard having the same shape and dimensions. The underlying relation is that the resonant frequency is the product of a shape factor and a physical factor. The shape factor includes length, width and thickness. The physical factor is a combination of modulus, density and Poisson's ratio.

Damping Measurement

Although dynamic resonance testing uses sustained forced vibrations, damping measurement uses the vibration's free decay.[11-13] The test object is isolated from external forces after excitation and either of two quantities can be measured: (1) the specific damping capacity or internal friction of the material or (2) a comparative structural damping factor of actual components.

Specific damping capacity D is a function of the logarithmic decrement d expressed in terms of the amplitude loss suffered by successive oscillations of a freely vibrating sample. The relation between D and d is:

$$(1) \quad D = 2d = 2 \ln \frac{A_N}{A_{N+1}}$$

where A_N is the amplitude of the Nth cycle (volts) and A_{N+1} is the amplitude of the next cycle (volts).[14]

Structural damping is not as sensitive as dynamic resonance to size, shape and other geometric factors. Although there are exceptions, damping values D tend to be small in most engineering materials.[9] Damping measurements are generally sensitive to discontinuities and damage, provided that extraneous damping from supports and fixtures is minimized. With simple excitation methods (point impulse), several simultaneous vibrational modes can be excited. These can be analyzed separately by computer for all frequency components and modes.

Applications of Dynamic Sonic Vibration

Dynamic sonic vibration techniques are suitable for studying microstructure dependent properties. Damping and resonant frequency measurements can be used to monitor phase transformations, plastic deformation, hardening, cold working and alloy composition effects.[15] Dynamic sonic and damping methods are used to evaluate porosity and density in ceramics, fiber-to-resin ratios in composites, bond strength in laminates,[16] nodularity and texture in metals[17] and strengthening by dispersoids in alloys.[18]

In its basic form, dynamic resonance affords a quick and convenient check for determining whether an object has appropriate mechanical properties or has undergone loss of elasticity or tensile strength. Elastic moduli and dynamic constants of structural materials can be assessed for predicting dynamic response, as discussed below.

Acoustic Emission Techniques

Acoustic emission is a passive phenomenon relying on spontaneous, transient, usually inaudible ultrasonic signals such as those released during mechanical deformation or thermal stressing (see the *Nondestructive Testing Handbook: Acoustic Emission Testing*). Acoustic emission frequencies range from the audible (sonic) to several megahertz (ultrasonic). Acoustic emission can arise when a material undergoes metallurgical transformations (twinning) or dislocation movements, plastic yielding or microcracking.[19]

Passive sensors are fixed to the surface of a test object and are selected to ensure sensitivity to signals generated at some distance by microdisturbances and other weak sources. Operational methods include event counts, ringdown counts, energy or amplitude distribution analysis, waveform analysis and frequency spectrum analysis.[20,21]

Applications

The objective of acoustic emission testing is the detection and location of incipient discontinuities. The spontaneous stress waves that constitute acoustic emission can be analyzed to obtain information concerning discontinuities' characteristics, location, abundance and distributions during the loading or proof testing of structures.[22,23] Acoustic emission testing monitors the presence and severity of growing cracks, plastic deformation or delaminations.

The acoustic emission technique also affords a means for monitoring structural integrity and dynamic response and for inferring the current internal condition or state of degradation in structural components. Examples of in-process monitoring of materials are available in the literature,[24,25] especially for solidification processes such as spot welding and heavy section welding.

Another objective of acoustic emission testing is source characterization.[26] This is hampered by signal modifications in transducers, instrumentation and especially the material. Signal modification by material microstructure, texture, diffuse discontinuity populations, mode conversions and reflections at boundary surfaces make it inherently difficult to quantitatively infer the exact nature of emitting sources.[27] Because source characteristics are usually unknown, acoustic emission is not used for quantitative characterization of microstructure or material properties.

Pulse Echo Technique

The ultrasonic pulse echo technique is a key method for materials characterization. It is widely used for making precise measurements of ultrasonic speed and attenuation. These two measurements are the bases for accurately evaluating elastic moduli, characterizing microstructure and for assessing mechanical properties.

The pulse echo technique uses a broad band, buffered piezo transducer that emits and collects ultrasonic signals. The transducer is held in contact with the test object at normal incidence. Contact with the test object is generally preferred over separation by a liquid buffer or immersion coupling medium. A solid buffer rod with low attenuation (usually quartz or fused silica) is integrated into the transducer case and provides the means for isolating a series of back echoes. The buffer delays front surface echoes and prevents them from becoming confused with reverberations in the piezoelectric crystal. The length of the buffer is dictated by the test object thickness and the number of echoes that need to be included within the buffer time delay. The frequency range for most engineering solids is from about 300 kHz to about 400 MHz.

Constraints on Pulse Echo Technique

Ideally, the test object must have smooth, flat, parallel opposing surfaces and should meet the constraints for precise signal analysis prescribed in Table 3. In addition, sufficient force on the transducer is required to squeeze out excess couplant between it and the test object.[28,29] The transducer collects a set of echoes returned by the front and back surfaces of the test object. Signal acquisition, processing and analysis methods are described in this volume and in the literature.[4,30-34]

Many kinds of test objects are appropriate for pulse echo ultrasonics, including rectangular components, sheet stock, bar stock and cylindrical rods. For complex objects, the need for perpendicular alignment of the transducer's axis with a test object's surface may demand certain design accommodations to satisfy the constraints in Table 3.

Note that direct, normal incidence reflections may *not* occur even if test object shape and boundaries meet the conditions given in Table 3. If the material is anisotropic, is orthotropic or contains microstructural gradients,[4] there may be multiple skewed quasilongitudinal and quasitransverse wave paths.

Pulse Echo Signal Processing

For speed measurements, the objective is to establish the exact time interval needed for a signal to travel between the front and back surface of a test object. Signal analysis yields the group speed and frequency dependent phase speeds (the speed dispersion characteristics of the material). For attenuation measurements, the objective is to determine the energy loss experienced by signals that traverse a test object. Signal analysis yields the attenuation coefficient as a function of frequency (the attenuation spectrum unique to the material). Using computers, both measurements can be made at once by collecting a series of echoes returned by the back surface of the test object.

Signal analysis can be done in either the time domain or the frequency domain depending on need and convenience. The simplest and usually least accurate measurements use time domain records of voltage (A-scans). Either analog or digitized records can be used for estimating speed and attenuation. The preferred method is to use digital fourier transforms to determine the frequency dependence of speed and attenuation over a broad frequency range. Generally, data needed for materials characterization are likely to be deficient unless they are based on broad band phase speed and attenuation spectrum analysis.

Speed Measurement

The four primary approaches to speed measurement using the pulse echo technique are the peak detection and echo overlap methods[30] or the cross correlation and phase measurement methods.[35]

Peak detection and echo overlap are sufficiently accurate if the echoes are not seriously distorted by dispersion effects. The cross correlation method gives group speed and is most useful with noisy signals such as those found in coarse materials and fiber reinforced composites. The phase method is used to determine the phase speed as a function of frequency.[35-38]

The cross correlation or group speed of the first two echoes B_1 and B_2 is given by:

$$(2) \quad v = \frac{2X}{\tau_0}$$

where X is the test object thickness (meter) and τ is the time shift (second).

TABLE 3. Constraints on the test object necessary to ensure precise ultrasonic attenuation and speed measurements.

Recommended Constraints	Ambiguities Eliminated
Normal incidence probing	Miscalculation of texture, anisotropy or wave paths
Clean, smooth surfaces	Poor transducer coupling and couplant reverberations
Flat, parallel surfaces	Deflected or distorted signals and oblique signal paths
Geometrically simple shapes	Signal path untraceability
Minimum thickness and length	Excess attenuation losses and low signal-to-noise ratios
Precise physical dimensions	Significant attenuation and speed measurement errors
Large test object-to-transducer area	Sidewall and edge effects
Accessibility of key areas[a]	Inability to characterize critical zones or volumes
Absence of overt discontinuities[b]	Spurious signals unrelated to material properties

a. Actual test objects may not lend themselves to precise characterization unless design accommodations are made to facilitate testing.
b. It is assumed that appropriate nondestructive testing has been applied to screen out objects with overt discontinuities that can interfere with materials characterization.

The value of τ in Eq. 3 is $-\infty \le \tau \le \infty$ and is determined by the maximum value of Eq. 3:

$$(3) \quad \tau_n = \left| \int_{-\infty}^{+\infty} B_1(t) B_2(t-\tau) dt \right|$$

The phase speed is given by:

$$(4) \quad v(f) = \frac{4 X \pi f}{\Delta B}$$

where:

$$(5) \quad \Delta B = B_2 - B_1$$

$$(6) \quad B_1(f) = \tan^{-1} \frac{I_m \left[B_1(f) \right]}{R_e \left[B_1(f) \right]}$$

$$(7) \quad B_2(f) = \tan^{-1} \frac{I_m \left[B_2(f) \right]}{R_e \left[B_2(f) \right]}$$

where f is frequency (hertz), I_m is an imaginary number and R_e is a real number.

Attenuation Measurement

The quantities B_1, B_2, I_1, I_2 and R are functions of frequency (fourier transforms of corresponding time domain quantities). The quantities B_1, B_2, I_1 and I_2 are spectra of corresponding waveforms. The reflection coefficient R of the front surface is generally also a function of frequency.

The reflection coefficient can be defined either in terms of energy (intensity) or amplitude (pressure).[39] Taking R as the reflection coefficient and T as the transmission coefficient across an interface from medium 1 to medium 2, the definition for energy is:

$$(8) \quad R + T = 1$$

$$(9) \quad R = \left(\frac{z_1 - z_2}{z_1 + z_2} \right)^2$$

$$(10) \quad T = \frac{4 z_1 z_2}{\left(z_1 + z_2 \right)^2}$$

where z_1 and z_2 are acoustic impedances of media 1 and 2:

$$(11) \quad z_1 = \rho_1 v_1$$

$$(12) \quad z_2 = \rho_2 v_2$$

where ρ_1 and ρ_2 are densities (kilogram per cubic meter) and v_1 and v_2 are phase speeds in the media (meter per second).

The preceding equations for reflection and transmission apply to ideal interfaces that have no thickness. When there is a finite thickness that greatly exceeds the transmitted ultrasonic wavelengths, the transmission and reflection coefficients are frequency dependent.[40] In general, the reflection coefficient as a function of frequency can be determined:

$$(13) \quad |R(f)| = \left| \frac{F_2(f)}{F_1(f)} \right|$$

where the fourier spectra of echoes from the end of the buffer are $F_1(f)$ and $F_2(f)$, with and without coupling to the test object, respectively.[41]

The reflection coefficient is unity (1) at the free back surface of the test object. Internal echo I_1 is the source of the signal B_1. A part of the energy of I_1 is reflected and appears as the second internal echo I_2 giving the reduced echo B_2, thus:

$$(14) \quad B_1 = G(1 - R) I_1$$

$$(15) \quad B_2 = G H R (1 - R) I_1$$

The quantity H represents a transfer function of the material defined in terms of the attenuation suffered by a pulse traveling twice the test object thickness X:

$$(16) \quad H = \exp(-2 X \alpha)$$

where α is the attenuation coefficient. Like B_1, B_2, G, R and T, α is a function of frequency and plots of α versus f are sometimes termed *attenuation spectra*.

The quantity G is a combination of transfer functions associated with instrumentation, signal transduction and other aspects of the signal acquisition system. In the pulse echo technique, G drops out of the expression for the attenuation coefficient found by solving the preceding equations. For example, the attenuation coefficient may be written as:[30,34]

$$(17) \quad \alpha = \frac{1}{2X} \ln \left(R \frac{B_1}{B_2} \right)$$

This equation is the deconvolution of echo B_1 with respect to B_2 as modified by the reflection coefficient function R.

Expressions for the attenuation coefficient can be derived by considering various energy loss mechanisms. Examples of the attenuation coefficient for different loss mechanisms are given in Table 4 for typical polycrystalline solids.

Pulse Echo Applications

The pulse echo technique is preferred for precise measurements of attenuation and velocity spectra that can in turn be used for quantitative characterization of microstructure and assessment of material properties. Mechanical properties and morphological conditions that can be evaluated by the pulse echo method are listed in Table 5.[5] The variables R, T, B_1, B_2 and hence attenuation and velocity spectra are affected by the properties of

bulk microstructures, interfaces, bonds, substrates, coatings and like factors that govern material response and integrity (see the discussion of microstructure and diffuse discontinuities, below).

Backscatter Technique

The backscattering of ultrasonic waves is caused by discontinuities in density and speed, that is, by the jump in acoustic impedance $\Delta \rho v$ encountered at phase and grain boundaries in metals or fiber matrix interfaces in composites. In the backscatter technique, the appearance of random stochastic reflections (between B_1 and B_2 or between the front surface echo and B_1) is of interest. The two key parameters that govern the nature and magnitude of scattering are $\Delta \rho v$ and $a \cdot \lambda^{-1}$. These include changes in acoustic impedance and ratio of scatterer size a to wavelength λ used to characterize microstructure. By using time domain waveforms or frequency domain spectra, it is possible to infer mean grain size, presence and distribution of inclusions.

The usual application of backscattering measurements is for nondestructive grain size determination.[42-44] The backscatter approach has also proved useful for measuring global heterogeneities such as those from segregations and inclusions in metals and ceramics. In addition, backscatter measurements can be applied to surfaces and substrates to determine relative roughness,[45] to measure case hardening depth,[46] to rank adhesive bond quality[47] and to monitor texture and porosity in metals and composites.[48,49]

TABLE 4. Theoretical ultrasonic attenuation coefficients for semilinear elastic polycrystalline solids.

Wavelength Relation	Attenuation Mechanism	Attenuation Coefficient ($Np \cdot m^{-1}$)
—	True absorption	$\alpha_a = C_a f$
$\lambda \gg \pi D$	Rayleigh scatter	$\alpha_r = C_r D^3 f^4$
$\lambda \cong \pi D$	Phase scatter	$\alpha_p = C_p D f^2$
$\lambda \ll \pi D$	Diffusion scatter	$\alpha_d = C_d D^{-1}$

D = nominal or mean grain size (μm)
λ = wavelength (m)
f = frequency (Hz)
α = attenuation coefficient ($Np \cdot m^{-1}$)
C = experimental constants (may include grain, geometric anisotropy, elastic anisotropy, density, longitudinal speed and transverse speed)

TABLE 5. Properties and conditions that can be monitored with ultrasonic techniques. (Ultrasonic measurements give indirect indications of mechanical property variations and morphological conditions. Empirical correlations and calibrations must be established for each material even where theoretical bases exist.)

Mechanical Properties	Morphological Conditions
Tensile modulus	Texture and anisotropy
Shear modulus	Grain size and distribution
Bulk modulus	Microvoid or porosity distribution
Lame constant	Phase composition
Tensile strength	Case hardening depth
Shear strength	Precipitation hardening
Yield strength	Residual stresses
Interlaminar bond strength	Overaging effects
Hardness and ductility	Undercuring and cure state
Impact resistance	Fatigue and impact damage
Impact strength	Fiber or whisker alignment
Fracture resistance	Degree of recrystallization
Fracture toughness	Alloy matrix supersaturation
Adhesive bond strength	Composite matrix crazing

Dual-Transducer Techniques

Dual-transducer techniques involve transducer pairs that are usually positioned so that signals are directed along well defined paths. Either contact or immersion coupling may be used at normal or oblique incidence. As in the case of the pulse echo technique, there are constraints that need to be met to produce and acquire meaningful signals. Three dual-transducer techniques for materials characterization are described here: (1) through-transmission, (2) pitch catch and (3) acoustoultrasonic.

Through-Transmission Technique

Through-transmission techniques use two transducers (sending and receiving) usually facing each other on opposite sides of a test object. The object that occupies the space between the transducers is either in contact with them or is separated by immersion in a fluid coupling medium. The acoustic beam is directed at normal incidence to test object surfaces that meet the constraints suggested in Table 3. Alternatively, with immersion coupling, the test object can be rotated between the transducers. Oblique incidence can be used to characterize material properties with transverse waves or surface (rayleigh) waves that are generated when fluid borne longitudinal waves meet a surface at an angle.

Through-transmission techniques are often used for making comparative property measurements with time-of-flight speed measurements and relative attenuation measurements.[30] Single-transit, through transmission is used if there is high signal attenuation because of test object thickness. This technique is often used in a comparator configuration where the test object's transit time delay is compared with the transit time delay in a reference standard, as when measuring relative changes in elastic moduli.

To ensure precise attenuation measurements in a through-transmission technique, the transducer pair must be perfectly matched or fully characterized. Signal modulation properties of the instrumentation, transducers and interfaces must be eliminated experimentally or taken into account with signal processing. This can be avoided by using the single-transducer pulse echo method where transducer related coupling and impedance mismatch factors can be better accounted for in analytical expressions.

Through transmission also lends itself to forward scattering measurements. The transducer on the opposite side of the test object collects wave energy scattered out of the main beam. Inverse analysis is used to infer size and distribution data.[50]

Pitch Catch Technique

The dual-transducer pitch catch technique uses a pair of transducers displaced from each other by a fixed distance, on the same side or opposite sides of a test object, as in the leaky lamb wave method (Fig. 1). The transducers may be in direct contact at either normal or oblique alignment. In the latter case, the transducers may be coupled by angle beam fixtures to excite transverse or rayleigh waves.

In a fluid medium, the pitch catch technique can be accomplished with a single focused transducer operating with self-generated and self-intercepted rayleigh waves (see Fig. 2).

The usual objective with pitch catch testing is discontinuity location and characterization. The technique can also characterize material properties. In either case, the positions of the transducers are calculated to recover specific signals that have traversed well defined paths along the surface or in the bulk. The paths usually involve simple reflections from the back surface or surface waves that are intercepted by the strategically placed receiving transducer. The pitch catch technique often uses surface waves and guided waves, such as rayleigh waves and plate waves, respectively. Lamb waves and

FIGURE 1. Pitch catch dual-transducer technique using leaky lamb wave effect.

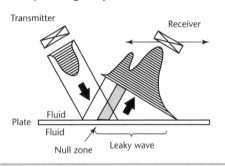

FIGURE 2. Pitch catch technique using focused transducer: (a) wave from rim of lens hits test object surface at critical angle producing surface waves that return to lens; (b) resulting waveform.

(a)

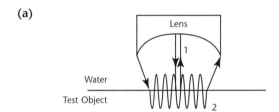

(b)

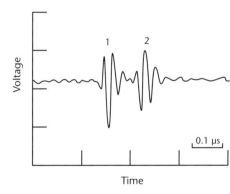

Legend
1. Direct reflection.
2. Rayleigh wave.

leaky lamb waves are used to evaluate bonds and interfaces by using angle beam immersion tests.[51] Variations in bonding are observed through variations in the spacing of null zones over a range of frequencies.

Acoustoultrasonics

The word *Acoustoultrasonics* may be taken as a contraction of *acoustic emission simulation with ultrasonic sources*. In contrast to acoustic emission techniques, the idea in acoustoultrasonic testing is to keep the nature and location of the source of ultrasonic radiation known and fixed. The idea is to introduce stress waves in the material and establish the change in waveform. The test is not concerned with source location and characterization but with characterization of the material medium between the source and receiver. The acoustoultrasonic approach uses analysis of simulated stress waves for detecting and mapping variations and the collective effects of diffuse discontinuities and material anomalies.[52,53]

Unlike the through-transmission or pitch catch technique, the acoustoultrasonic technique imposes no demand on having particularly well defined propagation paths. Indeed, typical applications are with materials that are so heterogeneous and anisotropic that it would be futile to demand well defined signal trajectories. The usual applications are with laminated fiber composites and coarse grained, highly textured materials.

The source may be any means for periodically exciting ultrasonic waves, usually a piezo transducer. A second transducer receives the signals. Both the sender and receiver are coupled to the test object surface at normal incidence. Although this arrangement resembles the pitch catch technique, the underlying approach is considerably different. Once launched in the test object, ultrasonic waves are modified by multiple reflections and stochastic processes. In this respect the acoustoultrasonic method most resembles the forward scatter technique. The acoustoultrasonic approach simulates the propagation of stress waves that might normally arise under acoustic emission testing.

Laser Techniques

Dual-transducer techniques increasingly use laser ultrasonics. Laser ultrasonic testing involves laser-in, laser-out excitation and detection without contact or immersion in a coupling medium. It allows high speed scanning and convenient test object contour following. Laser ultrasonic techniques provide good attenuation and speed measurements for materials characterization.[54,55]

Applications

There exists a wide range of applications for materials characterization using dual-transducer techniques. These include monitoring of metallurgical processes,[55] assessment of porosity,[56] measurement of elastic constants,[57] evaluation of fatigue damage,[58] interlaminar strength,[59] adhesive bond strength[60,61] and cure state.[62,63]

Ultrasonic Spectroscopy

Ultrasonic spectroscopy is done with single-transducer or dual-transducer configurations. The objective is to analyze modulations of ultrasonic waves caused by variations in microstructure and morphology. Ultrasonic spectroscopy presupposes unique signal modulations by the material. The pulse echo technique described above uses a form of spectroscopy in that a pair of back echoes are deconvolved to obtain an attenuation spectrum (attenuation as a function of frequency). The deconvolution step is not always necessary nor readily accomplished. As an alternative, the spectrum of a once-through signal (as in through-transmission) may be analyzed. The resulting spectral signature can be compared with that taken from a reference standard.

Spectrum analysis is an excellent approach for comparing subtle and often significant variations in material microstructures. Digital fast fourier transform methods are necessary to obtain quantitative results.[64-67] Ultrasonic spectrum analysis is used routinely in pulse echo, acoustoultrasonic and related testing techniques. Appropriate analytical procedures include spectrum analysis, spectral partitioning, regression analysis and the method of moments.[53,68] The latter uses statistical parameters to describe spectral signatures. Additional data processing techniques include pattern recognition and adaptive learning network theory.[52,69-77]

Ultrasonic spectroscopy is comparative and relies on a repertoire of spectral signatures for a wide range of material and boundary conditions.

Applications of Ultrasonic Spectroscopy

Ultrasonic spectroscopy has been widely used for both qualitative and quantitative microstructure characterization.[45,78] Attenuation spectra provide a powerful way to assess mean grain size in polycrystalline solids.[32,34,79,80] In addition, porosity and other morphological factors can be assessed with ultrasonic spectroscopy.[81]

Analysis of ultrasonic spectral features can yield quantitative correlations with material properties that are governed in turn by microstructure. These correlations include the ultimate strength and interlaminar strength of composite laminates[82,83] and toughness in metals.[84,85]

Ultrasonic Imaging Techniques

Several ultrasonic imaging techniques have a major role in materials characterization: (1) immersion macroscanning, (2) acoustic microscopy and (3) multiparametric scanning.

Acoustic microscopy and multiparametric scanning impose restrictions on the size and geometry of the test objects. These restrictions are often similar to those imposed in conventional optical microscopy in association with test object size, shape and mode of preparation. Magnified images, at very high resolution to submicrometer levels, can be formed with acoustic microscopy in the megahertz and gigahertz range by scanning minute areas of a surface or substrate.

Immersion Macroscanning

For large test objects, immersion scanning is the standard C-scan method, using assorted pulse echo, through-transmission or pitch catch configurations. The frequency range for immersion macroscanning is usually from 0.5 to about 25 MHz. It is universally applied for discontinuity detection but can be used to map relative global variations in material properties.

These variations can be related to material microstructure, texture or other extrinsic properties provided that the return signals are not also subject to changes in surface properties or thickness, curvature and similar boundary or geometric factors.

Acoustic Microscopy

Acoustic microscopy reveals density, texture and microelastic variations.[86] Images are generated by pulsed or continuous wave ultrasound, usually in the range from 50 MHz to 1 GHz. The images are produced either by pulse echo or thorough-transmission techniques. There are a number of acoustic microscopy methods, each with specific applications, including: (1) scanning

acoustic microscopy, (2) scanning laser acoustic microscopy, (3) scanning electron acoustic microscopy and (4) photoacoustic microscopy.

Scanning acoustic microscopy can take either of two forms. The first is simply a miniature C-scan or C-scanning acoustic microscopic technique that uses a focused transducer, a stepper driven scanner and a small immersion tank containing the test object (Fig. 3). The second form uses a raster vibrated scanning acoustic microscopic focused transducer coupled to the test object with a bead of fluid. Both methods operate in the focused pulse echo reflection mode with the option of using rayleigh wave imaging of surface features.[87]

C-scanning acoustic microscopy usually operates in the 50 to 200 MHz range whereas vibrated scanning acoustic microscopy operates in the 1 to 2 GHz range and requires metallographically polished surfaces. Either of these two forms of scanning acoustic microscopy is useful for imaging the elastic microstructure at surfaces and substrates. Pulse echo or rayleigh wave modes are used to reveal microstructure to depths of about 4 µm (at frequencies of about 4 GHz) to about 4 mm (at frequencies of 50 to 400 MHz). The field of view is 100 to 700 µm² for vibrated scanning acoustic microscopy and 2 to 15 mm² for C-scanning acoustic microscopy, giving image magnifications from roughly 2500× to 100×.

Scanning laser acoustic microscopy uses through-transmission continuous waves at specific frequencies, usually in

FIGURE 3. Scanning acoustic microscopy system for C-scan imaging.

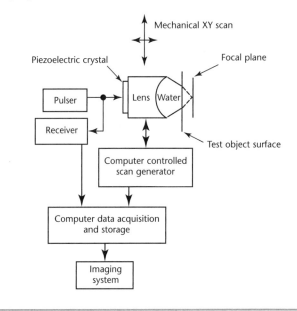

the 30 to 100 MHz range as dictated by the material attenuation and test object thickness.[88,89] Waves that pass through the test object set up perturbations on the opposite surface that are read by a raster scanning laser beam (Fig. 4). Reflected laser energy is sensed by a photooptical detector to generate a video image. This requires the scanned surface to be specularly reflective or coupled to a reflective cover slip. For typical metal and ceramic test objects, the thickness may be several millimeters. The scanning laser acoustic microscopic image reveals microstructural variations in the volume illuminated by the piezo transducer (usually about 4 mm² in area). The image is magnified about 100 times on the video monitor.

Scanning electron acoustic microscopy is accomplished by electron beam heating of the test object surface (Fig. 5). This requires that the test object be enclosed in a vacuum chamber. In fact, scanning electron acoustic microscopy is done with slightly modified scanning electron microscopy equipment and shares the scanning electron microscopy envelope.

The scanning electron microscopy electron beam is modulated (chopped) while it raster scans a small area that is typically a few millimeters square.[90-92] Acoustic signals generated at each point heated by the beam are sensed by a piezoelectric transducer attached to the bottom of the test object. The result of the raster scanning is displayed on a video screen. Both a conventional scanning electron microscopic and a scanning electron acoustic microscopy image can be viewed for the same area on the test object. As in the case of scanning acoustic microscopy, microelastic variations can be imaged using scanning electron acoustic microscopy. The scanning electron acoustic microscopy imaging depth depends on thermal diffusion length in the solid.

Photoacoustic microscopy uses a raster scanning laser beam to thermally excite acoustic waves (Fig. 6). The test object is enclosed in a pressure tight cell that contains a window through which the laser beam impinges on the test object.[88,89,93] Thermally generated acoustic waves are picked up by a miniature microphone in the cell. Images are created by displaying the intensity of the sound waves against the current coordinates of the laser beam. In an alternative configuration, a piezoelectric crystal is attached to the test object. In either case, the acoustic wave intensity values are used to image microstructural variations within the volume scanned (usually several millimeters in area and to depths of several millimeters, depending on the thermal diffusion length of the material).

FIGURE 5. Essential features of scanning electron acoustic microscope with typical parameters showing representative wavelengths.

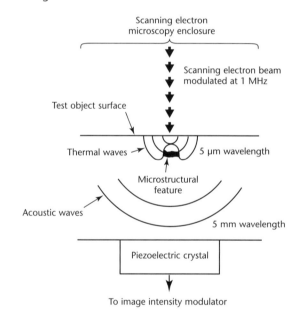

FIGURE 4. Diagram of scanning laser acoustic microscopy system.

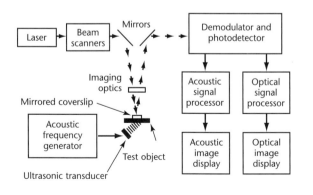

FIGURE 6. Diagram of photoacoustic microscopy system.

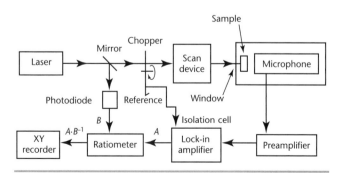

Multiparametric Scanning

Multiparametric scanning goes beyond producing images of material microstructure and microelastic domains. The goal is to collect an assortment of raw ultrasonic data and analyze them to give numerical values to a wide range of parameters. Selected parameters that can be mapped against the test object image include phase and group speeds, attenuation at selected frequencies, surface and internal reflection coefficients, and elasticity and stress values. Multiparametrics also comprises measurement of ultrasonic interactions with other forms of energy (thermal or magnetic).

Immersion noncontact C-scan approaches are fairly common for multiparametric mapping.[94] Contact scanning with a single-pulse echo transducer affords a means for obtaining more precise multiparametric data. In both cases, the test object is systematically scanned to collect sets of broad band (usually several hundred megahertz) echo waveforms.[95] When scanning is done with a contact transducer, the test object must have a flat, polished surface so that the transducer can be readily moved about. This movement is done by intermittently relaxing the coupling pressure as the transducer slides to the next position, using the couplant as lubricant. Although there are practical limits, large areas may be scanned with this method if the constraints in Table 3 are met.

Front surface and back surface echoes are collected for each of several hundred to several thousand equally spaced grid points on the test object. The data are stored and retrieved under computer control to generate attenuation and speed spectra for each point. The test object should have uniform thickness so that the speed and attenuation measurements can be compared from point to point. Mapping of attenuation and speed variations at selected frequencies can be generated from stored waveform data for the test object area being tested (Figs. 7 and 8).

Applications of Ultrasonic Imaging Techniques

For materials characterization, acoustic microscopy (particularly scanning acoustic microscopy) has capabilities that complement optical microscopy. Acoustic microscopy reveals grain, grain boundary and subgrain details without the need for special techniques such as etching to enhance contrast. In addition, acoustic microscopy can image subsurface microstructure features. Because ultrasonic waves are used, the image contains microelasticity information that does not appear in photomicrographs.

Scanning electron acoustic microscopy complements scanning electron microscopy because the former is based on thermal waves that penetrate below the surface to reveal subsurface features. Scanning laser acoustic microscopy images are projections of internal features imprinted on the laser scanned surface and therefore contain information on internal microelastic variations and other internal heterogeneities. Acoustic microscopy and multiparametric scanning can be applied to laboratory test objects for characterizing microstructure and elastic properties. Potential research and industrial applications include assessment of elastic anisotropy; surface and internal stress states; and mechanical, thermal and chemical damage.

Although C-scan imaging is widely used for materials characterization, the potential of acoustic microscopy and multiparametric scanning is still being developed. The applicability of acoustic microscopy techniques has been demonstrated on metals, ceramics and composites for evaluating grain structure, texture, porosity, fatigue damage, solid state weld bonding and fiber/matrix interface quality.[87-89,95,96]

FIGURE 7. Mapping speed variations in monolithic silicon carbide disk: (a) image; (b) speed profile along diameter.

(a)

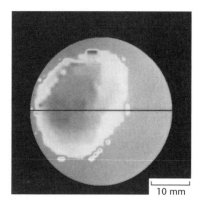

10 mm

(b)

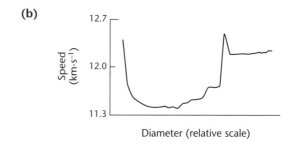

Speed (km·s^{-1})

12.7
12.0
11.3

Diameter (relative scale)

(a)

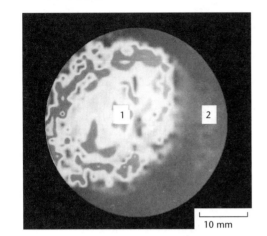

(b)

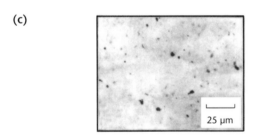

(c)

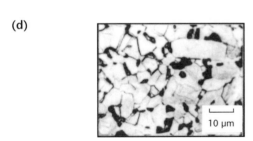

(d)

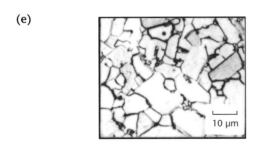

(e)

Analytical versus Imaging Techniques

Although the distinctions may not always be clear, there are differences between analytical and imaging ultrasonic testing. Analytical ultrasonic testing addresses the need to quantify factors such as speed and attenuation and their interrelation with material properties. Imaging ultrasonic testing is usually dedicated to revealing discontinuities, their location, orientation and microstructure. Imaging also addresses the spatial distribution of discontinuity populations and material anomalies such as porosity, texture and density variations.

Analytical and imaging ultrasonic testing are combined in multiparametric scanning where quantities like reflection coefficient, attenuation coefficient and phase speed are spatially mapped against a test object's outline.

PART 3. Measurement of Elastic Properties

Fundamental Elastic Property Relations

The measurement of elastic properties is basic to understanding and predicting the behavior of engineering materials. Ultrasonic wave propagation measurements afford a nondestructive means for determining elastic constants, texture and stress states. This can be done by introducing longitudinal and transverse waves in test objects and measuring the corresponding wave speeds.[57] Interrelations among these speeds and elastic moduli are shown in Table 6.

Anisotropic Materials

Real materials, even when they have simple shapes, rarely exhibit uniform and linear elastic properties assumed in the equations given for elastic moduli. Internal variations exist because of thermomechanical processing (solidification, densification and cold working) that can cause anisotropy and texture.[4] The distribution of toughening particles, whiskers and fibers can vary considerably (but not necessarily conspicuously) in ceramic and metal matrix composites. These factors lead to the need for measuring elastic properties that are direction dependent and that vary globally in the material volume.

Porous Solids

If solids are porous as in the case of cast metals, ceramics and most composites, then relations between elastic moduli and speed are more complex than indicated in Table 6. As discussed below, even if the solids are linearly elastic and isotropic, the moduli become functions of pore size, shape and orientation.[97] Moreover, other microstructural factors such as grain shape, grain boundaries, texture and precipitates can have pronounced effects on relations between speed and moduli.

Dynamic Resonance

Vibrational Modes

When determining elastic moduli of solids from resonance frequencies, the type of vibration may be longitudinal (extensional), transverse (flexural) or torsional.[10] The first two modes give Young's modulus and the last gives the shear modulus.

The way to obtain the best test results is to choose a geometry, such as a rectangle or cylinder, with simple boundary conditions. The dynamic resonance method is based on the standing waves in an object. If the object is undergoing longitudinal or torsional vibration, its length ℓ contains an integral number n of half wavelengths, $0.5\ \lambda$:

$$(18) \quad \ell \ = \ n\frac{\lambda}{2}$$

and the wave speed is:

$$(19) \quad v \ = \ \lambda f_r \ = \ 2\frac{\lambda f}{n}$$

where f_r is the resonant frequency. The equation does not apply to flexural resonance.

Longitudinal Vibration

If the object is a cylindrical rod or rectangular bar, Young's modulus E in pascal can be approximated from longitudinal resonances for $n = 1$:

$$(20) \quad E \ = \ \left(\rho G_\ell\right)\left(2\frac{\ell f_r}{n}\right)^2$$

$$= \ \rho G_\ell v^2$$

TABLE 6. Relations among elastic constants and ultrasonic wave speeds in fully dense linear elastic isotropic solids.

Elastic Constant (Pa)	Relation
Longitudinal modulus	$L = \rho v_\ell^2$
Shear modulus	$S = \rho v_t^2$
Bulk modulus	$K = L - 4S/3$
Young's modulus	$E = 3S - S^2(L - S)$
Lamé constant	$\lambda = L - 2S$

v_ℓ = longitudinal speed (meter per second)
v_t = transverse speed (meter per second)
ρ = density (kilograms per cubic meter)

---

where ρ is density (kilogram per cubic meter) and G_ℓ is a geometric factor containing object size and shape and Poisson's ratio.

Flexural Vibration

Flexural vibrations are easier to generate than longitudinal vibrations, especially for thin objects. Flexural vibration modes are more practical and more widely used for determining Young's modulus from:

$$(21) \quad E = \rho G_f \left(2\pi \ell^2 f_r \right)^2$$

where G_f is a factor that contains test object size, shape, Poisson's ratio, radius of gyration and a mode of vibration constant.

Torsional Vibration

The general equation that relates shear modulus S and torsional resonant frequency is:

$$(22) \quad S = 4\rho G_t \frac{\left(\ell f_r \right)^2}{n}$$

where G_t is a shape factor that depends on the test object's shape and cross section. The value of n is 1 for the fundamental mode and 2 for the first overtone.

Speed and Elastic Moduli

Dynamic resonance is an approach to measuring ultrasonic propagation speed by means of resonant frequencies — that is, by the ℓf_r factor in the previous equations. This approach is useful for calculating moduli and for inferring global changes in elastic moduli and associated mechanical properties. Applications of dynamic resonance are for test objects that do not lend themselves to direct measurement of speed because of inconvenience, geometric complexity or low signal-to-noise ratios (high attenuation).

Ultrasonic Measurements

Direct measurement of longitudinal v_ℓ and transverse v_t speeds give the fundamental longitudinal L and shear S moduli, respectively. Young's modulus is obtained from combinations of L and S given in Table 6:

$$(23) \quad L = \rho v_\ell^2$$

and:

$$(24) \quad S = \rho v_t^2$$

These relations assume that speed measurements are on test objects with dimensions much greater than the wavelength of the ultrasound. Otherwise, when wavelengths are comparable to dimensions, frequency dependent modes are generated.

For linear elastic isotropic solids, the moduli L and S are sufficient to completely define elastic behavior, given interconnecting relations with other moduli. Anisotropic solids present a more complicated situation because the principal moduli assume different values according to the direction of wave propagation. In general, the elastic characterization of a solid depends on nine separate speed measurements.[2] Transversely isotropic materials such as fiber reinforced lamina need five independent speed measurements.[98]

Effect of Porosity

There is considerable variability in the effects of porosity (and impurities) on the elastic properties of structural materials such as ceramics and composites. Expressions interrelating elastic properties, ultrasonic speed and porosity have been mostly empirical. Numerous theoretical and semitheoretical expressions have been derived to incorporate the effects of pore size, shape orientation and distribution conditions on various moduli (bulk, shear and Young's).[97] For example, the effect of porosity on Young's modulus has been expressed as:

$$(25) \quad E = E_0 \exp \left(-bP \right)$$

or

$$(26) \quad E = E_0 \left\{ 1 - \exp \left[-b \left(1 - P \right) \right] \right\}$$

where b is an adjustable porosity factor, E_0 is Young's modulus with no porosity (full density) and P is volume fraction of porosity.

The first equation is for P values less than 50 percent. Equation 26 is for P values greater than 50 percent.

The consequence of porosity is that speed is no longer a simple decreasing function of density as implied by the previous equations for L and S. Instead, speed is related to the porosity factors and also to grain size, shape and orientation factors peculiar to a given material. For most porous solids, speed is found to be an increasing function of density.[99] Mechanical strength and fracture behavior of structural ceramics have an important and complicated dependence on porosity, impurities and grain structure.

Elastic Moduli and Temperature

Speed and elastic moduli are functions of temperature. This temperature dependence is important because elastic moduli are related to interatomic forces that determine embrittlement at low temperatures. At cryogenic temperatures, the temperature variation of the longitudinal modulus L and shear modulus S tend to follow the relation:

$$(27) \quad L \text{ or } S = \frac{c - s}{\exp\dfrac{t}{T} - 1}$$

where c is the value of L or S as T approaches 0 K and T is the absolute temperature (kelvin).[100]

Variables c, s and t are adjustable parameters that depend on the material. The longitudinal and shear moduli usually vary linearly with temperature at room temperature. Empirical investigations have been conducted on both low (cryogenic) and high temperature variations of elastic moduli using ultrasonic speed.[101,102]

Acoustoelasticity

Acoustoelasticity is the term applied to changes in speed or attenuation wrought by applied or residual stress.[103-105] In practice, it is easier to measure speed changes although speed is a weak function of stress.

Effect of Stress

Relative changes in wave speed of only 10^{-5} per megapascal are typical for steel and aluminum so that precise speed measurements are needed. The simplest case can be represented by the linear expression:

$$(28) \quad \frac{\Delta v}{v_0} = A\sigma$$

where A is the acoustoelastic constant, v_0 is speed in the absence of stress (meter per second) and $\Delta v = (v_0 - v_\sigma)$ where σ is the induced stress.

Fundamentally, acoustoelastic constants apply to single crystals but empirical relations exist connecting acoustoelastic constants to polycrystalline aggregates. In most engineering solids, nonlinear relations between $\Delta v \cdot v^{-1}$ and σ may arise because of anisotropy or texture.[106]

Birefringence

Generally, there are two transverse wave speeds v_{tx} and v_{ty} polarized in two perpendicular directions corresponding to two principal stresses, σ_x and σ_y, so that:

$$(29) \quad \frac{\Delta v}{v_0} = \frac{v_{tx} - v_{ty}}{v_{t0}} = B_t\left(\sigma_x - \sigma_y\right)$$

The birefringent coefficient B_t is related to the second and third order elastic constants of the unstressed solid in which the transverse speed is v_{t0}.[105] Speed along the axes of principal stress are equal only if the principal stresses are equal and there is no texture.

Effect of Texture

In orthotropic and most polycrystalline solids there is an initial birefringence from anisotropy and texture such as nonrandom grain orientation. Induced or residual stresses result in secondary birefringence. For isotropic untextured materials, the initial, unstressed birefringence is zero. For slightly orthotropic solids, the birefringence is given by:

$$(30) \quad \frac{\Delta v}{v_0} = B_0 + B_t\left(\sigma_x - \sigma_y\right)$$

The birefringent constant B_t depends on the original (unstressed) anisotropy. In some materials, the initial birefringence caused by texture may be greater than that due to stresses as great as yield.[107-109] The previous expressions may be valid for determining stresses in an elastically deformed body but might produce large errors in residual stress measurements.[104]

Effect of Temperature

It has been established that ultrasonic speed varies linearly with temperature and, as indicated above, tends to vary linearly with stress. Externally induced elastic stress also affects the temperature dependence of ultrasonic speed. The relation is expressed by:

$$(31) \quad \frac{\left(\dfrac{dv}{dT}\right)_0 - \left(\dfrac{dv}{dT}\right)_\sigma}{\left(\dfrac{dv}{dT}\right)_0} = \pm K\sigma$$

where $dv \cdot (dT)_0^{-1}$ is the temperature dependence of ultrasonic speed at zero stress, $dv \cdot (dT)_\sigma^{-1}$ is the temperature dependence at an induced stress of σ and K is a material constant.[110]

Effect of Magnetization

Acoustoelastic speed changes can be magnetically induced in ferromagnetic materials. When an ultrasonic wave propagates through a ferromagnetic material, there is rotational vibration of magnetic domains due to magnetoelastic interactions that affect speed:

$$(32) \quad v = \sqrt{\frac{\sigma_u}{\rho c}} = v_e \frac{1 - c_m}{2 c_e}$$

where c is the overall strain due to σ_u, c_e is the ordinary elastic strain, c_m is the magnetostrictive strain, v_e is the purely acoustoelastic value of speed obtained in the absence of magnetostrictive strain (meter per second), ρ is material density (kilogram per cubic meter) and σ_u is the stress of the ultrasonic wave (pascal).[111]

The speed in a ferromagnetic material at zero magnetic field and zero stress is smaller than the purely elastic value by about $v_e \cdot c_m \cdot (2c_e)^{-1}$. The speed first increases rapidly with application of a magnetic field and then approaches the purely elastic value for high fields.

Application of Speed Measurements

The practical use of speed to determine elastic constants and stresses is hampered by two factors: (1) the effects of test object geometry and (2) the effects of texture, porosity and other microstructural variations. Geometric simplicity is needed for valid and accurate measurements of speed and speed changes wrought by temperature and acoustoelastic factors.[112,113]

Calibration reference standards can open possibilities for using speed and acoustoelastic effects to assess microstructural anomalies and nonuniformities such as those associated with porosity and texture. Ultrasonic speed measurements can detect volume and surface stresses but the problem is to separate the influence of texture and other microstructural factors.[106]

Elastic Constants

Because they are related to interatomic forces, elastic moduli indicate maximum attainable strengths. Elastic moduli also appear in equations for strain energy release rate and are related to stress wave propagation properties associated with impact shock, crack growth and fracture.[7] There are incentives for convenient, nondestructive means for measuring elastic constants, especially for materials at extreme conditions and test objects not

amenable to conventional mechanical inspection methods.

Brittle materials present a special problem for measuring elastic constants by conventional means such as tensile or bending tests. Ceramics in particular are amenable to the use of ultrasonics for elasticity measurements. Other test methods produce poor results because ceramics and other brittle solids are vulnerable to fracture from very small strains.

Elastic constants at extreme temperatures are most readily determined with speed measurements. Longitudinal, shear modulus, bulk modulus and Poisson's ratio have been measured for a series of stainless steels down to 5 K.[114] Laser ultrasonic techniques have been used to determine elastic constants of cermets to temperatures from 500 to 1000 °C (900 to 1800 °F).[102] Ultrasonic measurement of elastic constants for refractory metals to near melting point have been determined using self-heated wires.[115]

Stress and Texture

It is convenient to measure stress states and texture with birefringence because it requires only the measurement of transit time differences and is independent of errors in length measurements. These measurements can be aided by independent ultrasonic techniques for determining texture and anisotropy.[116-118]

The frequency dependence of transverse wave birefringence, ultrasonic attenuation and thermoelastic effects can be used to characterize grain structure and thus separate effects due to texture and anisotropy.[103] Experimental evidence indicates independent correlations between ultrasonic attenuation and stress in aluminum crystals subjected to uniaxial compression.[4] The temperature dependence of longitudinal and transverse waves has been used to produce calibration curves for measuring induced stress in steel.[119] It has also been shown that stress and texture can be independently inferred from the angular dependence of polarized plate mode speeds.[120]

In ferromagnetic materials, an external magnetic field can help unambiguously determine the stress dependence of speed changes.[121-122] Magnetically induced speed changes can be used to measure the effects of internal stresses by longitudinal or transverse waves and surface stresses by surface waves. Magnetoelasticity can be used to determine magnitude, sign and direction of tensile and compressive or residual stresses.[111]

Practical uses of acoustoelasticity for stress state measurements have been applied to stainless steel sheet, plate and piping[106,123] and to railroad wheels, rails and aircraft landing gear.[124,125] However, extraordinary precision is required to measure changes in acoustoelastic wave speeds. Because of this, it is advantageous to combine instrumentation with digital processing of the ultrasonic data.[66] Fourier transform techniques greatly improve not only speed but accuracy in speed phase delay measurements for residual stress determination.[126,127]

PART 4. Microstructure and Diffuse Discontinuities

Overview of Microstructure and Ultrasonic Methods

Microstructure and Morphology

Mechanical properties are controlled by composition, microstructure and morphology. Because these factors also influence ultrasonic wave propagation, ultrasonic characterization of material properties is possible. Modulations of ultrasonic waves by material variables determine ultrasonic correlations with strength, hardness, toughness and other mechanical properties governed by the same variables.

Diffuse Discontinuity Populations

The need for nondestructive materials characterization arises when the presence, identity and distribution of minute discontinuities can only be assessed statistically. In some materials, discontinuities can be so microscopic, numerous and widely dispersed that it is impractical to resolve them individually. Porosity in ceramics, crazing in composites, fatigue and creep damage in metals are examples of such anomalies.

Large populations of subcritical microscopic discontinuities in association with morphological anomalies produce degraded bulk mechanical properties and strength deficiencies. Although structures may be free of single critical discontinuities, they may still be susceptible to failure because of inadequate or degraded mechanical properties.

Fundamental Microstructure Quantities

Mean Grain Size

A universally cited quantity for characterizing polycrystalline microstructures is the mean grain size. This quantity is used despite difficulties inherent in measuring or assigning values to it, especially in materials that exhibit complex microstructures (subgrains,

second phases or precipitates). Moreover, heating and forming processes tend to result in nonuniform grain sizes and in nonrandom crystallographic orientations such as columnar grain growth. Therefore, most real polycrystalline solids possess what is known as *texturing*.[4]

There are many polycrystalline aggregates having microstructures with readily defined mean grain sizes.[128] For example, single-phase polycrystalline aggregates with uniform microstructures tend to exhibit a well defined mean grain size. In these cases, mean grain size can be determined from grain size distribution functions (histograms) based on photooptical (metallographic) analyses by using standard computer based techniques.[128,129]

Grain Boundaries

From a purely physical standpoint, grain interfaces, facets and surface areas should influence mechanical properties of polycrystalline and noncrystalline aggregate solids. This is certainly true of properties that depend on the surface energy of grains, properties affected by the grain boundary thickness, properties for which grain boundaries are obstacles and properties connected with grain and phase boundary migrations and obliterations.

Generally, grain boundaries of polycrystalline solids exhibit an abrupt change in acoustic impedance because the crystallites have different speeds in different principal directions. Similar changes in acoustic impedance and wave propagation occur in particulate toughened and fiber reinforced materials, such as those at fiber matrix or whisker matrix interfaces in ceramic and metal matrix composites.

Elastic Anisotropy

Elastic anisotropy and the impedance mismatch at grain boundaries influence wave propagation and scattering. Elastic anisotropy K for cubic crystallites is:

$$(33) \quad K = \left(\frac{c_{11} - \langle c_{11} \rangle}{\langle c_{11} \rangle} \right)^2$$

where c is the elastic tensor coefficient (compression modulus); and $\langle c \rangle$ is its average value.

For cubic crystallites, the elastic anisotropy may also be expressed in terms of acoustic impedance:

$$(34) \quad K = \left(\frac{z_2 - z_1}{z_2 + z_1} \right)^2$$

where the acoustic impedances $z = \rho v$ are based on principal longitudinal speeds. The equation is exactly the same for the reflection coefficient R at the boundary between two materials as described above.

Speed and Attenuation

Changes in wave propagation speed and energy losses from interactions with material microstructure are the two key factors in ultrasonic determination of material properties. Ultrasonic speed and attenuation measurements are basic. Relatively small variations of speed and attenuation are often associated with significant variations in microstructural characteristics and mechanical properties.

Single-frequency, continuous wave ultrasound is used in those cases where unique relations exist at a specific frequency but speed and attenuation are both functions of frequency. With transducers that emit broad band pulsed ultrasound, signals have a wide frequency spectrum. Generally, each spectral component is affected differently as the ultrasound propagates in a material.

In polycrystalline solids, each frequency component and wavelength is affected differently according to grain size, morphology, inclusions, texture and elastic anisotropy. Frequency dependence of speed and attenuation are very important in the ultrasonic characterization of material microstructures, porosity and diffuse discontinuities. It is precisely because of these interrelations that ultrasonic measurement can assess elastic, microstructural and hence mechanical properties of materials.

Ultrasonic Speed and Microstructure

Ultrasonic speed in many engineering solids (metals, ceramics or linearly elastic materials) is directly related to elastic constants and density (see Table 6). Elastic properties in turn can depend strongly on porosity and may also depend on precipitates and other impurities. Although elastic moduli have no basic dependence on grain size, they do depend on elastic anisotropy and therefore on grain orientation and microstructural texture. Because the size, shape and distribution of diffuse discontinuities and microporosity often correlate with grain size and shape orientation, there can be second order correlations among elastic properties, speed, grain shape and aspect ratio.

Effect of Porosity

The equations given to connect propagation speeds with elastic moduli and density (Eqs. 23 and 24) lead to the expectation that speed is an inverse function of density. The converse is true in porous solids where speed increases, usually linearly, with density. Speed depends on the elastic moduli, Poisson's ratio and density: $v = f(L,S,\mu,\rho)$. The moduli L and S are in turn dependent on pore volume fraction and pore size, shape, orientation and spacing factors.[97]

Group and Phase Speed

Neither v_ℓ nor v_t can be measured unambiguously as unique quantities except in the case of a nondispersive material. A medium may be dispersive because of its geometric boundaries or internal morphology or both. For example, speed dispersion occurs in wires and thin rods or plates when the wavelength nearly equals the thickness.

The bandwidth or main frequency content of a pulse traversing a dispersive medium is altered and may carry information on the medium's macrostructure and microstructure. In most solids, the speed dispersion is usually less than a few percent. By accounting for phase speed dispersion, measurements of subtle property variations can be made.[30,130]

For each phase or frequency component of an ultrasonic pulse, there is a particular phase speed v. The pulse (energy) travels with a group speed u.

$$(35) \quad v(f, \lambda) = f\lambda$$

and

$$(36) \quad u(f, \lambda) = \lambda^2 \frac{\partial f}{\partial \lambda}$$

where f is frequency (hertz) and λ is wavelength (meter).

The group speed u varies with frequency depending on the particular values assumed by $df \cdot d\lambda^{-1}$, which is in turn a function of the phase speed v. Dispersion or variation of speed with frequency occurs in the case of lamb or plate waves and with guided waves whenever wavelengths are comparable to the plate or waveguide dimensions. Techniques of measuring group and phase speeds are described below and elsewhere.[36]

Ultrasonic Attenuation and Microstructure

Attenuation measurements are pivotal for establishing correlations between microstructure and mechanical properties. Mechanical property characterization depends on precise attenuation measurements.[131,132]

Scattering and absorption are the energy loss mechanisms that govern ultrasonic attenuation in the frequency ranges of interest for characterizing most engineering solids. Diffusion, rayleigh and stochastic (phase) scattering losses are extrinsic whereas absorption losses from dislocation damping, anelastic hysteresis, relaxation and thermoelastic effects are intrinsic to individual grains such as crystallites.

There are other losses associated with techniques for measuring attenuation. These are geometric losses such as those from diffraction effects and beam divergence, which are not inherent to material microstructures. These losses can be controlled or eliminated from attenuation measurements by experimental and data reduction procedures[130] to get the true attenuation coefficient as a function of frequency.

Attenuation Coefficient

Attenuation from scattering and other mechanisms is measured by an attenuation coefficient α usually expressed in terms of the intensity I of sound after traversing a distance X through a material:

$$(37) \quad I = I_0 \exp(-\alpha X)$$

where I_0 is the initial intensity and $I_0 - I$ is the loss in intensity over distance X.

Extrinsic Mechanisms

Scattering usually accounts for the greatest portion of losses in engineering solids. The scatter attenuation coefficient α is a function of frequency f. In polycrystalline aggregates (metals and ceramics), there are three scatter attenuation processes defined by the ratio of mean grain size D to the dominant wavelength λ (see Table 4). For the rayleigh scattering process where $\lambda \gg \pi D$:

$$(38) \quad \alpha_r = C_r D^3 f^4$$

For the stochastic (phase) scattering process where $\lambda \cong \pi D$:

$$(39) \quad \alpha_p = C_p D f^2$$

For the diffusion scattering process where $\lambda \ll \pi D$:

$$(40) \quad \alpha_d = C_d D^{-1}$$

The constants C_d, C_p and C_r contain geometric factors, longitudinal and transverse speeds, density and elastic anisotropy factors.[28,133-136]

Intrinsic Mechanisms

Absorption losses due to dislocation damping, hysteresis and thermoelastic effects are intrinsic to grains (crystallites) and involve direct conversion of acoustic energy to heat. These attenuation mechanisms are essentially independent of grain size, shape and volume. For hysteresis, the absorption losses are:[11,137]

$$(41) \quad \alpha_h = C_h f$$

For thermoelastic effects, absorption losses are:[138]

$$(42) \quad \alpha_t = C_t f^2$$

Hysteresis losses arise when acoustic waves cause stress-strain dampening. Hysteresis losses with a first power frequency dependence are usually observed in single crystals, amorphous solids and with difficulty in polycrystalline solids.[98] Frequency dependent thermodynamic losses arise when longitudinal waves produce heat flow from dilatation to compression regions.

Viscous losses[139] also exhibit a second power frequency dependence but are generally negligible in solids. Models for absorption losses caused by dislocation vibrations, relaxation effects and internal friction predict second power frequency dependence down to frequency independence.[28,140,141] Absorption losses due to electrons or photons comprise special cases involving ferromagnetic materials, very high frequencies or cryogenic temperatures. Magnetoelastic absorption (due to magnetic domains) tends to occur at frequencies on the order of 5 to 10 MHz in structural steels.[142]

Combined Expressions

Total attenuation coefficients are usually written as sums of coefficients for scattering and absorption. For example, equations for hysteresis and stochastic attenuation are combined to form an expression for the total attenuation coefficient:

$$(43) \quad \alpha_{hp} = C_h f + C_p D f^2$$

Equations for hysteresis and rayleigh scattering are combined to produce:

$$(44) \quad \alpha_{hr} = C_h f + C_r D^3 f^4$$

Combined expressions are convenient for fitting experimental data and for analyzing the contributions of attenuation mechanisms and underlying microstructural factors.[80]

Scattering Centers

Scattering theories used to derive the previous equations usually consider ensembles of scattering centers embedded in a featureless continuum. Current theories for polycrystalline materials account only for scattering by equiaxed grains, neglecting effects of texture, anisotropy and grain size variations. Well formulated theories for attenuation exist only for: (1) the simple case of single-phase polycrystalline solids with virtually identical, equiaxed grains; and (2) frequencies that satisfy the conditions $ka \ll 1$ or $ka \gg 1$, where k is wave number and a is mean scatterer size.

Fourth and second power relations given in the previous equations have been experimentally confirmed only for special cases.[143] The fourth power relation for rayleigh scattering was realized by measuring scattering due only to sparsely distributed scatterers or minority phases (carbon nodules and inclusions) in polycrystalline aggregates.[144-147]

Grain Size Distribution

For most polycrystallines, the overall experimentally determined frequency dependence of attenuation is not an integral power even in the rayleigh or stochastic processes. There are a variety of reasons for this, including the fact that premises underlying scatter attenuation equations are not met in engineering solids that tend to exhibit a wide distribution in grain size and textured, quasielastic microstructures. Various investigations suggest approaches for handling the effects of grain size distributions. One method is to include a probabilistic distribution function in scatter attenuation coefficients.[34,148-150]

Empirical Correlations

There are special cases where it is possible to fit attenuation data with expressions that allow the exponent of frequency to be an experimentally determined variable.[5,32] The simplest expressions of this kind are:

$$(45) \quad >\alpha< = c f^m$$

In Eq. 45, $f_1 < f < f_2$ and $>\alpha<$ denotes that α is empirically defined only in a limited frequency range. The quantities c and m assume noninteger values and change with microstructural changes that affect attenuation (mean grain size or size distribution). Experimental results show that the previous equation is statistically valid for fitting attenuation data over a frequency range that spans the rayleigh scattering process for a variety of polycrystalline materials.[84,85,151,152]

Applications in Microstructure Characterization

Selected examples are given below for a variety of potential applications of ultrasonics for characterizing microstructure. These include the measurements of mean grain size, texture, recrystallization, cure state, porosity and diffuse discontinuity populations. The examples show that simple pulse echo speed or attenuation measurements often suffice to establish correlations with microstructure.

Speed and attenuation, usually at a single and sometimes arbitrarily selected frequency, correlate well with certain microstructural factors in some cases. This does not mean that the methodologies are simple, as can be appreciated by consulting the references cited. There are other cases where empirical correlations depend very strongly on making ultrasonic measurements with broad band waveforms (100 to 200 MHz bandwidths), followed by detailed comparative analyses of amplitude and phase spectra.

Mean Grain Size

Perhaps the most underused yet well proven capability of ultrasonics is the estimation of mean grain size in simple polycrystalline solids. Literature surveys show that there has been extensive work dedicated to ultrasonic assessment of grain size.[79,153] Abundant data exist showing the capability of ultrasonics for assigning photomicrographically confirmable values to the mean grain size in polycrystalline solids.[42-44,154-155]

Strong incentives exist for in-process monitoring of grain size and microstructure in materials research and development and in manufacturing environments.[156,157] There is strong interest in ultrasonic assessment of microstructural quantities like grain size because of their role in governing mechanical properties, such as strength and toughness. Many empirical correlations that demonstrate relations between grain size and strength properties can be exploited in research and industry.[155,158]

Techniques for ultrasonic grain size determination use both speed and attenuation measurements. Theoretical bases for speed correlations with grain size are virtually nonexistent compared with the equations connecting attenuation and grain size given previously. Speed depends on elastic properties that have no basic dependence on grain size.[2,97] Still, in most polycrystalline aggregates, elastic properties and speed are affected by grain boundary impurities and grain orientation. Consequently, there are examples of empirical correlations between speed and mean grain size in polycrystalline solids (see Fig. 9).[5]

Attenuation spectrum analysis is fundamental for developing correlations with grain structure. Pulse echo and backscatter are methods used for attenuation spectrum analysis.[30,42,43] Excellent correlations between attenuation and mean grain size in polycrystalline materials are obtained in the rayleigh scattering frequency process using the pulse echo technique and broad band spectrum analysis (see Fig. 10).[80,147,149,153,159] In addition, noncontact laser generation and detection techniques have been used for measuring frequency dependent attenuation and forward scattering to assess microstructure.[54] Characterization of anisotropic and textured metals and composites presents special problems. Directional speed variations and acoustoelasticity are appropriate for microstructure and texture characterization of these materials. In the case of texture characterization, there remains the problem of separating the combined effects of texture and residual stress. Surface wave birefringence, speed dispersion and speed slowness curves have been proposed for separating effects of texture and stress in textured monolithic and composite materials.[160-162]

Tests of rolled aluminum plate have illustrated the use of rayleigh waves for measuring subsurface texture. The results compared well with various texture coefficients obtained by X-ray pole figures.[163] Columnar grain structure and

FIGURE 9. Relation between speed and grain size at frequency of 30 MHz for titanium alloy.[184]

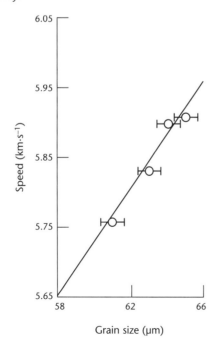

FIGURE 10. Calibration curves for mean grain size and its effect on attenuation spectra for heat treated copper and nickel samples: (a) 99.99 percent pure copper; (b) 99.5 percent pure nickel, Unified Numbering System N02200.[34]

(a)

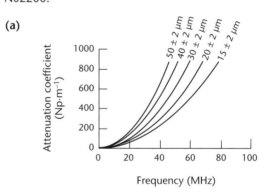

(b)

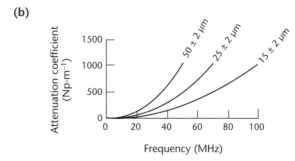

elastic anisotropy in cast stainless steel has been determined even in thick walled components by speed measurements.[164] A key factor was the measurement of ultrasonic beam skewing by the crystalline texture. The beam skewing was found only in columnar and not in equiaxed microstructures.[118]

Recrystallization and Precipitation

One method for controlling metallic properties is to apply thermomechanical processing such as cold working and aging to increase strength. After cold working, there is usually a need for annealing to relieve residual stresses and to soften the metal by recrystallization. Changes in the slope (first derivatives) of broad band attenuation spectra were found to correlate quite well with stages of recrystallization in nickel.[165]

In the case of rapidly solidified powders, it has been shown that both attenuation and backscatter measurements reveal the onset of recrystallization and grain growth.[48] Amorphous materials such as glassy metals and alloys revert to a crystalline structure and lose advantageous properties under certain thermomechanical conditions. Clear changes in longitudinal speed have been shown to accompany transitions from the amorphous to the crystalline state in metallic glass ribbons produced by melt spinning.[55,166]

Precipitation hardening or aging is also an important metallurgical process for improving the strength of structural metals. Strength improvements depend on spacing, size, shape and distribution of precipitated particles. Ultrasonic speed and attenuation correspond to microstructural changes that increase both hardness and strength during the aging process of aluminum alloys.[55]

Porosity and Density

The strength lowering effects of porosity affect all structural materials, from powder metallics to monolithic ceramics, polymers and their composites. The presence of porosity can be determined by speed or attenuation measurements. The goals are (1) to characterize mean pore size and (2) to distinguish porosity from grain structure in metals or ceramics and from fiber content in composites. Complementary use of radiography can help make this distinction. In most porous solids, speed varies linearly and inversely with porosity and directly with density (Fig. 11).[99] For polyethylene, an important commercial material, compressional and transverse wave speeds strongly correlate with density, although the correlation is nonlinear.[167]

Complementary speed and attenuation spectral measurements can also help to differentiate density and grain structure effects in polycrystalline solids (Fig. 12 and Table 7).[168] Attenuation spectra are useful for differentiating porosity variations from roughly 0.2 to 5 percent in an aluminum alloy.[169] Spectral analysis of backscatter radiation is used to characterize porosity in a fiber reinforced composite.[67] The approach uses spectral signal analysis to reveal both fiber related ordered structure and random pore distribution.

Using a powder metallurgy alloy as a model has provided a demonstration of the viability of both attenuation and backscatter spectra for characterizing porosity.[50] The results show that the dominant cause of attenuation and therefore backscatter is a dense distribution (100 per cubic millimeter) of micropores (10 μm radius). The porosity is beyond the ability of the technique to

FIGURE 11. Correlation between ultrasonic speed and material density for monolithic sintered alpha silicon carbide.[99]

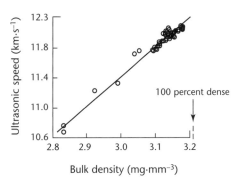

FIGURE 12. Representative attenuation spectra for three samples of monolithic silicon carbide with deliberately varied microstructures.[168]

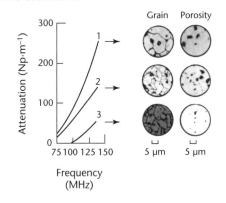

TABLE 7. Representative speed and density data for three samples of monolithic silicon carbide with deliberately varied microstructures (see Fig. 12).

| Sample | Sintering Conditions | | | Mean Density (kg·m⁻³) | Mean Grain Size (μm) | Mean Speed (km·s⁻¹) |
	Temperature (°C)	Time (h)	Pressure (atm)			
1	2300	1.0	1	3054	12	11.65
2	2150	4.0	1	3058	4	11.67
3	2200	0.5	1	3117	6	11.80

resolve individual pores. This is an example of nonimaging analytical ultrasonics for characterizing microporosity.

Diffuse Discontinuity Populations

In a sense, diffuse discontinuity populations define material properties and dynamic response just as microstructure does. Diffuse discontinuities are either inherent to the material from processing or are introduced by thermomechanical degradation. Examples are porosity that results from sintering of ceramics or microcracking that results from fatiguing of metals and composites.

In both cases, the discontinuities consist of diffuse populations of small discontinuities that exist globally or in localized colonies and it is impractical to attempt to resolve them individually. Because no one discontinuity is dominant, it is virtually impossible to characterize any one as a potential fracture origin. Instead, the problem is to characterize the population in terms of mean size, number per unit volume or nature (void or inclusion).

Part 5. Ultrasonic Testing for Mechanical Properties

Determination of mechanical properties like strength and toughness is conventionally done with destructive tests. At the expense of material and manufacturing costs, destructive tests provide data that cannot be duplicated by nondestructive methods. Destructive testing in the laboratory is the basis for establishing ultrasonic correlations with mechanical properties. In-process and continuous monitoring of mechanical properties is a strong incentive for nondestructive materials characterization.[155,157]

Empirical correlations between speed and attenuation and various mechanical properties have been reported in the literature. However, theoretical foundations for the correlations are not well developed. In some instances, the correlations appear fortuitous and depend on conditions peculiar to individual materials. Nevertheless, theoretical models predict correlations between ultrasonic and mechanical properties.

Theoretical foundations and examples of experimental validations are presented below for ultrasonic assessments of several key mechanical properties: strengths (tensile, yield and shear), fracture toughness and hardness. The examples consist primarily of laboratory demonstrations of ultrasonic measurements and indicate the capabilities of ultrasonic material property assessment on the basis of calibrations derived from destructive test measurements.

Ultrasonics and Mechanical Properties

Wave speeds are directly related to material moduli (Table 6). Because moduli are in turn directly related to interatomic forces, attempts have been made to link speed to material strength. But material strength is not dependent only on moduli or elastic spring constants. For example, although some alloys can be processed to increase their fracture toughness by a factor of ten or more, elastic moduli such as Young's modulus remain essentially constant.

In polycrystalline solids, microstructure and morphology play important roles in determining extrinsic mechanical properties like strength and toughness. Strength and fracture toughness are extrinsic to elastic properties of individual crystallites or grains. Ultimate tensile and yield strength, ductility, toughness and other mechanical properties are governed by microstructural factors that include dislocation densities; grain size, aspect ratio and orientation; grain interface properties; impurities; phase structure; and other features in aggregate. Although speed can be correlated with some of these factors, attenuation measurements are much more sensitive to the microstructural factors that govern strength, toughness and other mechanical properties. For example, in metallic polycrystallines, the pivotal factors appear to be grain structure, morphology and dislocation density, all of which have strong effects on attenuation.

To establish correlations with microstructural factors that govern mechanical properties, precise ultrasonic measurements based on the pulse echo approach are necessary. Attenuation spectra (attenuation coefficient versus frequency curves) need to be carefully determined for each material. Subtle but important variations in the microstructure appear as changes in slope and other parameters that define the attenuation spectrum.

The emphasis on attenuation does not preclude speed or other basic measurements for obtaining correlations with mechanical properties. Certainly, any approach sensitive to microstructural variables should be invoked and studied. For example, wave speeds have been shown to correlate with age hardening of steels.[55] The ductility of diffusion bonds in titanium has been assessed using ultrasonic reflection coefficients.[170] Mechanical strengths of gray cast irons and cobalt cemented tungsten carbides can be inferred from internal friction damping measurements.[171]

Tensile and Yield Strength

Griffith Model

Relations between strength and grain size can be derived from the griffith criterion, which relates strength σ to crack size:

(46) $\sigma = \dfrac{K_{Ic}}{\sqrt{\pi c}}$

where c is half the length of a semicircular surface crack or notch (meter) and K_{Ic} is the plane strain fracture toughness (pascal root meter). Equation 46 has been modified to give a grain size dependence of strength:

(47) $\sigma = \dfrac{A}{\sqrt{D}}$

where A is a stress intensity constant for the material's grain structure (pascal root meter) and D is mean grain size (meter).

In this modification of the griffith criterion, grains are assumed to act as edge or crack discontinuities. The quantity A depends on composition, phase structure, texture and other morphological factors. In carbon steel, A depends on the percent of pearlite.[156]

Hall-Petch Model

The hall-petch model further modifies Eq. 47 to give:

(48) $\sigma = \sigma_i + \dfrac{A}{\sqrt{D}}$

where σ_i is a yield stress. The hall-petch model assumes that dislocation motions in a grain are arrested by grain boundaries and that any tensile stresses associated with dislocation pileups are sufficient to cause fracture. In this case, σ_i is the yield stress of the metallic grain.[172-174]

Investigations have shown that yield strength obeys the hall-petch relation and that yield strength has the predicted dependence on grain size for plain carbon steels (see Fig. 13).[156,158] Although tensile strength also obeys the hall-petch relation, it is less sensitive to grain size and the quantity A for tensile strength is about half of that for yield strength. The hall-petch relation is not necessarily limited to tensile or yield strength. Any property that depends on dislocation motions and grain structure may in principle be characterized by the hall-petch relation. Such properties include hardness, fatigue limit, impact and ductile brittle transition temperatures.[175-178]

Nondestructive prediction of grain size dependent properties is based on relations between extrinsic attenuation and mean grain size (see the discussion of microstructure and diffuse discontinuities). The predictions depend on attenuation measurements primarily in the rayleigh scattering process. From variations in attenuation spectra, it is possible to infer mean grain size for the hall-petch equation.[80,149,178,179] It should be remembered that factors other than grain structure (porosity, for instance) influence both attenuation and mechanical properties. These other factors may dominate both attenuation spectra and strength and lead to ambiguities in ultrasonic property correlation.

Although the preceding equations apply fairly well to polycrystalline metals, they require modification for brittle materials. For ceramics, either maximum grain size or discontinuity size must be substituted for D in the griffith equation to predict flexural strength.[180] That is, discontinuities rather than grain size govern the strength of monolithic brittle materials. In ceramics, large numbers of discontinuities may be distributed throughout a component's volume so that large grains, microvoids or microcracks can appear as diffuse discontinuity populations. In this case, mean discontinuity size needs to be substituted for D in the griffith relation to predict strength.

Hardness

Tensile strength, yield strength and hardness are interrelated in polycrystalline metals. Because it is simple and essentially nondestructive, microhardness indentation testing is often used to estimate tensile and yield strengths.[181] Hardness measurements can also be accomplished by a resonant vibration method related to microindentation. The resonance method uses a piezoelectric transducer mechanism to measure hardness.[10]

FIGURE 13. Measured yield strength for plain carbon steel versus yield strength calculated from hall-petch relation and metallographically measured grain size. Standard error is 15.4 MPa (2.234×10^3 $lb_f \cdot in.^{-2}$).[158]

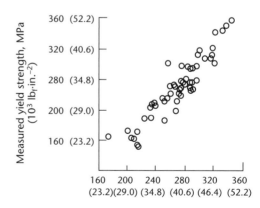

Nondestructive methods for unambiguous determination of hardness are in high demand. Ultrasonic techniques can form a basis for inferring strength from hardness and can provide continuous monitoring of hardness in production control.

Experimental evidence shows that pulse echo speed and attenuation measurements can uniquely determine hardness (within limits that depend on the material). This experiment was conducted with variously age hardened specimens of an aluminum copper alloy.[55] Although speed varies parabolically with hardness in the alloy, attenuation varies linearly and inversely with hardness (Fig. 14).

In another investigation, an angle beam pulse echo backscatter method was used to estimate case depth in hardened steel.[46] Case hardening has also been measured by dispersion of rayleigh (surface) waves.[182] Depth of hardness in various steel grades was found to relate to a break in the slopes of speed change versus wavelength curves.

Fracture Toughness

Fracture toughness is (1) an extrinsic material property that depends on microstructure and (2) a measure of a material's fracture resistance. Fracture toughness quantifies the critical stress intensity at which a crack of particular size becomes unstable and grows catastrophically.[7] Governed by more than mean grain size, fracture toughness is determined in polycrystalline solids by grain boundaries, shapes, aspect ratios, subgrain structure, dislocation densities and other morphological factors.

FIGURE 14. Linear correlation of ultrasonic attenuation with age hardening of samples of Unified Numbering System A92024 heat treatable wrought aluminum alloy, temper 351.[55]

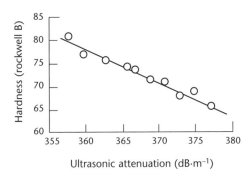

Stress Wave Interaction Model

The basis for ultrasonic assessment of fracture toughness is the concept of stress wave participation in the fracture process during catastrophic crack growth. The concept assumes that the attenuation properties of a material microstructure are important in the fracture process.

A stress wave interaction model based on this concept helps explain existing correlations between ultrasonic attenuation and fracture toughness.[153,183] By using the stress wave interaction model in conjunction with fracture mechanics precepts, it is possible to derive relations between fracture toughness and attenuation factors.[184-187]

Toughness and Ultrasonic Factors

The key relation derived from the stress wave interaction model expresses the ratio of fracture toughness to yield strength as a function of speed and attenuation spectrum parameters:

$$(49) \quad \left(\frac{K_{Ic}}{\sigma_y} \right)^2 = M \sqrt{\frac{v_\ell \beta_\delta}{m}}$$

where K_{Ic} is plane strain fracture toughness (pascal root meter), M is a material constant, m is the exponent on frequency f in the equation for the rayleigh scattering process attenuation coefficient $\alpha = cf^m$, v_ℓ is longitudinal velocity (meter per second), σ_y is yield strength (pascal) and β_δ is the derivative.

$$(50) \quad \beta_\delta = \left. \frac{d\alpha}{df} \right|_\delta$$

where $d\alpha \cdot (df)^{-1}$ is evaluated at a frequency that corresponds to a *critical* ultrasonic wavelength λ_δ in the material. This wavelength is defined by the critical dimension δ, which may be the mean grain size or another feature that participates in crack nucleation and deformation processes.

The quantity $(K_{Ic} \cdot \sigma_y^{-1})^2$ is known as the *characteristic length* and is also a measure of fracture toughness.[188] It is proportional to the size of the crack blunting zone at an active crack tip. This assumes a material in which plastic deformation or some similar micromechanism exists for absorbing stress wave energy at a crack front, such as occurs in a polycrystalline metal.

The preceding equation for characteristic length can be rewritten as:

(51) $\left(\dfrac{K_{Ic}}{\sigma_y}\right)^2 = M\sqrt{\delta\alpha_\delta}$

where α_δ is specific (phase) attenuation for the critical microstructural feature.[132] It is true that this critical feature and its mean size δ must be presupposed to evaluate the characteristic length in either of the preceding equations. However, in theory δ can be deduced from attenuation spectra because it is defined in terms of the mean (phase) wavelength at which

stochastic scattering begins.[80,149,179,184] A second relation that can be derived from the stress wave interaction model is:

(52) $\sigma_y = AK_{Ic} + B\beta_1 + C$

where A, B and C are material constants. The ultrasonic factor β_1 is the slope of the attenuation a versus frequency f curve evaluated at $\alpha = 1$.[84,184]

Experimental Results

The foregoing relations between fracture toughness, yield strength and ultrasonic speed and attenuation have been verified.[84,85,189] As expected, even large changes in fracture toughness produced only slight changes in speed. By contrast, fracture toughness, yield strength and characteristic length $(K_{Ic} \cdot \sigma_y^{-1})^2$ appear to be strongly influenced by stress wave attenuation properties of the tested materials. As a practical matter for some polycrystalline materials, it is unnecessary to determine the critical microstructural feature δ to calculate β_δ. This is because correlations with fracture toughness can usually be obtained by directly comparing it to the attenuation coefficient measured at the highest frequency within rayleigh or stochastic scattering, at 100 MHz for example (see Figs. 15 and 16).[152]

Figures 17 and 18 show results for two maraging steels and a titanium alloy where the critical microstructural factor δ

FIGURE 15. Correlation between ultrasonic attenuation factor and toughness for three heats of low carbon steel; photomicrographs show decreasing grain size associated with increased toughness and attenuation.[132]

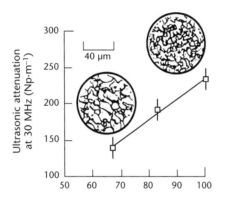

FIGURE 16. Correlation between ultrasonic attenuation factor and toughness for cobalt cemented tungsten carbide. Photomicrographs show that toughness and attenuation increase with cobalt binder content. Toughness measured by palmquist technique is directly proportional to fracture toughness.[152]

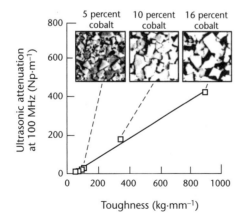

FIGURE 17. Experimental results showing predicted correlation of ultrasonic attenuation factor and fracture toughness characteristic length factor for two maraging steels and titanium alloy.[84]

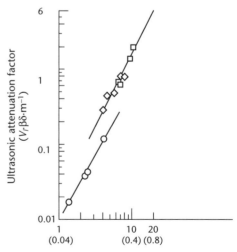

Legend
◇ = Unified Numbering System K92820 nickel alloy maraging steel
□ = Unified Numbering System K92890 nickel alloy maraging steel
○ = titanium beta alloy (8Mo, 8V, 6Cr, 4Mo, 4Zr)

was determined from photomicrographs using the ASTM line intercept method. Figure 18 shows that the well known inverse relation between fracture toughness and yield strength becomes more coherent when yield strength is compared with the expression:

$$(53) \quad a = B_1 + \frac{A}{B} K_{Ic}$$

which is based on Eq. 52. The slopes of the lines in Fig. 18a depend on whether the material fractures in a brittle or ductile manner.[184]

In the case of a titanium alloy with a two phase alpha/beta subgrain structure, there are several possible critical features. As demonstrated in Fig. 19, regression analysis of the data indicates that the beta phase component has the greater dislocation density and is the critical microstructural feature. The alpha phase

component is comparable to the beta component but has a smaller correlation coefficient.[85] Although the ultrasonic data show the beta component to be critical for plastic yielding, the ultrasonic data do not conflict with fractographic data indicating that the alpha component adds to toughness by increasing crack path deflections. The results in Fig. 19 are based on using photomicrographically measured alpha and beta phase platelet thicknesses for a series of test objects heat treated to achieve different toughnesses. The phase thicknesses were taken as the critical microstructural dimensions for calculating β_δ.

These results infer that higher attenuation leads to greater toughness. But the results predicted by Eqs. 49 and 51 and shown in Figs. 17 and 19 apply to materials that exhibit plastic deformation. In brittle materials (ceramics) that do not provide for plastic absorption of stress wave energy, higher attenuation corresponds to lower toughness.

FIGURE 18. Experimental results showing predicted relations among yield strength and ultrasonic factor incorporating fracture toughness and attenuation for titanium alloy and maraging steel: (a) yield strength versus the ultrasonic factor $\beta_1 + (A \cdot B^{-1}) K_{Ic}$ (toughness modified by attenuation) (b) conventional plot of yield strength versus toughness.[184]

(a)

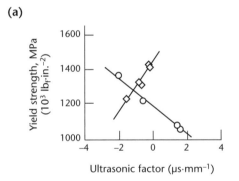

(b)

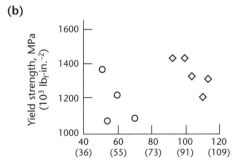

Legend
◇ = Unified Numbering System nickel alloy steel (Ni 200)
○ = titanium beta alloy (8Mo, 8V, 6Cr, 4Mo, 4Zr)

FIGURE 19. Comparison of toughness (characteristic length = $[K_{Ic}/\sigma_y]^2$) and attenuation factors for critical microstructural factors in a two-phase titanium alloy. Best correlation is with the beta phase which, along with the alpha phase, governs fracture toughness: (a) alpha phase thickness with correlation factor of 0.977; (b) beta phase thickness with correlation factor of 0.998.[85]

(a)

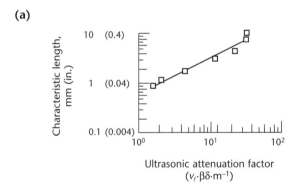

(b)

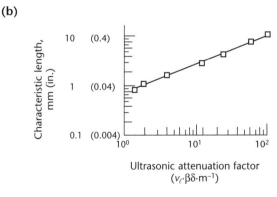

Interrelated Factors

Figure 19 exemplifies an important idea in the nondestructive testing of mechanical properties and microstructure. Any evaluation is incomplete unless three complementary factors are tied together: ultrasonic nondestructive testing measurements, microstructure characteristics and mechanical properties. Conventional destructive methods in materials characterization usually attempt to uncover only correlations between microstructure and destructive test results.

It has been shown that ultrasonic testing is an alternative means for microstructure characterization. Moreover, the results cited above indicate that ultrasonic measurements can not only correlate with destructively measured mechanical properties but can also help identify microstructural features that govern those properties. Figure 19 is an example of a case where three factors are tied together by means of ultrasonic testing.[132]

General Applicability

These examples of ultrasonic tests of mechanical properties are special cases that require constraints on the test object as itemized in Table 3. The close correlations found between ultrasonic measurements and mechanical properties depend on high precision in the determination of speed and attenuation spectra. This is not universally possible even when monolithic materials and composite materials add further difficulties.

Precision ultrasonic methods are not always necessary. Typically, continuous fiber reinforced and woven fiber composites are highly attenuating and heterogeneous. They do not typically lend themselves to precise ultrasonic measurements in the appropriate frequency ranges. Therefore, some alternative approaches have been developed, including the acoustoultrasonic method. With this method, precision measurements of absolute attenuation and speed are not necessary. Instead, relative stochastic wave propagation effects are used to assess mechanical properties.[52]

Composite and Bond Strengths

The relations among grain size, strength and toughness properties do not apply to fiber reinforced composites or fiber matrix, laminated and bonded interfaces. Theoretical foundations are being developed to better explain correlations between ultrasonic measurements and mechanical properties of composite materials and bonded interfaces. For fiber reinforced composites, the efficiency of stress wave energy propagation appears to underlie strength correlations.[53]

The concept is that more efficient stress wave energy transfer (higher speed, lower attenuation) leads to better transmission of dynamic strain, better load distribution and consequently to greater strength, impact resistance and fracture resistance. This generalization leads to ultrasonic methods that place emphasis on waveform analysis to extract information relating to the combined effect of microstructural factors and diffuse discontinuity populations that influence mechanical strength, toughness and dynamic response (as in composites and structures with bonded interfaces). Examples of methods that use this concept are given below.

Interface and Bond Strengths

Ultrasonic assessment of cohesive and adhesive bond and interface strengths is generally based on interface reflectivity variations associated with bond quality.[47] Assuming good mechanical or chemical bonding, there is no overt discontinuity but there is usually a definite jump in acoustic impedance. This results in different reflection coefficients according to the nature of the joined materials and the bond quality. If the bond line is of finite thickness, it may contain microporosity or other diffuse microstructural discontinuities that cause lower strength.

A theoretical basis for ultrasonic bond strength assessment has been proposed in which transverse waves are used to test the cohesive shear strength of the bond line or interface adhesive strength.[62] This requires the introduction of interface or guided lamb waves using oblique incidence pitch catch techniques. Interface waves arise when bonded adherent thicknesses are much greater than the wavelengths used. Guided lamb wave modes arise when the bond line or adherent thicknesses are comparable to the wavelengths used. One approach is to use speed measurements to estimate shear strength from shear modulus. Another approach uses attenuation measurements to estimate strength by sensing morphological variations in bondlines.

Composite Strengths

Ultrasonic tests can form the basis for measuring energy transfer efficiency and for ranking composite components according to strength. Ultrasonic attenuation and speed vary with the combined effects of fiber matrix interface quality, matrix porosity, fiber and ply orientation and other microstructural factors.

These same factors govern mechanical properties (ultimate tensile strength, interlaminar strength, impact strength and toughness). Ultrasonic attenuation in polymer matrix composite laminates correlates with ultimate strength, interlaminar shear strength and stiffness. The measurements can be accomplished by through-transmission, pulse echo backscatter and acoustoultrasonic methods.[51,52,61,190-192]

PART 6. Acoustoultrasonic Tests for Mechanical Properties

The acoustoultrasonic approach to characterization of composite and bond strengths is highlighted below. Examples are given of applications to composite panels and adhesive bonds. In both cases, the acoustoultrasonic signal consists primarily of the superposition of multiple reverberations of waves reflected by bounding surfaces and internal interfaces. The waveforms usually result from stochastic interactions and have the general nature of burst waveforms found in acoustic emission.[19]

In the acoustoultrasonic method, the stress wave factor is used to quantify the signal. Lower values of the stress wave factor generally correspond to higher attenuation.

The stress wave factor may be defined in a variety of ways based primarily on acoustic emission practice: ringdown count, peak voltage or root mean square energy of the time domain signal (see Fig. 20).[20,53,61] Spectral analysis and partitioning of acoustoultrasonic signals are additional means for assigning values to the stress wave factor and for comparing the relative strength of composite test objects (Fig. 21).[52,59,74,75,190,191,193,194]

Typical acoustoultrasonic waveforms are shown in Fig. 22 for two unidirectional composite panels and transducers to illustrate the effect of fiber

FIGURE 20. Diagram of two basic techniques for quantifying of acoustoultrasonic stress wave factor: (a) peak voltage (SWF) = $E_v = V_{max}$; (b) ringdown count $E_c = PRC$, corresponding to positive threshold crossings.[20]

(a)

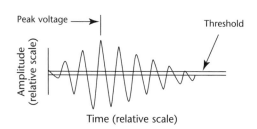

(b)

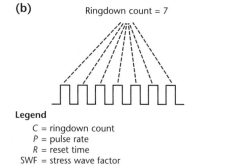

Legend
C = ringdown count
P = pulse rate
R = reset time
SWF = stress wave factor

FIGURE 21. Alternative approaches to acoustoultrasonic stress wave factor quantification.[53]

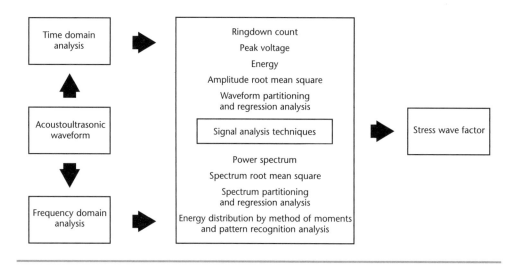

direction relative to the sending and receiving transducer. It is apparent that significant changes in the waveform occur as ply orientation changes from axial to transverse. The changes in waveform include signal strength, shape, speed and frequency content. The net change can often be quantified by a simple ringdown count to calculate stress wave factor values parallel and perpendicular to the fiber direction.

The stress wave factor measurements were made on a series of laminated composite panels with a variety of ply orientations (various fiber directions). The results in Fig. 23 show that the normalized stress wave factor correlates with ultimate tensile strength as governed by ply orientation.[82]

Interlaminar Shear Strength

There are other means for evaluating the stress wave factor when simple ringdown counts produce poor correlations. Information contained in the acoustoultrasonic signal can be exploited by alternative analysis methods. One of these is waveform (or spectrum) partitioning in which that part of the waveform (or spectrum) that best correlates with a particular property is determined by regression analysis.[59] The result given in Fig. 24 is an example of this approach, where regression analysis showed the partition of the acoustoultrasonic waveform giving the best correlation with interlaminar shear strength. In this case, a relative stress wave factor was defined as:

$$(54) \quad SWF = \int_{t_1}^{t_2} V^2 dt$$

This is the integral of voltage squared over the time zone of the partition t_1 to t_2.

FIGURE 23. Stress wave factor versus ultimate tensile strength for series of graphite fiber, epoxy matrix composite laminate samples with various ply orientations. Stress wave factor calculated from ringdown count.[82]

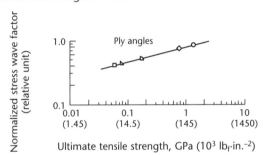

Legend
◻ = 1.57 rad (90 deg)
▲ = 0.18 rad (10 deg)
◺ = ±0.79 rad (±45 deg)
◇ = 0 ± 0.79 rad (0 ± 45 deg)
○ = 0 rad

FIGURE 22. Typical waveforms for acoustoultrasonic signals that have traveled in unidirectional composite panels:
(a) waveform for travel parallel to fibers;
(b) waveform for travel perpendicular to fibers.

(a)

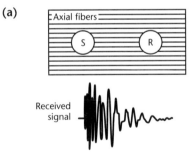

(b)

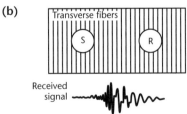

Legend
S = sending piezotransducer coupled to panel surface
R = receiving piezotransducer coupled to panel surface

FIGURE 24. Stress wave factor versus interlaminar shear strength for filament wound graphite epoxy composite bend test objects. Stress wave factor is the integral of voltage squared over a partitioned zone of the waveform. Correlation factor is 0.968.[59]

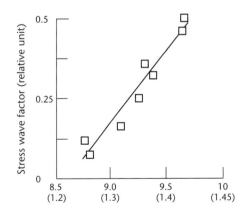

Poor correlations or indeterminate results were found in other time partition zones or over the entire time window of the waveform.

Adhesive Bond Strength

An alternative approach to defining the stress wave factor was found useful in establishing a correlation with the shear strength of adhesively bonded steel plates.[61] For the results given in Fig. 25, the stress wave factor was expressed as a voltage weighted ringdown count:

$$(55) \quad SWF = \sum_i^p V_i \left(C_i - C_{i+1} \right)$$

where C_i is the number of counts at the ith level, V_i is the threshold voltage at the ith level and V_p is the peak voltage of the waveform.

In this case, the entire raw waveform above a preselected minimum voltage threshold was used to quantify the stress wave factor. However, conditions may dictate that the best correlation depends on first filtering the raw waveform and dealing only with that portion of the signal within a preselected bandwidth or frequency zone.[195]

FIGURE 25. Stress wave factor versus shear strength of adhesively bonded steel test objects for range of test temperatures. Stress wave factor was calculated as voltage weighted ringdown count with correlation factor of 0.964.[61]

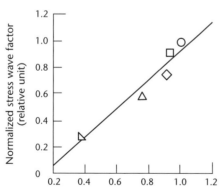

Legend

○ = 30 °C (85 °F)
□ = 60 °C (140 °F)
◇ = 90 °C (190 °F)
△ = 120 °C (250 °F)
◁ = 150 °C (300 °F)

Modulus Degradation

Another alternative for defining the stress wave factor is given with respect to measuring changes in modulus (stiffness) associated with cyclic fatiguing and associated microcracking (see Fig. 26).[196] In this case, the stress wave factor was defined as the root mean square value of the power spectrum of the acoustoultrasonic waveform.[190]

Note that the stress wave factor is about ten times more sensitive to the effects of fatigue damage than the secant modulus measurement. Moreover, the slopes of the two curves in Fig. 26 differ in detail because, although the secant modulus refers to the length of the entire test object, the stress wave factor measurements represent only part of it.

Limitations of Acoustoultrasonic Techniques

Acoustoultrasonic testing represents a generalized approach for materials characterization and carries both the capabilities and the limitations found in a variety of kindred techniques. Beyond the limitations common to all discontinuity detection methods, the ultrasonic characterization of subtle discontinuities and material properties is also subject to circumstances that affect sensitivity and signal reproducibility.[197]

Both the acoustoultrasonic and pulse echo technique are vulnerable to transducers misalignment and couplant variations. With pulse echo ultrasonic testing, it is common to misread attenuation by a factor of ten or more.

FIGURE 26. Covariation of stress wave factor and secant modulus with fatigue degradation in graphite epoxy fiber composite laminate. Stress wave factor is the root mean square of the power spectrum.[190, 196]

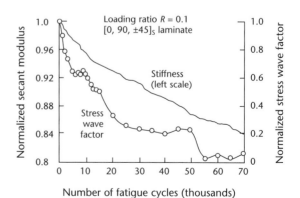

This magnitude of error can occur if the transducer is not literally ground onto the test object surface.[28] This error is particularly common at high frequencies (over 20 MHz) where couplant thickness variations, bubbles, surface porosity and reflection coefficient anomalies can have serious effects.[29,33]

Factors Affecting Test Results

Acoustoultrasonic measurements are affected by several factors associated with the attachment of the transducer to the test object: (1) applied pressure, (2) type and amount of couplant, (3) object surface roughness, (4) transducer alignment, (5) spacing between transducers and (6) exact location of transducers on the object.

Even if these are optimized, a further problem remains. In practice, acoustoultrasonic measurements must be repeatable over the test object surface. This may require lifting and recoupling the transducers or inventing transducers that can scan while remaining in contact with the surface.

The coupling problems associated with scanning may be avoided by using noncontact laser ultrasonics. However, laser ultrasonics introduces other problems that can limit signal control and readout. Such problems arise from surface roughness, reflectivity and other factors.

The selection of sending and receiving transducers, their bandwidth, their resonance frequencies and their internal damping all have an effect on test results, primarily because ringdown in an undamped transducer can be confused with reverberations. In testing composite panels, it is useful to select transducer frequencies that introduce wavelengths less than the panel thickness. Or, in the case of continuous fiber reinforced composites, it is helpful to cover the frequency range likely to be transmitted by both the composite and fibers acting as waveguides.

These two considerations dictate transducer spacing, which must be small enough to avoid losing the reception of high frequency signal components. However, general guidelines for selecting transducer frequency, bandwidth and instrumentation parameters cannot be prescribed for all cases. The best approach is to use the successful examples cited here and to experimentally seek the optimum conditions for particular applications. This approach can be facilitated by waveform (or spectrum) partitioning and by regression analysis to identify the portion of the signal that best correlates with the material property of interest.

Closing

Ultrasonic nondestructive material property characterization can be divided into several categories.

1. Elastic moduli are determined through measurements of ultrasonic speed or dynamic vibration.
2. Some methods depend on speed and attenuation measurements to characterize residual stress, grain size, porosity, texture and other microstructural factors of material behavior. Sometimes these microstructural factors can be used to predict values or variations of mechanical properties such as strength or toughness.
3. Ultrasonic measurements can be correlated with mechanical properties: speed with hardness or attenuation with toughness. This category generally includes empirical correlations that have been found to apply only to specific materials, usually in the form of laboratory specimens.

Precise ultrasonic measurements must be made on test objects with specific size, shape, thickness and surface condition. Or, for the measurements to have at least relative significance, geometric properties of the test objects must be held constant, as in damping measurements to obtain relative modulus changes. This leads to an alternative approach to materials characterization in which greater emphasis is placed on signal analysis to extract information on relative changes in material properties. In this approach, ultrasonic wave propagation, energy transfer and signal modulation properties of a material are used to assess relative variations in mechanical properties: ultimate strength or bond strength.

Empirical correlations between ultrasonic measurements and mechanical properties have important roles in industry. There are likely to be ambiguities concerning the exact nature and influence of underlying microstructural factors being measured. This is true in the case of complex, heterogeneous, anisotropic, textured and composite materials where several variables can simultaneously affect wave propagation. These factors introduce complex relations among microstructure, mechanical properties and load response (deformation and fracture modes).

The inferring of material properties often depends on the use of two or more corroborative and complementary test methods, some of which are neither widely applied nor widely accepted in industry. The biggest challenge in ultrasonic materials characterization has been to apply the techniques to practical field work.

Wider use of ultrasonic methods has expanded through significant improvements in computers, instrumentation and materials themselves, particularly with respect to electronic materials and nanotechnology. The literature describing these advancements has continued to grow.[198-207]

References

1. Vary, A. Section 12, "Material Property Characterization." *Nondestructive Testing Handbook,* second edition: Vol. 7, *Ultrasonic Testing.* Columbus, OH: American Society for Nondestructive Testing (1991): p 383-431.

2. Green, R.E. *Ultrasonic Investigation of Mechanical Properties. Treatise on Materials Science and Technology.* Vol. 3. Saint Louis, MO: Elsevier/Academic Press (1973).

3. Green, R.E. "Ultrasonic Attenuation Detection of Fatigue Damage." *Ultrasonics International 1973.* Guildford, United Kingdom: Elsevier (1973): p 187-193.

4. Green, R.E. "Ultrasonic Nondestructive Materials Characterization." *Materials Analysis by Ultrasonics.* Park Ridge, NJ: Noyes Data Corporation (1987): p 1-29.

5. Vary, A. "Ultrasonic Measurement of Material Properties." *Research Techniques in Nondestructive Testing.* Vol. 4. London, United Kingdom: Academic Press (1980): p 159-204.

6. Manderscheid, J.M. and J.P. Gyekenyesi. "Fracture Mechanics Concepts in Reliability Analysis of Monolithic Ceramics." *Nondestructive Testing of High-Performance Ceramics* [Boston, MA, August 1987]. Columbus, OH: American Ceramics Society (1987): p 59-72.

7. Kanninen, M. and C. Popelar. *Advanced Fracture Mechanics.* Oxford, United Kingdom: Oxford University Press (1985): p 392-432.

8. Cawley, P. and R. Adams. "The Mechanics of the Coin-Tap Method." *Journal of Sound and Vibration.* Vol. 122, No. 2. Amsterdam, Netherlands: Elsevier (1988): p 299-316.

9. Adams, R.D. and P. Cawley. "Vibration Techniques in Nondestructive Testing." *Research Techniques in Nondestructive Testing.* Vol. 8. London, United Kingdom: Academic Press (1985): p 303-360.

10. Uygur, E. "Nondestructive Dynamic Testing." *Research Techniques in Nondestructive Testing.* Vol. 4. London, United Kingdom: Academic Press (1980): p 205-244.

11. Nowich, A. and B. Berry. *Anelastic Relaxation in Crystalline Solids.* London, United Kingdom: Academic Press (1972).

12. Tittmann, B. "Apparatus for Measuring High Internal Friction Q-Factors." *Review of Scientific Instruments.* Vol. 47. Melville, NY: American Institute of Physics (1976): p 1516.

13. Smith, C., ed. *Internal Friction and Ultrasonic Attenuation in Solids: Proceedings of the European Conference on Internal Friction and Ultrasonic Attenuation* [July 1980]. Oxford, United Kingdom: Pergamon Press (1980).

14. Cawley, P. and R. Adams. "Vibration Techniques." *Non-Destructive Testing of Fibre-Reinforced Plastic Composites.* Vol. 1. London, United Kingdom: Elsevier Applied Science (1987): p 151-200.

15. Deka, M. and N. Eberhardt. "Internal Friction of Fe-Based Binary Alloys at High Frequency." *Nondestructive Methods for Material Property Determination* [Hershey, PA, April 1983]. New York, NY: Plenum (1984): p 135-148.

16. DiCarlo, J. and J. Maisel. "Measurement of the Time-Temperature Dependent Dynamic Mechanical Properties of Boron/Aluminum Composites." *Composite Materials: Testing and Design.* Special Technical Publication 674. West Conshohocken, PA: ASTM International (1979): p 201-227.

17. Papadakis, E.P. and B. Kovacs. "Theoretical Model for Comparison of Sonic-Resonance and Ultrasonic Velocity Techniques for Assuring Quality in Nodular Iron Parts." *Materials Evaluation.* Vol. 38, No. 6. Columbus, OH: American Society for Nondestructive Testing (May 1980): p 25-30.

18. Shiori, J., O. Furuta and K. Satoh. "Analysis of Elevated Property of Heat Resistant Materials by Internal Friction." *Nondestructive Characterization of Materials II* [Montreal, Canada, July 1986]. New York, NY: Plenum (1987): p 325-333.

19. Matthews, J.R., ed. *Acoustic Emission.* New York, NY: Gordon and Breach Science Publishers (1983).

20. Kline, R.A. "Acoustic Emission Signal Characterization." *Acoustic Emission*. New York, NY: Gordon and Breach Science Publishers (1983): p 105-138.
21. Arrington, M. "Acoustic Emission." *Non-Destructive Testing of Fibre-Reinforced Plastic Composites*. Vol. 1. London, United Kingdom: Elsevier Applied Science (1987): p 25-63.
22. Liptai, R.G., D.O. Harris and C.A. Tatro. *Acoustic Emission*. Special Technical Publication 505. West Conshohocken, PA: ASTM International (1972).
23. Spanner, J. *Acoustic Emission: Techniques and Applications*. Evanston, IL: Intex Publishing (1974).
24. Wadley, H.N.G. and R. Mehrabian. "Acoustic Emission for In-Process Monitoring and Microstructure Control?" *Nondestructive Methods for Material Property Determination* [Hershey, PA, April 1983]. New York, NY: Plenum (1984): p 207-236.
25. *Nondestructive Testing Handbook*, second edition: Vol. 5, *Acoustic Emission Testing*. Columbus, OH: American Society for Nondestructive Testing (1986).
26. Scruby, C. "Quantitative Acoustic Emission Techniques." *Research Techniques in Nondestructive Testing*. Vol. 8. London, United Kingdom: Academic Press (1985): p 141-210.
27. Green, R.E. "Basic Wave Analysis of Acoustic Emission." *Mechanics of Nondestructive Testing*. New York, NY: Springer (1980): p 55-76.
28. Truell, R., C. Elbaum and B. Chick. *Ultrasonic Methods in Solid State Physics*. Saint Louis, MO: Elsevier/Academic Press (1969).
29. Vary, A. "Simulation of Transducer-Couplant Effects on Broadband Ultrasonic Signals." *International Advances in Nondestructive Testing*. Vol. 8. New York, NY: Gordon and Breach (1980): p 167-200.
30. Papadakis, E.P. "Ultrasonic Velocity and Attenuation: Measurement Methods with Scientific and Industrial Applications." *Physical Acoustics: Principles and Methods*. Vol. 12. Saint Louis, MO: Elsevier/Academic Press (1976): p 277-374.
31. Vary, A. "Computer Signal Processing for Ultrasonic Attenuation and Velocity Measurement for Material Property Characterization." *Proceedings of the Twelfth Symposium on Nondestructive Evaluation* [San Antonio, TX, April 1979]. San Antonio, TX: Southwest Research Institute (1979): p 33-46.
32. Vary, A. "Concepts and Techniques for Ultrasonic Evaluation of Material Mechanical Properties." *Mechanics of Nondestructive Testing*. New York, NY: Plenum (1980): p 123-141.
33. Generazio, E.R. "The Role of the Reflection Coefficient in Precision Measurement of Ultrasonic Attenuation." *Materials Evaluation*. Vol. 45, No. 8. Columbus, OH: American Society for Nondestructive Testing (July 1985): p 995-1004.
34. Vary, A. and H. Kautz. "Transfer Function Concept for Ultrasonic Characterization of Material Microstructures." *International Advances in Nondestructive Testing*. Vol. 13. New York, NY: Gordon and Breach (1988): p 193-249.
35. Hull, D., H. Kautz and A. Vary. "Measurement of Ultrasonic Velocity Using Phase-Slope and Cross-Correlation Methods." *Materials Evaluation*. Vol. 43, No. 11. Columbus, OH: American Society for Nondestructive Testing (October 1985): p 1455-1460.
36. Sachse, W. and Y. Pao. "On the Determination of Phase and Velocity of Dispersive Waves in Solids." *Journal of Applied Physics*. Vol. 39. Melville, NY: American Institute of Physics (1978): p 4320.
37. Tittmann, B., H. Nadler, V. Clark, L. Ahlberg and T. Spencer. "Frequency Dependence of Seismic Dissipation in Rocks." *Geophysical Research Letters*. Vol. 8. Washington, DC: American Geophysical Union (1981): p 36-88.
38. Winkler, K. "Frequency Dependent Ultrasonic Properties of High Porosity Sandstones." *Journal of Geophysical Research*. Vol. 88. Washington, DC: American Geophysical Union (1983): p 9493-9499.
39. Krautkrämer, J. and H. Krautkrämer. *Ultrasonic Testing of Materials,* fourth edition. New York, NY: Springer-Verlag (1990).
40. Kinsler, L.E., A.R. Frey, A.B. Coppens and J.V. Sanders. *Fundamentals of Acoustics*, fourth edition. New York, NY: Wiley (1999).
41. Papadakis, E.P. "Buffer Rod System for Ultrasonic Attenuation Measurements." *Journal of the Acoustical Society of America*. Vol. 44, No. 5. Melville, NY: American Institute of Physics, for the Acoustical Society of America (1968): p 1437-1441.

42. Goebbels, K. "Structural Analysis by Scattered Ultrasonic Radiation." *Research Techniques in Nondestructive Testing.* Vol. 4. London, United Kingdom: Academic Press (1980): p 87-157.

43. Theiner, W.A. and H.H. Willems. "Determination of Microstructural Parameters by Ultrasonic NDE." *Nondestructive Methods for Material Property Determination* [Hershey, PA, April 1983]. New York, NY: Plenum (1984): p 249-258.

44. Willems, H. and K. Goebbels. "Characterization of Microstructure by Backscatter Ultrasonic Waves." *Metal Science.* London, United Kingdom: Metals Society (1981): p 549-553.

45. Fitting, D.W. and L. Adler. *Ultrasonic Spectral Analysis for Nondestructive Evaluation.* New York, NY: Plenum (1981).

46. Good, M.S. and J.L. Rose. "Measurement of Thin Case Depth in Hardened Steel by Ultrasonic Pulse-Echo Technique." *Nondestructive Methods for Material Property Determination* [Hershey, PA, April 1983]. New York, NY: Plenum (1984): p 189-203.

47. Segal, E. and J. Rose. "Nondestructive Testing Techniques for Adhesive Bond Joints." *Research Techniques in Nondestructive Testing.* Vol. 7. London, United Kingdom: Academic Press (1980): p 275-316.

48. Telschow, K.L. and J.E. Flinn. "Ultrasonic Characterization of Consolidated Rapidly Solidified Powders." *Nondestructive Characterization of Materials II* [Montreal, Canada, July 1986]. New York, NY: Plenum (1987): p 149-157.

49. Qu, J. and J. Achenbach. "Analytical Treatment of Polar Backscatter from Porous Composites." *Review of Progress in Quantitative Nondestructive Evaluation.* Vol. 6B. New York, NY: Plenum (1987): p 1137-1146.

50. Tittmann, B., L. Ahlberg and K. Fertig. "Ultrasonic Characterization of Microstructures in Powder Metal Alloy." *Materials Analysis by Ultrasonics.* Park Ridge, NJ: Noyes Data Corporation (1987): p 30-46.

51. Bar-Cohen, Y. "Ultrasonic NDE of Composites — A Review." *Solid Mechanics Research for Quantitative Non-Destructive Evaluation* [Evanston, IL, September 1985]. Dordrecht, Netherlands: Martinus Nijhoff (1987): p 187-201.

52. Duke, J.C., Jr., ed. *Acousto-Ultrasonics: Theory and Applications* [Blacksburg, VA, July 1987]. New York, NY: Plenum (1988).

53. Vary, A. "The Acousto-Ultrasonic Approach." *Acousto-Ultrasonics: Theory and Applications* [Blacksburg, VA, July 1987]. New York, NY: Plenum (1988): p 1-21.

54. Scruby, C., R. Smith and B. Moss. "Microstructural Monitoring by Laser Ultrasonic Attenuation and Forward Scattering." *NDT International.* Vol. 19, No. 5. Guildford, Surrey, United Kingdom: Butterworth Scientific Limited (1986): p 307-313.

55. Rosen, M. "Analytical Ultrasonics for Characterization of Metallurgical Microstructures and Transformations." *Materials Analysis by Ultrasonics.* Park Ridge, NJ: Noyes Data Corporation (1987): p 79-98.

56. Tittmann, B., L. Ahlberg, J. Richardson and R. Thompson. "Determination of Physical Property Gradients from Measured Surface Wave Dispersion." *Transactions on Sonics and Ultrasonics.* Vol. 34, No. 5. New York, NY: Institute of Electrical and Electronics Engineers (1987): p 500-507.

57. Schreiber, E., O. Anderson and N. Soga. *Elastic Constants and Their Measurement.* New York, NY: McGraw-Hill (1973).

58. J.C. Duke, Jr., and E.G. Henneke, II. "Analytical Ultrasonics for Evaluation of Composite Material Response." *Materials Analysis by Ultrasonics.* Park Ridge, NJ: Noyes Data Corporation (1987): p 148-163.

59. Kautz, H. *Acousto-Ultrasonic Verification of the Strength of Filament Wound Composite Material.* NASA Technical Memorandum 88827. Washington, DC: National Aeronautics and Space Administration (1986).

60. Dos Reis, H. and H. Kautz. "Nondestructive Evaluation of Adhesive Bond Strength Using the Stress Wave Factor Technique." *Journal of Acoustic Emission.* Vol. 5, No. 4. Los Angeles, CA: Acoustic Emission Group (1986): p 144-147.

61. Fahr, A., S. Lee, S. Tanary and Y. Haddad. "Estimation of Strength in Adhesively Bonded Steel Specimens by Acousto-Ultrasonic Technique." *Materials Evaluation.* Vol. 45, No. 2. Columbus, OH: American Society for Nondestructive Testing (February 1989): p 233-239.

62. Rokhlin, S.I. "Characterization of Composites and Adhesive Cure by Ultrasonic Waves." *Nondestructive Characterization of Materials II* [Montreal, Canada, July 1986]. New York, NY: Plenum (1987): p 105-113.

63. Rokhlin, S.I. "Adhesive Joint Evaluation by Ultrasonic Interface and Lamb Waves." *Materials Evaluation by Ultrasonics*. Park Ridge, NJ: Noyes Data Corporation (1987): p 299-310.

64. Bracewell, R.N. *The Fourier Transform and Its Applications,* third edition. New York, NY: McGraw-Hill (1999).

65. Kline, R.A. "Measurement of Attenuation and Dispersion Using an Ultrasonic Spectroscopy Technique." *Journal of the Acoustical Society of America*. Vol. 76, No. 2. Melville, NY: American Institute of Physics, for the Acoustical Society of America (1984): p 498-504.

66. Kline, R. and D. Egle. "Applications of Digital Methods to Ultrasonic Materials Characterization." *NDT International*. Vol. 19, No. 5. Guildford, Surrey, United Kingdom: Butterworth Scientific (1986): p 341-347.

67. Roberts, R. "Porosity Characterization in Fiber-Reinforced Composites by Backscatter." *Review of Progress in Quantitative Nondestructive Evaluation*. Vol. 6B. New York, NY: Plenum (1987): p 1147-1156.

68. Henneke, E.G., II, J.C. Duke, Jr. and R.C. Stiffler. "Characterization of the Damage State of Composite Laminates via the Acousto-Ultrasonic Technique." *Solid Mechanics Research for Quantitative Non-Destructive Evaluation* [Evanston, IL, September 1985]. Dordrecht, Netherlands: Martinus Nijhoff (1987): p 217-235.

69. Andrews, H.C. *Introduction to Mathematical Techniques in Pattern Recognition*. New York, NY: Wiley-Interscience (1972).

70. Johnson, R.A. and D.W. Wichern. *Applied Multivariate Statistical Analysis,* fifth edition. Upper Saddle River, NJ: Prentice Hall (2002).

71. Oppenheim, A.V., A.S. Willsky and S.H. Nawab. *Signals and Systems,* second edition. Upper Saddle River, NJ: Prentice Hall (1996).

72. Gammell, P. "Coherent Processing of the Full Analytical Signal Information of Ultrasonic Waveforms." *International Advances in Nondestructive Testing*. Vol. 10. New York, NY: Gordon and Breach (1984): p 183-266.

73. Karagülle, H., J.H. Williams and S.S. Lee. "Application of Homomorphic Signal Processing to Stress Wave Factor Analysis." *Materials Evaluation*. Vol. 43, No. 11. Columbus, OH: American Society for Nondestructive Testing (October 1985): p 1446-1454.

74. Williams, J.H., S.S. Lee and H. Karagülle. "Input-Output Characterization of an Ultrasonic Testing System by Digital Signal Analysis." *Materials Analysis by Ultrasonics*. Park Ridge, NJ: Noyes Data Corporation (1987): p 302-330.

75. Williams, J.H. and S.S. Lee. "Pattern Recognition Characterizations of Micromechanical and Morphological Material States via Analytical Ultrasonics." *Materials Analysis by Ultrasonics*. Park Ridge, NJ: Noyes Data Corporation (1987): p 193-206.

76. Weaver, R. "Diffuse Field Decay Rates for Material Characterization." *Solid Mechanics Research for Quantitative Non-Destructive Evaluation* [Evanston, IL, September 1985]. Dordrecht, Netherlands: Martinus Nijhoff (1987): p 426-434.

77. Weaver, R. "Diffuse Waves for Materials NDE." *Acousto-Ultrasonics: Theory and Applications* [Blacksburg, VA, July 1987]. New York, NY: Plenum (1988): p 35-43.

78. Gericke, O. "Ultrasonic Spectroscopy." *Research Techniques in Nondestructive Testing*. London, United Kingdom: Academic Press (1970): p 31-62.

79. Serabian, S. "Ultrasonic Material Property Determinations." *Materials Analysis by Ultrasonics*. Park Ridge, NJ: Noyes Data Corporation (1987): p 211-224.

80. Smith, R. "Ultrasonic Materials Characterization." *NDT International*. Vol. 20, No. 1. Guildford, Surrey, United Kingdom: Butterworth Scientific Limited (1987): p 23-28.

81. Tittmann, B., B. Hosten and M. Abdel-Gawad. "Ultrasonic Attenuation in Carbon-Carbon Composites and the Determination of Porosity." *Proceedings of the 1986 IEEE Ultrasonics Symposium*. New York, NY: Institute of Electrical and Electronics Engineers (1986).

82. Vary, A. and R. Lark. "Correlation of Fiber Composite Tensile Strength with the Ultrasonic Stress Wave Factor." *Journal of Testing and Evaluation*. Vol. 7, No. 4. Philadelphia, PA: American Society for Testing and Materials (1979): p 185-191.

83. Vary, A. and K. Bowles. "Ultrasonic Evaluation of the Strength of Unidirectional Graphite/Polyimide Composites." *Proceedings of the Eleventh Symposium on Nondestructive Evaluation*. San Antonio, Texas: Southwest Research Institute (1977): p 242-258.

84. Vary, A. "Correlations among Ultrasonic Propagation Factors and Fracture Toughness Properties of Metallic Materials." *Materials Evaluation*. Vol. 36, No. 7. Columbus, OH: American Society for Nondestructive Testing (June 1978): p 55-64.

85. Vary, A. and D. Hull. "Interrelation of Material Microstructure, Ultrasonic Factors and Fracture Toughness of a Two-Phase Titanium Alloy." *Materials Evaluation*. Vol. 41, No. 3. Columbus, OH: American Society of Nondestructive Testing (March 1982): p 309-314.

86. Briggs, A. *An Introduction to Scanning Acoustic Microscopy*. London, United Kingdom: Oxford University Press, for the Royal Microscopical Society (1986).

87. Nikoonahad, M. "Reflection Acoustic Microscopy for Industrial NDT." *Research Techniques in Nondestructive Testing*. Vol. 7. London, United Kingdom: Academic Press (1984): p 217-257.

88. Birnbaum, G. and G. White. "Laser Techniques in Nondestructive Evaluation." *Research Techniques in Nondestructive Testing*. Vol. 7. London, United Kingdom: Academic Press (1984): p 259-365.

89. Yuhas, D. and M. Oravecz. "Microstructure Characterization of Titanium by Acoustic Microscopy." *Nondestructive Methods for Material Property Determination* [Hershey, PA, April 1983]. New York, NY: Plenum (1984): p 259-270.

90. Rosencwaig, A. *Photoacoustics and Photoacoustic Microscopy*. New York, NY: Wiley (1980).

91. Rosencwaig, A. "Thermal-Wave Imaging in a Scanning Electron Microscope." *International Advances in Nondestructive Testing*. Vol. 10. New York, NY: Gordon and Breach (1985): p 105-174.

92. Ringermacher, H. and C. Kitteredge. "Photoacoustic Microscopy of Ceramics." *Review of Progress in Quantitative Nondestructive Evaluation*. Vol. 68. New York, NY: Plenum (1987): p 1231-1240.

93. Thomas, R.L., L.D. Favro and P.K. Kuo. "Thermal Wave Imaging for Quantitative Non-Destructive Evaluation." *Solid Mechanics Research for Quantitative Non-Destructive Evaluation* [Evanston, IL, September 1985]. Dordrecht, Netherlands: Martinus Nijhoff (1987): p 239-253.

94. Gruber, J., J. Smith and R. Brockelman. "Ultrasonic Velocity C-Scans for Ceramics and Composites." *Materials Evaluation*. Vol. 46, No. 1. Columbus, OH: American Society for Nondestructive Testing (January 1988): p 90-96.

95. Generazio, E.R., D.J. Roth and G.Y. Baaklini. "Acoustic Imaging of Subtle Porosity Variations in Ceramics." *Materials Evaluation*. Vol. 46, No. 10. Columbus, OH: American Society for Nondestructive Testing (September 1988): p 1338-1343.

96. Briggs, G.A.D. and M.G. Smoekh. "Acoustic Microscopy of Surface Cracks: Theory and Practice." *Solid Mechanics Research for Quantitative Non-Destructive Evaluation* [Evanston, IL, September 1985]. Dordrecht, Netherlands: Martinus Nijhoff (1987): p 155-169.

97. Rice, R. "Microstructure Dependence of Mechanical Behavior of Ceramics." *Treatise on Materials Science and Technology*. Vol. 11. New York, NY: Academic Press (1977): p 199-381.

98. Mason, W.P. *Physical Acoustics and the Properties of Solids*. Princeton, NJ: D. Van Nostrand Company (1958).

99. Klima, S. and G.Y. Baaklini. "Ultrasonic Characterization of Structural Ceramics." *Materials Analysis by Ultrasonics*. Park Ridge, NJ: Noyes Data Corporation (1987): p 112-121.

100. Varshini, Y.P. *Physical Review*. Vol. 2. Melville, NY: American Institute of Physics (1970): p 3952-3955.

101. Ledbetter, H. and D. Read. "Low Temperature Elastic Properties of a 300-Grade Maraging Steel." *Metallurgical Transactions*. Vol. 8A. Materials Park, OH: ASM International (1977): p 1805-1808.

102. Monchalin, J.-P., R. Héon, J.F. Bussière and B. Farahbakhsh. "Laser Ultrasonic Determination of Elastic Constants at Ambient and Elevated Temperatures." *Nondestructive Characterization of Materials II* [Montreal, Canada, July 1986]. New York, NY: Plenum (1987): p 717-723.

103. Allen, D., W. Cooper, C. Sayers and M. Silk. "The Use of Ultrasonics to Measure Residual Stress." *Research Techniques in Nondestructive Testing*. Vol. 6. London, United Kingdom: Academic Press (1982): p 151-209.

104. Pao, Y., W. Sachse and H. Fukuoka. "Acoustoelasticity and Ultrasonic Measurement of Residual Stress." *Physical Acoustics*. Vol. 17. Saint Louis, MO: Elsevier/Academic Press (1984): p 61-143.

105. Pao, Y.-H. "Theory of Acoustoelasticity and Acoustoplasticity." *Solid Mechanics Research for Quantitative Non-Destructive Evaluation* [Evanston, IL, September 1985]. Dordrecht, Netherlands: Martinus Nijhoff (1987): p 257-273.

106. Droney, B.E. "Use of Ultrasonic Techniques to Assess the Mechanical Properties of Steels." *Nondestructive Methods for Material Property Determination* [Hershey, PA, April 1983]. New York, NY: Plenum (1984): p 237-248.

107. Hsu, N. "Acoustic Birefringence and Use of Ultrasonic Waves for Experimental Stress Analysis." *Experimental Mechanics*. Vol. 14, No. 5. Bethel, CT: Society for Experimental Mechanics (1974): p 169-176.

108. Okada, K. "Stress-Acoustic Relations for Stress Measurements by Ultrasonic Techniques." *Journal of the Acoustical Society of Japan*. Vol. 1, No. 3. Tokyo, Japan: Acoustical Society of Japan (1980): p 193-200.

109. Mignogna, R.B., A.V. Clark, B.B. Rath and C.L. Vold. "Effects of Rolled Plate Thickness on Anisotropy with Applications to Acoustic Stress Measurement." *Nondestructive Methods for Material Property Determination* [Hershey, PA, April 1983]. New York, NY: Plenum (1984): p 339-351.

110. Salama, K. and C.K. Ling. "The Effect of Stress on the Temperature Dependence of Ultrasonic Velocity." *Journal of Applied Physics*. Vol. 51. Melville, NY: American Institute of Physics (1980): p 1505.

111. Kwun, H. "Measurement of Stress in Steels Using Magnetically Induced Velocity Changes for Ultrasonic Waves." *Nondestructive Characterization of Materials II* [Montreal, Canada, July 1986]. New York, NY: Plenum (1987): p 633-642.

112. Bell, J. and J. Chen. "Pulse-Echo Method of Determining the Elastic Constants of Rectangular Strips and Square Plates." *NDT International*. Vol. 14, No. 6. Guildford, Surrey, United Kingdom: Butterworth Scientific (1981): p 325-327.

113. Blessing, G.V., N.N. Hsu and T.M. Proctor. "Ultrasonic Shear Wave Measurements of Known Residual Stress in Aluminum." *Nondestructive Methods for Material Property Determination* [Hershey, PA, April 1983]. New York, NY: Plenum (1984): p 353-363.

114. Ledbetter, H. "Stainless Steel Elastic Constants at Low Temperatures." *Journal of Applied Physics*. Vol. 52, No. 3. Melville, NY: American Institute of Physics (1981): p 1587-1589.

115. Lynnworth, L., E.P. Papadakis and K. Fowler. "Ultrasonic Propagation Measurements and Applications." *International Advances in Nondestructive Testing*. Vol. 5. New York, NY: Gordon and Breach (1977): p 71-115.

116. Tittmann, B., G. Alers and L. Graham. "Use of the Impulse Technique for Rapid Texture Evaluation in Commercial Tube and Plate Materials." *Metallurgical Transactions*. Vol. 7A. Materials Park, OH: ASM International (1976): p 229.

117. Schneider, E., S. Chu and K. Salama. "Influence of Texture on the Variations of Temperature Dependence of Ultrasonic Wave Velocities with Stress." *Proceedings of Ultrasonics International*. Guildford, Surrey, United Kingdom: Butterworth Scientific (1985): p 133-138.

118. Kupperman, D.S. "Analytical Ultrasonics for Structural Materials." *Materials Analysis by Ultrasonics*. Park Ridge, NJ: Noyes Data Corporation (1987): p 99-111.

119. Chandrasekaran, N. and K. Salama. "Relationship between Stress and Temperature Dependence of Ultrasonic Shear Velocity." *Nondestructive Methods for Material Property Determination* [Hershey, PA, April 1983]. New York, NY: Plenum (1984): p 393-403.

120. Thompson, R., J. Smith and S. Lee. "Inference of Stress and Texture from Angular Dependence of Ultrasonic Plate Mode Velocities." *Materials Analysis by Ultrasonics*. Park Ridge, NJ: Noyes Data Corporation (1987): p 164-175.

121. Heyman, J. and M. Namkung. "Residual Stress Measurements in Carbon Steel." *Materials Evaluation by Ultrasonics*. Park Ridge, NJ: Noyes Data Corporation (1987): p 61-74.

122. Namkung, M., D. Utrata, J.S. Heyman and S.G. Allison. "Low-Field Magnetoacoustic Residual Stress Measurements in Steel." *Solid Mechanics Research for Quantitative Non-Destructive Evaluation* [Evanston, IL, September 1985]. Dordrecht, Netherlands: Martinus Nijhoff (1987): p 301-318.

123. Husson, D., S.D. Bennett and G.S. Kino. "Rayleigh Wave Measurement of Surface Stresses in Stainless Steel Piping." *Nondestructive Methods for Material Property Determination* [Hershey, PA, April 1983]. New York, NY: Plenum (1984): p 365-375.

124. Egle, D.M. and D. Bray. "Measurement of Acousto-Elastic and Third Order Elastic Constants for Rail Steel." *Journal of the Acoustical Society of America*. Vol. 60, No. 3. Melville, NY: American Institute of Physics, for the Acoustical Society of America (1976): p 741-744.

125. Fukuoka, H. "Ultrasonic Measurement of Residual Stress." *Solid Mechanics Research for Quantitative Non-Destructive Evaluation* [Evanston, IL, September 1985]. Dordrecht, Netherlands: Martinus Nijhoff (1987): p 275-299.

126. Allen, D. and W. Cooper. "A Fourier Transform Technique that Measures Phase Delays of Ultrasonic Pulses with Accuracy for Determining Residual Stress in Metals." *NDT International*. Vol. 16, No. 4. Guildford, Surrey, United Kingdom: Butterworth Scientific (1983): p 205-217.

127. Mott, G. and M. Tsao. "Acoustoelastic Effects in Two Structural Steels." *Nondestructive Methods for Material Property Determination* [Hershey, PA, April 1983]. New York, NY: Plenum (1984): p 377-392.

128. Schuckler, F. "Grain Size." *Quantitative Microscopy*. New York, NY: McGraw-Hill (1968): p 201-265.

129. DeHoff, R. "The Statistical Background of Qualitative Metallography." *Quantitative Microscopy*. New York, NY: McGraw Hill (1968): p 11-44.

130. Papadakis, E.P. "Ultrasonic Diffraction from Single Apertures with Application to Pulse Measurements and Crystal Physics." *Physical Acoustics: Principles and Methods*. Vol. 11. Saint Louis, MO: Elsevier/Academic Press (1975): p 152-211.

131. Green, R.E. "Effect of Metallic Microstructure on Ultrasonic Attenuation." *Nondestructive Evaluation: Microstructural Characterization and Reliability Strategies*. Warrensdale, PA: Metallurgical Society of the American Institute of Mechanical Engineers (1981): p 115-132.

132. Vary, A. "Concepts for Interrelating Ultrasonic Attenuation, Microstructure and Fracture Toughness in Polycrystalline Solids." *Materials Evaluation*. Vol. 46, No. 5. Columbus, OH: American Society for Nondestructive Testing (April 1988): p 642-649. Erratum, Vol. 46, No. 8 (July 1988): p 1118.

133. Mason, W. and H. McSkimmin. "Attenuation and Scattering of High Frequency Sound Waves in Metals and Glasses." *Journal of the Acoustical Society of America*. Vol. 19, No. 3. Melville, NY: American Institute of Physics, for the Acoustical Society of America (1947): p 464-473.

134. Mason, W. and H. McSkimmin. *Journal of Applied Physics*. Vol. 19, No. 10. Melville, NY: American Institute of Physics (1948): p 940-946.

135. Lifsitz, I. and G. Parkomovskii. *Zhurnal Eksperimental'noi i Teoreticheskoi Fiziki*. Vol. 20. Moscow, Russia: Izdatel'stvo Nauka. Melville, NY: American Institute of Physics (1950): p 175-182.

136. Merkulov, L. "Investigation of Ultrasonic Scattering in Metals." *Soviet Physics. Technical Physics*. Vol. 1, No. 1. Melville, NY: American Institute of Physics (1957): p 59-69.

137. Kolsky, H. *Stress Waves in Solids*. New York, NY: Dover (1963).

138. Lücke, K. "Ultrasonic Attenuation Caused by Thermoelastic Heat Flow." *Journal of Applied Physics*. Vol. 27. Melville, NY: American Institute of Physics (1956): p 1433-1438.

139. Auld, B. *Acoustic Fields and Waves in Solids*. Vol. 1. New York, NY: John Wiley and Sons (1973).

140. Granato, A.V. and K. Lücke. "Theory of Mechanical Damping Due to Dislocations." *Journal of Applied Physics*. Vol. 27, No. 6. Melville, NY: American Institute of Physics (1956): p 583-593.

141. Seeger, A. and P. Schiller. "The Formation and Diffusion of Kinks As the Fundamental Process of Dislocation Movement in Internal Movement Friction Measurements." *Acta Metallurgica*. Vol. 10. Elmsford, NY: Pergamon Press (1962): p 348-357.

142. Langlois, P. and J.F. Bussière. "Magnetoelastic Contribution to Ultrasonic Attenuation in Structural Steels." *Nondestructive Characterization of Materials II* [Montreal, Canada, July 1986]. New York, NY: Plenum (1987): p 291-298.

143. Winkler, K. and W. Murphy. "Scattering in Glass Beads: Effects of Frame and Pore Fluid Compressabilities." *Journal of the Acoustical Society of America.* Vol. 76, No. 3. Melville, NY: American Institute of Physics, for the Acoustical Society of America (1984): p 820-825.

144. Papadakis, E.P. "Ultrasonic Attenuation Caused by Rayleigh Scattering by Graphite Nodules in Nodular Cast Iron." *Journal of the Acoustical Society of America.* Vol. 70, No. 3. Melville, NY: American Institute of Physics, for the Acoustical Society of America (1981): p 782-787.

145. Sayers, C. "Scattering of Ultrasound by Minority Phases in Polycrystalline Metals." *Wave Motion.* Vol. 7. Amsterdam, Netherlands: Elsevier Science Publications (1985): p 95-104.

146. Evans, A., B. Tittmann, L. Ahlberg, B. Khuri-Yakub and G. Kino. "Ultrasonic Attenuation in Ceramics." *Journal of Applied Physics.* Vol. 49, No. 5. Melville, NY: American Institute of Physics, for the Acoustical Society of America (1978): p 2669-2679.

147. Perkeris, C. "Note on the Scattering of Radiation in an Inhomogeneous Medium." *Physical Review.* Vol. 71, No. 4. Melville, NY: American Institute of Physics (1947): p 268-270.

148. Roney, R. *The Influence of Metal Grain Structure on the Attenuation of an Ultrasonic Acoustic Wave.* Dissertation. Pasadena, CA: California Institute of Technology (1950).

149. Serabian, S. and R.S. Williams. "Experimental Determination of Ultrasonic Attenuation Characteristics Using the Roney Generalized Theory." *Materials Evaluation.* Vol. 36, No. 8. Columbus, OH: American Society for Nondestructive Testing (July 1978): p 55-62.

150. Smith, R. "The Effect of Grain Size Distribution on the Frequency Dependence of the Ultrasonic Attenuation in Polycrystalline Materials." *Ultrasonics.* Vol. 22, No. 9. Saint Louis, MO: Elsevier (1982): p 211-214.

151. Bozorg-Grayeli, N. *Acoustic Nondestructive Evaluation of Microstructure.* Dissertation. Stanford, CA: Stanford University (1981).

152. Vary, A. and D. Hull. TM-83358, *Ultrasonic Ranking of Toughness of Tungsten Carbide.* Washington, DC: National Aeronautics and Space Administration (1983).

153. Serabian, S. "Frequency and Grain Size Dependency of Ultrasonic Attenuation in Polycrystalline Materials." *British Journal of Non-Destructive Testing.* Vol. 22, No. 2. Northampton, United Kingdom: British Institute of Non-Destructive Testing (1980): p 69-77.

154. Kopec, B. and V. Hanak. "Use of Ultrasonic Attenuation to Investigate Anomalies in the Structure of Railway Axles." *NDT International.* Vol. 17, No. 5. Saint Louis, MO: Elsevier (1984): p 265-268.

155. Bussière, J.F. "Application of Nondestructive Evaluation to Processing of Metals." *Review of Progress in Quantitative Nondestructive Evaluation.* Vol. 6B. New York, NY: Plenum (1987): p 1377-1393.

156. Klinman, R., G. Webster, F. Marsh and E. Stephenson. "Ultrasonic Prediction of Grain Size, Strength and Toughness in Plain Carbon Steel." *Materials Evaluation.* Vol. 38, No. 10. Columbus, OH: American Society for Nondestructive Testing (September 1980): p 26-32.

157. Yada, H. and K. Kawashima. "Important Metallurgical Parameters That Must be Determined to Control the Properties of Steels during Processing." *Nondestructive Characterization of Materials II* [Montreal, Canada, July 1986]. New York, NY: Plenum (1987): p 195-209.

158. Klinman, R. and E. Stephenson. "Ultrasonic Prediction of Grain Size and Mechanical Properties in Plain Carbon Steel." *Materials Evaluation.* Vol. 39, No. 12. Columbus, OH: American Society for Nondestructive Testing (November 1981): p 1116-1120.

159. Generazio, E.R. "Ultrasonic Verification of Microstructural Changes Due to Heat Treatment." *Materials Analysis by Ultrasonics.* Park Ridge, NJ: Noyes Data Corporation (1987): p 200-210.

160. Goebbels, K. and S. Hirsekorn. "A New Method for Stress Determination in Textured Materials." *NDT International.* Vol. 17, No. 6. Saint Louis, MO: Elsevier (1984): p 337-341.

161. Hosten, B., M. Deschamps and B. Tittmann. "Inhomogeneous Wave Generation and Propagation in Lossy Anisotropic Solids — Composites Characterization." *Journal of the Acoustical Society of America.* Melville, NY: American Institute of Physics, for the Acoustical Society of America (1986-1987).

162. Sayers, C. "Ultrasonic Determination of Texture and Residual Stress in Polycrystalline Metals." *Solid Mechanics Research for Quantitative Non-Destructive Evaluation* [Evanston, IL, September 1985]. Dordrecht, Netherlands: Martinus Nijhoff (1987): p 319-333.

163. Mignogna, R., P.P. Delsanto, A.V. Clark, B.B. Rath and C.L. Vold. "Ultrasonic Measurements on Textured Materials." *Nondestructive Characterization of Materials II* [Montreal, Canada, July 1986]. New York, NY: Plenum (1987): p 545-553.

164. Kupperman, D.S., K.J. Reimann and J. Abrego-Lopez. "Ultrasonic NDE of Cast Stainless Steel." *NDT International*. Vol. 20, No. 3. Saint Louis, MO: Elsevier (June 1987): p 145-152.

165. Generazio, E.R. "Ultrasonic Determination of Recrystallization." *Review of Progress in Quantitative Nondestructive Evaluation*. Vol. 6B. New York, NY: Plenum (1987): p 1465-1475.

166. Friant, C.L. and M. Rosen. "Ultrasonic Materials Characterization of Melt Spun Metallic Ribbons." *Nondestructive Methods for Material Property Determination* [Hershey, PA, April 1983]. New York, NY: Plenum (1984): p 301-314.

167. Piché, L. "Application of Ultrasonics to the Characterization of Composites: A Method for the Determination of Polyethylene Density." *Nondestructive Characterization of Materials II* [Montreal, Canada, July 1986]. New York, NY: Plenum (1987): p 79-87.

168. Vary, A., E.R. Generazio, D.J. Roth and G.Y. Baaklini. "Ultrasonic NDE of Structural Ceramics for Power and Propulsion Systems." *Non-Destructive Testing: Proceedings of the Fourth European Conference* [London, United Kingdom, September 1987]. Vol. 2. Oxford, United Kingdom: Pergamon Press (1988): p 1299-1307.

169. Adler, L. and S. Wang. "Ultrasonic Measurement of Porosity in Casts and Welds." *Materials Analysis by Ultrasonics*. Park Ridge, NJ: Noyes Data Corporation (1987): p 72-78.

170. Tittmann, B. "Ultrasonic Measurements for the Prediction of Mechanical Strength." *NDT International*. Vol. 11. Guildford, Surrey, United Kingdom: Butterworth Scientific Limited (1978): p 17.

171. Schaller, R., J.J. Ammann and P. Millet. "Mechanical Properties of Composite Materials by Internal Friction." *Nondestructive Characterization of Materials II* [Montreal, Canada, July 1986]. New York, NY: Plenum (1987): p 345-353.

172. Petch, N. "The Cleavage Strength of Polycrystals." *Journal of the Iron and Steel Institute*. Vol. 174. Materials Park, OH: ASM International (1953): p 25.

173. Hall, E. "Deformation and Aging of Mild Steel III: Discussion and Results." *Proceedings of the Physical Society*. Vol. 64. London, United Kingdom: Physical Society (1951): p 747.

174. Hall, E. *Yield Point Phenomena in Metals and Alloys*. New York, NY: Plenum (1970).

175. Armstrong, R. "The Influence of Polycrystalline Grain Size on Several Mechanical Properties." *Metallurgical Transactions*. Materials Park, OH: ASM International (1970): p 1169-1176.

176. Armstrong, R. "The Influence of Polycrystal Grain Size on Mechanical Properties." *Advances in Materials Research*. Vol. 4. New York, NY: Wiley (1970): p 101-146.

177. Smith, R. and W. Reynolds. "The Correlation of Ultrasonic Attenuation, Microstructure and Ductile to Brittle Transition Temperature in Low Carbon Steels." *Journal of Materials Science*. Vol. 17. London, United Kingdom: Chapman and Hall (1982): p 1420-1426.

178. Smith, R.L., K.L. Rusbridge, W.N. Reynolds and B. Hudson. "Ultrasonic Attenuation, Microstructure and Ductile to Brittle Transition Temperature in Fe-C Alloys." *Materials Evaluation*. Vol. 41, No. 2. Columbus, OH: American Society for Nondestructive Testing (February 1983): p 219-222.

179. Smith, R. "Materials Characterization by Ultrasonic Attenuation Spectral Analysis." *Review of Progress in Quantitative Nondestructive Evaluation*. Vol. 6B. New York, NY: Plenum (1987): p 1475-1483.

180. Alford, N., K. Kendall, W. Clegg and J. Birchall. "Strength/Microstructure Relation in Alumina and Titania." *Advanced Ceramic Materials*. Vol. 3, No. 2. Westerville, OH: American Ceramic Society (1988): p 113-117.

181. Shabel, B.S. and R.F. Young. "A New Procedure for Rapid Determination of Yield and Tensile Strength from Hardness Tests." *Nondestructive Characterization of Materials II* [Montreal, Canada, July 1986]. New York, NY: Plenum (1987): p 335-343.

182. Rivenez, J., A. Lambert and C. Flambard. "Nondestructive Determination of Hardening Depths with Ultrasonic Surface Waves." *Nondestructive Characterization of Materials II* [Montreal, Canada, July 1986]. New York, NY: Plenum (1987): p 373-380.

183. Vary, A. "Ultrasonic Nondestructive Evaluation, Microstructure and Fracture Toughness Interrelations." *Solid Mechanics Research for Quantitative Non-Destructive Evaluation* [Evanston, IL, September 1985]. Dordrecht, Netherlands: Martinus Nijhoff (1987): p 135-152.

184. Vary, A. "Correlations between Ultrasonic and Fracture Toughness Factors in Metallic Materials." *Fracture Mechanics*. Special Technical Publication 677. West Conshohocken, PA: ASTM International (1979): p 563-578.

185. Fu, L. "Mechanical Aspects of NDE by Sound and Ultra-Sound." *Applied Mechanics Reviews*. Vol. 55, No. 8. New York, NY" ASME International (1982): p 1047-1057.

186. Fu, L. "On Ultrasonic Factors and Fracture Toughness." *Engineering Fracture Mechanics*. Vol. 18, No. 1. New York, NY: Pergamon (1983): p 59-67.

187. Fu, L. "Micromechanics and Its Application to Fracture and NDE." *Developments in Mechanics*. Vol. 12. Iowa City, IA: University of Iowa Press (1983): p 263-265.

188. Hahn, G., M. Kanninen and A. Rosenfeld. *Annual Reviews of Materials Science*. Vol. 2. Palo Alto, CA: Annual Reviews (1972): p 381-404.

189. Canella, G. and M. Taddei. "Correlation Between Ultrasonic Attenuation and Fracture Toughness of Steels." *Nondestructive Characterization of Materials II* [Montreal, Canada, July 1986]. New York, NY: Plenum (1987): p 261-269.

190. Govada, A., J.C. Duke, Jr., E.G. Henneke, II, and W. Stinchcomb. CR-174870, *A Study of the Stress Wave Factor Technique for the Characterization of Composite Materials*. Washington, DC: National Aeronautics and Space Administration (1985).

191. Govada, A., E.G. Henneke, II, and R. Talreja. "Acousto-Ultrasonic Measurements to Monitor Damage during Fatigue of Composites." *Advances in Aerospace Sciences and Engineering* [New Orleans, LA, December 1984]. New York, NY: ASME International (1984): p 55-60.

192. Duke, J.C., Jr., E.G. Henneke, II, and W. Stinchcomb. CR-3976, *Ultrasonic Stress Wave Characterization of Composite Materials*. Washington, DC: National Aeronautics and Space Administration (1986).

193. Williams, J.H. and N. Lampert. "Ultrasonic Evaluation of Impact-Damaged Graphite Fiber Composite." *Materials Evaluation*. Vol. 38, No. 12. Columbus, OH: American Society for Nondestructive Testing (November 1980): p 68-72.

194. Williams, J.H. and S.S. Lee. "Pattern Recognition Characterization of Micromechanical and Morphological Materials States via Analytical Quantitative Ultrasonics." *Materials Analysis by Ultrasonics*. Park Ridge, NJ: Noyes Data Corporation (1987): p 187-199.

195. Tanary, S. *Characterization of Adhesively Bonded Joints Using Acousto-Ultrasonics*. Thesis. Ottawa, Province of Quebec, Canada: University of Ottawa (1988).

196. Duke, J.C., Jr., E.G. Henneke, II, W. Stinchcomb and K. Reifsnider. "Characterization of Composite Materials by Means of the Ultrasonic Stress Wave Factor." *Proceedings of the Second International Conference on Composite Structures*. London, United Kingdom: Applied Science Publishers (1984): p 53-60.

197. Russell-Floyd, R. and M.G. Phillips. "A Critical Assessment of Acousto-Ultrasonics As a Method of Nondestructive Examination." *NDT International*. Vol. 21, No. 4. Guildford, Surrey, United Kingdom: Butterworth Scientific (1988): p 247-257.

198. Thompson, R.B. "Determination of Texture and Grain Size in Metals: An Example of Materials Characterization." *Topics on Nondestructive Evaluation:* Vol. 1, *Sensing for Materials Characterization, Processing, and Manufacturing*. Columbus, OH: American Society for Nondestructive Testing (1998): p 23-45.

199. Rohklin, S.I. and A.I. Lavrentyev. "Ultrasonic Characterization of Thin Surface and Interphase Layers." *Topics on Nondestructive Evaluation:* Vol. 1, *Sensing for Materials Characterization, Processing, and Manufacturing*. Columbus, OH: American Society for Nondestructive Testing (1998): p 47-83.

200. Hsu, D.K. "Ultrasonic Sensors for Robotics and Field Operation." *Topics on Nondestructive Evaluation*: Vol. 4, *Automation, Miniature Robotics, and Sensors for Nondestructive Testing and Evaluation*. Columbus, OH: American Society for Nondestructive Testing (2000): p 165-173.

201. Sherrit, S., Y. Bar-Cohen and X. Bao. "Ultrasonic Materials, Actuators, and Motors (USM)." *Topics on Nondestructive Evaluation*: Vol. 4, *Automation, Miniature Robotics, and Sensors for Nondestructive Testing and Evaluation*. Columbus, OH: American Society for Nondestructive Testing (2000): p 215-231.

202. Rogers, W.P. "Elastic Property Measurement Using Rayleigh-Lamb Waves." *Research in Nondestructive Evaluation*. Vol. 6. Columbus, OH: American Society for Nondestructive Testing (1995): p 185-208.

203. Roth, D.J., J.D. Kiser, S.M. Swickard, S.A. Szatmary and D.P. Kerwin. "Quantitative Mapping of Pore Fraction Variations in Silicon Nitride Using an Ultrasonic Contact Scan Technique." *Research in Nondestructive Evaluation*. Vol. 6. Columbus, OH: American Society for Nondestructive Testing (1995): p 125-168.

204. Kawamoto, S., J.H. Muehl and R.S. Williams. "Use of Acousto-Ultrasonic Techniques to Determine Properties of Remanufactured Particle Boards Made Solely from Recycled Particles." *Third International Workshop on Green Composites* [Kyoto, Japan, March 20005]. Tokyo, Japan: Japanese Society for Nondestructive Inspection (2005): p 184-189.

205. Kautz, H.E. NASA TM-1998-208410, *Noncontact Acousto-Ultrasonics for Material Characterization*. Washington, DC: National Aeronautics and Space Administration (1998).

206. Kautz, H.E. NASA CR-2002-211881, *Acousto-Ultrasonics to Assess Material and Structural Properties*. Washington, DC: National Aeronautics and Space Administration (2002).

207. Finlayson, R.D., M. Friesel, M. Carlos, P. Cole and J.C. Lenain. "Health Monitoring of Aerospace Structures with Acoustic Emission and Acousto-Ultrasonics." *Insight*. Vol. 43, No. 3. Northampton, United Kingdom: British Institute of Non-Destructive Testing (March 2001): p 155-158.

Bibliography

Achenbach, J. and Y. Rajapakse. *Solid Mechanics Research for Quantitative Non-Destructive Evaluation* [Evanston, IL, September 1985]. Dordrecht, Netherlands: Martinus Nijhoff (1987).

Allen, D.R. and C.M. Sayers. "The Influence of Stress on the Principal Polarisation Directions of Ultrasonic Shear Waves in Textured Steel Plates." *Journal of Physics D: Applied Physics*. Vol. 17, No. 7. Melville, NY: American Institute of Physics (1984): p 215-222.

Allen, D.R. and C.M. Sayers. "Ultrasonic SH Waves in Textured Aluminum Plates." *Ultrasonics*. Vol. 23. Guildford, Surrey: IPC Science and Technology Press (1984): p 215-222.

AMD, Vol 234: ASME International Mechanical Engineering Congress and Exposition [Nashville, TN, November 1999]. NDE, Vol. 17: *On the Recent Advances of the Ultrasonic Evaluation and Composite Material Characterization*. New York, NY: ASME International (1999).

ASTM E 1736, *Standard Practice for Acousto-Ultrasonic Assessment of Filament-Wound Pressure Vessels*. West Conshohocken, PA: ASTM International (2005).

Bar-Cohen, Y. and D.E. Chimenti. "Detection of Porosity in Composite Laminates by Leaky Lamb Waves." *11th World Conference on Nondestructive Testing*. Vol. 3. Columbus, OH. American Society for Nondestructive Testing (1985): p 1661-1668.

Betz, D.C., G. Thursby, B. Culshaw and W.J. Staszewski. "Acousto-Ultrasonic Sensing Using Fiber Bragg Gratings." *Smart Material Structures*. Vol. 12, No. 1. Melville, NY: American Institute of Physics (February 2003): p 122-128.

Bhatia, A.B. *Ultrasonic Absorption: An Introduction to the Theory of Sound Absorption and Dispersion in Gases, Liquids, and Solids*. New York, NY: Dover (1967, 1985).

Chang, M., R. Chang and C. Shu. "The Application of Ultrasonic Attenuation Measurements to Estimate Corrosion in Pipeline at Support Structures." *Materials Evaluation*. Vol. 60, No. 5. Columbus, OH: American Society for Nondestructive Testing (May 2002): p 631-634.

Chen, C.-H. *Nonlinear Maximum Entropy Spectral Analysis for Signal Recognition*. New York, NY: Research Studies Press (1982).

Dos Reis, H. "Acousto-Ultrasonic Non-Destructive Evaluation of Wire Rope Using the Stress Wave Factor Technique." *British Journal of Non-Destructive Testing.* Vol. 28, No. 3. Northampton, United Kingdom: British Institute of Non-Destructive Testing (1986): p 155-156.

Dos Reis, H., L. Bergman and J. Bucksbee. "Adhesive Bond Strength Quality Assurance Using the Acousto-Ultrasonic Technique." *British Journal of Non-Destructive Testing.* Vol. 28, No. 6. Northampton, United Kingdom: British Institute of Non-Destructive Testing (1986): p 357-358.

Ganesan, V., P. Palanichamy and B. Raj. "Elastic Modulus Determination as a Potential Tool for Predicting Embrittlement in a Ferritic Steel." *Materials Evaluation.* Vol. 62, No. 2. Columbus, OH: American Society for Nondestructive Testing (February 2004): p 137-142.

Hahn, H.T. "Application of Ultrasonic Technique to Cure Characterization of Epoxies." *Nondestructive Methods for Material Property Determination* [Hershey, PA, April 1983]. New York, NY: Plenum (1984): p 315-326.

Haines, N., J. Bell and P. McIntyre. "The Application of Broadband Ultrasonic Spectroscopy to the Study of Layered Media." *Journal of the Acoustical Society of America.* Vol. 64, No. 6. Melville, NY: American Institute of Physics, for the Acoustical Society of America (1978): p 1645-1651.

Hemann, J.H., P. Cavano, H.E. Kautz and K. Bowles. "Trans-Ply Crack Density Detection by Acousto-Ultrasonics." *Acousto-Ultrasonics: Theory and Applications* [Blacksburg, VA, July 1987]. New York, NY: Plenum (1988): p 319-325.

Heyman, J., S. Allison and K. Salama. "The Effect of Carbon Concentration and Plastic Deformation on Ultrasonic Higher Order Elastic Constants." *Ultrasonics International Conference Proceedings.* Surrey, United Kingdom: Butterworth Scientific Limited (1985): p 786-791.

Hinrichs, R. and J. Thuen. *Control System for Processing Composite Materials.* United States Patent 4 455 268 (1984).

Höller, P. "Nondestructive Analysis of Structure and Stresses by Ultrasonic and Magnetic Methods." *Nondestructive Characterization of Materials II* [Montreal, Canada, July 1986]. New York, NY: Plenum (1987): p 211-225.

Hosten, B., L. Alberg, B. Tittmann and B. Springarn. "Ultrasonic Characterization of Diffusion Bonds." *Review of Progress in Quantitative Nondestructive Evaluation.* Vol. 6B. New York, NY: Plenum (1987): p 1701-1706.

Kline, R.A. and D. Hashemi. "Ultrasonic Guided-Wave Monitoring of Fatigue Damage Development in Bonded Joints." *Materials Evaluation.* Vol. 45, No. 9. Columbus, OH: American Society for Nondestructive Testing (September 1987): p 1076-1082.

Kumar, A., T. Jayakumar, B. Raj and K.K. Ray. "Ultrasonic Time Domain Technique for Frequency Dependent Attenuation Measurement for Microstructural Characterization of a Titanium Alloy." *Materials Evaluation.* Vol. 61, No. 12. Columbus, OH: American Society for Nondestructive Testing (December 2003): p 1321-1326.

Kumar, A., V. Shankar, T. Jayakumar, G. Srinivasan and B. Raj. "Nondestructive Measurement of Coating Thickness Using Through Thickness Ultrasonic Velocity Measurements." *Materials Evaluation.* Vol. 60, No. 6. Columbus, OH: American Society for Nondestructive Testing (June 2002): p 791-794.

Kutty, T., K. Chandrasekharan, J. Panakkal, S. Ghosal and P. De. "Use of Ultrasonic Velocity for Nondestructive Evaluation of Ferrite Content in Duplex Stainless Steel." *NDT International.* Vol. 20, No. 6. Guildford, Surrey, United Kingdom: Butterworth Scientific Limited (1987): p 359-361.

Ledbetter, H. "Texture in Stainless Steel Welds: an Ultrasonic Study." *Journal of Materials Science.* Vol. 20. London, United Kingdom: Chapman and Hall (1985): p 1720-1724.

Lin, L., X.M. Li and J.S. Zhang. "Nondestructive Differentiation of Three Transformation Products in Low Alloy Steel Using Two Ultrasonic Methods." *Materials Evaluation.* Vol. 61. No. 4. Columbus, OH: American Society for Nondestructive Testing (April 2003): p 512-516.

MacCrone, R., ed. *Treatise on Materials Science and Technology.* Vol. 11. Saint Louis, MO: Elsevier/Academic Press (1977).

Massines, F. and L. Piché. "Ultrasonic Characterization of Polymers in Their Evolution from Solid to Liquid State." *Nondestructive Characterization of Materials II* [Montreal, Canada, July 1986]. New York, NY: Plenum (1987): p 49-60.

Monchalin, J.-P. and J.F. Bussiére. "Measurement of Near-Surface Ultrasonic Absorption by Thermo-Emissivity." *Nondestructive Methods for Material Property Determination* [Hershey, PA, April 1983]. New York, NY: Plenum (1984): p 289-297.

Nondestructive Testing Handbook, second edition, Volume 5: Acoustic Emission Testing. Columbus, OH: American Society for Nondestructive Testing (1986).

Palanichamy, P. and M. Vasudevan. "Ultrasonic Testing of Annealing Behavior and Texture and Determination of Texture Coefficients in Stainless Steel." *Materials Evaluation.* Vol. 61, No. 9. Columbus, OH: American Society for Nondestructive Testing (September 2003): p 1020-1025.

Papadakis, E.P. "From Micrograph to Grain-Size Distribution with Ultrasonic Applications." *Journal of Applied Physics.* Vol. 35. Melville, NY: American Institute of Physics (1964): p 1586-1594.

Papadakis, E.P. "Revised Grain-Scattering Formulas and Tables." *Journal of the Acoustical Society of America.* Vol. 37, No. 4. Melville, NY: American Institute of Physics, for the Acoustical Society of America (1965): p 703-710.

Papadakis, E.P. "Ultrasonic Attenuation in SAE 3140 and 4150 Steel." *Journal of the Acoustical Society of America.* Vol. 32, No. 12. Melville, NY: American Institute of Physics, for the Acoustical Society of America (1960): p 1628-1639.

Papadakis, E.P. "Ultrasonic Attenuation and Velocity in SAE 52100 Steel Quenched from Various Temperatures." *Metallurgical Transactions.* Vol. 1. Materials Park, OH: ASM International (1970): p 1053-1057.

Papadakis, E.P. "Ultrasonic Attenuation and Velocity in Three Transformation Products in Steel." *Journal of Applied Physics.* Vol. 35. Melville, NY: American Institute of Physics (1964): p 1474-1482.

Papadakis, E.P. "Ultrasonic Attenuation Caused by Scattering in Polycrystalline Metals." *Journal of the Acoustical Society of America.* Vol. 37, No. 4. Melville, NY: American Institute of Physics, for the Acoustical Society of America (1965): p 711-717.

Phani, K.K. and N.R. Bose. "Application of Acousto-Ultrasonics for Predicting Hygrothermal Degradation of Unidirectional Glass-Fiber Composites." *Acousto-Ultrasonics: Theory and Applications* [Blacksburg, VA, July 1987]. New York, NY: Plenum (1988): p 327-336.

Piché, L. and A. Hamel. "Characterization of Isotropic Composites Containing Inclusions of Specific Shapes by Ultrasonics." *Nondestructive Characterization of Materials II* [Montreal, Canada, July 1986]. New York, NY: Plenum (1987): p 95-103.

Razvi, S., P. Li, K. Salama, J. Cantrell and W. Yost. "Nondestructive Characterization of Aluminum Alloys." *Review of Progress in Quantitative Nondestructive Evaluation.* Vol. 6B. New York, NY: Plenum (1987): p 1403-1408.

Rebello, C. and J.C. Duke, Jr. "Factors Influencing the Ultrasonic Stress Wave Factor Evaluation of Composite Material Structures." *Journal of Composites Technology and Research.* Vol. 8, No. 1. West Conshohocken, PA: ASTM International (1986): p 18-23.

Reed, R.W. and A.L. Bertram. "Ultrasonic Measurements of Elastic Moduli of Thermally Cycled Metal Matrix Composite Precursor Wires." *Nondestructive Methods for Material Property Determination* [Hershey, PA, April 1983]. New York, NY: Plenum (1984): p 327-336.

Reynolds, W. and R. Smith. "Ultrasonic Wave Attenuation Spectra in Steels." *Journal of Physics D: Applied Physics.* Vol. 17, No. 1. Melville, NY: American Institute of Physics (1984): p 109-116.

Rokhlin, S.I., A. Baltazar, B. Xie, J. Chen and R. Reuven. "Method for Monitoring Environmental Degradation of Adhesive Bonds." *Materials Evaluation.* Vol. 59, No. 6. Columbus, OH: American Society for Nondestructive Testing (June 2002): p 795-801.

Ruud, C.O. and R.E. Green, eds. *Nondestructive Methods for Material Property Determination* [Hershey, PA, April 1983]. New York, NY: Plenum (1984).

Scott, W. and P. Gordon. "Ultrasonic Spectrum Analysis for Nondestructive Testing of Layered Composite Materials." *Journal of the Acoustical Society of America.* Vol. 62, No. 1. Melville, NY: American Institute of Physics, for the Acoustical Society of America (1977): p 108-116.

Shukla, S. and S. Yun. "Ultrasonic Attenuation in GaAs." *Journal of the Acoustical Society of America*. Vol. 70, No. 6. Melville, NY: American Institute of Physics, for the Acoustical Society of America (1981): p 1713-1716.

Srivastava, V. and R. Prakash. "Fatigue Prediction of Glass Fiber Reinforced Plastics Using the Acousto-Ultrasonic Technique." *International Journal of Fatigue*. Vol. 9, No. 3. Amsterdam, Netherlands: Elsevier (1987): p 175-178.

Srivastava, V. and R. Prakash. "Prediction of Material Property Parameter of FRP Composites Using Ultrasonic and Acousto-Ultrasonic Techniques." *Composite Structures*. Vol. 8. Barking, Essex, United Kingdom: Applied Science (1987): p 311-321.

Vary, A. "Acousto-Ultrasonic Characterization of Fiber Reinforced Composites." *Materials Evaluation*. Vol. 40, No. 6. Columbus, OH: American Society for Nondestructive Testing (May 1982): p 650-654.

Vary, A., ed. *Materials Analysis by Ultrasonics — Metals, Ceramics, Composites*. Park Ridge, NJ: Noyes Data Corporation (1987).

Willems, H. "Investigation of Creep Damage in Alloy 800H Using Ultrasonic Velocity Measurements." *Nondestructive Characterization of Materials II* [Montreal, Canada, July 1986]. New York, NY: Plenum (1987): p 471-479.

Willems, H., W. Bendick and H. Weber. "Nondestructive Evaluation of Creep Damage in Service Exposed 14 MoV 6 3 Steel." *Nondestructive Characterization of Materials II* [Montreal, Canada, July 1986]. New York, NY: Plenum (1987): p 451-459.

Williams, J.H., H. Yuce and S.S. Lee. "Ultrasonic and Mechanical Characterization of Fatigue States of Graphite Epoxy Composite Laminates." *Materials Evaluation*. Vol. 40, No. 5. Columbus, OH: American Society for Nondestructive Testing (June 1982): p 560-565.

CHAPTER

Ultrasonic Testing of Advanced Materials[1]

Yoseph Bar-Cohen, Jet Propulsion Laboratory, Pasadena, California

Ajit K. Mal, University of California at Los Angeles, Los Angeles, California

Donald J. Roth, National Aeronautics and Space Administration, Cleveland, Ohio

PART 1. Ultrasonic Testing of Advanced Structural Ceramics

The high temperature thermal, mechanical and physical properties of structural ceramics suit them for applications such as advanced engines, enabling higher combustion temperatures and therefore higher thermodynamic efficiencies. The relatively low fracture toughness of structural ceramics and the corresponding critical discontinuity size require significantly higher sensitivities than those of nondestructive test techniques commonly used for detection of discontinuities in metals.

Ultrasonic techniques for testing ceramics use high frequency elastic waves to probe both green state and sintered ceramic bodies. Discontinuities smaller than 25 μm (0.001 in.) have been detected in monolithic and composite ceramics at depths of about 3 mm (0.1 in.) in alumina, silicon carbide and silicon nitride and at depths of about 5 mm (0.2 in.) in zirconia. Described below are procedures for the rapid determination of attenuation as a function of frequency for studies of microstructural variation. Both frequency dependent and frequency independent corrections are incorporated to yield the true material attenuation. An example of the detection of whisker clumping in composite ceramics by variations in the attenuation characteristic is also described.

Discontinuity Detection in Ceramics

Critical discontinuities can be detected in most structural metals with ultrasonic wave frequencies from 1 to 10 MHz. Consequently, most research and development in ultrasonics has concentrated on this frequency range, with little activity above 15 MHz. In conventional monolithic ceramics, the critical discontinuity size is often 20 μm (0.0008 in.) or less and frequencies of 50 MHz and higher are required.

In addition, detection of such small discontinuities at reasonable depths requires focused ultrasound, and the propagation of such energy through the ceramic surface introduces severe beam aberrations. This condition is made worse by the very high index of refraction of typical ceramics, thus limiting to a few millimeters the depth at which effective focus can be maintained. For these reasons, testing ceramics requires new techniques to optimize available energy and permit detection and characterization of discontinuities as small as 20 μm (0.0008 in.).

In addition to the important task of detecting critical discontinuities in structural ceramics, there is also a need to develop predictive capability for some of the mechanical properties, based on easily measured material characteristics. This has been achieved for some metals, where a correlation has been found between the fracture toughness and attenuation of elastic waves.[2]

Green State Ceramics

An intermediate step in the processing of structural ceramics is the fabrication of green state bodies. At this first stage of component shaping (such as through powder compaction), uncontrolled conditions can lead to less than optimum material and component properties. Discovery and elimination of these conditions through process optimization, rejection or repair of the green bodies could lead to significant cost savings.

Several characteristics of green state bodies have been identified as important to the production of reliable structural ceramic components. These include (1) selection and composition of binders and sintering aids, (2) techniques of form removal and interactions with powders, (3) elemental composition, (4) mechanical properties and (5) discontinuities such as porosity and surface condition. For some of these characteristics, ultrasonic measurements and test procedures have proven useful. The green state body has much lower density than the final sintered product because of its distributed porosity. Variations in properties of the finished component may result from variations in the spatial distribution and size distribution of pores and the attendant effect on density uniformity in the green state. Characterization of the size and spatial distribution of porosity and density variations is an important part of process control.

To determine the feasibility of nondestructive discontinuity detection in green ceramics, many laboratory studies have been conducted: radiographic, ultrasonic, nuclear magnetic resonance and small angle neutron scattering techniques.

Studies of Green State Applications

Despite some difficulties, ultrasonic techniques have been studied for testing green state ceramics.[3] It was determined that the low density and porous nature of the green state limits the applicable frequencies to less than 10 MHz (depending on test object thickness) because of attenuation. The wavelength associated with the range of frequencies limits the test sensitivity to discrete discontinuities approaching 1 mm (0.04 in.).

Correlation was observed between measurements of ultrasonic velocity and material density. Ultrasonic couplants such as water or glycerol are generally absorbed by green state ceramics, eliminating the coupling effect and potentially affecting subsequent fabrication. In some cases, applying pressure to the transducer without supplementary couplant has allowed adequate transmission into the test object. Care must be taken to avoid damage to the test object. In addition, velocity data vary with transducer pressure.

An alternate coupling technique in which the green ceramic is placed in an evacuated film enclosure also has been successful.[4] Through-transmission, immersion ultrasonic techniques using a 10 MHz transducer allowed (1) detection of isolated inclusions with diameters on the order of 500 μm (0.02 in.) and (2) mapping of velocity differences attributed to density differences correlated with X-ray tomography.

Sintered Ceramics

Heating or sintering is typically the final fabrication stage for many ceramic components (in some cases, a grinding operation may be needed for surface preparation or sizing). Because sintering often completes the fabrication process, proper discontinuity characterization is important to ensure that the desired integrity and quality is achieved and maintained.

A number of critical characteristics affect the service life of ceramic components. These include local density variations, microstructure, mechanical properties, physical properties, surface properties (affected by machining), elemental composition and distribution. For some of these characteristics, ultrasonic techniques are used with production quantities or with sampling tests during process development.

Density

Sintering of preformed, green state ceramic bodies at high temperatures reduces or eliminates voids and increases density. Localized variations in the attained density of ceramic shapes after sintering are undesirable because of the effects on structural performance. Radiographic and ultrasonic nondestructive tests offer the potential for detecting and measuring density variations.

Investigations have been made into the feasibility of using ultrasonic velocity measurements[5-7] to determine bulk density in sintered alpha silicon carbide with densities varying from 2.8 to 3.2 mg·mm^{-3}. Using 20 MHz frequencies and commercial ultrasound equipment, the nominal bulk density could be estimated within 1 percent.

Bulk Material and Mechanical Properties

Common practice for determining sintered ceramics' mechanical properties (such as strength or fracture toughness) is to perform destructive tests on large numbers of specially prepared reference standards (three and four point bending standards for strength determination and short rod, notched beam standards for fracture toughness). Performance proof tests can also be made on objects that represent actual components. However, these destructive tests are expensive and time consuming when providing statistical data on materials under development.

The acceptable performance of a ceramic material in service may depend as much on the basic bulk material and mechanical properties of the individual component as on the presence of discrete discontinuities. For that reason, nondestructive testing of these properties on the actual item is a very powerful tool for predicting a newly fabricated component's serviceability or for determining the residual life of a component after service.

Measuring Correlated Properties

Ultrasonic technology for discontinuity detection can be used for measuring parameters that correlate with desired material properties. The ultrasonic velocity is a function of the elastic properties of the material, and ultrasonic attenuation can be related to bulk microstructure and to structural discontinuities (both microscopic and macroscopic). Laboratory studies by several investigators confirm the feasibility of techniques for making such measurements.

Ultrasonic longitudinal and transverse wave velocities have been measured in different directions in hot pressed silicon nitride.[8] Anisotropy was observed and velocities perpendicular to the hot pressing direction were about 5 percent higher than velocities parallel to it. Ultrasonic attenuation measured with both longitudinal and transverse waves in the 30 to 130 MHz frequency range exhibits a frequency dependent characteristic proportional to the square of the frequency.

Work on siliconized silicon carbide tubes indicated that the velocity of sound changed as a function of the volume fraction of silicon and this may offer a technique for indicating silicon content.[9] The feasibility of using ultrasonic techniques to measure elastic moduli, microstructure, hardness, fracture toughness and strength has been demonstrated for a wide range of materials, including metals, ceramics and fiber composites.[10,11] Ultrasonic techniques are particularly useful because they involve mechanical elastic waves modulated by some of the morphological factors that govern mechanical strength and dynamic failure processes.

Ultrasonic Attenuation Studies

Ultrasonic attenuation has also been studied for testing microstructural properties.[12] To measure the attenuation rapidly over a wide frequency range, a broad band elastic wave was transmitted through a sample and a material transfer function was computed from digitized records of the input and transmitted signals. A commercial 150 MHz ultrasonic system with an integral high speed (2 ns) peak detector and four-bit digitizer was assembled for the tests. This system used an immersion tank that included an integral three-axis scanning system controlled by a dedicated computer.

Although pure backscattering measurements might appear preferable for investigating the microstructure of ceramics, through-transmission measurements (or pulse echo, using the backwall reflection) were used because of the difficulty in obtaining repeatable results from pure backscatter. The literature details problems attendant to backscattering measurements and offers some hope for improving the accuracy and repeatability of this test.[13] Although through-transmission measurements are affected by damping losses and scattering losses in the test object, this turned out to

be advantageous in whisker reinforced ceramic composites, as described below.

The transducer chosen for attenuation studies was a 100 MHz center frequency, plane wave unit having a 20 dB bandwidth ranging from 30 to 120 MHz. This transducer had a quartz delay line and was coupled to the sample with a very thin layer of water.

For the measurements to reflect the intrinsic attenuation, the data must be corrected for nonmaterial losses. Two effects are impedance mismatch losses at the sample interfaces and beam spreading or diffraction losses. Both of these losses are often much larger than the intrinsic material losses and, if uncorrected, will corrupt the measurements. Correction for beam spread losses is made and all corrections are then combined in a program that acquires the needed data, deconvolves the input and output data, determines and applies the appropriate corrections and plots the resulting transfer curve.[14]

Initial results indicated sharply increasing attenuation above 30 MHz in all samples, even those for which the grain size was too small (1 μm) to produce measurable scattering at these frequencies. Comparison of the signals from the end of the delay line with the transducer coupled to the test object and with the transducer in air indicated that the reflection coefficient was much higher than assumed from the acoustic impedances of the coupled materials.

This effect was shown to be caused by the water coupling layer, whose effect is entirely negligible at frequencies below about 20 MHz.[15] The condition was subsequently analyzed as a three-layer problem and an expression was obtained for the reflection and transmission coefficient as a function of frequency, for both normal and nonnormal incidence on the interface. These results were incorporated in the analysis, which then determined the thickness of the coupling layer (and thus the frequency dependent reflection coefficient) from the digitized delay line signals in air and coupled to the test object.

A value for thickness is determined at each frequency within the pass band of the transducer, including computation of gaussian summary statistics. Experience with this program has indicated that slight (less than 1 μm [4×10^{-5} in.]) wedging of the transducer can easily be detected from the standard deviation of the measurements.

A typical value for the water layer thickness is 0.5 μm (2×10^{-5} in.) and Fig. 1 shows the reflection coefficient as a function of frequency for this thickness. With the latest corrections, transfer curve results are highly repeatable, are independent of sample thickness and appear to reflect frequency dependent losses commensurate with those expected from scanning electron microscope observations of the microstructure. A least squares fit to the experimental data was found to coincide with theory.

Figure 2 shows results obtained on a monolithic alumina. The solid line is the experimental data and the dashed line is a least squares fit to these data. The coefficients of fit indicate that a linear fit was optimum. This is not surprising, for the average grain size in this material is

about 1 μm (4.0×10^{-5} in.). For such a small source, frequencies of more than 1 GHz are necessary before scattering losses become important. The dominant losses in the range shown in Fig. 2 appear to be damping losses, linear with frequency.

The constant term in Fig. 2, term 1 under coefficient of fit, is 0.345 dB·mm^{-1} and is generally considered to be a measure of the viscous damping loss in the material. Unfortunately, this term is also affected by several error sources, such as attenuator errors, that are difficult to determine. The repeatability of this term is not particularly good, even for the same test object. However, the linear term is extremely repeatable for a single object or for different objects produced by a common process and is useful for characterization.

Figure 3 shows the transfer curve obtained from partially stabilized zirconia. For this material, the average grain size is about 100 μm (0.004 in.) and scattering becomes important even for frequencies as low as 10 MHz. This is shown in the transfer curve, where losses increase approximately as the square of the frequency. No data are shown for frequencies greater than 60 MHz because those losses exceed the dynamic range of the measuring system.

Because the transfer curve is highly repeatable for a given material and indicative of its microstructure, it would appear to be an excellent variable for correlation with fracture properties.

FIGURE 1. Reflection coefficient at quartz silicon carbide interface coupled by 0.5 μm (2×10^{-5} in.) of water.

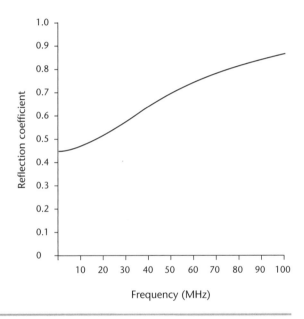

FIGURE 2. Transfer curve of monolithic alumina with length of 9.4 mm (0.37 in.) and acoustic impedance of 43.02 g·cm^{-2}·s^{-1}. Coefficient of fit at term 1 is 0.345 dB·mm^{-1} and at term 2 is 0.007 dB·mm^{-1}·MHz^{-1}.

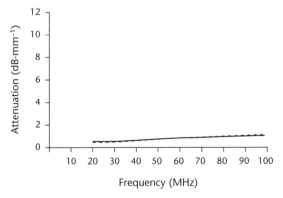

Legend
——— = experimental data
- - - - - = least squares fit

FIGURE 3. Transfer curve of magnesia stabilized zirconia with length of 2.6 mm (0.1 in.) and acoustic impedance of 39.88 g·cm^{-2}s^{-1}. Coefficient of fit at term 1 is 2.971 dB·mm^{-1}, at term 2 is –0.109 dB·mm^{-1}·MHz^{-1} and at term 3 is 0.003 dB·mm^{-1}·MHz^{-1}.

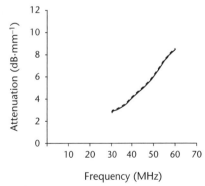

Legend
——— = experimental data
- - - - - = least squares fit

Microstructure in Whisker Reinforced Ceramics

Whisker reinforced ceramics consist of typical ceramic matrices in which ceramic whiskers are dispersed. A whisker is typically 0.5 μm (2×10^{-5} in.) in diameter, 20 to 30 μm (0.0008 to 0.001 in.) long and is too small to be detected by the frequencies available in a commercial ultrasonic test system. The major problem with these materials is whisker clumping rather than voids or inclusions in the matrix. Clumping causes the matrix material to be very sparse in large regions, on the order of 100 to 200 μm (0.004 to 0.008 in.) in diameter, thus forming an effective void on the scale of the clump.

These clumps are easily detectable by ultrasonic scanning but the approach is relatively time consuming. The transfer curve can be obtained in just a few seconds and, if sensitive to whisker clumping, is a valuable preliminary test that could obviate detailed scanning for voids.

Figure 4 shows the test results obtained from a whisker reinforced alumina known to contain severe clumping. The presence of clumps was established by ultrasonic scanning and by scanning electron microscope analysis of a fracture surface.

The transfer curve shows a linear characteristic, which is reasonable in light of the fact that the density of whisker clumps is probably too low to measurably increase the scattering losses for plane wave insonification. However, the linear term is about seven times that obtained for the same material with no whiskers. A number of whisker reinforced samples were tested with a constant ratio of whiskers to volume but with various degrees of clumping as determined with scanning electron microscopy. One of the samples had no demonstrable clumping and this was confirmed by ultrasonic testing. The transfer curve's linear term for this test object was about three times that of the monolithic material. Other objects' curves fell between the clump free component and the one with severe clumping.

While this study was not definitive, it appears that, in whisker reinforced alumina, there is a relationship between the degree of whisker clumping and the damping losses, as determined by the ultrasonic attenuation characteristic.

Detection of Discontinuities

Various Techniques

Several nondestructive testing methods have been studied for detection of discontinuities in sintered ceramics. These methods include ultrasonic, radiographic, small angle neutron scanning, acoustic emission, infrared, liquid penetrant, photoacoustic microscopic and microwave testing. The minimum detectable size of discrete discontinuities or distributed discontinuities varies significantly among the various methods.

Ultrasonic techniques for discontinuity detection include (1) traditional pulse echo techniques for detecting reflections from discrete discontinuities and (2) measurement of ultrasonic attenuation and velocity as a function of frequency with correlation to distributed discontinuity size. The literature includes reports on a 50 MHz C-scan imaging system for discontinuity detection in silicon nitride and a high frequency (150 to 450 MHz) A-scan system for discontinuity characterization and matrix testing.[16-19] Signal processing schemes include temporal and spatial averaging, filtering and corrections for diffraction and for attenuation.

Backscattering Techniques

Difficulties have been encountered in discontinuity characterization with single backscattering measurements. For high frequency systems, special transducers and filtering techniques have been developed, allowing comparison of time domain backscattered signals from inclusions with calculations from theory. Good agreement

FIGURE 4. Transfer curve of silicon carbon whisker reinforced alumina (numerous whisker clumps), with length of 2.9 mm (0.11 in.) and acoustic impedance of 40.49 g·cm^{-2}·s^{-1}. Coefficient of fit at term 1 is 0.192 dB·mm^{-1}·MHz^{-1} and at term 2 is –0.047 dB·mm^{-1}·MHz^{-1}.

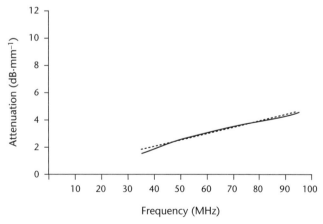

Legend
——— = experimental data
- - - - - = least squares fit

was observed for 100 μm (0.004 in.) inclusions in silicon nitride.

Synthetic aperture imaging at 50 MHz has been studied to obtain three-dimensional images of discontinuities. Computer simulations based on theoretical discontinuity models have been implemented. Longitudinal and transverse wave ultrasonic pulse echo techniques have been investigated in silicon nitride and silicon carbide ceramics at frequencies between 25 and 45 MHz for detection of pores and inclusions in the range of 10 to 130 μm (0.0004 to 0.005 in.).

Transverse wave techniques are more sensitive than longitudinal wave techniques for tests of ceramics. Sensitivity to discontinuities as small as 25 μm (0.001 in.) has been demonstrated. Objects that had subsequent failure at detected discontinuities showed lower strengths.[20,21]

Scanning Laser Techniques

Several investigators have reported studies with a scanning laser acoustic microscope. In one study, a frequency of 100 MHz was used to detect and display pores and inclusions from 50 to 100 μm (0.002 to 0.004 in.) in silicon nitride disks.[22,23] Distributed porosity smaller than 50 μm (0.002 in.) was detected because of its effect on ultrasonic attenuation rather than by discrete indications.

Statistical studies have been conducted to determine the probability of detecting surface and internal voids using 100 MHz scanning laser acoustic microscopy in sintered components of silicon carbide and silicon nitride.[24,25] Surface voids as small as 100 μm (0.004 in.) in diameter were reliably detected in polished test objects. If close to the surface, internal voids as small as 30 μm (0.0012 in.) in silicon nitride and 60 μm (0.0024 in.) in silicon were detected. Larger voids were reliably detected at greater depths. Ultrasonic techniques have been applied up to 45 MHz and show potential for detecting clusters of subsurface discontinuities near 25 μm (0.001 in.) in hot pressed silicon nitride.[26]

Similar studies in reaction bonded silicon nitride show the potential for detecting clusters in the 125 μm (0.005 in.) range. Silicon rich inclusions are difficult to detect when less than 250 to 500 μm (0.01 to 0.02 in.). A 36 MHz pulse echo ultrasonic technique and scanning laser techniques have been applied to the detection of intentionally seeded discontinuities in the range of 50 to 125 μm (0.002 to 0.005 in.) and 150 to 250 μm (0.006 to 0.010 in.) in silicon carbide disk thicknesses ranging from 2.5 to 130 mm (0.1 to 5 in.).[27] The seeded

discontinuities (as well as others) were successfully detected. In this case, the critical strength limiting discontinuities were complex shaped, three-dimensional voids 75 to 200 μm (0.003 to 0.008 in.) in size and two-dimensional surface cracks less than 150 μm (0.006 in.) deep.

An acoustic microscopy technique has been developed using high frequency (50 MHz) focused ultrasonic transducers and fast signal processing to rapidly scan silicon carbide heat exchanger tubes for discontinuities and to display the results in real time.[28] The system can acquire data as fast as 2800 data points per second and has demonstrated the ability to detect and image seeded discontinuities as small as 0.05 mm (0.002 in.).

Techniques for Very Small Discontinuities

Both theoretical and experimental studies have been used in developing techniques for very small critical discontinuities.[12] Reliable detection of discontinuities as small as 20 μm (0.0008 in.) cannot be achieved simply by increasing the interrogating frequency until the wavelength is comparable to the discontinuity size. The reason for this is that the amount of energy intercepted by such a discontinuity is a negligible fraction of the total transducer energy for a typical plane wave transducer.

In addition, the intensity of scattering from a small discontinuity illuminated by plane wave radiation decreases approximately as $(a \cdot d^{-1})^2$, where a is the discontinuity radius and d is the depth of the discontinuity, assuming that the wavelength is small compared to the discontinuity. Therefore, discontinuities can be detected much smaller than the transducer size only at relatively shallow depths for plane wave insonification. To reliably detect 20 μm (0.0008 in.) discontinuities at depths of several millimeters (0.1 in.), sharply focused transducers are typically required. Focusing in turn dictates a small scan index with its attendant large scan time. Unfortunately, the propagation of energy through the ceramic surface under these conditions introduces into the beam severe spherical aberration that partially offsets the benefits of focusing.

Spherical Void Measurement

In monolithic ceramics, one of the common discontinuities is a quasispherical void, so the typical scattering center is modeled as a spherical cavity. Although detection is not restricted to this shape, scattering data are interpreted in the light of this model, unless there are valid reasons for suspecting otherwise. Models have been developed for other discontinuity shapes such as planar cracks that commonly occur in ceramics.[29]

There is also an analytical model for the spherical cavity[30] and Fig. 5 shows the theoretical response from such a cavity in silicon nitride. Here k is the wave vector of the ultrasound and a is the radius of the cavity. The scattering is characterized by a rapid increase in cross section with frequency (the rayleigh region), followed by a transition to an oscillatory cross section at about $ka = 1$. These oscillations are caused by interference between direct and creeping waves and are often missing in real discontinuities because of their surface irregularities. In this case, the scattering response is characterized by the rayleigh tail and a transition to a cross section nearly constant with frequency.

Figure 6 shows experimental data obtained from a natural discontinuity in tetragonal zirconia polycrystalline (TZP), a fine grained zirconia. The transducer and system response have been removed from the data by deconvolution and the results depend only on the discontinuity characteristics. If the turning point in the response at about 89 MHz is equated with the theoretical transition at $ka = 1$, a discontinuity diameter of about 25 μm (0.001 in.) is estimated. Smaller discontinuities can be detected at higher frequencies.

With these capabilities, discontinuities on the order of 20 μm (0.0008 in.) can be detected at depths up to 3 mm (0.1 in.) in alumina or silicon nitride and at depths up to 5 mm (0.2 in.) in tetragonal zirconia polycrystalline. In coarse grained materials, severe scattering losses increase the minimum discontinuity detection threshold but the critical discontinuity size is also larger in these materials.

Detection of Other Discontinuity Types

Figure 7 shows numerous indications obtained in three modulus-of-rupture (MOR) bars. Note the high density of indications near the ends of two of the bars. These indications are equivalent to 100 μm (0.004 in.) and larger diameter voids. The variations among the indications are more visible in color enhanced displays.

Figure 8 shows the results obtained from a 650 mm² (1 in.²) piece of monolithic silicon nitride. The smallest

FIGURE 5. Theoretical scattering from spherical void.

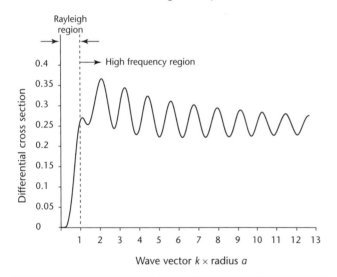

FIGURE 6. Experimental scattering from a 25 μm (0.001 in.) discontinuity in tetragonal polycrystalline zirconia.

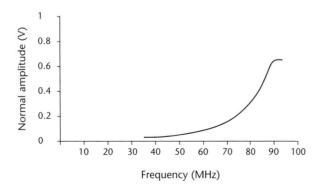

FIGURE 7. Gray scale presentation of discontinuities in zirconia modulus-of-rupture bars.

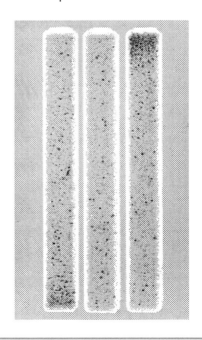

indications probably correspond to voids with diameters of 20 μm (0.0008 in.) and lie at a depth of 3 mm (0.1 in.).

Figure 9 shows the results obtained from whisker reinforced alumina known to contain clumping. The indications are from clumps on the order of 100 to 200 μm (0.004 to 0.008 in.) in diameter. Similar results were obtained from whisker reinforced silicon nitride. However, a monolithic sample prepared from the same powder was virtually free of indications.

Advanced Ceramics

Ceramic matrix composites developed for advanced aerospace propulsion to save weight, to improve reuse capability and to increase performance provide a challenge for accurate discontinuity detection and microstructural characterization. Mechanical and environmental loads applied to ceramic matrix composites can cause degradation in the form of discrete discontinuity nucleation and distributed microscopic damage that plays a significant role in reduction of desirable physical properties. Categories of microscopic damage include fiber-to-matrix disbonding (interface failure), matrix microcracking, fiber fracture and buckling, oxidation and second phase formation. An ultrasonic guided wave scan system was developed to characterize various microstructural and discontinuity conditions in ceramic matrix composite samples: (1) silicon carbide fiber in silicon carbide matrix and (2) carbon fiber in silicon carbide matrix (Figs. 10 to 12).[31]

Guided wave ultrasonic testing is generally thought to be an attractive alternative to scanning because guided waves can be excited at one location of a structure by a single transducer or line of transducers with returning or received echoes indicating the presence of

FIGURE 8. Threshold presentation of discontinuities in silicon nitride (frequency is 50 MHz).

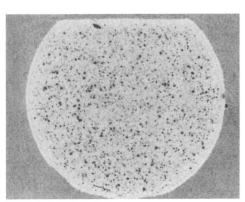

FIGURE 9. Photomicrograph of whisker clumps in silicon carbide whisker reinforced alumina.

FIGURE 10. Ultrasonic guided wave test system: (a) scanner hardware; (b) typical waveform.

(a)

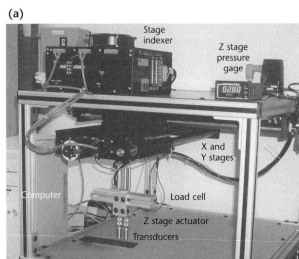

(b)

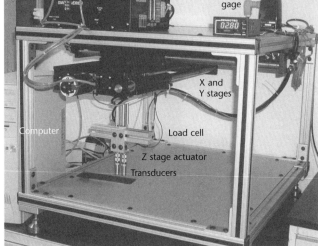

discontinuities. This type of test has detected discontinuities and material degradation in many types of materials and components — in some applications over significant distances. The guided wave signal in raw form is very complex (many dispersive and interfering modes, traveling at different velocities) with significant coherent noise that cannot be averaged out. As a result, guided wave techniques seem to be most successful for discontinuity detection when tuning for a minimally or nondispersive mode of ultrasound, at a particular excitation frequency, in one direction, to control coherent noise. One guided wave technique takes a different approach by using the total, multiple-mode ultrasonic response, using separate sending and receiving transducers, doing so in a scanning configuration and using specialized signal processing routines to extract parameters of the time domain and frequency domain signals.[31] These parameters have proven sensitive to changes in microstructural conditions and to the presence of discontinuities and appear promising at monitoring degradation in ceramic matrix composites. There may be several further advantages of using guided wave scanning over conventional ultrasonic techniques.

1. Guided wave scanning can be performed directionally, allowing correlations between ultrasonic parameters and directionally dependent material properties, such as for unidirectional composites or to test the premise of nondirectionality of properties.
2. The sample under test does not have to be immersed in fluid as for most conventional ultrasonic characterization.
3. Guided wave scanning can be applied to components with mildly curved surfaces.
4. Guided wave scanning can be more versatile in characterizing local modulus changes than resonant frequency techniques that require nodal excitation and generation and are thus not applicable for scanning.

Typical experimental setup parameters when scanning ceramic composites include broad band ultrasonic transducers with center frequencies f ranging from 1 to 3.5 MHz (both sender and receiver of the same frequency). Ultrasound is coupled to the material via elastic coupling pads. The distance between sending and receiving transducers is 25 mm (1 in.). Analog-to-digital sampling rates used are 10 MHz to 25 MHz. A measurement is made (contact load = 35.6 ± 2.3 N [8 ± 0.5 lb]), the sender receiver pair is lifted, moved to the next location,

lowered to be in contact with the sample, and another measurement is made. This routine is repeated to perform raster scans. Scan increments vary between 1 and 5 mm (0.05 and 0.25 in.). Images constructed included those calculated from centroid mean time, time-versus-distance skew factor, zeroth moment and frequency centroid of the power spectrum, frequency dependent ultrasonic decay rate and frequency dependent energy density initial value.

Figure 11 shows an ultrasonic guided wave scan image showing delamination within a silicon carbide fiber composite in a silicon carbide matrix. The delamination was most easily discriminated in the centroid mean time image (whitish areas in image). Centroid mean time can be thought of as the time in the raw waveform demarcating the location of energy balance. Time domain waveforms associated with the delaminated area and a nondelaminated area are shown in the figure. The shift in centroid mean time away from the origin is quite apparent for the delamination when viewing the waveforms.

Figure 12 shows the ability of guided wave scanning to detect cracking perpendicular to wave travel in such a fiber matrix.

FIGURE 11. Silicon carbide fiber in silicon carbide matrix: (a) centroid mean time image with delamination showing as white area; (b) time domain waveforms.

(a)

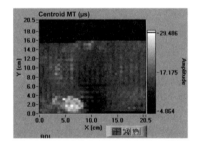

(b)

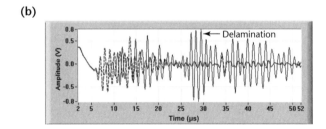

Detection of Surface Properties

The integrity of a sintered ceramic surface is critical because of the small critical discontinuity size, the tensile stress concentrations possible on the object surface during service and the potential for damage during fabrication (during grinding or other machining, for example). For these reasons, surface testing is useful in demonstrating ceramic performance.

Several different methods have been used to accomplish high resolution, high sensitivity tests, including optical techniques, ultrasonics, penetrants and others. Some of the technology used for detection of discontinuities in the microstructure is also applicable for surface testing.

High frequency ultrasonic surface waves have been studied by several investigators and shown to be useful for the detection of small surface discontinuities. A 45 MHz ultrasonic surface wave technique has been developed for detecting surface discontinuities less than 100 µm (0.004 in.) deep in silicon nitride and silicon carbide.[32,33] The technique was found to be sensitive to surface conditions such as grinding damage as well as to discontinuities. Flexural strength was correlated qualitatively with ultrasonic response to machining damage. Sensitivity to discontinuities is limited by the depth of machining damage and the focal spot size of the ultrasonic beam. For the 5.8 mm (0.230 in.) focal spot, the smallest verified discontinuity was a semicircular crack with a depth of 30 µm (0.0012 in.).

Surface acoustic waves in ceramics have also been studied for detecting individual cracks with depths as small as 60 µm (0.0024 in.).[33,34] Detectability is affected by the size distribution of adjacent background microcracks (such as those caused by grinding).

A preliminary correlation has been observed between attenuation of the surface wave and the extremes of the crack size distribution. In the studies particularly addressed to machining damage (suspected of being a major cause of test object failure), a measurement technique was developed to find the microcracks and a long wavelength

FIGURE 12. Value images of carbon fiber in silicon carbide matrix: (a) zeroth energy density after 14 h; (b) frequency dependent energy initial density after 14 h; (c) zeroth energy density after 16 h; (d) frequency dependent energy initial density after 16 h. Note the white indication in both 16 h images at X = 100 to 110 mm, which was not apparent after 14 h of testing and which was at the eventual failure location.

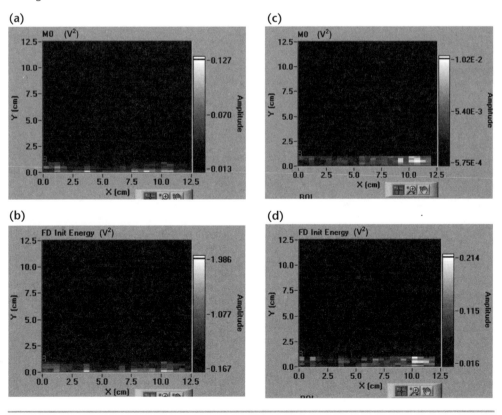

scattering theory was proposed for predicting size. The techniques are affected by variations in the plastic zone and by the crack closure at the surface resulting from residual stresses. Fracture stress prediction may be possible if the long wavelength criterion is met and the size of the plastic zone is correctly estimated.

The long wavelength (low frequency) showed good agreement between predicted and actual fracture stresses in silicon nitride test objects containing semicircular surface cracks with radii (depths) ranging from 50 to 275 μm (0.002 to 0.011 in.).[35] The scattered ultrasonic radiation patterns from surface cracks show that modulation of the ultrasonic frequency spectrum is related to crack length and aspect ratio (geometric crack parameters important for failure prediction).[36-39]

PART 2. Ultrasonic Testing of Adhesive Bonds

Adhesives are used to maintain structural integrity and to transfer loads between the components of an assembly. For adhesives in discontinuity sensitive structures with complex configurations, there is a need for highly reliable nondestructive testing techniques for evaluating bond performance.

The capability of ultrasonic tests of bond quality in structural components is described below. Also discussed is the limitation of other nondestructive tests for providing quantitative results, along with the details of a joint theoretical and experimental research program using leaky lamb waves on laboratory test objects. The leaky lamb wave technique is shown to have advantages over other nondestructive tests.

Characteristics of Adhesive Bonds

The condition of a bond can be evaluated best only with a test that detects unbonds, characterizes them and determines the properties of the adhesive. Nondestructive determination of the strength of a bonded joint provides the most meaningful information about bond quality. To this end, material parameters that might be sensitive to strength have been sought by many investigators.[40] Limited success was achieved for cases in which material variables were carefully controlled and where there was a direct relationship between the average strength and a single property of the adhesive material, such as thickness.

In practice, it is difficult to correlate nondestructive test data with the strength of a bond. Bond strength is not a physical property but a structural parameter, an indication of the highest stress that a specific structure's weakest spot can bear. Generally, there is no nondestructive test method that can search systematically through a structure to identify all the weak points and then determine which is the weakest.

Furthermore, bonding is particularly sensitive to interface characteristics, difficult to determine nondestructively. Therefore, even though it may be possible to estimate the average strength of a bonded system, the usefulness of this measure is questionable. A bond fails when the stress exceeds the material strength in its weakest spot, not when a stress exceeds the average bond strength, which may be substantially higher.

Bond Strength

The mechanical strength of an adhesive bond depends on two factors, cohesion and adhesion. Cohesion is the attraction between the molecules of the adhesive layer. Cohesive strength is determined by the type of adhesive, its elastic properties and its thickness. Limited information can be obtained about these parameters when using nondestructive test methods.

Adhesion is the molecular attraction between dissimilar bodies in physical contact or the bond between an adhesive and the adherends. Adhesion quality is critical to the performance of a bond between components of an assembly. Because a bond interface layer is often a fraction of a micrometer thick, it is very difficult to characterize it nondestructively. Weakness of this layer can be caused by poor surface preparation and is not detectable by contemporary nondestructive test methods. In cases such as diffusion bonding and steel-to-rubber bonding, weak adhesion can also result from many minute separations over a certain area. This type of unbond can be measured nondestructively for the average degree of separation rather than for the weakness of the bond.

Because of these limitations, nondestructive testing is used to detect and characterize unbonds rather than to determine bond strength. Acoustics and ultrasonics are the primary means for nondestructive testing of unbonds. Resonance, pulse echo, through-transmission and ultrasonic spectroscopy are the most widely used techniques and are reviewed below. The leaky lamb wave technique reportedly has potential for nondestructive testing of bonds and is discussed later in this section.

Tap Testing

The simplest and most common adhesive bond test is called *tap testing*. The inspector strikes the test object, typically with a metal implement such as a hammer or coin, and listens to the characteristics of the resulting sound. This is a qualitative, sonic technique rather than an ultrasonic technique and, although fast and simple, it can only detect gross unbonds.

A systematic study has been made of the tap testing method by examining the input force.[41] The study found that the characteristics of the force input by a tap are changed by an unbond. Furthermore, the impact duration increases and the peak input force of the impact decreases as the discontinuity becomes larger.

Even though this study resulted in a substantial improvement in the reliability and detectability of tapping, the method is still limited to thin layers less than 1 mm (0.04 in.) thick. The smallest unbond detectable with tapping is 10 mm (0.4 in.) in diameter in typical test objects.

Resonance Tests

The resonance method can be used to test adhesive bonding by accessing the test object from one side using broad band or swept frequency excitation. Resonance testing is based on establishing a standing wave in the material when the effective thickness of the material is equal to an integral number of half wavelengths.[42] The effective thickness of the test material is inversely related to the resonant frequency. An unbonded material gives rise to a higher resonant frequency than the resonance frequency of the bonded structure.

The shift in frequency can be determined by measuring its loading effect on piezoelectric transducers. This effect can be analyzed using transmission line theory, where the test material serves as a termination or load. The transducer's electrical impedance and its resonant frequency are affected by the load. Their values for bonded materials can be used as a reference when searching for unbonds.

To determine the effect of the unbond on the induced ultrasonic wave, the wave behavior must be analyzed. At low frequencies (in the kilohertz range), the attenuation in the test material can be neglected. Assuming an incident plane wave, the acoustic pressure can be related to particle velocity through acoustic impedance z:[43]

$$(1) \quad z = \rho v \tan h \left[\alpha + i(\beta + kd) \right]$$

where d is the distance (millimeter), k is the wave number, v is acoustical velocity (millimeter per second), α is the reflectivity constant, β is the change in

phase and ρ is the material density (gram per cubic millimeter).

The change in the acoustic impedance because of unbond also changes the electric impedance of the transducer loaded by the material. The change in the load depends on the distance traveled by the acoustic energy in the material (the effective thickness) causing an appropriate change in z. A proper selection of the test frequency allows an increase in the response to unbond and this is done during instrument calibration.

Applications of Resonance Tests

Resonance techniques for nondestructively detecting unbonds are based on the difference in characteristic response between bonded and unbonded areas. Commercial instruments developed for this application are typically calibrated by using the response from a bonded or an unbonded area as a reference.

One of these instruments displays the transducer's electrical impedance at a selected frequency as a point on the complex plane. Figure 13 shows typical responses to transducer loading by bonded and unbonded metal-to-metal areas of a reference standard. In this figure, three impedance points are displayed: (1) air loading, where the transducer is not loaded, (2) an unbonded layer of aluminum and (3) a bonded system of two aluminum plates. The transducer's impedance changes with loading.

The other type of bond tester displays the impedance amplitude and phase as a function of frequency on two different indicators, thereby providing additional data. Using this system, it has been shown that a change in each of these parameters is related to a change in adhesive layer thickness.[44,45] Because the thickness of the adhesive can be correlated to the bond strength, the instrument can be used as an indirect means of bond strength measurement. This application was widely used during the 1960s but is not reliable for general adhesives.

FIGURE 13. Display of transducer impedance and changes caused by changes in loading.

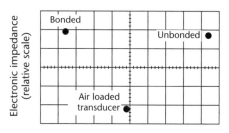

Ultrasonic Pulse Echo and Through-Transmission Tests

An elastic wave traveling from one material to another is partially reflected and partially transmitted through the interface. The relative amount of energy of each of the two generated wave components is determined by the degree of mismatch in the acoustic impedance between the two materials.

The reflection coefficient R and transmission coefficient T for an incident wave normal to an interface may be determined:

$$(2) \quad R = \left(\frac{z_1 - z_2}{z_1 + z_2} \right)^2$$

and

$$(3) \quad T = 1 - R$$

where z_1 and z_2 are the acoustic impedances of the two materials, defined through the relation:

$$(4) \quad z_j = p_j v_j$$

where $j = 1$ or 2. The larger the impedance mismatch between the two materials, the higher the reflection coefficient. As an example, if aluminum is bonded to an adhesive layer of epoxy, then $R = 0.48$. If the aluminum is not bonded, then at the interface of aluminum and air, $R \cong 1$ and total reflection occurs.

On the other hand, if water penetrates the unbonded area during a standard ultrasonic test, then $R < 0.71$ and the sensitivity to the unbond decreases. This analysis can be applied to through-transmission by using Eq. 2. In the case of an unbond, the discontinuity causes a complete blockage of the wave transmission, because $T = 0$ for an interface of aluminum and air.

These two ways of identifying an unbond are the nondestructive techniques known as pulse echo and through-transmission. For such tests, short ultrasonic pulses are used at frequencies higher than the resonance technique (0.5 to 10 MHz). For pulse echo tests, a single transducer is used and access to only one side of the test object is required. For through-transmission tests, two transducers are required (one on each side of the test material) and must be maintained along the wave path. To improve on the detectability of discontinuities in a through-transmission test, a reflector plate can be used to reflect the transmitted signal back to the transducer. Thus, a single transducer is used and the effect of attenuation is increased by doubling the wave path.

Using the through-transmission technique in field conditions is sometimes difficult because of the required access to both sides, the alignment of the two transducers during testing and the need to maintain water columns for coupling. The pulse echo technique, on the other hand, provides information about the bonded areas without these difficulties. Pulse echo tests can be used to determine whether the unbond is above or below the adhesive layer or, in the case of composites, if it is an unbond or delamination. When the delamination is detected, its depth can be determined with an accuracy of ±0.1 mm (±0.004 in.) in typical test objects.[46]

Typical pulse echo data for a relatively thick aluminum plate and the results of theoretical calculations are shown in Fig. 14. The agreement between data and theory is excellent.

Examples of response when using pulse echo and through-transmission techniques in more complex test objects

FIGURE 14. Comparison of typical pulse echo data with theory for unbonded aluminum: (a) pulse echo response for wrought aluminum alloy at 5 MHz; (b) theoretical response for same test object. The first pulse represents reflection from the front surface of the aluminum plate immersed in water; all other pulses are from the back of the plate.

(a)

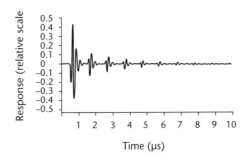

(b)

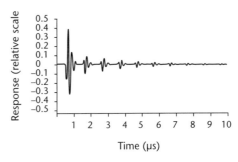

are shown in Figs. 15 and 16. For through-transmission testing (Fig. 15), the difference between bonded and unbonded areas is related to the amplitude of the received signal after traveling through the test object. This technique is widely used because it inspects the entire volume of an object in one test.

Detected discontinuities are accepted or rejected by comparing the response from a discontinuity to the response from a reference standard defined by the material specifications. It is common to define levels of quality that depend on the discontinuity size with letters *A, B* and *C*, where *A* identifies the highest quality used for primary structures and *C* identifies the lowest quality.[45]

The detectability of unbonds using either of the two methods is critically dependent on the unbond gap. If the gap is much smaller than the wavelength of the ultrasound, then both bonded and unbonded areas have the same response. Assuming that a layer of foreign material is sandwiched between two half spaces of the same material. The transmission coefficient *T* for normal incidences is given by:[47]

$$(5) \quad T = \frac{2m}{\sqrt{4m^2 + \left(1 - m^2\right)^2 \sin^2 kd}}$$

where is *d* is the thickness of the gap (millimeter), *k* is the wave number in the gap and *m* is the degree of impedance mismatch ($z_1 \cdot z_2^{-1}$).

The transmission coefficient *T* of the air gap between two aluminum half spaces is shown in Fig. 17. The ultrasonic frequency times the gap thickness is on the logarithmic abscissa. As shown for 1 MHz, a gap of 5 µm (0.0002 in.) allows very little transmission. However, if the frequency is reduced to 10 kHz, then about 25 percent transmission occurs and the detectability of the discontinuity is substantially reduced. This shows that

FIGURE 16. Pulse echo from graphite-to-epoxy [0,90]$_{2S}$, glass-to-epoxy layer bonded with adhesive to aluminum honeycomb: (a) bonded sample; (b) delamination between fourth and fifth layers of the graphite-to-epoxy skin; (c) unbond between glass-to-epoxy and adhesive layers.

(a)

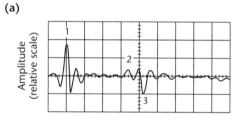

Time (relative scale)

(b)

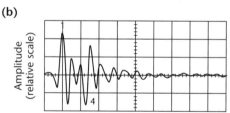

Time (relative scale)

(c)

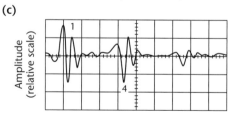

Time (relative scale)

Legend
1. Front surface reflection.
2. Reflection from interface of graphite epoxy to glass epoxy.
3. Reflection from adhesive honeycomb interface.
4. Disbond or delamination.

FIGURE 15. Through-transmission response of sandwich structure made of graphite-to-epoxy skin and metallic honeycomb: (a) bonded sandwich; (b) unbonded sandwich.

(a)

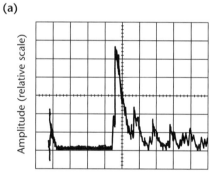

Time (relative scale)

(b)

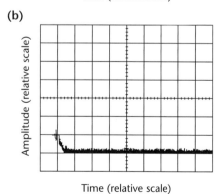

Time (relative scale)

unbonds can best be detected using frequencies with wavelengths sufficiently smaller than the suspected unbond gap.

Ultrasonic Spectroscopy

Data signals measured by pulse echo or through-transmission are usually examined in the time domain using a broad band signal. The ultrasonic spectroscopy technique is based on analyzing the received signal in the frequency domain. For this purpose, the signal is transformed to the frequency domain using a fast fourier transformation algorithm.

The advantage of spectroscopy is its ability to reveal frequency dependent features that cannot be easily identified in time domain signals. Furthermore, the signal can be processed and enhanced to improve its detection of discontinuities. Examples of such processes include filtering, convolution and correlation. This technique is called *ultrasonic spectroscopy* and was studied as a potential nondestructive testing tool during the 1970s.[48]

The technique is based on the analysis of the spectral response of the bonded test object compared to the response from an unbonded reference standard. The frequency dependent reflection and transmission coefficients can be determined for any given number of elastic, isotropic and homogeneous layers, by means of several well established techniques.[49] A plane longitudinal wave is assumed to propagate normal to these layers.

The reflection coefficient has a frequency dependence related to the thickness and the elastic properties of each layer of the bonded medium. The attenuation in each layer and specifically in the adhesive layer can be taken into account by assuming that the wave number and the acoustic impedance are complex. Efficient computer codes have been developed for the calculation of the frequency dependent reflection coefficient.[50]

This analysis can be useful when examining the effect of the bonded and unbonded materials on the reflection coefficient. As an example, consider a test object consisting of two identical aluminum plates bonded by a layer of epoxy. Assume that the aluminum layers are 1 mm (0.04 in.) thick and the epoxy layer is 0.1 mm (0.004 in.) thick and with attenuation of 10 dB·mm^{-1}·MHz^{-2}. The calculated reflection coefficients as a function of frequency for several possible cases are shown in Fig. 18.

FIGURE 18. Amplitude spectra of calculated reflection at 0 rad: (a) perfectly bonded aluminum plate; (b) plate with complete disbonding at lower epoxy-to-aluminum interface; (c) plate with complete disbonding at upper interface.

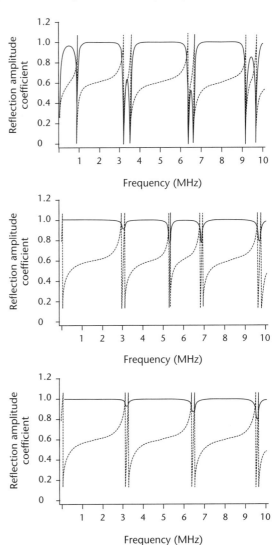

FIGURE 17. Transmission response for air gap between two aluminum half spaces. (X axis is logarithmic scale.)

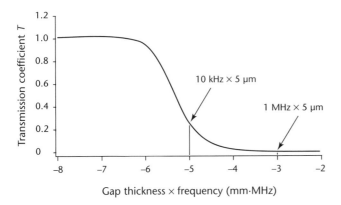

The predicted spectra can be compared with measured responses to determine if the aluminum layers are bonded. The bonded system has six minima within the frequency range of 1 to 10 MHz. The unbonded aluminum layer has only three minima. The minima are the result of destructive interference of the waves within the test object. In the time domain, a large number of minima are associated with fewer reflections in a given time. Multiple reflections with a short time of flight identify unbonded aluminum plate and are used in a test called the *ringing technique*.

The spectral representation of the pulse echo results in Fig. 19a are shown in Fig. 19b. There is general agreement between the theoretical and measured spectra but a number of detailed features of the theoretical predictions are not reproduced in the measured spectra.

Leaky Lamb Waves

In the techniques discussed above, the ultrasonic waves were incident normal to the test object. The leaky lamb wave technique is based on insonification of the test object at an oblique angle, where the wave is refracted and mode converted to induce plate waves. When excited, these waves propagate along the plate and are strongly affected by the properties of the bond.[50,51]

The leaky lamb wave technique uses two transducers in a pitch catch arrangement. The test object is typically immersed in a water tank or a water column is maintained between the transducers and the object surface. For a fixed angle of insonification, the acoustic waves are mode converted to lamb waves at specific frequencies, resulting in leakage of acoustic radiation into the fluid.

When a leaky wave is introduced, the field of the specularly reflected wave (reflection from a half space) is distorted. The specular component of the reflected wave and the leaky wave interfere, a phase cancellation occurs and two components are generated with a null between them.[52] A schematic diagram of the leaky lamb wave technique using a plate immersed in fluid is shown in Fig. 20. A typical pulsed schlieren image of the leaky lamb wave response using a glass epoxy laminate is shown in Fig. 21.

Figures 22 and 23 show the spectral response of a uniform aluminum plate and a bonded aluminum epoxy plate immersed in water and insonified at 0.34 rad (19.5 deg). The minima often are associated with the excitation of leaky lamb wave modes in the test object. The agreement between theory and experiment is excellent for the unbonded plate and reasonably good for the bonded plate, indicating a need for further study.

The possible lamb modes at various angles of incidence are shown by dispersion curves. Figure 24 shows the calculated dispersion curves for the three possible cases of a bonded aluminum plate. The dispersion curves in Fig. 24c show good agreement between theory and experiment for unbonded plate. The agreement is good for the bonded plate, except at high frequencies and high phase velocities.

FIGURE 19. Measured data from joint in thin bonded aluminum plates immersed in water. Epoxy layer is 0.1 mm (0.004 in.) thick and plate is 0.8 mm (0.032 in.) thick: (a) time domain data; (b) spectral data.

(a)

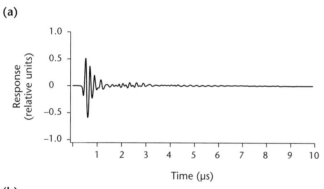

(b)

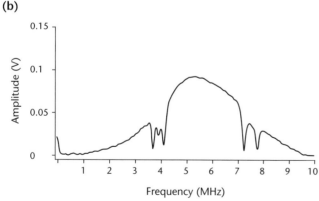

FIGURE 20. Schematic diagram of leaky lamb wave field.

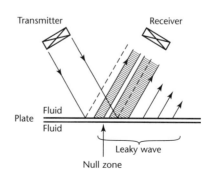

Generally, a bonded structure can give rise to many possible modes that are modifications of those for a single layer. For a bonded system, the excitation of the spectral response predicted for a single layer is an indication of unbonding in the tested area. Leaky lamb waves can be used for nondestructive testing of bonds by scanning an assembly and detecting areas at which the leaky lamb wave modes appear. These modes are different from those of the bonded assembly.

Leaky Lamb Wave Characteristics

Leaky lamb wave phenomena have two characteristics that make them useful for nondestructive tests of bonds. First, phase cancellation in the null zone of the leaky lamb wave field is sensitive to changes in interface conditions. The presence or absence of bonding as well as the change in the properties of the adhesive significantly alter the leaky lamb wave response.

Furthermore, two types of stress (compression and shear, corresponding to longitudinal and transverse waves) are encountered simultaneously when a lamb wave travels in a plate. Only one type of

FIGURE 21. Pulsed schlieren image of leaky lamb wave mode for tone burst signal before and after impinging on glass-to-epoxy sample: (a) incident beam; (b) reflected and transmitted beams.

(a)

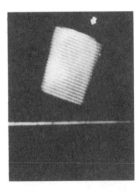

(b)

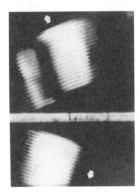

FIGURE 22. Leaky lamb wave spectra from unbonded aluminum plate (0.8 mm [0.032 in.]) immersed in water with incidence angle of 0.34 rad (19.5 deg): (a) measured spectrum; (b) calculated reflection spectrum.

(a)

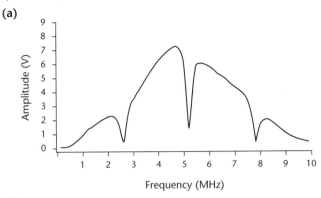

(b)

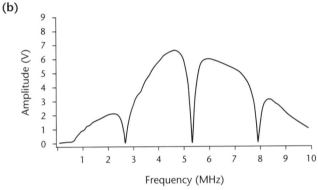

FIGURE 23. Leaky lamb wave reflection spectra from bonded aluminum plate [0.8 mm (0.032 in.)] immersed in water with incidence angle of 0.34 rad (19.5 deg). Epoxy layer 0.1 mm (0.004 in.): (a) measured spectrum; (b) calculated spectrum.

(a)

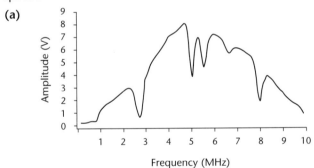

(b)

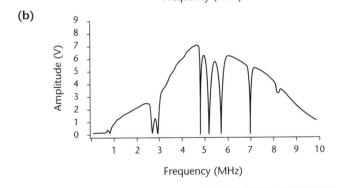

stress is involved in other ultrasonic tests. Because the two types of stress are affected differently by different material and discontinuity parameters, the lamb wave technique can potentially provide better diagnostics of interfacial bonds.

An example of the influence of bonding layer properties on leaky lamb waves is given in Fig. 25. In Figs. 25a to 25c, the reflected amplitude spectra from a single layered half space are shown for three possible cases: perfect bonding, a weak bond and complete disbond at the interface. The strong influence of bond

quality on the location of the minima in the spectra is shown. In Fig. 25d, the dispersion curves for the same bonded system are shown.

The influence of the bonding layer's elastic properties on the lamb wave phase velocity is significant over a specific frequency range. An inversion technique has been developed to extract the elastic properties of the adhesive from the bonded joint dispersion curve.[53]

FIGURE 24. Calculated dispersion curves for lamb waves: (a) in bonded plate of 1 mm (0.04 in.) aluminum, 0.1 mm (0.004 in.) epoxy and 1 mm (0.04 in.) aluminum; (b) with disbonding at lower interface of plate with 1 mm (0.04 in.) aluminum and 0.1 mm (0.004 in.) epoxy; (c) with disbonding at upper interface of 1 mm (0.04 in.) aluminum plate.

(a)

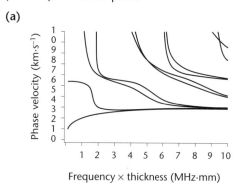

(b)

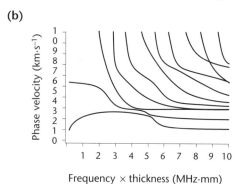

(c)

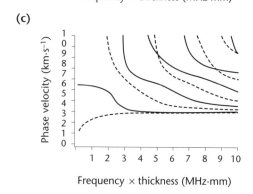

FIGURE 25. Influence of bond properties on leaky waves in single-layered medium (titanium bonded to beryllium substrate): (a) perfect bonding; (b) thin low velocity interfacial layer; (c) complete disbonding at interface; (d) frequency versus wave speed.

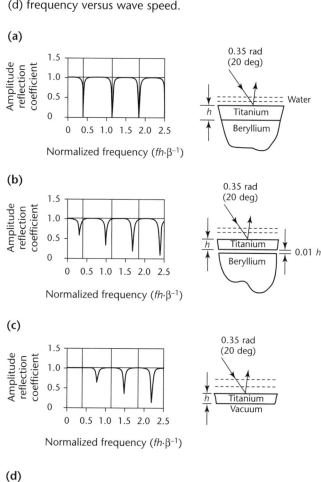

(d)

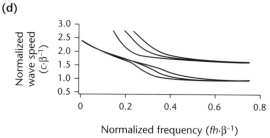

Legend
f = frequency (MHz)
h = thickness (mm)
β = transverse wave speed in titanium (mm·s⁻¹)

Applications of Leaky Lamb Wave Tests

Various applications of the leaky lamb wave phenomenon have been investigated for nondestructive tests of bonds. For studies of composites, a precured sandwich was prepared, containing [0,90]$_{2S}$ carbon epoxy skins with a 13 mm (0.5 in.) high, 3.2 mm (0.13 in.) polyamide paper, phenolic honeycomb cell and simulated unbonds made of synthetic fluorine wafers of 25, 19, 13 and 6.4 mm (1, 0.75, 0.5 and 0.25 in.) diameter.[54] The reference standard was insonified at 0.26 rad (15 deg) and the leaky lamb wave modes were measured.

A C-scan system was connected to the leaky lamb wave setup and the amplitude was recorded as a function of location. Initially, a frequency sweep was made and the minima associated with the leaky lamb wave modes were recorded. The test was conducted at 5.31 MHz, which represents one of the leaky lamb wave modes in the unbonded skin. The test results are shown in Fig. 26, where the unbonds are clearly identified — the generation of a leaky lamb wave mode creates a null detected by the receiver.

Detection of unbonds between metals and rubber is another difficult nondestructive test application. The problems result from the low acoustic impedance of rubber and the large mismatch in acoustic impedance between rubber and metals. This makes the difference in the reflected signal from bonded and unbonded rubber relatively small. Because the leaky lamb wave technique is based on measurement of the amplitude of the null due to a phase cancellation, the technique is very sensitive to changes in boundary conditions.[55] A 6.4 mm (0.25 in.) thick steel plate bonded to a 3.2 mm (0.13 in.) thick rubber mat has been tested with the pulse echo technique at 10 MHz and with the leaky lamb wave technique at 4.63 MHz. The results are shown in

Fig. 27. The pulse echo technique shows a relatively small difference, at the level of the material variations across the bonded area. On the other hand, the unbond is clearly indicated when using leaky lamb waves.

Assessment of Ultrasonic Tests of Bonds

Technology does not provide a physical parameter that can be directly correlated with bond strength for a practical test method. Nondestructive test techniques are more capable of detecting unbonds either at the adhesive layer or at its interface with the adherend. Because adhesive bond strength strongly depends on surface preparation, a nondestructive means for determining surface quality (the presence of contamination, for instance) is essential.[56]

FIGURE 26. Leaky lamb wave C-scan showing disbonds in substrate of graphite epoxy sandwich.[54]

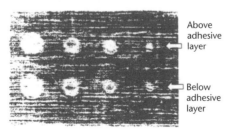

Above adhesive layer

Below adhesive layer

FIGURE 27. C-scan images of steel-to-rubber bonds: (a) leaky lamb wave image from 4 to 2 V in 15-color scale; (b) pulse echo image from 0.55 to 0.25 V in 15-color scale, showing 13 mm (0.5 in.) unbond.[54]

(a)

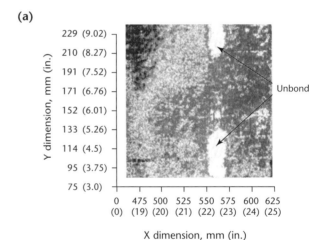

Unbond

(b)

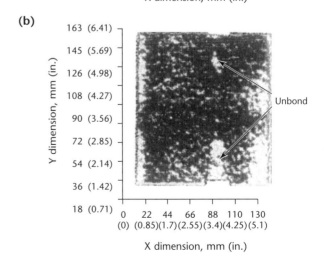

Unbond

Ultrasonic techniques can provide information about adhesive bond properties but some relevant parameters in the detected signals may be unused. An increase in the signal acquisition speed, an improvement in signal processing techniques and an increase in the size and speed of access to computer memory are expected to improve the capability of the technique. Improved techniques should allow several parameters to be captured while a bonded area is being scanned and this should enable an accurate assessment of bond quality.

One approach assesses the durability of commercial epoxy adhesive bonds by measuring ultrasonic reflection from an interphase region between the adhesive and the adherend.[57] The technique uses a specimen geometry that overcomes the drawbacks of the conventional adhesive sandwich. The interphase region is modeled with spring boundary conditions. The normal and tangential spring constants are determined as a function of epoxy degradation, from normal incidence longitudinal and from transverse wave measurements. Obliquely incident transverse waves are also measured with a dual-sensor thermoplastic (polyvinyllidene difluoride) transducer. An efficient angular spectrum approach was used to model the oblique incidence measurements, and the predictions of the model are compared with the measurements for various levels of degradation.

Pulse echo and through-transmission have traditionally been the most widely used production ultrasonic techniques for tests of adhesive bonding. Resonance and pulse echo are used in field conditions. However, leaky lamb waves have been used because of superiority in cases such as steel-to-rubber and composite bonds. Related techniques have been used for interphase characterization.[58]

For composites, the leaky lamb wave technique has been found useful for laminates with limited types of fiber orientation. Development of theoretical analysis of wave propagation in anisotropic, multilayered media would lead to a better understanding of wave behavior.[59-63] Such a development has led to an increased use of leaky lamb waves for nondestructive testing of bonded composites (the methods are presently too complex to interpret for multilayered laminates). Another area that benefits from ultrasonic testing is analysis of the bond between steel and rubber.

Assessment of Ultrasonic Tests of Coatings

Coatings require ultrasonic testing for verification of integrity in high temperature thermal barrier coatings and in some cases, evaluation of the process itself.[64] Coating means include plasma spray, chemical vapor deposition and physical vapor deposition. For instance, the chemical vapor deposition environment for silicon nitride reacts with carbon-to-carbon surfaces at 1400 °C (2550 °F). Oxidation barriers require noncontact measurement of coating thickness and modulus while undergoing deposition in real time. A laser ultrasonics system was successfully implemented for monitoring this process. This methodology for determining reaction parameters in situ also provides the opportunity to develop a system model of the process so that production runs are always controlled in the same way for repeatable coatings.

Rayleigh wave velocities have been measured in metallic coatings electrodeposited on steel and an experimental correlation was found between hardness and velocity.[65] This result suggests that surface wave velocity measurements can be used to evaluate coating hardness over regions inaccessible to conventional hardness tests. A laser ultrasonic system was set up with a chromium coating on a steel right circular cylinder. Laser generation of the surface wave and detection was accomplished using a plastic wedge with a 5 MHz broad band transducer. Dispersion curves were calculated using a wavelet decomposition for time versus frequency. The correlation was made using calibration data from these measurements.

The elastic constants of zirconia air plasma sprayed thermal barrier coatings were studied using two 15 MHz transducers in a water immersion tank.[66] Data were taken at various incident angles and fitted to a calculated theoretical transfer function for an unlimited isotropic plate with plane waves. The average longitudinal and transverse wave velocities are 2560 m·s^{-1} and 1710 m·s^{-1} respectively with variation lower than 3 percent over a wide refraction angle range, 0 to 1.1 rad (0 to 60 deg). Young's modulus was measured to be 33 GPa in comparison to compact zirconia at 241 GPa, indicating a high void count of 15 percent in the presence of a microcrack network. In another application, the elastic constants obtained from bulk wave measurements were used to assess the quality of thermal barrier coatings, which may develop a substantial amount of porosity if the process is not controlled properly.[67]

Short pulse scanning acoustic microscopy has been developed to investigate the structure, properties and geometry of highly absorptive multilayered polymer media.[68] The evaluation and visualization of internal layers having three percent of the total thickness have been demonstrated. The approach also included a time domain digital algorithm to provide the precision needed. The polymer sample was an advanced material for gas storage tanks consisting of high density polyethylene, an upper layer of the same high density polyethylene with a black pigment filler, a barrier layer of ethylene vinyl alcohol copolymer and an adhesive layer of polyethylene based modified polyolefin adhesive resins.

Testing can be implemented remotely to detect discontinuities of large metallic pipes, tubes and plates with a surface coating added for corrosion protection or insulation.[69] Because the coatings are usually viscoelastic, the guided wave ranges may be severely reduced unless a proper mode and an adequate frequency range are selected. To overcome this limitation, a hybrid finite element boundary element method which explicitly includes the attenuating properties of the coating was used to determine the lamb and transverse horizontal mode conversion factors at the corrosion discontinuities under the coating. Monotonic variations of the primary mode conversion factors with discontinuity depth enabled weakly attenuated modes to be inspected.

Part 3. Ultrasonic Tests of Composite Laminates

Composites are useful structural materials because of their high ratios of strength to weight and moduli to weight. Composites are multilayered, heterogeneous and anisotropic on both macroscopic and microscopic levels. Most discontinuities in composites are different from those in metals, and the fracture mechanisms are much more complex.

Various discontinuities or combinations of discontinuities can have specific degradation effects on the performance of a given composite and these effects are determined by several factors: discontinuity characteristics (such as dimensions and location), geometry, composition and other properties of the host composite, the type and magnitude of the applied stress and the environment to which the structure is exposed during service.

For many discontinuities, the specific mechanisms of degradation and the effects of the above factors are not well understood. The anticipated durability of composite structural components can be confirmed by efficient, reliable and cost effective ultrasonic tests. These techniques should allow the determination of performance levels and serviceability at an acceptable probability of detection.

Described below are (1) the life cycle of a composite, (2) the type of discontinuities that can be induced at each stage of the life cycle and (3) the ultrasonic techniques in use or under development for tests of composites. Although the tests described here are applicable to a wide variety of composite materials, including metal matrix composites, the following discussion concentrates on fiber reinforced plastic composites, particularly those used for aircraft structures. The fiber materials include graphite, glass and boron. Epoxy resin is the usual matrix material. Boron epoxy was the first material to be used for primary composite structures but was replaced by graphite epoxy because of cost.

Sources of Discontinuities

Fiber reinforced plastic components are commonly made by curing preimpregnated fibers stacked in layers of a certain orientation. The sequence of stacking is determined by design requirements and can be done in manual layup or by automated filament winding. Different types of discontinuities can be introduced during the production of preimpregnated fibers: (1) not enough resin, (2) inclusions and contaminations, (3) excessive variability in fiber or resin properties, (4) nonuniform hardener content and (5) fiber misalignment.

To make a composite, the preimpregnated layup or the filament wound structure is cured by exposure to elevated temperature and pressure in a predetermined procedure. A vacuum is maintained in the curing environment to eliminate porosity in the resin. Resin is cured in three stages: (1) the fluid stage (the resin is liquid and its molecules combine to form a reactive polymerizable material), (2) the polymerization stage (polymers of long chains are formed) and (3) the hardening stage (polymeric chains cross link to produce a three-dimensional network).

The progressive physical condition of the curing resin determines the duration of each stage and the times when various temperatures and pressures are applied. The resin condition must therefore be within specifications to ensure the final quality.

Once curing is completed, the composite is postcured to relieve stresses. These stresses are induced mainly by a mismatch of thermal expansion coefficients between the various layers of the composite and between the fibers and the matrix. The laminate or filament wound structure might contain several types of discontinuities, depending on the production process. Each of these discontinuities degrades the performance of the host composite structure and its durability in service. Possible discontinuities induced by fabrication include (1) delamination, broken fibers and matrix cracking, (2) fiber misalignment, (3) inclusions and contaminations, (4) inadequate volume ratio of fiber to resin, (5) wrong layup order, (6) overlap or the gap between the fiber bundles in a layer, (7) insufficient curing or overcuring, (8) excessive porosity or voids and (9) knots or missing roving of the winding fibers.

Aircraft composite structures are assembled using adhesive bonds to join combinations of composite laminates to metallic or other composite structures such as honeycomb. Two basic fabrication concepts, precure and cocure, are used to build up a composite assembly. In precuring, skins made of laminates with the required layup order are cured first and then bonded to an adherend. In cocure, the assembly is prepared by stacking the adhesive layers over the adherend, laying up laminate plies at the required sequence and then curing the complete structure.

These processes can induce discontinuities such as unbonds, porosity and voids as well as contamination of the adhesive joint. Other means of assembly include rivets or bolts, but these can initiate cracking and delaminations near the fastener hole.

In service, structural composites are exposed to conditions that can induce discontinuities different from those produced during fabrication. These include environmental degradation, erosion and damage from impact, weather and fatigue. In the case of aircraft components, impact damage is typically caused by dropped tools, birds or debris encountered during taxiing or landing, military action or weather conditions during flight. Erosion is caused by rain, hail, dust or sand. These damage sources degrade the performance of the composite skins, the adhesive and the adherend.

In some cases, the mechanism of degradation is not well understood or predictable. The response of composite materials to fatigue conditions depends on the layer's orientation, on the stacking order and on the nature of the applied loads. Fatigue can cause matrix cracking and crazing, fiber failure, delamination and disruption of the bond between fibers and matrix.

Impact damage is a primary concern to users of composite materials because the damage can appear at any location over the structure and at any time. This is in contrast to fatigue damage, which can be induced only at high stress concentration areas after exposure to a sufficiently large number of mechanical loading cycles. Even low levels of impact damage can be serious over time because of growth resulting from stress concentration.

Role of Ultrasonic Testing

Ultrasonic techniques play a major role in the nondestructive testing of composites, both in research and in practical applications. Ultrasound provides many parameters that can be used to detect and characterize discontinuities and to determine the elastic properties of the composite. Anomalies and property variations affect the intensity, velocity, scattering, mode conversion and reflection characteristics of an ultrasonic beam that insonifies the test object.

Different types of information can be obtained when the incident acoustic wave is normal or at an angle to the material surface. To understand wave behavior and to predict its characteristics in composite material, a theory for the analysis of the wave behavior in anisotropic layered media is needed. A general theory of wave propagation in multilayered composite laminates has been presented in the literature.[60] The fundamental features of the theory are briefly described below.

Theory of Wave Propagation in Composites

In a general test configuration for composite materials, the composite laminate contains N layers (called *laminae*) and is of total thickness H. Each lamina is a unidirectional fiber reinforced layer and may have different orientations, depending on the design requirements of the laminate. The laminae are assumed to be perfectly bonded at their interfaces.

In many multiple-orientation laminates, the interfacial zones are matrix rich and therefore have material properties that may be significantly different from those of the adjacent laminae. In such cases, the interfacial zone should be represented by an additional layer of material with certain assumed properties and the solution procedure can still be applied to the resulting problem. The laminate is assumed to be immersed in water and insonified by a plane acoustic wave at an incidence angle θ. The incident wave can be either time harmonic or pulsed. The theory of wave propagation in multilayered composite laminates has been presented in the literature.[1,57] The equations are well behaved at all frequencies and can be solved by means of standard techniques.[70]

This general treatment of wave propagation in composites can be applied for any angle of incidence, including normal incidence at which composites behave as a layered isotropic medium. The main interest of ultrasonic testing is the reflection coefficient R as a function of the frequency and incident angle. For this purpose, the order of the system of equations that need to be solved can be somewhat reduced. Also, by treating k_0 as the unknown wave number, the dispersion equation for guided wave propagation in the medium can be derived.

Testing Composites at Normal Incidence

In most ultrasonic tests, a longitudinal beam is incident normal to the composite surface. Under these conditions, the effect of material anisotropy can be neglected and the approach is similar to tests of isotropic media. Even though the material behaves as if it were isotropic, its layers cause extraneous reflections and increase attenuation.

Two basic testing modes of normal incidence are commonly performed. In through-transmission tests, the attenuation is determined from the amplitude of the wave after it has traveled through the test object. In pulse echo tests, several parameters can be evaluated: (1) changes in the back reflection amplitude, (2) amplitude of extraneous reflections and (3) variations in time of flight measured from the front reflection to the back reflection or the extraneous reflection.

Attenuation

Attenuation is relatively high in composites, primarily because of scattering by the fibers and isothermal absorption in the resin. High attenuation can be reduced by using the through-transmission mode, passing through the test object only once. For thick composites, the attenuation needs to be reduced further by using lower frequencies (0.5 to 2.25 MHz) and sacrificing resolution or by using high power signals. The through-transmission technique and C-scan systems are widely used for detection of delaminations, voids, resin rich and resin starved areas and other anomalies that significantly affect attenuation.[71]

The use of attenuation as a characterization parameter is hampered by variables such as surface roughness or wave coupling and their effects are difficult to deconvolve from the data. In addition, the transducer and instrument characteristics are difficult to control in a reproducible manner. Therefore, attenuation measurements are applied mainly to identify a significant deviation of material response from an average attenuation value for the tested laminate.

Time of Flight

The depth of discontinuities in composite laminates can be determined with relatively high precision by measuring time of flight. For this purpose, short duration pulses are used in the pulse echo mode (Fig. 28) and the test procedure is similar to those for metallic objects. Using 100 ns pulses, this technique has detected 1 mm (0.04 in.) diameter delaminations in graphite epoxy laminates with ±0.2 mm (±0.008 in.) depth accuracy.[72]

The accuracy of assessing depth depends on (1) the consistency of the ultrasonic velocity across the material and (2) the similarity of velocity in the test material to velocity in a reference material. In composites, this accuracy is limited because of elastic property variations within the materials and between various components. These property variations are caused by nonuniform volume ratios of resin to fiber, by differences in polymerization levels and by variations in material content between batches of the same composite.[73]

Velocity Measurements

Using time-of-flight measurements, the ultrasonic velocity of a given mode along the material can be determined. Studies of both longitudinal and transverse wave velocities can be used to determine some of the elastic constants of a composite. The anisotropic nature of composites is evident when examining the ultrasonic velocities of various modes parallel and normal to the fibers. Use of these measurements with lamb waves has also been shown to provide the capability to monitor fatigue and thermal damage in aerospace composite materials.[73,74]

Theoretical velocity curves for models of graphite epoxy and glass epoxy

FIGURE 28. Pulse echo response from 24-layer unidirectional graphite-to-epoxy laminate: (a) without discontinuities; (b) with discontinuities.

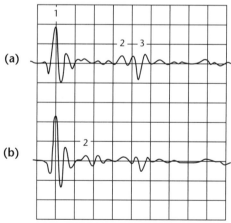

Legend
1. Front surface reflection.
2. Delamination.
3. Reflection from graphite-to-epoxy layer.

composites are shown in Fig. 29. As the figure shows, graphite epoxy is much more anisotropic than glass epoxy. Studies indicate that velocity calculations can be applied for fiber reinforced plastic materials containing matrix voids.[75] The same studies also indicate the feasibility of predicting fiber volume fraction, assuming low frequencies or small fiber diameter. Deviation from these conditions gives rise to velocity dispersion. This dispersion is most noticeable for boron fiber because it has ten times greater diameter than glass or graphite fibers.[77]

FIGURE 29. Theoretical velocity curves for three basic modes of propagation (longitudinal horizontal transverse, vertical transverse) in: (a) unbounded graphite-to-epoxy composite at 0.62 fiber volume fraction; (b) unbounded glass-to-epoxy composite at 0.4 fiber volume fraction.[70]

(a)

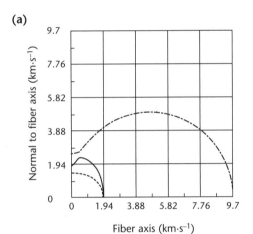

Fiber axis (km·s^{-1})

(b)

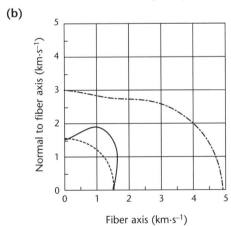

Fiber axis (km·s^{-1})

Legend
······· = horizontal transverse
—·—·— = longitudinal
——— = vertical transverse

Resonance

Resonance conditions are established in a composite plate when the thickness is a numeric multiple of half the wavelength. For this purpose, low frequencies are used to reduce the effect of attenuation on the measurements. Generally the resonance technique is used to test bonded structures or to detect delaminations.

The resonance technique can also be used to measure the depth of discontinuities but is not as practical as other techniques. Depth testing requires fabrication of a large set of calibration standards with controlled discontinuity size and depth. In addition, test results are significantly affected by pressure on the transducer, variations in the material surface roughness and variations in the elastic properties of the test object.

Spectroscopy

Conventional ultrasonic tests are based on studies of the time domain acoustic intensity integrated over the transducer area.[78] If these data are analyzed in the frequency domain using signal processing techniques, frequency dependent features can be determined. The interaction between ultrasonic waves and discontinuities — for example, scattering, absorption and, in particular, interference of wavelets scattered from various parts of discontinuities — depends on the wave frequency. The frequency dependence of the signal, detected by a wideband transducer, contains useful information for characterizing discontinuities. Using spectral analysis, discontinuities such as delaminations have been studied by several investigators.[79]

Spectral analysis is finding limited application for discontinuity testing because of the large number of factors (coupling and surface roughness) affecting the spectrum and the fact that their effects cannot be predetermined. Deconvolution methods have been used to extract the relevant signal from the characteristic signal of the transducer,[80] thus reducing the number of factors contaminating the signal scattered from the discontinuity. It remains difficult, however, to evaluate the scattered field from discontinuities in composites as a function of frequency.

Testing Composites at Oblique Incidence

The behavior of an acoustic wave impinging at an angle on a composite is significantly affected by the layered, heterogeneous and anisotropic nature of a composite. Oblique incidence is used to test composites in two modes. First is the backscattering mode, where a single transducer is used. Scattering sources in the composite are identified as a function of fiber orientations.

Second is the leaky lamb wave mode, where two transducers are used in a pitch catch arrangement. The transducers can be on the same side or on opposite sides of the laminate. The leaky lamb wave receiver is placed at the null zone caused by the interference of the specular reflection and the leaky wave components. As detailed below, many discontinuities are detectable by these two oblique incidence modes.

Backscattering

When a composite half space or a plate is insonified at an angle, a specular reflection occurs. The characteristics of reflection depend on the material and the fluid loading. While an unperturbed specular reflection is observed along the fiber direction, strong scattering takes place as the wave propagates normal to the fibers. A schlieren image of this behavior is shown in Fig. 30.[81,82] Many investigators have tried to develop theories to predict this scattered field from the fibers but none of the proposed models has been corroborated by experiment with composites.

The scattered field has been studied extensively at different frequencies.[81,82] An experimental setup was prepared with a transmitter set in a fixed location normal to the sample and rotating with it on a turntable. To eliminate the side lobes, transducers with a gaussian directivity were used. The laminate was placed so that the fibers were parallel to the axis of rotation and its front surface matched this axis. The receiver was placed in a stationary position outside the turntable to allow measuring the scattered wave amplitude as a function of the angle.

The measured field consists of side lobes that strongly depend on the frequency but do not present any consistent trend. The side lobes are dominated by local variations and irregularities in the order of the fibers within the laminate. Even when the fiber volume fraction is high, as in the case of graphite epoxy, the diffracted field is strongly perturbed by local variations.

Although it is difficult to obtain a typical or characteristic scattered field, backscattering measurements using pulses and spatial averaging have been highly successful. Because a single transducer is used, the number of variables associated with the test setup is limited, making such a setup more practical. Another advantage of the backscattering method is

FIGURE 31. Acoustic backscattering from [0,±45,90]s graphite-to-epoxy laminate: (a) setup; (b) as function of rotation angle β for 0.5 rad (30 deg) incident angle.[71]

(a)

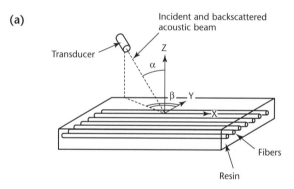

(b)

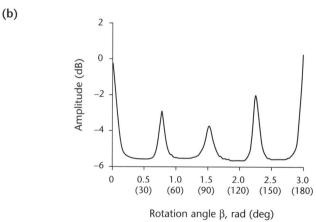

Rotation angle β, rad (deg)

Legend
α = angle of incidence
β = angle between Y axis and transmitter beam trajectory on layer plane

FIGURE 30. Schlieren image of incident and reflected waves from unidirectional glass-to-epoxy laminate: (a) along fiber direction; (b) normal to fiber direction.[70]

(a)

(b)

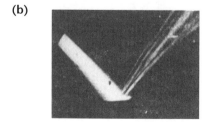

that the scattered wave is physically separated from the specular reflection.

Using the setup shown in Fig. 31a,[83] it was observed that backscattering occurs only when the angle of insonification is normal to the fiber axis.[81] As shown in Fig. 31b, a laminate with a [0,±45,90]$_S$ layup (0 indicates symmetric) gives rise to a maximum backscatter each time the beam is normal to the fibers. The finite width of the angular spectrum is determined by the transducer directivity.

In another study, the signals were spatially averaged to reduce the effects of local variations and small discontinuities.[83] Tests were conducted in the frequency range from 1 to 25 MHz. Using pulses and a boxcar averager, the peak amplitude of the backscattering was measured.

Backscattering at the plane normal to the fibers, measured as a function of incident angle, showed two maxima at the critical angles. The mechanism of generating a maximum at the critical angles is not clear and is not explained by documented theories. Note that the wave number length ka (k is the wave number and a is the fiber diameter) is relatively small and reaches only about 0.2 mm (0.008 in.) at 25 MHz for graphite epoxy.

Fiber orientations and stacking order determine the final properties of structural composites. Fiber layup is identified as follows: fiber orientations are identified in square brackets, an index indicates the number of times these orientations are repeated and an S subscript denotes that the layup is symmetric. Using backscattering measurements, fiber orientation can be determined ultrasonically by measuring the spatial distribution of intensity for a constant angle of incidence.[83] This has been implemented with the aid of a polar C-scan system. As shown in Fig. 32, the fiber orientations of graphite epoxy laminates in several layups are easily resolved. It was also shown that backscattering can be used to determine fiber misalignment and to detect ply gaps.

Matrix cracking is common in composite materials. It is induced by mechanical and thermoelastic stresses and serves as an initiation site for delaminations under interlaminar shear stresses. The cracks typically extend through the total thickness of a lamina (a stack of layers of a given orientation within a laminate) and are at least an order of magnitude larger than the fiber diameter.

For example, the thickness of a graphite ply is about 125 μm (0.005 in.) and the diameter of a graphite fiber is about 5 μm (0.0002 in.). The backscattering from transverse cracks is more than 30 dB higher than scattering from the 1.57 rad (90 deg) fibers in a [0,±45,90]$_S$ laminate. This fact allows the detection and imaging of transverse cracks, using a C-scan system, by discriminating the scattering amplitude of the cracks from that of the fibers. An example image of transverse cracks in graphite epoxy is shown in Fig. 33.

Porosity is another discontinuity for which backscattering provides unique information. Generally, porosity tends to accumulate between the layers of

FIGURE 32. Backscattering characterization for the orientation of graphite-to-epoxy layers:[71] (a) [0]$_8$; (b) [0,±45,90]$_S$; (c) [0,90]$_{2S}$.

(a)

(b)
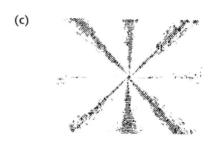

(c)

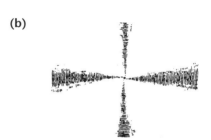

FIGURE 33. Acoustic backscattering images of transverse cracking in graphite-to-epoxy laminate: (a) fatigued sample; (b) statically loaded sample.[70]

(a)
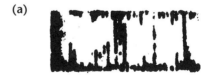

(b)
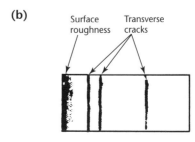

composites. To simulate porosity, a $[0,90]_{2S}$ laminate was prepared using microscopic balloons 40 µm (0.0015 in.) in diameter and a 2 µm (8×10^{-5} in.) shell thickness, spread in a thin coat between the first and second layers. Because porosity as randomly spread spheres does not have any preferred orientation, it generates backscattering of equal amplitude for all angles of insonification.

This behavior is shown in Fig. 34 where porosity causes an increase in scattering for angles not normal to the fiber axes. This behavior generates a spatial window in the backscattering field through which discontinuities of different scattering directivity can be detected and characterized. With limited success, attempts have been made to develop a theoretical model for the relation between porosity and backscattering.[84,85]

Leaky Lamb Wave Applications

Leaky lamb waves have been applied to the nondestructive testing of composites.[82,86] The technique can provide an excellent nondestructive test for detecting and characterizing various discontinuities, including delamination, porosity, ply gaps and variations in resin content.[81]

The phenomena of leaky lamb waves are described above, with reference to adhesive bonding. The leaky lamb wave field for a typical composite laminate is shown schematically in Fig. 35. The technique is applicable even with relatively thick laminates. Leaky lamb waves are not widely used, however,

because of (1) insufficient understanding of this subtle interference phenomenon and (2) the complexity of its associated acoustic field. In particular, it is difficult to interpret the received wave for laminates with multiple orientations. Extensive research has been conducted to corroborate a theoretical model for determining wave behavior.[87]

Leaky Lamb Wave Theory

For the analysis of leaky lamb wave behavior in composite materials, a matrix technique can be used.[1] A pitch catch setup has been used to verify the theory: a receiver was placed at the null zone of the leaky wave field for testing at various angles of incidence. Pairs of flat broad band transducers examined the leaky lamb wave field in the frequency range of 0.1 to 15 MHz.

Tone burst signals, with durations sufficiently long to establish a steady state condition in the test laminates, were induced with the aid of a function generator. The received signals were amplified and two aspects of the leaky lamb wave phenomenon were examined: the reflection coefficient and the dispersion curve.

At specific angles of incidence, the amplitude is acquired as a function of frequency. These experimental results were then compared with the theoretical reflection coefficient for a graphite epoxy AS4/3501-6 $[O]_8$ laminate tested at 0, 0.79 and 1.57 rad (0, 45 and 90 deg). In testing along the fibers, at 0.26 rad (15 deg) angle of incidence, the theoretical data have been convolved with the transducer characteristic response. A relatively good agreement of theory and experiment was observed.

The phase velocity of the leaky lamb wave modes was recorded as a function of the frequency for incidence angles in the range of 0.2 to 1.1 rad (10 to 60 deg) at 35 mrad (2 deg) increments. These data allowed the preparation of characteristic

FIGURE 34. Backscattering from $[0,90]_{2S}$ glass-to-epoxy laminate with and without porosity.[70]

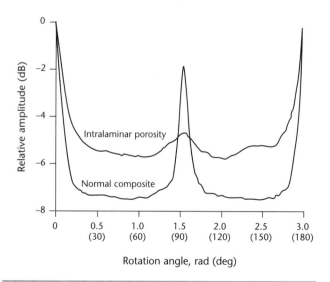

FIGURE 35. Schematic diagram of leaky lamb wave acoustic field for immersed laminate.

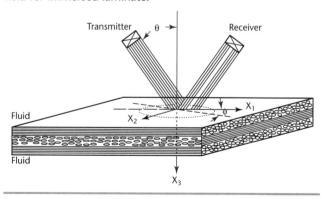

dispersion curves for lamb waves propagating at 0, 0.79 and 1.57 rad (0, 45 and 90 deg) to the fiber orientation. The results were then compared to theoretical predictions for a $[O]_8$ graphite epoxy laminate. The agreement of the theory and the experiment is excellent at lower frequencies and acceptable at higher frequencies.

This theory has also been successfully applied to multiple-layered multiple-orientation laminates, including interfacial matrix rich layers.[88,89] The agreement between theoretical and experimental dispersion curves for a $[0,90]_{2S}$ graphite epoxy laminate is excellent at lower frequencies and acceptable at higher frequencies.

Leaky Lamb Wave Portable Immersion Fixture

The leaky lamb wave method requires a fluid medium between the transducers and the test object. With this constraint, leaky lamb wave tests cannot be used in the field without a device that maintains a water column between the transducers and the laminate.[90] As is evident in the dispersion curves of composites, leaky lamb wave modes are relatively constant for angles of incidence below 0.35 rad (20 deg). Therefore, using a device (known as a *bubbler*) with an angle of incidence lower than 0.35 rad (20 deg) can reduce sensitivity to surface curvature of the test object.

The bubbler can be provided with a means of positioning the receiver at the null zone by simultaneously adjusting the ultrasonic frequency and the height of the transducers until the measured amplitude is at minimum. The height adjustment replaces changing the distance between transducers and needs to be done only once at calibration. Generally, responses obtained with a bubbler are similar to those obtained with the test object immersed in water. The small changes observed in the measured values are attributed to the difference in boundary conditions, namely the presence of a stress free back surface when using the bubbler.

Signal Processing of Leaky Lamb Wave Response

Leaky lamb wave tests for discontinuities can be performed in two ways: (1) by evaluating amplitude changes at a tone burst frequency that induces a leaky lamb wave mode in a discontinuity free sample or (2) by evaluating changes in the spectral response while sweeping through a given frequency range. Both of these techniques are very sensitive to small variations in elastic properties or plate thickness, making it difficult to discriminate between insignificant variations and the presence of discontinuities.

To reduce the sensitivity of the leaky lamb wave phenomenon to insignificant changes and to take advantage of the information available in a broad frequency range, a forward fast fourier transform is used.[91] In this process, a periodic minimum in the frequency domain is characterized by a single peak value representing the inverse of the period of leaky lamb wave excitation modes.

Using this procedure, a substantial increase in the signal-to-noise ratio (more than 20 dB) has been achieved and discontinuity detection is significantly improved. To perform such a test, a signal analyzer can be programmed to perform the fast fourier transform of the leaky lamb wave spectral response at the null zone. Relatively high noise contaminated the signal (1) after the process of obtaining the spectrum and (2) after the fast fourier transform of the spectrum. To reduce this noise, a cross correlation was applied between the resulting fast fourier transform and the discontinuity free reference signal.

The location of the peak depends on the depth of the delamination. The closer a delamination is to the upper surface of a laminate, the smaller the value of the transformed frequency (abscissa of the fast fourier transform graph) of the associated peak.

Leaky Lamb Wave Time Domain Analysis

Although a forward fast fourier transform of the leaky lamb wave spectra allows a significant improvement in sensitivity to discontinuities, it is time consuming and requires relatively complex equipment. Generally, a fourier transform of a periodic function either forward or backward leads to a similar functional result. This means that a transform of the leaky lamb wave spectrum to the time domain (backward) or to the transformed frequency domain (forward) effectively produces the same data. Time domain response is the commonest form of signal presentation on commercial ultrasonic instruments.

Time domain leaky lamb wave techniques require placing the receiver in the null zone of the reflected wave using a tone burst transmitter. Once this positioning is properly established, the pulsing transmitter is substituted to induce short pulses instead of tone bursts. The reflected signal can be processed very rapidly for C-scan or computer analysis and is associated with a very high signal-to-noise ratio when compared to the forward fast fourier transform process.

The advantages of the Using time domain approach, a C-scan image can be made for improved sensitivity over previously documented results.[90]

Time domain leaky lamb wave tests in the radiofrequency form provide significant information about composite laminates. Several unidirectional laminates were examined along the fibers at 0, 0.79 and 1.57 rad (0, 45 and 90 deg) propagation and at 0.26 and 0.35 rad (15 and 20 deg) incidence. The responses along the fibers and normal to the fibers show repetitive reflections with a constant time of flight between them. The time duration between the reflections is determined by the thickness of the laminate. This result conforms with the results from the forward fast fourier transform process, where the location of the peak correlates well with the thickness.

When testing the sample normal to the fiber, the reflections pattern is significantly different from the one obtained along the fibers. The time duration between the reflections is no longer constant and the second reflection appears closer than expected in the case of the internal specular reflection of a longitudinal wave. If this were a longitudinal mode, it would have been three times slower and would have appeared much later.

When testing a unidirectional laminate at 0.79 rad (45 deg) from the fiber orientation, reflections beyond the first one are weak and complex. On the other hand, at this direction of wave propagation, discontinuities produce significant reflection amplitude with the time of flight correlated to discontinuity depth.

Generally, it is determined that the leaky lamb wave behavior, as a function of the fiber orientation, is responsible for the above phenomena. In a pulsed form, these phenomena are sensitive to changes in boundary conditions. For example, a delamination (a stress free surface) completely changed the response at 0.79 rad (45 deg).

This technique has been used with a C-scan setup and a time gate placed over the range beyond the position of the specular reflection to produce a C-scan image. The host computer acquired the peak-to-peak value of the maximum reflection as well as the time-of-flight value. Figure 36a shows a C-scan image presenting the amplitude variations obtained within the time gate. As can be seen, all three types of imbedded discontinuities (delaminations, ply gap and porosity) are clearly distinguishable.

In addition, changes in the resin-to-fiber ratio significantly affected the amplitude.

The variations of the time-of-flight values for the $[O]_{24}$ sample can also be recorded on a C-scan image (Fig. 36b). While all the embedded discontinuities have been detected, they are observed with a sensitivity superior to the one obtained with tone burst leaky lamb wave tests. The dark lines along the C-scan image are parallel to the fiber orientation and are a result of the migration of the porosity 40 μm (0.0016 in.) from the center of the object during the cure of the laminate. A close look at the image shows that the porosity also migrated through the plies during cure.

Different colors were assigned to the various time-of-flight ranges, thus presenting the depth of the discontinuities in the sample. The depth distribution of the trapped clusters of porosity can be identified by the color of pixels around the porosity. The leaky lamb wave theory has been applied to corroborate time domain results. Using convolution of the transducer impulse response in the frequency domain and a fast fourier transform, the frequency dependent, complex valued reflection coefficient was transformed to the time domain. The theoretical pulse responses

FIGURE 36. C-scan image of $[0]_{24}$ graphite-to-epoxy laminate tested with pulsers at 0.75 rad (45 deg) to fiber orientation: (a) amplitude; (b) time of flight.

(a)

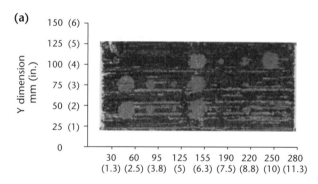

X dimension, mm (in.)

(b)

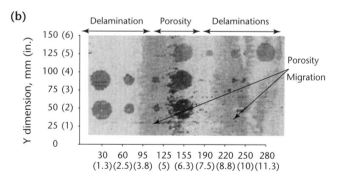

X dimension, mm (in.)

for various propagation orientations with the fibers agree with experimental data.

A technique for determining elastic constants of laminar composite materials using line focused acoustic microscopic experiments is based on time domain response studies.[92] The microscopy response is complicated by multiple reflections in the layers and also by the anisotropic nature of the material. The model used is based on a stable, recursive, stiffness matrix algorithm that can be applied to the interpretation of the time resolved acoustic microscopy signature. It has been shown that the fluid load has a significant effect on the leaky surface waves in these materials, increasing the wave speed above that for the slow transverse wave. This results in its absence from the microscopy signature of the surface wave. Time resolved acoustic microscopy has been applied to the determination of elastic constants of a unidirectional composite or of one lamina of a cross ply composite. The lateral waves and multiple reflections of bulk waves appearing in the microscopy signature are used for the elastic properties reconstruction. The reconstruction results can then be compared to the data obtained by the self-reference, double-through-transmission bulk wave technique.

Other advances in high resolution acoustical imaging and quantitative acoustical microscopy for advanced material evaluation based on leaky surface lamb waves (sometimes called *simply leaky surface acoustic waves*) have been demonstrated. The most popular quantitative technique in acoustic microscopy is the $V(z)$ technique, in which the acoustic velocity and attenuation of the leaky surface acoustic waves can be determined from the output signal V of the transducer, which is acquired as a function of specimen displacement relative to the ultrasonic sources and receiver.[93,94] The output voltage is recorded as a function of the distance between the focus and the surface of the specimen. The phase velocity and propagation attenuation of the leaky surface acoustic waves, as well as the reflectance function for the specimen-to-liquid coupling interface, can be obtained from the recorded amplitude data. The experimental configuration as shown in Fig. 37 is called the $V(z)$ system. In this arrangement, the leaky surface lamb waves are generated by a ray incident on the liquid-to-solid interface at the critical angle θ_R. A surface wave propagates along the interface reradiating back to the liquid at the same angle θ_R. As the transducer is moved toward the specimen, one of the reradiated rays is effectively received by the transducer.

Only a leaky wave whose critical angle θ_R is less than the half-aperture angle θ_m of the transducer, $\theta_R < \theta_m$, can be excited and detected in this scheme. The time delay Δz in the responses to the ray R is directly related to the velocity C_R of the leaky surface lamb waves:[95,96]

$$(6) \quad C_R = \cfrac{1}{\sqrt{\cfrac{\Delta t}{C \cdot \Delta z} - \cfrac{1}{4} \cdot \left(\cfrac{\Delta t}{\Delta z} \right)}}$$

The maximum value of Δz is limited by the focal distance of the lens and the half aperture angle θ_m. Thus $\Delta z < F \cdot \cos(\theta_m)$. The maximum value of F is usually limited by the sound attenuation in the liquid. It is also possible to obtain better accuracy by decreasing θ_m, but this is not desirable because of the reduction in the critical angle range. However, the accuracy does increase with increasing Δz. Extensions of the $V(z)$ technique have been described for another configuration in which the received voltage $V(x,t)$ is acquired during relative translation along the specimen surface.[96] Angular resolution of the measurements in the $V(x,t)$ technique is better than the $V(z)$ technique for small incident angles.

Computerized Testing

Nondestructive testing of composites and other advanced materials requires gathering many data, statistically processing them using numerical techniques and comparing them with a reference data bank. These tasks are time consuming and can include human error if done manually, so they are ideally

FIGURE 37. Ray model of the $V(z)$ technique for high resolution acoustic imaging.

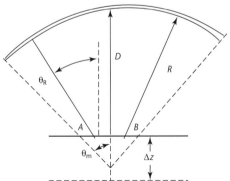

Legend
A = ray of reflected wave
B = ray of reflected wave
D = ray of normal incidence
θ_m = half-aperture angle
θ_R = critical angle
Δz = time delay related to test object thickness

handled by computers. Computer technologies are increasingly being adapted to ultrasonic research and applications, mainly because of a significant reduction in computer cost and size with substantial increases in speed, memory and performance.

Digital systems with standard communication interfaces have become widely available. Use of computerized systems has contributed significantly to the ability to acquire a large volume of data and to process, display and store it in an automatic, reliable and fast way.[97] Computerized C-scan systems are commercially manufactured and widely used for automated testing, research and development. Test results are presented on a video display in color or grayscale on high resolution monitors. This technology is assisted by developments in related fields such as X-ray tomography and image processing.

Ultrasonic parameters can be evaluated with computerized systems to provide detailed information about discontinuities. One such approach includes a features mapping technique developed to characterize various discontinuity types.[98]

Conclusion

Although ultrasonic nondestructive tests of composites are a relatively well established technology, reliability is hampered by the anisotropic, heterogeneous, layered nature of the test object. These material characteristics are not properly accounted for in conventional ultrasonic methods.

Ultrasonic nondestructive testing plays an important role in the development and application of composites as raw materials for primary structures, specifically for modern aircraft. Generally, ultrasonic nondestructive testing is used (1) for detection of discontinuities and determination of characteristics, such as type, dimension and location, and (2) for determination of mechanical properties such as stiffness.

The results of an ultrasonic test can be used to predict the performance and serviceability of the composite. However, the high variance in material properties, surface roughness and the heterogeneous, anisotropic and layered nature of composites places severe constraints on the development of effective ultrasonic nondestructive tests. In particular, the constraints make it more difficult to define and produce reliable reference standards. Statistical techniques can be used to help solve these problems.

In the past, ultrasonic testing has been considered an empirical science because of the limited capability of quantitative techniques, especially for composites. In many investigations, researchers have looked for correlations between material properties or discontinuity characteristics and a specific physical parameter. Some of the research results contributed significantly to the effort to ensure the quality of composite structures.

However, factors that can affect the measured nondestructive test parameters and are not related to the evaluated properties are not always taken into account. Sometimes, the effect of these factors is unpredictable. A correlation not properly founded on a scientific basis may result in failure of a test's predictions.

One of the most applicable nondestructive test parameters in ultrasonics is attenuation. It has served in studying numerous phenomena, including fatigue damage, weathering degradation, porosity content and resin-to-fiber volume ratios. The results of these studies may be useful in assessing the change in material properties from reference conditions but test results must be evaluated carefully. Such results can serve as data for the development of theoretical models to obtain a quantitative methodology or to monitor changes in an individual composite exposed to experimental conditions. Before high reliability and confidence can be obtained, it has been necessary to develop analytical tools that support experimental testing data. Important progress was achieved with the growing understanding of wave behavior, both empirically and theoretically.[99,100] The field has been advanced by a number of studies not referenced above.[101-111] This progress can be attributed to nondestructive test research in an increasing number of universities and scientific institutes.

The need for reliable and cost effective ultrasonic test techniques has become more critical in all areas of technology. It is widely recognized that nondestructive testing can make a significant contribution in energy savings and effective use of raw materials. As a result, government agencies and industry have invested more resources in the development of nondestructive testing in general and for composites in particular.

There is much promise in several areas: (1) phenomena such as ultrasonic backscattering and leaky lamb waves, (2) signal processing, (3) incorporation of several techniques in one test system through computer controls, (4) fast, lightweight and inexpensive computers and (5) the development of quantitative nondestructive test techniques based on proven theory. All of these developments have been addressing the obstacles that limit the ultrasonic testing of composites.

References

1. Bar-Cohen, Y., D.R. Johnson, A.K. Mal, R.W. McClung and W. Simpson, Jr. Section 15, "Ultrasonic Testing Applications in Advanced Materials and Processes." *Nondestructive Testing Handbook*, second edition: Vol. 7, *Ultrasonic Testing*. Columbus, OH: American Society for Nondestructive Testing (1991): p 505-549.
2. Vary, A. "Ultrasonic Nondestructive Evaluation, Microstructure, and Fracture Toughness Interrelations." *Solid Mechanics Research for Quantitative Nondestructive Evaluation*. Dordrecht, Netherlands: Kluwer, Martinus Nijhoff (1987): p 135-152.
3. Kupperman, D.S., H.B. Karplus, R.B. Poeppel, W.A. Ellingson, H. Berger, C. Robbins and E. Fuller. ANL/FE-83-25, *Applications of NDE Methods to Green Ceramics: Initial Results*. Argonne, IL: Argonne National Laboratory (1984).
4. Roberts, R.A., W.A. Ellingson and M.W. Vannier. "A Comparison of X-Ray Computed Tomography, Through-Transmission Ultrasound, and Low kV X-Ray Imaging for Characterizing Green State Ceramics." *Proceedings of the Fifteenth Symposium on Nondestructive Evaluation*. San Antonio, TX: Southwest Research Institute (1985).
5. Klima, S., G.K. Watson, T.P. Herbell and T.J. Moore. NASA TM 82765, DOE/NASA/51040-35, "Ultrasonic Velocity for Estimating Density of Structural Ceramics." *Proceedings of the Automotive Technology Development Contractor Meeting*. Washington, DC: National Aeronautics and Space Administration (1981).
6. Generazio, E.R., D.B. Stang and D.J. Roth. NASA TM 10 1340, *Dynamic Porosity Variations in Ceramics*. Cleveland, OH: National Aeronautics and Space Administration, Lewis Research Center (1988).
7. Klima, S.K. and H.E. Kautz. TM 101489, *Nondestructive Evaluation of Advanced Ceramics*. Cleveland, OH: National Aeronautics and Space Administration, Lewis Research Center (1988).
8. Iwasaki, H. and M. Izumi. "Acoustic Characterization of Si_3N_4 Ceramics." *Journal of the Society of Materials Science*. Vol. 30, No. 337. Tokyo, Japan: Society of Materials Science (1981): p 1044-1050.
9. ANL/MSD-79-7, *Nondestructive Evaluation Techniques for High-Temperature Ceramic Components*. Argonne, IL: Argonne National Laboratory (1979).
10. Vary, A. NASA-TM-B1530, *Quantitative Ultrasonic Evaluation of Engineering Properties in Metals, Composites, and Ceramics*. Washington, DC: National Aeronautics and Space Administration (1980).
11. Vary, A. *Quantitative Ultrasonic Evaluation of Mechanical Properties of Engineering Materials*. NASA-TM-78905. Washington, DC: National Aeronautics and Space Administration (1978).
12. Simpson, W.A., Jr. and R.W. McClung. "NDE of Advanced Structural Ceramics." *Nondestructive Testing of High-Performance Ceramics: Conference Proceedings* [Boston, MA, August 1987]. Westerville, OH: American Ceramic Society (1987): p 290-303.
13. Nagy, P.B. and L. Adler. "Surface Roughness Induced Attenuation of Reflected and Transmitted Ultrasonic Waves." *Journal of the Acoustical Society of America*. Vol. 82. Melville, NY: American Institute of Physics, for the Acoustical Society of America (1987): p 193-197.
14. Rogers, P.H. and A.L. Van Buren. "An Exact Expression for the Lommel Diffraction Correction Integral." *Journal of the Acoustical Society of America*. Vol. 55, No. 4. Melville, NY: American Institute of Physics, for the Acoustical Society of America (1974): p 724-728.

15. Generazio, E.R. "The Role of the Reflection Coefficient in Precision Measurement of Ultrasonic Attenuation." *Review of Progress in Quantitative Nondestructive Evaluation* [San Diego, CA, July 1984]. Vol. 4B. New York, NY: Plenum (1985): p975-989.

16. Chou, C.H., B.T. Khuri-Yakub, K. Liang and G.S. Kino. "High-Frequency Bulk Wave Measurements of Structural Ceramics." AFWAL-TR-80-4078, *Review of Progress in Quantitative Nondestructive Evaluation* [La Jolla, CA, July 1979]. Wright Patterson Air Force Base, OH: United States Air Force (1980): p663-670.

17. Chou, C.H., K. Liang, B.T. Khuri-Yakub and G.S. Kino. "Bulk Defect Characterization Using Short Wavelength Measurement." *New Procedures in Nondestructive Testing.* New York, NY: Springer (1983): p337-354.

18. Kino, G.S., B.T. Khuri-Yakub, Y. Murakami and K.H. Yu. "Defect Characterization in Ceramics Using High-Frequency Ultrasonics." AFML-TR-78-205, *Review of Progress in Quantitative Nondestructive Evaluation* [La Jolla, CA, July 1978]. Springfield, VA: National Technical Information Service (1979): p242-245.

19. Khuri-Yakub, B.T., C.H. Chou, K. Liang and G.S. Kino. "NDE for Bulk Defects in Ceramics." AFML-TR-81-4080, *Review of Progress in Quantitative Nondestructive Evaluation* [La Jolla, CA, July 1980]. Springfield, VA: National Technical Information Service (1981): p137-143.

20. Derkacs, T. "High-Frequency Longitudinal and Shear Wave Inspection of Gas Turbine Ceramics." AFML-TR-78-55, *Proceedings of the ARPA-AFML Review of Progress in Quantitative NDE* [San Diego, CA, 1977]. Springfield, VA: National Technical Information Service (1978): p 251-256.

21. Derkacs, T., I.M. Matay and W.D. Brentnall. TRW-ER-7798-F, *Nondestructive Evaluation of Ceramics.* Cleveland, OH: TRW Corporation (1976).

22. Kessler, L.W. and D.E. Yuhas. "High Resolution Real Time Acoustic Microscopy." AFML-TR-78-55, *Proceedings of the ARPA/AFML Review of Progress in Quantitative Nondestructive Evaluation* [San Diego, CA, 1977]. Springfield, VA: National Technical Information Service (1978): p 241-244.

23. Yuhas, D.E., T.E. McGraw and L.W. Kessler. "Scanning Laser Acoustic Microscope Visualization of Solid Inclusions in Silicon Nitride." AFWAL-TR-80-4078, *Proceedings of the DARPA/AFML Review of Progress in Quantitative Nondestructive Evaluation* [La Jolla, CA, July 1979]. Springfield, VA: National Technical Information Service (1980): p 683-690.

24. Roth, D.J., S.J. Klima, J.D. Kiser and G.Y. Baaklini. NASA TM 87035, *Reliability of Void Detection in Structural Ceramics Using Scanning Laser Acoustic Microscopy.* Washington, DC: National Aeronautics and Space Administration (March 1985).

25. Roth, D.J. and G.Y. Baaklini. NASA TM 87222, *Reliability of Scanning Laser Acoustic Microscopy for Detecting Internal Voids in Structural Ceramics.* Washington, DC: National Aeronautics and Space Administration (January 1986).

26. Schuldies, J.J. and T. Derkacs. "Ultrasonic NDE of Ceramic Components." MCIC-78-36, *Proceedings of the DARPA/NAVSEA Ceramic Gas Turbine Demonstration Engine Program Review* [Castine, ME, August 1977]. Springfield, VA: National Technical Information Service (1978): p 429-448.

27. Srinivasan, M., D. Lawler, D. Yuhas, L.J. Inglehart and R.L. Thomas. "The Application of the State of the Art NDE Techniques to Defect Detection in Silicon Carbide Structural Ceramics." *Review of Progress in Quantitative Nondestructive Evaluation* [Boulder, CO, August 1981]. Vol. 1. New York, NY: Plenum (1982): p269-278.

28. Briggs, G.A., C.W. Lawrence and C.B. Scruby. ADD337529, *Acoustic Microscopy of Ceramic-Fibre Composites.* Springfield, VA: National Technical Information Service (1993).

29. Simpson, W.A., Jr. "Time-Domain Deconvolution: A New Technique to Improve Resolution for Ultrasonic Flaw Characterization in Stainless Steel Welds." *Materials Evaluation.* Vol. 44, No. 8. Columbus, OH: American Society for Nondestructive Testing (July 1986): p 998-1003.

30. Ying, C.F. and R. Truell. "Scattering of a Plane Longitudinal Wave by a Spherical Obstacle in an Isotropically Elastic Solid." *Journal of Applied Physics.* Vol. 27. New York, NY: American Institute of Physics (1956): p1086.

31. Roth, D.J., M.J. Verrilli, L.M. Cosgriff, R.E. Martin and R.T. Bhatt. "Microstructural and Discontinuity Characterization in Ceramic Composites Using an Ultrasonic Guided Wave Scan System." *Materials Evaluation.* Vol. 62, No. 9. Columbus, OH: American Society for Nondestructive Testing (September 2004): p 948-953.

32. Derkacs, T. and I.M. Matay. "Ultrasonic Detection of Surface Flaws in Gas Turbine Ceramics." AFWAL-TR-80-4078, *DARPA/AFML Review of Progress in Quantitative Nondestructive Evaluation* [La Jolla, CA, July 1979]. Springfield, VA: National Technical Information Service (1980): p 691-699.

33. Khuri-Yakub, B.T., G.S. Kino and A.G. Evans. "Acoustic Surface Wave Measurements of Surface Cracks in Ceramics." *Journal of the American Ceramic Society.* Vol. 63, Nos. 1-2. Westerville, OH: American Ceramics Society (January-February 1980): p 65-71.

34. Khuri-Yakub, B.T., G.S. Kino, K. Liang, J. Tien, C.H. Chou, A.G. Evans and D.B. Marshall. "Nondestructive Evaluation of Ceramics." *Review of Progress in Quantitative Nondestructive Evaluation* [Boulder, CO, August 1981]. Vol. 1. New York, NY: Plenum (1982): p 601-605.

35. Tien, J., B.T. Khuri-Yakub and G. Kino. "Acoustic Surface Wave Probing of Ceramics." AFWAL-TR-80-4078, *DARPA/AFML Review of Progress in Quantitative Nondestructive Evaluation* [La Jolla, CA, July 1979]. Wright Patterson Air Force Base, OH: United States Air Force (1980): p 671-677.

36. Tittman, B.R., O. Buck, L. Ahlberg, M. de Billy, F. Cohen-Tenoudji, A. Jungman and G. Quentin. "Surface Wave Scattering from Elliptical Cracks for Failure Prediction." *Journal of Applied Physics.* Vol. 51, No. 1. Melville, NY: American Institute of Physics (January 1980): p 142-150.

37. Whaley, H.L. and K.V. Cook. "Ultrasonic Frequency Analysis." *Materials Evaluation.* Vol. 28, No. 3. Columbus, OH: American Society for Nondestructive Testing (March 1970): p 61-66.

38. Whaley, H.L. and L. Adler. United States Patent 3 776 026, *Ultrasonic Flaw Determination by Spectral Analysis* (December 1973).

39. Adler, L., K.V. Cook and W.A. Simpson. "Ultrasonic Frequency Analysis." *Research Techniques in Nondestructive Testing.* Vol. 3. London, United Kingdom: Academic Press (1977): p 1-49.

40. Rose, J.L. and P.A. Meyer. "Ultrasonic Procedures for Predicting Adhesive Bond Strength." *Materials Evaluation.* Vol. 31, No. 6. Columbus, OH: American Society for Nondestructive Testing (June 1973): p 109.

41. Cawley, P. and R.D. Adams. "The Mechanics of the Coin-Tap Method of Non-Destructive Testing." *Journal of Sound and Vibration.* Vol. 122, No. 2. New York, NY: Academic Press (1988): p 299-316.

42. Botsco, R.J. and R.T. Anderson. "Ultrasonic Impedance Plane Analysis of Aerospace Laminates." *Adhesives Age.* Atlanta, GA: Channel Communications (June 1984): p 22-25.

43. Report 2100, *Ultrasonic Physics of the Bondascope.* Huntington Beach, CA: NDT Instruments (March 1982).

44. Cagle, C.V. "Ultrasonic Testing of Adhesive Bonds Using the Fokker Bondtester." *Materials Evaluation.* Vol. 24, No. 7. Columbus, OH: American Society for Nondestructive Testing (July 1966): p 362-370.

45. Hagemaier, D.J. Paper 6652, *NDT of Adhesive Bonded Structure.* Long Beach, CA: Douglas Aircraft Company (1977).

46. Bar-Cohen, Y., U. Arnon and M. Meron. "Defect Detection and Characterization in Composite Sandwich Structures by Ultrasonics." *SAMPE Quarterly.* Vol. 14, No. 1. Covina, CA: Society for the Advancement of Material and Process Engineering (1978): p 4-8.

47. Krautkrämer, J. and H. Krautkrämer. *Ultrasonic Testing of Materials,* fourth edition. New York, NY: Springer (1990).

48. Chang, F.H., P.L. Flynn, D.E. Gordon and J.R. Bell. "Principles and Application of Ultrasonic Spectroscopy in NDE of Adhesive Bonds." *Transactions on Sonics and Ultrasonics.* Vol. SU-23, No. 5. New York, NY: Institute of Electrical and Electronics Engineers (1976): p 334-338.

49. Brekhovskikh, L.M. *Waves in Layered Media,* second edition. New York, NY: Academic Press (1980).

50. Mal., A.K., P.C. Xu and Y. Bar-Cohen. "Analysis of Leaky Lamb Waves in Bonded Plates." *International Journal of Engineering Science*. Vol. 27, No. 7. Oxford, United Kingdom: Pergamon (1989): p 770-791.

51. Xu, P.C., A.K. Mal and Y. Bar-Cohen. "Inversion of Leaky Lamb Wave Data to Determine Cohesive Properties of Bonds." *International Journal of Engineering Science*. Vol. 28, No. 4. Oxford, United Kingdom: Pergamon (1990): p 331-346.

52. Schoch, A. "Sound Transmission in Plates." *Acustica*. Vol. 2, No. 1. Stuttgart, Germany: S. Hirzel (1952): p 1-17.

53. Bar-Cohen, Y. and A.K. Mal. "Characterization of Adhesive Bonding Using Leaky Lamb Waves." *Review of Progress in Quantitative Nondestructive Evaluation* [Brunswick, ME, July 1989]. Vol. 9B. New York, NY: Plenum (1990): p 1271-1277.

54. Bar-Cohen, Y. and D.E. Chimenti. "NDE of Composite Laminates by Leaky Lamb Waves." *Review of Progress in Quantitative Nondestructive Evaluation* [Williamsburg, VA, June 1985]. Vol. 5B. New York, NY: Plenum (1986): p 1199-1206.

55. Bar-Cohen, Y., A.K. Mal and P.C. Xu. Paper 8055, "Ultrasonic NDE of the Cohesive and Adhesive Properties of Bonded Joints Using Leaky Lamb Waves." Long Beach, CA: Douglas Aircraft Company (1989).

56. Hart-Smith, L.J. AFWAL-TR-82-4172, *Adhesive Layer Thickness and Porosity Criteria for Bonded Joint*. Wright Patterson Air Force Base, OH: United States Air Force (1982).

57. Moidu, A.K., A.N. Sinclair and J.K. Spelt. "Nondestructive Characterization of Adhesive Joint Durability Using Ultrasonic Reflection Measurements." *Research in Nondestructive Evaluation*. Vol. 11. Columbus, OH: American Society for Nondestructive Testing (1999): p 81-95.

58. Roklin, S.I. and A.I. Lavrentyev. "Ultrasonic Characterization of Thin Surface and Interphase Layers." *Topics on Nondestructive Evaluation*: Vol. 1, *Sensing for Materials Characterization, Processing, and Manufacturing*. Columbus, OH: American Society for Nondestructive Testing (1998): p 47-83.

59. Lavrentyev, A.I. and S.I. Rokhlin. "Ultrasonic Study of Environmental Damage Initiation and Evolution in Adhesive Joints." *Research in Nondestructive Testing*. Vol. 10, No. 1. Columbus, OH: American Society for Nondestructive Testing (1998): p 17-41.

60. Mal, A.K. "Wave Propagation in Layered Composite Laminates under Periodic Surface Loads." *Wave Motion*. Vol. 10. Amsterdam, Netherlands: Elsevier Science (1988): p 257-266.

61. Nayfeh, A.H. and D.E. Chimenti. "Fluid-Coupled Wave Propagation in Orthotropic Plates with Application to Fibrous Composites." *Journal of Applied Mechanics*. Vol. 55. New York, NY: ASME International (1988): p 863-870.

62. Heller, K., L.J. Jacobs and J. Qu. "Characterization of Adhesive Bond Properties Using Lamb Waves." *NDT&E International*. Vol. 33. Kidlington, United Kingdom: Elsevier Science (2000): p 555-563.

63. Miyasaka, C., B.R. Tittmann and S. Tabaka. "Stress Characterization of a Ceramic/Metal Jointed Interface by Collimated X-Ray Beam Radiography and Scanning Acoustic Microscopy." *NDT&E International*. Vol. 18. Kidlington, United Kingdom: Elsevier Science (2003): p 131-148.

64. Ringermacher, H.I. and A.D.W. McKie. "Laser Ultrasonics for the Evaluation of Composites and Coatings." *Materials Evaluation*. Vol. 53, No. 12. Columbus, OH: American Society for Nondestructive Testing (December 1995): p 1356-1361.

65. Abbate, A., J.F. Cox, S.S. Schroeder, B. Knight and J. Frankel. "Rayleigh Velocities for the Evaluation of Coating Hardness." *1996 IEEE Ultrasonics Symposium* [San Antonio, TX, November 1996]. New York, NY: Institute of Electrical and Electronics Engineers (1996): p 1017-1020.

66. Crutzen, H.P., F. Lakestani and J.R. Nicholls. "Ultrasonic Characterization of Thermal Barrier Coatings." *1996 IEEE Ultrasonics Symposium* [San Antonio, TX, November 1996]. New York, NY: Institute of Electrical and Electronics Engineers (1996): p 731-734.

67. Cheeke, J.D.N., Z. Wang and M. Viens. "Thermal Sprayed Coatings Characterization by Acoustic Waves." *1996 IEEE Ultrasonics Symposium* [San Antonio, TX, November 1996]. New York, NY: Institute of Electrical and Electronics Engineers (1996): p 749-752.

68. Maev, R.G., E.Y. Maeva and K.I. Maslov. "Ultrasonic Measurements of Thickness of Thin Internal Layers in Highly Absorbtive Layered Polymer Composite Based on Time Domain Inversion Algorithm." *Topics on Nondestructive Evaluation: Vol. 3, Advances in Signal Processing for NDE of Materials.* Columbus, OH: American Society for Nondestructive Testing (1998): p 33-37.

69. Galan, J.M. and R. Abascal. "Remote Characterization of Defects in Plates with Viscoelastic Coatings Using Guided Waves." *Ultrasonics.* Vol. 42. Guildford, Surrey, United Kingdom: IPC Science and Technology (April 2004): p 877-882.

70. Kundu, T. and A.K. Mal. "Acoustic Material Signature of a Layered Plate." *International Journal of Engineering Science.* Vol. 24, No. 4. Oxford, United Kingdom: Pergamon (1986): p 1819-1829.

71. Martin, B.G. "Ultrasonic Attenuation Due to Voids in Fiber-Reinforced Plastics." *NDT International.* Vol. 9, No. 5. Guildford, Surrey, United Kingdom: Butterworth Scientific (1976): p 242-246.

72. Bar-Cohen, Y., U. Arnon and M. Meron. "Defect Detection and Characterization in Composite Sandwich Structure by Ultrasonics." *SAMPE Quarterly.* Vol. 14, No. 1. Covina, CA: Society for the Advancement of Material and Process Engineering (1978): p 4-9.

73. Seale, M.D., B.T. Smith and W.H. Prosser. "Lamb Wave Assessment of Fatigue and Thermal Damage in Composites." *Journal of the Acoustical Society of America.* Vol. 103, No. 5. Melville, NY: American Institute of Physics, for the Acoustical Society of America (1998): p 2416-2424.

74. Shih, J.-H., A.K. Mal and M. Vemuri. "Plate Wave Characterization of Stiffness Degradation in Composites during Fatigue." *Research in Nondestructive Testing.* Vol. 10, No. 3. Columbus, OH: American Society for Nondestructive Testing (1998): p 147-162.

75. Reynolds, W.N. and S.J. Wilkinson. "The Analysis of Fiber-Reinforced Porous Composite Materials by the Measurement of Ultrasonic Wave Velocities." *Ultrasonics.* Vol. 16, No. 4. Guildford, Surrey, United Kingdom: Elsevier (1978): p 159-163.

76. Sve, C. "Elastic Wave Propagation in Porous Laminated Composites." *International Journal of Solids and Structures.* Vol. 9. Amsterdam, Netherlands: Elsevier (1973): p 937-950.

77. Nayfeh, A., R.L. Crane and W.C. Hoppe. "Reflection of Acoustic Waves from Water/Composite Interfaces." *Journal of Applied Physics.* Vol. 55, No. 3. Melville, NY: American Institute of Physics (February 1984): p 685-689.

78. Bar-Cohen, Y., E. Harnik, M. Meron and R. Davidson. "Ultrasonic Nondestructive Evaluation Method for the Detection and Identification of Defects in Filament Wound Glass Fiber-Reinforced Plastic Tubes." *Materials Evaluation.* Vol. 37, No. 8. Columbus, OH: American Society for Nondestructive Testing (July 1979): p 51-55.

79. Gericke, O.R. and B.L. Monogle. "Detection of Delaminations by Ultrasonic Spectroscopy." *Transactions on Sonics and Ultrasonics.* Vol. SU-23, No. 5. New York, NY: Institute of Electrical and Electronics Engineers (1976): p 292-299.

80. Furgason, E.S., R.E. Twyman and V.L. Newhouse. "Deconvolution Processing for Flaw Signatures." AFML-TR-78-55, *Proceedings of the ARPA/AFML Review of Progress in Quantitative NDE.* Springfield, VA: National Technical Information Service (1978): p 312-318.

81. Bar-Cohen, Y. "Ultrasonic NDE of Composites — A Review." *Solid Mechanics Research for Quantitative NDE.* Boston, MA: Marinus Nijhoff (1987): p 187-201.

82. Bar-Cohen, Y. and S.S. Lih. "Experimental Enhancements of Leaky Lamb Wave Dispersion Data Acquisition and Implementation Challenges in Composites." *Materials Evaluation.* Vol. 58, No. 6. Columbus, OH: American Society for Nondestructive Testing (June 2000): p 801-806.

83. Bar-Cohen, Y. and R.L. Crane. "Nondestructive Evaluation of Fiber Reinforced Composites with Acoustic Backscattering Measurements." *Composite Materials: Testing and Design (Sixth Conference)*. Special Technical Publication 787. Philadelphia, PA: American Society for Testing and Materials (1981): p 343-354.

84. Qu, J. and J.D. Achenbach. "Backscatter from Porosity in Cross-Ply Composites." *Review of Progress in Quantitative Nondestructive Evaluation* [Williamsburg, VA, June 1987]. Vol. 7B. New York, NY: Plenum (1988): p 1029-1036.

85. Blodgett, E.D., L.J. Thomas and J.G. Miller. "Effects of Porosity on Polar Backscatter from Fiber Reinforced Composites." *Review of Progress in Quantitative Nondestructive Evaluation* [Williamsburg, VA, June 1985]. Vol. 5B. New York, NY: Plenum (1986): p 1267-1274.

86. Bar-Cohen, Y. "NDE of Fiber Reinforced Composites — A Review." *Materials Evaluation*. Vol. 44, No. 4. Columbus, OH: American Society for Nondestructive Testing (July 1986): p 446-454.

87. Bar-Cohen, Y. and A.K. Mal. "Leaky Lamb Waves in Multiorientation Composite Laminates." *Review of Progress in Quantitative Nondestructive Evaluation* [Brunswick, ME, July 1989]. Vol. 9B. New York, NY: Plenum (1990): p 1-7.

88. Mal, A.K. and Y. Bar-Cohen. "Wave Propagation in Structural Composites." *Proceedings of the Joint ASME/SES Applied Mechanics and Engineering Sciences Conference* [Berkeley, CA, June 1988]. New York, NY: ASME International (1988): p 1-16.

89. Mal, A.K., M.R. Karim and Y. Bar-Cohen. "Determination of Dynamic Elastic Moduli of Composite Materials by Leaky Lamb Wave Experiment." *International Advances in Nondestructive Testing*. Vol. 16. Philadelphia, PA: Gordon and Breach (1990): p 77-101.

90. Bar-Cohen, Y. and D.E. Chimenti. "NDE of Composite Laminates by Leaky Lamb Waves Using Bubbler." *Nondestructive Characterization of Materials II*. New York, NY: Plenum (1987): p 89-93.

91. Chimenti, D.E. and Y. Bar-Cohen. "Signal Analysis of Leaky Lamb Wave Spectra for NDE of Composites." *Proceedings of the Ultrasonics Symposium* [Williamsburg, VA, November 1986]. New York, NY: Institute of Electrical and Electronics Engineers (1986): p 1028-1031.

92. Wang, L. and S. Rokhlin. "Time Resolved Line Focus Acoustic Microscopy of Layered Anistropic Media: Application to Composites." *IEEE Transactions on Ultrasonics, Ferroelectrics and Frequency Control*. Vol. 49, No. 9. New York, NY: Institute of Electrical and Electronics Engineers (September 2002): p 1231-1244.

93. Maev, R.G. "New Development in High Resolution Acoustic Imaging for Materials Evaluation." *World Conference on Ultrasonics* [Paris, France, September 2003]. Paris, France: Société Française d'Acoustique (2003): p 287-293.

94. Yamanaka, K. "Surface Acoustic Waves Measurements Using an Impulsive Converging Beam." *Journal of Applied Physics*. Vol. 5. Melville, NY: American Institute of Physics (1983): p 4323-4329.

95. Xiang, D., N.N. Hsu and G.V. Blessing. "The Design, Construction and Application of a Large Aperture Lens-less Line Focus PVDF Transducer." *Ultrasonics*. Vol. 34, No. 6. Amsterdam, Netherlands: Elsevier Science (August 1996): p 641-647.

96. Titov, S.A. and R.G. Maev. "V(X,T) Acoustic Microscopy Method for Leaky Surface Acoustic Waves Parameters Measurements." *Ultrasonics Symposium*. New York, NY: Institute of Electrical and Electronics Engineers (2000): p 607-610.

97. Proakis, J.G. and D.K. Manolakis. *Digital Signal Processing*, fourth edition. Upper Saddle River, NJ: Prentice Hall (2004).

98. Nestleroth, J.B., J.L. Rose, M. Baslyam and K. Subramanian. "Physically Based Ultrasonic Feature Mapping for Anomaly Classification in Composite Materials." *Materials Evaluation*. Vol. 43, No. 5. Columbus, OH: American Society for Nondestructive Testing (April 1985): p 541-546.

99. Mal, A.K. and Y. Bar-Cohen. "Stress Waves in Layered Composite Laminates." *Proceedings of the Fourth Japan-United States Conference on Composite Materials* [Washington, DC, June 1988]. Lancaster, PA: Technomic, for the American Society for Composites (June 1988).

100. Chimenti, D.E. and A.H. Nayfeh. "Experimental Ultrasonic Reflection and Guided Waves Propagation in Fibrous Composite Laminates." *Proceedings of the Fourth Japan-United States Conference on Composite Materials* [Washington, DC, June 1988]. Lancaster, PA: Technomic, for the American Society for Composites (June 1988).

101. Roth, D.J., M.R. DeGuire, L.E. Dolhert and A.F. Hepp. "Spatial Variations in A.C. Susceptibility and Microstructure for the $YBa_2Cu_3O_{7-x}$ Superconductor and Their Correlation with Room-Temperature Ultrasonic Measurements." *Journal of Materials Research.* Vol. 6, No. 10. Warrendale, PA: Materials Research Society (June 1991): p 2041-2053.

102. Roth, D.J., D.B. Stang, S.M. Swickard, M.R. DeGuire and L.E. Dolhert. "Review, Modeling and Statistical Analysis of Ultrasonic Velocity–Pore Fraction Relations in Polycrystalline Materials." *Materials Evaluation.* Vol. 49, No. 7. Columbus, OH: American Society for Nondestructive Testing (July 1991): p 883-888.

103. Roth, D.J., J.D. Kiser, S.M. Swickard, S.A. Szatmary and D.P. Kerwin. "Quantitative Mapping of Pore Fraction Variations in Silicon Nitride Using an Ultrasonic Contact Scan Technique." *Research in Nondestructive Evaluation.* Vol. 6, No. 3. Columbus, OH: American Society for Nondestructive Testing (1995): p 125-168.

104. Chu, Y.C. and S.I. Rokhlin. "Effective Elastic Moduli of Fiber-Matrix Interphases in High-Temperature Composites." *Metallurgical Transactions A: Physical Metallurgy and Materials Science.* Vol. 27A. Materials Park, OH: ASM International (1996): p 165-182.

105. Rokhlin, S.I. and T.E. Matikas. "Ultrasonic Characterization of Surfaces and Interphases." *MRS Bulletin.* Vol. 21, No. 10. Warrendale, PA: Materials Research Society (1996): p 22-29.

106. Degtyar, A.D. and S.I. Rokhlin. "Comparison of Elastic Constant Determination in Anisotropic Materials from Ultrasonic Phase and Group Velocity Data." *Journal of the Acoustical Society of America.* Vol. 102, No. 6. Melville, NY: American Institute of Physics, for the Acoustical Society of America (1997): p 3458-3466.

107. Degtyar, A.D., W. Huang and S.I. Rokhlin. "Wave Propagation in Stressed Composites." *Journal of the Acoustical Society of America.* Vol. 104, No. 4. Melville, NY: American Institute of Physics, for the Acoustical Society of America (1998): p 2192-2199.

108. Rokhlin, S.I. and L. Wang. "An Efficient Stable Recursive Algorithm for Elastic Wave Propagation in Layered Anisotropic Media." *Journal of the Acoustical Society of America.* Vol. 112, No. 3. Melville, NY: American Institute of Physics, for the Acoustical Society of America (2002): p 822-834.

109. Wang, L. and S.I. Rokhlin. "Ultrasonic Waves in Layered Anisotropic Media: Characterization of Multidirectional Composites." *International Journal of Solids and Structures.* Vol. 39. Amsterdam, Netherlands: Elsevier (2002): p 4133-4149.

110. Wang, L., A.I. Lavrentyev and S.I. Rokhlin. "Beam and Phase Effects in Angle-Beam-Through-Transmission Method of Ultrasonic Velocity Measurement." *Journal of the Acoustical Society of America.* Vol. 113, No. 3. Melville, NY: American Institute of Physics, for the Acoustical Society of America (2003): p 1551-1559.

111. Wang, L. and S.I. Rokhlin. "Ultrasonic Wave Interaction with Multidirectional Composites: Modeling and Experiment." *Journal of the Acoustical Society of America.* Vol. 114, No. 5. Melville, NY: American Institute of Physics, for the Acoustical Society of America (2003): p 2582-2595.

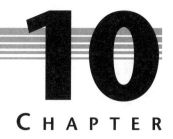

CHAPTER

Metals Applications of Ultrasonic Testing

Hormoz Ghaziary, Advanced NDE Associates, San Diego, California (Part 2)

Howard R. Hartzog, The Timken Company, Canton, Ohio (Part 3)

Part 1. Ultrasonic Tests of Steel and Wrought Alloys[1]

Primary mill products, such as bar, plate and tubes are the intermediate forms from which finished components are made. Bar products are typically machined or hot worked to a finished condition. Plate and tubular products are machined or formed to a finished condition.

In all cases, the soundness of the finished component depends on the soundness of the intermediate product. Ultrasonic testing is the most effective nondestructive method of detecting subsurface discontinuities commonly found in bar, plate and tubes. The capabilities of several ultrasonic techniques are discussed below.

Discontinuities Originating in Ingot

Segregation

The elements in cast steel or alloy are seldom distributed uniformly. Complex alloys (such as nickel based, cobalt based and high alloy stainless steels) are more susceptible to segregation than low alloy or unalloyed metals. Impurities known as *tramp elements* or dissolved gases may also cause segregation.

Segregation is found in solidified ingot and is defined as localized variations in composition resulting in nonuniform material properties. Nonuniform properties can lead to problems during hot working of the ingot and may result in rejectable discontinuities in the product.

Nonmetallic Inclusions

Nonmetallic inclusions are usually oxides, nitrides, sulfides or other compounds that have very low solubility. Such inclusions are typically entrapped in the metal during solidification, after the initial melting.

Because some of these inclusions are products of reactions within the metal, they are considered normal constituents of the finished metal: conventional melting practices cannot completely eliminate them. Nonmetallic inclusions can cause rupture during hot working and may contribute to service failures.

Ingot Pipe

A common discontinuity in ingots is the shrinkage cavity known as *pipe*. This cavity is found in the upper part of the ingot and is formed during solidification. Solidification occurs from the ingot surface toward the center and from bottom to top. As it proceeds, there may be insufficient liquid metal available near the top to feed the ingot's solidified form and a cavity may then occur.

Hydrogen Entrapment

Hydrogen in steel originates from moisture trapped during melting and casting. The presence of hydrogen in steel can cause small cracks known as *flakes*. Dissolved hydrogen may also cause large discontinuities during the hot working stages used to produce bar, plate and tubes.

Discontinuities Caused by Processing

Discontinuities that may occur during hot reduction of the ingot or billet include internal bursts and surface discontinuities such as laps seams, slivers, rolled-in scale, ferrite stringers, fins, overfills and underfills.

Bursts

Where the worked metal is weak (possibly from pipe, segregation, porosity or inclusions), the tensile stresses produced in the hot working process can be high enough to tear the metal. Tearing can occur if the hot reduction is severe or if the hot working temperature is too high. Hot working temperature may be limited by low melting phases caused by segregation.

Surface Discontinuities

The hot working process may combine with ingot or billet surface conditions to produce surface discontinuities in bars and plates. Ingots are normally forged or rolled to intermediate sized billets. The surface discontinuities in the intermediate billet must be removed by overhauling the surface before further forging or rolling, to avoid an unsatisfactory product.

Improper hot working can also produce surface discontinuities. Too much hot reduction in each pass over the hammer, press or rolls can cause hot bursts on the billet surface. Improper hot rolling can result in overfills (fins) that must be removed before further hot working to avoid formation of laps.

Ultrasonic Testing Procedures for Ingots

Ingot discontinuities such as shrinkage cavities and cold shuts are likely to weld during rolling. Inclusions in ingots are transferred to rolls but their shape and size change so much that it is difficult to predict whether they will produce defective or unacceptable plates. For these reasons, aluminum ingots intended for flat rolling are sometimes not tested ultrasonically.

However, it is often necessary to test the ingots in process control, as when new alloys or casting methods are used. Ultrasonic testing of ingots with rectangular cross section is similar to testing of aluminum plates. The ingots are placed in an immersion tank and scanned by a transducer mounted on a manipulator and scanning bridge. The transducers are typically 5 MHz but in rare cases 2.25 MHz transducers are used. Larger transducer diameters provide a good signal-to-noise ratio because of their smaller beam spread. Discontinuities down to 0.75 mm (0.03 in.) can be reliably detected.

Ingots with round cross section are tested in a rotary test system. The ingots are rotated as they move through a stationary multitransducer assembly. The coupling between the transducer and the ingot is accomplished by water jets. Two to four transducers may be used to provide the necessary coverage.

Ultrasonic pulse echo testing is the most widely used method for primary mill products, including steels, stainless steels, nickel, nickel alloys, cobalt, cobalt alloys and other nonferrous alloys.

Factors Affecting Ultrasonic Test

The surface roughness of the test material strongly influences the reliability and quality of the ultrasonic test. The more sensitive the test is to be, the smoother the material surface must be. Therefore, the test material's acceptance criteria dictate the surface condition that can be tolerated.

The grain structure of the test material determines the amount of noise, scatter and attenuation that occur during ultrasonic testing. The finer the grain size, the more sensitive is the test. In a more sensitive test, smaller discontinuities can be detected.

Equipment Qualification

Test system performance characteristics must be sufficient for the required test. To ensure suitability of the equipment, such characteristics may be evaluated in accordance with ASTM E 317, *Practice for Evaluating Performance Characteristics of Ultrasonic Pulse-Echo Testing Systems without the Use of Electronic Measurement Instruments.*[2]

The ultrasonic test frequency should be the highest that will give an adequate response (based on applicable specifications) from the reference standard in use. Typical frequencies range from 1 to 10 MHz. Specific frequencies are determined by the test criteria, grain structure and metal travel distance.

The choice of transducers is governed by the acceptance criteria and the type of testing needed. The transducer may be focused or nonfocused. The metal travel distances of the calibration reference standard and the metal cross section to be tested determine the type and size of the transducer.

Reference Standards

Reference standards are usually made from acoustically compatible materials of the same form and alloy type as the test material. Acoustic compatibility is determined by similarities in sound attenuation.

Standards that differ in attenuation from the test material by more than 6 dB or 50 percent are generally considered unsuitable. The compatibility may vary, depending on the required sensitivity. Differences in acoustic compatibility are usually compensated for by changing the instrument gain (decibel) controls.

Artificial Discontinuities

In most United States industries, the standard discontinuity for longitudinal wave (straight beam) testing is a flat bottom circular hole with a machined reflecting surface (Table 1). The common standard discontinuity for transverse wave (angle beam) testing is the *U* or *V* notch.

Immersion Ultrasonic Testing of Metals

Immersion testing is performed by placing the test object in an immersion tank or by passing the material through a water box (a relatively small tank that couples the ultrasound by means of seals around the test object).

Immersion tanks are suitable for testing rounds, squares, plates and large polygons. In an immersion tank, round bars are supported on drive rolls that rotate the materials as the transducer moves over the surface. Transducers are usually fixed in holders that ride on the surface of the product or are suspended from a carrier that rides on the tank (Figs. 1 to 3). The water in the immersion tank or water box must be free of visible air bubbles or other foreign material that could interfere with the ultrasonic test results. Suitable corrosion inhibiting agents may be used in the bath when necessary.

The sensitivity level, rejection criteria and scanning techniques are typically given by the specification in force.

TABLE 1. Calibration hole size for longitudinal wave tests of wrought metals.

Hole Number	Flat Bottom Hole Diameter	
	mm	(in.)
2	0.8	(0.03)
4	1.6	(0.06)
6	2.4	(0.09)
8	3.2	(0.13)
10	4.0	(0.16)
12	4.8	(0.19)
14	5.6	(0.22)
16	6.4	(0.25)
24	9.6	(0.38)

FIGURE 1. Transducers riding on surface of steel cylinder.

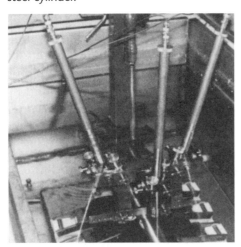

Ultrasonic Immersion Testing of Round Bars

Ultrasonic testing is usually performed after calibrating with flat bottom holes of standard diameters (Fig. 4 shows typical metal test distances). The hole size and test distance used are determined by the acceptance criteria.

Transverse wave ultrasonic testing is performed to detect transverse discontinuities when test distances are too great to perform end face longitudinal wave scanning. For tests of primary metals, the reference standards are usually at 1.05 rad (60 deg), including angle

FIGURE 2. Ultrasonic transducers suspended in immersion tank.

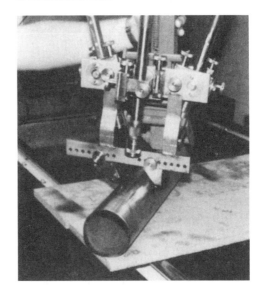

FIGURE 3. Transducer mounted on skid base for tests of plates.

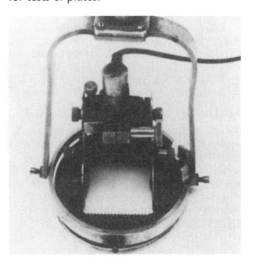

V notches. The standard notch depth is 3 percent of the cross section thickness with a length of 25 mm (1 in.) at full depth (Fig. 5).

Standard Test Block Material

High alloy austenitic materials such as stainless steels, nickel and nickel alloys, cobalt and cobalt alloys typically have greater sound attenuation than low alloy steels. For this reason, greater acoustic incompatibility between the standard and the test object must be permitted (acoustic compatibility within 75 percent is acceptable). If the acoustic compatibility is between 25 and 75 percent for austenitic materials, compensation is accomplished by changing the gain (decibel) controls to allow for the differences.

For steels and some low alloy materials, acoustic compatibility within 25 percent is acceptable. When acoustic compatibility is within 25 percent, typically no compensation is required. Requirements vary depending on specification.

Scanning Index and Speed

The scanning index or overlap changes according to specification criteria. The index may vary from 25 percent overlap to an overlap sufficient for rejecting the reference hole on two adjacent scans.

FIGURE 4. Typical reference standards for ultrasonic longitudinal wave tests of round bars: (a) flat bottom hole positions; (b) cross section showing distances.

(a)

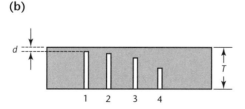

(b)

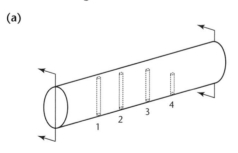

Legend
1. Distance d = 6.4 mm (0.25 in.).
2. d = thickness $T \div 8$.
3. $d = T \div 4$.
4. $d = T \div 23 + 13$ mm (0.5 in.).

A uniform scanning speed should be maintained consistent with the pulse repetition rate. The ability to reject the calibration reflector is demonstrated at the testing speed.

System Calibration

Single Flat Bottom Hole

The bottom of the reference hole should be normal to the test object surface. The equipment is adjusted so that the amplitude of the response from the flat bottom hole is between 25 and 100 percent of full linear screen height. At this gain setting, a line parallel to the sweep line at the selected amplitude height is drawn on the screen. This is known as the *reference line*. It should only be used for ranges close to the reference thickness.

Multiple Flat Bottom Holes

A distance amplitude curve may be established as follows. First, adjust the instrument gain so that the reference reflector producing the largest response is at least 80 percent of the full linear screen height. At this gain setting, record the responses from the other reference reflectors. The distance amplitude curve is constructed by joining the peak responses from each reference reflector with a straight line or a smooth curve.

The response from the hole at the greatest test metal distance should be at least twice the height of the material

---

FIGURE 5. Reference standard for axial transverse wave tests of round bars: (a) notch position; (b) cross section.

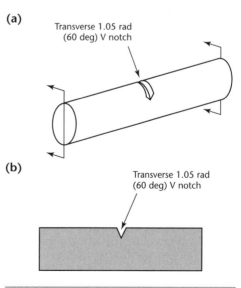

noise level and at least 20 percent of the instrument's linear response. It may be necessary to increase the instrument gain to obtain an amplitude response of at least 20 percent from the reference hole with the greatest test distance. The other points of the reference curve may be marked on the screen as a reference line.

The off-screen points of the reference curve are determined by making calibrated adjustments of the gain setting. The reference line is extended horizontally in front of the first point on the screen and after the last point.

Transverse Wave Calibration

Whenever possible, transverse wave calibration should be made at half-node and full-node test metal travel distances. The notch responses should be determined with the transducer in position on the top surface. The maximum indication from each notch should be obtained with the gain of the ultrasonic equipment adjusted so that the indication from the notch at the full-node test distance is at least 20 percent of the linear instrument range and at least twice the height of the material noise level.

If indications cannot be obtained from both notches, calibration is performed at half-node from both surfaces, with the gain of the equipment adjusted so that the indication from the notch in the opposite surface is at least 20 percent of the linear instrument range.

A line is drawn from the half-node to full-node peaks of the first reflections obtained from the two notches. This is the reference line. When testing with only one calibration notch, a line drawn parallel to the sweep line through the notch response serves as the reference line. When possible, the response from the calibration notches should be checked for symmetry by positioning the transducer in each opposing direction. If a difference is noted, the smaller signal amplitude is used to construct the reference line.

Tests of Other Metal Shapes

Squares, Rectangles and Other Polygons

Except for the scanning procedure, the testing technique for most metal shapes is the same as that for round bars. Multisided bars are stationary in the immersion tank and the transducers move in parallel paths with a suitable overlap. The overlap is usually 25 percent of the minimum effective beam width. The scanned surfaces are usually two adjacent surfaces for squares and rectangles and all surfaces of other polygons.

Tests of Plate

Testing of plate is typically the same as testing of bars except for the scanning procedure (Fig. 6). Plate is normally scanned on one surface only. The transducer movement is usually across the width of the plate. The scan path is indexed to provide a 25 percent overlap of the effective beam width. Clusters of transducers in system components known as *plate followers* are often used to minimize testing time.

Transverse wave scanning (Fig. 6b) is performed with the sound beam propagating in two opposite directions across the width and along the length, effectively scanning the surface four times.

Tests of Pipe and Tube

Pipe and tube are routinely tested by the transverse wave technique. The sound beam is propagated circumferentially in two opposite directions and axially in two opposite directions (Fig. 7).

Pipe and tube are ultrasonically tested at a frequency and beam angle able to detect inside and outside surface indications and subsurface discontinuities. The calibration standard is usually a tube or pipe of the same type, free of discontinuities, with the same nominal wall thickness and outside diameter as the test object. The standard should contain two longitudinal notches (one on the inside surface and one on the outside surface) and two circumferential notches

FIGURE 6. Beam directions for ultrasonic tests of plate on one surface: (a) longitudinal scan; (b) transverse scans.

(a)

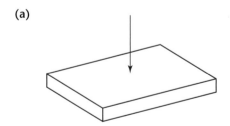

(b)

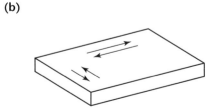

(one on the inside surface and one on the outside surface). The notches should be separated so that individual indications can be obtained from each notch.

Each notch should be a minimum of 25 mm (1 in.) away from the end of the reference standard. Unless otherwise specified, the notches should have a maximum depth of 3 percent of the nominal wall thickness or 0.1 mm (0.004 in.), whichever is greater. In addition, for tests of metals, other tolerances apply, including (1) a depth tolerance of ±0.012 mm (0.0005 in.) for notches 0.13 mm (0.005 in.) or less in depth and (2) a tolerance of ±10 percent of the specified depth for notches exceeding 0.13 mm (0.005 in.) in depth (Fig. 8). Notches (either U or V) are used for small diameter tubing and pipe. The notch lengths do not exceed 13 mm (0.5 in.) for wall thickness greater than 1.7 mm (0.065 in.).

The ultrasonic beam refracted angle is adjusted to equalize (to the maximum extent possible) the peak response from both the inside diameter (half-node) and outside diameter (full-node) notches.

Instrument settings are made so that indications from the notches are at least 50 percent (but not more than 90 percent) of linear full-screen amplitude. A line is drawn through the peaks of the reflections obtained from the inside diameter (half-node) and outside diameter (full-node) notches and serves as the reference line. For tests using automatic alarms, calibration is based on the notch producing the lower amplitude signal. The automatic alert level is based on this calibration.

Other Tube Test Parameters

The transducer overlap during scanning is adjusted to obtain a reject amplitude from the notches on two adjacent scans. The reference standard for contact testing is the same as that used for immersion testing. For couplants, petroleum based oils such those with viscosities of 65, 125 and 200 mPa·s (65, 125 and 200 cP), corresponding to SAE 10, SAE 20 and SAE 30,[3] have proven satisfactory for tests of metals. Other couplants are commercially available.

The selection of transducer frequencies described for immersion testing also applies to contact testing. The transducer is fitted with suitable wedges or shoes for curved test surfaces

Manual scanning speeds normally do not exceed 150 mm·s⁻¹ (6 in.·s⁻¹). The overlap of each scan path is typically 20 percent minimum.

Longitudinal wave calibration is the same as that described for longitudinal wave immersion testing. Transverse wave transducers are fitted with shoes or wedges to produce a 0.79 rad (45 deg) refracted angle in the test material. Calibration is the same as for transverse wave immersion testing.

FIGURE 7. Scan plan for transverse wave tests of tubes.

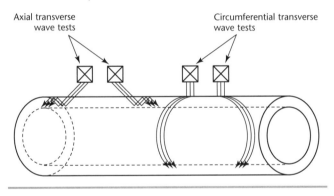

Axial transverse wave tests

Circumferential transverse wave tests

FIGURE 8. Notched reference standard for transverse wave tests of tubes.

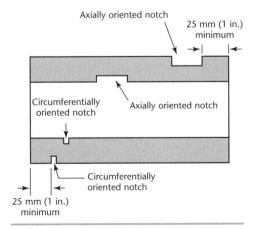

Axially oriented notch

25 mm (1 in.) minimum

Circumferentially oriented notch

Axially oriented notch

Circumferentially oriented notch

25 mm (1 in.) minimum

PART 2. Ultrasonic Testing of Primary Aluminum[1]

Most aluminum is produced as wrought products, particularly sheet, plate and foil. Bar, rod and forged materials are produced by further processing of aluminum slabs and billets.

Unlike steel, aluminum slabs can be ultrasonically tested even in the cast stage. This testing, to some degree, enables an aluminum producer to provide higher quality material for further processing. Subsequent tests are often necessary for wrought materials, depending on the required quality and the end use.

Aerospace industries have the highest acceptance standards for primary metal quality. Among the wrought products intended for use in the aerospace industries, sheet, plate and forged components are routinely tested by ultrasonic techniques. Stringent specifications set by the military and private aerospace organizations govern the ultrasonic test practices for plates and forged material.

Wrought aluminum for other applications (transportation or beverage industries) typically undergoes testing based on aerospace procedures and standards. Often, aerospace ultrasonic test practices and acceptance levels are downgraded for tests of materials with lower quality requirements. However, the ultrasonic test installation and instrumentation in aluminum production environments (rolling mills and forging plants) are for the most part set to meet aerospace requirements.

Typical Discontinuities in Rolled Aluminum Plates

Discontinuities that usually occur in aluminum plates are porosity, inclusions and, to a much lesser degree, cracks.

Porosity

Pores and cavities incurred during casting of ingots are normally closed during the rolling process. However, in medium and heavy gage plates, the effect of hot rolling is sometimes not enough to close or weld the pores.

These cavities vary in size from 50 to 200 μm (0.002 to 0.008 in.). Although a single pore might not influence the properties of a finished product, high densities of porosity may greatly reduce the fatigue life of many components.

Inclusions

Inclusions are nonaluminum particles trapped in aluminum alloy castings and wrought products. These particles can cause premature failure during metal processing or in service.

The following types of inclusions are likely to occur in aluminum plates.

1. Oxide films enter the ingot and consequently the plate as a result of aluminum oxide formation on surfaces. Oxides enter the molten metal during the casting process.
2. Spinels, mixed oxide inclusions of aluminum and magnesium, may form during the casting of aluminum magnesium alloys.
3. Refractory materials used in filters, furnaces and troughs are likely to enter aluminum plates as inclusions. Among these materials are tabular and calcined alumina.
4. Titanium diboride is used as a grain refiner and, because it has virtually no solubility in aluminum, can sometimes form inclusions.
5. Aluminum carbide precipitates out of the saturated liquid metal during cooling.
6. Graphite flakes are caused by dissolution of cast iron by molten aluminum and erosion of graphite assemblies.

Photomicrographs of common inclusions in aluminum plates are shown in Figs. 9 and 10.

FIGURE 9. Oxide layer with entrapped refractory inclusions in rolled aluminum.

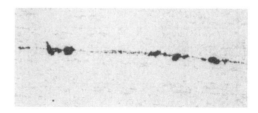

Ultrasonic Test Procedures for Aluminum

Ultrasonic Test Parameters

Frequency and sensitivity of the ultrasound used for tests of aluminum plates depend on several factors, including ultrasonic attenuation in the alloy, thickness of the material, minimum discontinuity size to be detected, grain structure of the test material, required front and back surface resolution and the ratio of signal to noise.

Ultrasound Attenuation in Aluminum

Unlike steel and other ferrous alloys, aluminum alloys differ only slightly in attenuation at frequencies typically used for ultrasonic tests. However, coarse grain structures in thick plates, ingots and cast materials cause considerable increase in attenuation, mainly because of scattering and diffraction at the grain boundaries. As a rule, ultrasonic beam intensity decreases exponentially with metal travel distance. Attenuation is also affected by the ultrasonic beam spread and by the acoustic impedance mismatch between the material and the interfacing medium.

The manner in which ultrasound attenuates in aluminum influences discontinuity detection and material characterization techniques. Therefore, in a primary aluminum production environment, it often becomes necessary to establish laboratory or on-line attenuation measurement practices.

The intensity of the ultrasound after traveling a distance X in a material is defined by:

$$(1) \quad I = I_0 \exp\left(-\alpha' X\right)$$

where I_0 is the intensity of the incident beam at $X = 0$, I is the intensity of the ultrasonic beam after traveling the distance X in the material, X is the metal travel distance (meter) and α' is the intensity attenuation coefficient (decibel per meter).

Ultrasonic amplitude can be conveniently measured in most ultrasonic test environments and is directly related to the acoustic pressure. The acoustic pressure is related to the ultrasound intensity by:

$$(2) \quad I = \frac{P^2}{2Z}$$

where Z is the acoustic impedance (gram per cubic meter second) of the material, and by:

$$(3) \quad P = P_0 \exp\left(-\frac{\alpha'}{2} X\right)$$

where P = acoustic pressure (pascal) at distance X and P_0 is acoustic pressure at $X = 0$.

The term $\alpha = \alpha'/2$ denotes the acoustic pressure attenuation coefficient:

$$(4) \quad P = P_0 \exp\left(-\alpha X\right)$$

The ultrasound amplitude is directly proportional to the acoustic pressure:

$$(5) \quad A = A_0 \exp\left(-\alpha X\right)$$

where A_0 and A are ultrasound amplitudes before and after traveling through the test material.

The ultrasonic attenuation coefficient for aluminum (or any solid material) is determined by measuring the ultrasonic transmission through prepared specimens of different thicknesses, using direct amplitude measurement. The attenuation coefficient is calculated from the following equation in neper per millimeter or in decibel per millimeter:

$$(6) \quad \alpha = \frac{\ln\left(\dfrac{A_0}{A}\right)}{X} \, \text{Np} \cdot \text{mm}^{-1}$$

$$= \frac{20 \log\left(\dfrac{A_0}{A}\right)}{X} \, \text{dB} \cdot \text{mm}^{-1}$$

The attenuation coefficient theoretically increases with frequency. To obtain accurate results, single-frequency ultrasound must be used and the attenuation coefficient can be obtained at that frequency. Corrections must be made for incomplete reflections at material interfaces, coupling losses, diffraction and beam spreading. In addition, the test

FIGURE 10. Fragments of grain refiner (titanium diboride) entrapped in oxide layer of rolled aluminum plate.

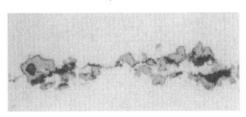

objects must have smooth parallel surfaces.

Several types of coupling and several transducer arrangements are possible. At least two signals are needed to calculate the attenuation coefficient: a reference signal and a succeeding echo signal. The reference signal should be an early echo. Using good coupling and a contact technique with a single transducer for source and receiver, the attenuation coefficient can be calculated from the following equation, in neper per millimeter:

$$(7) \quad \alpha = \frac{1}{2d} \ln\left(\frac{A_n}{A_{n+1}}\right)$$

where A_n and A_{n+1} are amplitudes (decibel) of the successive echoes and d is the test object thickness (millimeter).

A liquid coupling (usually water) may be used if the measurement requires only compressional waves. In the technique above, one or both faces of the test object and the transducer are immersed in water. To minimize the effect of beam divergence, both the reference signal and the echo signal should be in the near field of the transducer. If this is not possible, corrections for beam divergence are necessary. Furthermore, incomplete reflections at the couplant-to-material interface must be accounted for. If one of the faces of the test object is kept out of water, complete reflection may be assumed at that surface.

On-line measurements of attenuation coefficient are often used to obtain qualitative and quantitative information on the internal structure of primary aluminum, especially flat rolled products such as plates. These measurements may be made when the plates are placed in an immersion tank for ultrasonic discontinuity detection. Because plates are completely immersed in water, incomplete reflection of the ultrasound takes place at both front and back surfaces. Wave components for this arrangement are shown in Fig. 11.

For frequencies up to about 15 MHz and for short water travel distances, ultrasonic attenuation in water may be considered negligible.

In one measurement method, the amplitude of the first back surface echo serves as the reference signal, the nth succeeding echo is measured and the attenuation coefficient can be calculated from the following equation:

$$(8) \quad \alpha = \frac{1}{2d(n-1)} \\ \times \left[\ln\frac{A_r}{A_n} + 2(n-1)\ln R \right]$$

where A_n is the amplitude of the nth back surface echo, A_r is the amplitude of the reference signal (first back surface echo), d is the test material thickness (millimeter), R is $(1-\eta)\cdot(1+\eta)^{-1}$ or the amplitude reflection coefficient at the couplant-to-material interface, α is the attenuation coefficient (neper per millimeter) and η is the acoustic impedance ratio of the couplant to the test material.

If the first and second back surface echoes are used ($n = 2$), then the attenuation coefficient can be calculated:

$$(9) \quad \alpha = \frac{1}{2d}\left(\ln\frac{A_r}{A_n} + 2\ln R \right)$$

For example, for Unified Numbering System 97029 wrought aluminum alloy (heat treatable, temper 4), with a density of 2.78×10^3 kg·m^{-3} and acoustic velocity of 6.32×10^6 mm·s^{-1}, the attenuation coefficient is calculated:

$$(10) \quad \alpha = \frac{1}{2d}\left(\ln\frac{A_1}{A_2} - 0.3377 \right)$$

For thicker sections of aluminum and at ultrasonic frequencies above 10 MHz, it is often difficult to obtain a second back surface echo. In such cases, it is more convenient to use the signal reflected from the front surface of the test object as

FIGURE 11. Wave components for attenuation measurement in pulse echo technique.

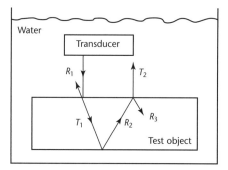

Legend
R_1 = reflection amplitude from first interface
R_2 = reflection amplitude from second interface
R_3 = reflection amplitude from third interface
T_1 = transmission amplitude from first interface
T_2 = transmission amplitude from second interface

the reference signal. The attenuation coefficient can then be calculated in neper per millimeter:

$$(11) \quad \alpha = \frac{\ln \dfrac{A_0}{A} - \ln T_1 - \ln T_2}{2d}$$

where $T_1 = 2 \cdot (1+\eta)^{-1}$ or the amplitude transmission coefficient at the interface of couplant to material and where T_2 is $2\eta \cdot (1+\eta)^{-1}$ or the amplitude transmission coefficient at the material-to-couplant interface.

For Unified Numbering System 97029 wrought aluminum alloy (heat treatable, temper 4), the attenuation coefficient can be calculated in neper per millimeter:

$$(12) \quad \alpha = \frac{\ln \dfrac{A_0}{A} - 1.2495}{2d}$$

Aluminum attenuation coefficients obtained by this procedure are typically between 0.0034 and 0.008 Np·mm^{-1} (0.03 and 0.07 dB·mm^{-1}) for frequencies between 5 and 20 MHz (without correcting for beam diffraction) and can be used only to obtain approximate values of attenuation. The approximation occurs because it is very difficult to correct for the effect of beam divergence and diffraction — frequency dependent quantities that may be calculated only for a monochromatic source of ultrasound.

Selection of Ultrasonic Frequency

The ultrasonic sensitivity to a discontinuity of a given size depends on, among other factors, the ratio of the ultrasound's wavelength to the reflector size. At higher frequencies (small ratios of wavelength to reflector size), the amount of sound energy scattered from the edges of the reflector is minimal. At normal incidence on a flat reflector, a good portion of the incident energy is reflected back to the transducer. As the ratio increases, more of the ultrasonic energy is scattered, resulting in reduced sensitivity and lower ratios of signal to noise. Therefore, higher ultrasonic frequencies are preferred for tests of aluminum.

However, because of frequency dependence of the attenuation coefficient (and the fact that attenuation increases exponentially with material thickness), the effect of ultrasonic attenuation becomes more pronounced at higher frequencies. Furthermore, in alloys with coarse grain structure, the portion of the ultrasonic energy scattered from the grain boundaries is considerably greater at higher frequencies.

Ultrasonic frequencies from 7.5 to 10 MHz are used for aluminum sections up to 75 mm (3 in.). For thicker sections up to 500 mm (20 in.), 5 MHz may be used. It is common to use 7.5 MHz for all the thicknesses up to 150 mm (6 in.).

Testing aluminum ingots of at least 500 mm (20 in.) thickness and very coarse grain structure may require the use of 2.25 MHz. At that frequency, it is difficult to detect discontinuities smaller than 1.3 mm (0.05 in.) with conventional test systems. Ingots up to 500 mm (20 in.) can be reliably tested with 5 MHz frequencies and discontinuities down to 0.75 mm (0.03 in.) can be detected.

Measurement of Discontinuity Size

In ultrasonic tests of wrought aluminum products, flat bottom holes are used to simulate natural discontinuities. The test instrument is calibrated using a series of reference standards, in the form of cylindrical blocks containing flat bottom holes of specified sizes at different depths. Discontinuity size is determined by comparing the reflected signal amplitude with that reflected by a flat bottom hole at a similar depth.

The size of a discontinuity in the form of a circular disk smaller than the cross section of the ultrasonic beam is related to the amplitude of the ultrasound reflected from it by the following equation:

$$(13) \quad A = A_0 \frac{S_s S_f}{d^2 \lambda^2} * \exp(-2\alpha d)$$

where A is amplitude of the sound beam reflected from the cylindrical disk (volt), A_0 is the amplitude of the ultrasound at the transducer (volt), d is the distance (millimeter) between the transducer and the circular disk, S_s is the surface area of the transducer (square millimeter), S_f is the surface area of the circular disk (square millimeter), α is the attenuation coefficient and λ is ultrasound wavelength (meter).

The distance d is assumed greater than the near field distance of the transducer and 100 percent reflection occurs at the circular disk.

If an aluminum section containing a flat bottom hole is immersed in water for the measurement of the discontinuity size, calculation of the reflector size becomes more complicated or even impractical. Complications occur because the amplitude of the sound reflected from the hole back to the source depends also on the ultrasonic beam divergence and reflection at the interface of water to aluminum.

In practice, however, reflector size can be obtained with a distance amplitude curve, produced by measuring the ultrasound amplitude reflected from flat bottom holes at different depths in a series of calibration blocks.

The common method of obtaining a distance amplitude curve is to set the echo signal of the flat bottom hole which provides the highest amplitude at 80 percent of the full screen scale by adjusting the instrument receiver gain. Then, without changing this adjustment, the signal amplitudes of all other flat bottom holes are measured and a graph of amplitude versus depth (metal travel distance) is generated.

To measure the size of a natural discontinuity, its signal amplitude is compared with that of the flat bottom hole at the corresponding metal travel distance. A typical distance amplitude curve is shown in Fig. 12.

Figure 12. Typical transducer distance amplitude curve.

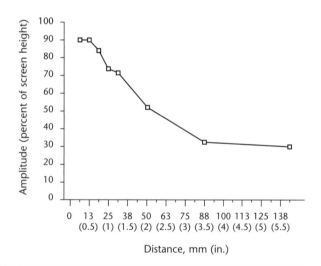

Effect of Transducer Size

The beam spread of a circular ultrasonic transducer is determined by the following equation:

$$(14) \quad \sin\frac{\theta}{2} \ = \ 1.22\frac{C}{f} * D \ = \ 1.22\frac{\lambda}{D}$$

where C is ultrasound velocity (meter per second), D is diameter of the transducer element (meter), f is ultrasound frequency (hertz), $\theta/2$ is the half-angle of beam divergence (degree) and λ is ultrasound wavelength (meter).

Higher frequencies and larger element sizes generate narrower sound beams and therefore a higher concentration of the ultrasonic energy over a given area. Higher frequencies lead to better sensitivity and higher signal-to-noise ratios. However, the near field distance (from source surfaces of equal size) also increases with increasing frequency. Generally, in nondestructive testing, it is desirable to test for discontinuities in the far field, at a distance beyond the near field of the transducer. Therefore, it is often necessary to choose the highest ultrasonic frequency and largest transducer size that provide a practical near field distance.

The beam divergence and the width of the test area covered at different depths are shown in Table 2 for a variety of transducers used in tests of aluminum sections.

Front and Back Surface Resolution

In the pulse echo technique, where a single transducer is used as a transmitter and receiver, a portion of the A-scan display is masked by the test material's front surface signal. In this area (often called the *dead zone*), discontinuities are concealed by the front surface indication and cannot be detected.

Table 2. Angle of ultrasonic beam spread and theoretical width of area covered by transducers of different frequency and size at different depths of aluminum.

Frequency (MHz)	Element Width (mm)	Half Angle mrad	Half Angle (deg)	Width (mm) of Covered Area At Depth 25 mm	At Depth 50 mm	At Depth 75 mm	At Depth 100 mm	At Depth 125 mm	At Depth 150 mm
10	6.4	120	(6.9)	6.0	12.0	18.0	24.2	30.2	36.3
10	13	61	(3.5)	3.0	6.0	9.0	12.2	15.3	18.3
7.5	6.4	162	(9.3)	8.1	16.3	24.5	32.7	41.0	49.1
7.5	13	80	(4.6)	4.0	8.0	12.0	16.0	20.0	24.1
5	13	120	(6.9)	6.0	12.0	18.0	24.2	30.2	36.3
5	19	80	(4.6)	4.0	8.0	12.0	16.0	20.0	24.1

Front surface resolution may be defined as the minimum distance between the front surface and a discontinuity (of a given size) that permits receiving a detectable first echo. To detect such a near surface discontinuity, it is necessary that the leading edge of the discontinuity signal be clearly separated from the front surface indication.

The amount of separation needed to make a near surface signal detectable depends in part on how the signal is monitored. In a basic test system, where signal indications are visually monitored by the operator, greater separation between front surface and discontinuity echoes is required. Most specifications governing ultrasonic tests of wrought aluminum, require a clear separation, down to at least 20 percent screen level. Electronic signal monitoring devices, on the other hand, require less separation between the two signals and enable the detection of discontinuities nearer the front surface.

Front surface resolution depends on (1) transducer characteristics such as center frequency, frequency bandwidth and damping, (2) instrument characteristics such as the shape of the initial pulse and (3) test conditions including roughness of the entry surface. To measure the front surface resolution, test conditions must be accurately simulated and the actual test parameters must be used.

Back surface resolution may be defined as the minimum distance between the back surface and a discontinuity of a known size that permits receiving an echo indication clearly separable from the back surface indication. A clear separation between the back surface indication and the trailing edge of the discontinuity signal is required.

Transducers for Tests of Wrought Aluminum Products

Transducer Characterization

Immersion transducers have a relatively short service life because of prolonged exposure to water. The epoxy protective layer on the transducer element is not permanently resistant to water penetration and can be expected to deteriorate gradually. The corresponding effects on the transducer are loss of sensitivity, lower resolution and inaccuracy in detecting discontinuities. It is therefore necessary to characterize transducers at the beginning of their service and at regular subsequent intervals

to monitor significant changes in their performance.

Transducer characterization procedures include measuring and recording a number of properties that are characteristic of a particular transducer. The procedure typically includes the following steps.

Acquire an unsaturated front surface signal and examine it for excessive ringdowns and pulse distortions.

Examine the frequency spectrum of the front surface waveform against side lobes and undesired components and measure characteristic values such as frequency bandwidth at different amplitude levels (–3 and –6 dB, for example) as well as peak and center frequencies.

Measure front and back surface resolution for the minimum flat bottom hole size that the transducer is intended to detect. This is generally done by setting the amplifier gain at a level sufficiently high to give an 80 percent screen level signal from the flat bottom hole at the highest metal travel distance intended for the transducer in question. Then, place the transducer over a calibration block containing near surface flat bottom holes. The depth of the hole nearest the front surface that can be clearly separated from the front surface echo is the indicator of the transducer's front surface resolution. Back surface resolution is determined by measuring the width of the signal acquired from a flat bottom hole at the highest metal travel distance (Fig. 13).

Acquire a distance amplitude curve. The distance amplitude curve is normally obtained at regular intervals during production and then compared with a measurement taken at the beginning of the transducer's service life. If significant changes are observed, one or several characteristic properties of the transducer must be retested.

Note that (1) higher ultrasonic frequencies provide better resolution, (2) pulse shape of the instrument pulser affects the front surface resolution and (3) front surface resolution is reduced by material surface roughness. Although broad band transducers provide better front and back surface resolution, their penetration power is considerably less than that of narrow band transducers. In addition, some frequency components of broad band ultrasound might not be desirable for testing coarse grain aluminum.

Paintbrush Transducers for Testing Aluminum

Broad beam rectangular transducer elements known as *paintbrush transducers* are commonly used for ultrasonic tests of large flat rolled aluminum products.

The width of the transducer element is similar to that of round transducers, 6.4 to 13 mm (0.25 to 0.5 in.). However, the length of paintbrush transducers varies from 25 to 75 mm (1 to 3 in.). These greater lengths provide much larger beam coverage and larger indexing distance for scanning plates and other flat rolled products. As a result, scan times for each plate can be reduced by more than 25 percent.

Discontinuity sizing is not very accurate with a paintbrush transducer and the accuracy of discontinuity location is limited to the length of the transducer element. For these reasons, paintbrush transducers must only be used for rough scanning. For accurate location and sizing, areas of the plate where discontinuity signals are observed are rescanned with a round transducer of smaller element size.

Beam Profile of Paintbrush Transducers

Paintbrush transducers are made from a variety of piezoelectric elements. Polarized ceramic crystals are most commonly used for testing aluminum flat rolled products. The crystal ends in a paintbrush transducer are shaped or masked with damping material for the following reasons: (1) to suppress excessive vibrations that typically occur at crystal ends and (2) to reduce the energy of the side lobes resulting from diffraction and interference of the ultrasonic field at the crystal ends.

There are several shapes for the crystal ends, including pointed, slant cut and half-oval. Although the proper shaping of the crystal ends can lead to a smoother and more uniform beam profile, it may also produce a narrowing effect on the ultrasonic beam in the long dimension of the transducer.

Furthermore, considerable reduction in beam length is caused by the phenomenon known as *quasifocus* along the length of the element. The near field distance and therefore the natural focus of a paintbrush transducer is generally determined by the width and frequency of its active element. For example, the natural focus of a 50 × 6.4 mm (2 × 0.25 in.) 7.5 MHz model is 50 mm (2 in.) in water. Along the longitudinal axis, however, there is also a *quasifocus point* at a distance determined by the length of the element and its frequency. This focal point for the transducer above is about 3 m (40 in.) in water and 730 mm (30 in.) in aluminum. As the beam converges on the quasifocus point, the effective beam length decreases.

Beam profile and reduction in beam length of typical paintbrush transducers are shown in Fig. 14. The effective beam length of the paintbrush transducer used in aluminum plate tests determines the index distance. As shown, the index distance decreases with metal travel distance.

FIGURE 13. Measurement of entry and back surface resolution in aluminum: (a) echo signal obtained at depth of 145 mm (5.75 in.) from 1.2 mm (0.05 in.) flat bottom hole; (b) without changing instrument receiver gain setting and energy conditions, echo signal from same hole size was acquired at 1 μs or 3 mm (0.13 in.) beyond start of front surface echo, so that is front surface resolution. Width of hole echo was 0.8 μs or 2.5 mm (0.1 in.), so that is back surface resolution.

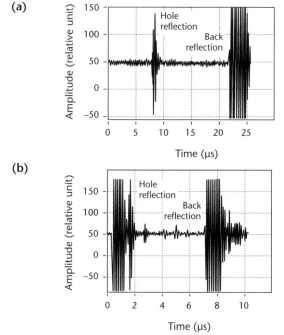

(a)

(b)

FIGURE 14. Variation of effective beam length of paintbrush transducer at different aluminum depths for 1.2 mm (0.05 in.) flat bottom hole.

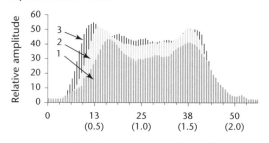

Transducer beam length mm (in.)

Legend
1. At 146 mm (5.75 in.) aluminum depth with effective beam length of 28 mm (1.1 in.) and maximum amplitude variation of 3.4 dB.
2. At 70 mm (2.75 in.) aluminum depth with effective beam length of 30 mm (1.2 in.) and maximum amplitude variation of 2.7 dB.
3. At 44 mm (1.75 in.) aluminum depth with effective beam length of 33 mm (1.3 in.) and maximum amplitude variation of 2.3 dB.

Variation from beam uniformity in a paintbrush transducer also influences the accuracy of ultrasonic tests. A variation of 10 percent or less over the length of the transducer must be allowed. More pronounced at higher metal depths, beam variations are sometimes unavoidable.

Measurement of transducer beam profile and uniformity must be done at the beginning of the transducer's service life and subsequently at regular intervals.

Paintbrush transducers are extremely sensitive to normalization in their length direction. Even a fraction of a degree of deviation from perpendicular produces a significant drop in signal amplitude. Figure 15 shows the effect of angular deviations in signal amplitude along the length and width of a paintbrush transducer.

Ultrasonic Testing of Aluminum Plates

The dominant ultrasonic test technique for aluminum plate is the pulse echo immersion technique, where water is used as the coupling medium. To perform the tests, aluminum plates are immersed in a tank containing water and scanned with an ultrasonic transducer. Aluminum plates can be as wide as 3.3 m (130 in.) and as long as 10 m (400 in.). A large facility is needed for handling the typical output of an aluminum rolling mill.

Plate thicknesses may vary from 6.4 to 200 mm (0.25 to 8 in.). Aluminum plate surfaces are normally parallel and reasonably smooth, enabling good transmission of ultrasound.

Plate Testing Installations

Aluminum plate testing installations are designed to perform high speed scanning of immersed plates. Typical systems include a bridge and a manipulator mounted over a water tank large enough to accommodate the plates. Drive power units move the bridge along the tank side rails while traversing power units move the manipulator from side to side along the bridge.

In conventional systems, the ultrasonic test instruments including the pulser/receiver unit and the display are mounted on the bridge. In newer systems, the ultrasonic instruments are stationary and located in a control pulpit along with computers and other electronics. To avoid signal distortion from long cable lengths, the received ultrasonic signal is preamplified at the transducer.

Scanning Head

The ultrasonic transducers for plate tests are mounted on an assembly called the *scanning head* that contains the electrical and mechanical connections as well as the transducer fixtures. The design of a single transducer head is simple and limited to a ultrahigh frequency connector and housing for electrical cables. The design of a multiple-transducer head can be much more complicated.

All electrical connections of the scanning head must be waterproof and the head must be resistant to corrosion in water.

Bridge, Carriage and Manipulator

The scanning head is mounted on a manipulator that enables the following movement: (1) vertical motion for the transducer (motion perpendicular to the plate surface) and (2) angular movement along two gimbal axes (allows accurate normal angularity).

The manipulator is mounted on a traversing mechanism on the bridge to allow movement across the tank. The bridge has a carriage unit at each end so that it can easily move along the tank side rails. A plate is scanned while immersed in the tank. Scanning is a combination of movements along the longitudinal and transverse plate axes. One of the following scan techniques is typically used.

Figure 15. Front surface signal amplitude drop from angulation along the length of 50 mm (2 in.) paintbrush transducer: (a) along length; (b) along width.

(a)

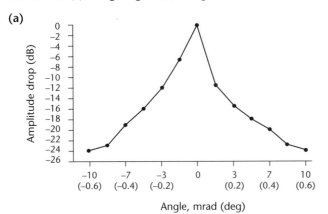

(b)

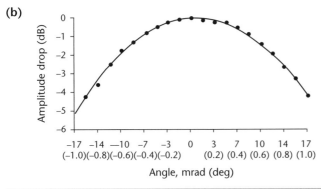

1. In the *transverse scanning technique,* the transducer moves across the width of the tank, then stops and moves in the longitudinal direction for a distance usually called the *index distance.* The index distance is determined by the transducer beam coverage. This motion is repeated until the entire plate is covered. The transverse scanning technique is made slower by the carriage's traveling a relatively short distance during each scan: a good portion of the time for each scan is used for acceleration and deceleration and the average scanning speed is much less than the maximum carriage speed. Also, the number of times that the scanner has to index is considerably greater in transverse scanning.
2. In the *longitudinal scanning technique,* the transducer scans a line along the length of the plate and indexes in the transverse direction. The scanner moves along the entire length of the plate for each scan line and can run at its maximum speed during most of each scan line. Average speeds are relatively close to the maximum speed in that direction.

One disadvantage of longitudinal scanning is that the bulk of the scanning bridge and the instruments mounted on it must move at high speeds and undergo a braking action at the end of each line. These abrupt starts and stops can produce considerable wear on the system's mechanical and electrical components.

Scanning Speed

The maximum speed of a scanning bridge system in each direction is determined by its design and the power of its motor drives. The scanning speed for tests of plates is related to the minimum discontinuity size and the thickness of the plate, as well as the ultrasonic instrumentation and the required pulse repetition rate.

In contact pulse echo testing, the time interval between consecutive ultrasonic pulses (the interpulse period) must be at least 60 times greater than the material travel time, the time required for a pulse to make a round trip in the material. This helps avoid interference from multiple echoes of previous pulses. Note that the maximum pulse repetition rate is determined by the plate thickness.

A typical ultrasonic instrument alarm system is activated after receiving a specified number of pulses. This prevents noise and inconsistent electrical pulses from activating the discontinuity gates. Alarms are typically adjusted to respond to three or more signals, so the scan speed at high pulse repetition rate should be slow enough so that a discontinuity of minimum size can be pulsed at least three times.

Considering all of these factors, there is a limited range of scanning speeds that can be used for a particular plate thickness and a given minimum discontinuity size.

Instrumentation for Tests of Aluminum

In conventional plate testing facilities, an ultrasonic pulse echo instrument is used. The instrument is generally mounted on the scanning bridge and connected through coaxial cables to the transducer. At least two discontinuity gates with alarm thresholds are used for plate tests. One gate is for discontinuities and the other is for monitoring the back surface echo signal.

A back echo attenuator enables an unsaturated back echo and helps with monitoring of its variations. Many discontinuity detectors are equipped with a *time correction gain* system that compensates for the reduction in echo amplitude caused by material attenuation.

Frequency filters (high and low pass filters) are necessary to eliminate the effect of undesired frequency components from the transducer.

Calibration

The ultrasonic transducer must be properly angulated before plate testing. This is done by acquiring a signal from the plate surface and maximizing the reflection by angulation.

Before starting the test, a set of distance amplitude calibration blocks are scanned and a distance amplitude curve is obtained. The instrument amplifier gain is set to bring the signal amplitude from the flat bottom hole corresponding to the lowest point of the distance amplitude curve to 80 percent screen scale. The discontinuity gate alarm threshold is set at half of this level. The beginning and the end of the discontinuity gate must correspond to the required entry and back surface resolutions.

The back echo signal is attenuated to 80 percent screen level and a negative alarm threshold is set at half of this level, for the back echo gate. A drop exceeding 50 percent in the back echo amplitude because of lack of perpendicularity or excessive material attenuation activates the alarm.

In most test systems, the alarm is directly connected to the bridge motion control system. This connection allows the bridge to stop immediately after a drop in back echo amplitude or after a discontinuity activates the alarm. The operator may then record the amplitude and depth of the discontinuity or investigate the cause of amplitude drop.

Data Recording

In a typical ultrasonic plate test system, the amplitude, depth, size and location of discontinuities are recorded in hardcopy and a copy of the record may accompany the plate through further processes.

Acceptance Levels

The size and number of the discontinuities as well as their proximity determine the acceptance level of the plate. Contracts specify acceptance classes for wrought products according to published industry standards or according to requirements for the products or systems being inspected.

Data Acquisition for Flat Rolled Aluminum

Computerized ultrasonic data acquisition systems offer many advantages for interpretation of test data. During the basic operation of such systems, the reflected ultrasonic signal is received by the transducer and amplified at the receiver. The signal is then fed into a peak detector that transfers the amplitude and time-of-flight information into computer memory. Positional information (the location where each signal is obtained) is provided by stepper drive motors or separate position encoders integrated in each motion axis of the scanning bridge. This information is transferred to the computer through special cabling.

The computer data processing programs finally process, integrate and store these data in proper format. The data (the combination of time, amplitude and position) may be further manipulated by image processing software to produce a C-scan of the plate. Amplitude and time-of-flight data are represented by colors or shades of gray. The function of gates, thresholds, filters and distance amplitude correction also may be performed by the computer software. A typical discontinuity map obtained by image processing of data from an aluminum plate is shown in Fig. 16.

The scanning bridge and the ultrasonic pulser/receiver may be controlled by computer motion control software. This software lets the user program several instrument settings and scan plans. Unlike conventional systems, there is no need for a computer controlled scanner to stop on discontinuities. After the scan, a graphic representation of the entire plate can be displayed for data analysis. When necessary, the scanner can return to suspected discontinuity locations for reevaluation of the data. A typical ultrasonic data acquisition system is shown in Fig. 17.

Because of the data handling capabilities of computerized systems, the use of multiple-array transducers has increased substantially. Simultaneous use of several paintbrush or regular transducers in one array can reduce the plate test time to a fraction of that with conventional ultrasonic systems.

Monitoring Porosity in Aluminum Sections

Centerline porosity occurs mostly in heavy gage flat rolled aluminum sections, mainly because the center of the plate receives considerably less mechanical work during rolling and may not achieve the levels needed to close the pores transferred from the ingot.

Individual pores do not produce distinguishable ultrasonic indications under production conditions. The ultrasonic indication of centerline porosity is typically in the form of noise or so-called grass in the center of the A-scan display. This makes it difficult to distinguish between porosity and large grain structure that is generally harmless and yet produces similar ultrasonic indications.

It is common practice to verify the presence of porosity by monitoring the noise level and the reduction in amplitude of the back echo signal. For example, if the noise level reaches 50 percent of the alarm threshold and the back echo is attenuated to 50 percent of its original amplitude, there is a good chance that porosity is present there.

FIGURE 16. Discontinuity map obtained by image processing of data from aluminum plate containing flat bottom holes of different sizes and depths.

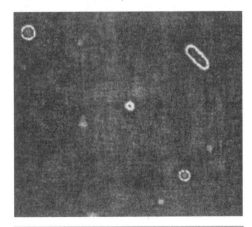

However, plates with large grain structure might produce a similar effect, resulting in rejection of good material.

Ultrasonic data acquisition systems offer digital filtering, which eliminates the frequency components of the incident ultrasound that might be particularly sensitive to the grain structure of the plate.

Signal processing techniques may be used to verify the presence of porosity more accurately and also to approximate the size and volume fraction. Changes in frequency dependence of the attenuation coefficient are measured by using a broad band transducer. The front and back surface signals of the plate are digitized. The frequency spectra of both signals are obtained by performing a fourier transform. The frequency dependence curve of the attenuation coefficient is then obtained by deconvolving the back surface echo spectrum by that from the front surface and making necessary corrections for geometric losses.

An attenuation coefficient value higher than normal indicates porosity. Quantitative measurements can be made by taking the slope of the attenuation curve or by comparing attenuation coefficient values with that from a reference standard.

Theoretical Inflection Point

Another valuable quantitative method uses an inflection point theoretically predicted and may appear on the attenuation versus frequency plot. For isometric materials, a fairly sharp peak appears in the derivative of the attenuation versus frequency curve. For example, in cast aluminum, the average pore size is theoretically related to the frequency at the inflection point by the following equation:

$$(15) \quad R = \frac{1.08}{f_p}$$

where f_p is the frequency at the inflection point (megahertz) and R is the average pore radius (millimeter).

The factor of 1.08 accounts for the Poisson's ratio of aluminum and the scattering cross section of the porosity. The average volume fraction of porosity C may be determined by measuring the attenuation coefficient at the inflection point and using the following equation:

$$(16) \quad C = 1.22 * \alpha_p R$$

where R is the average pore radius (millimeter) and α_p is the attenuation coefficient (neper per millimeter).

FIGURE 17. Typical ultrasonic data acquisition system.

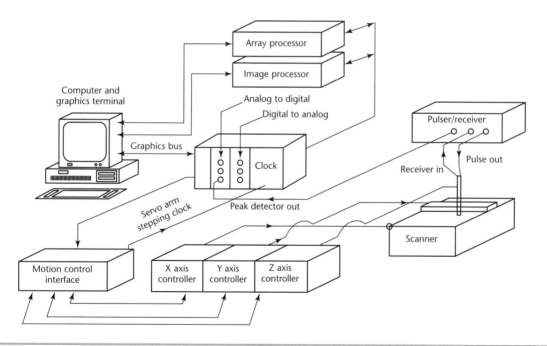

The factor of 1.22 is related to the average cross section of the porosity and to the Poisson's ratio of aluminum. Figure 18 shows the attenuation coefficient frequency curves in an aluminum plate.

Ultrasonic Tests of Forgings

For aluminum forgings, the ultrasonic immersion technique is commonly used. The favorable surface conditions of aluminum forgings enable the detection of small discontinuities, including minute cracks. Tests of forgings with simple shapes and configurations use immersion tanks, bridges and manipulators similar to but smaller than those used in plate tests.

For more complex components, the transducer is guided underwater by an exchangeable pipe attached to provide spacing support. The front edge of the pipe may be shaped to match curved test surfaces. The results from this test have good reproducibility.

FIGURE 18. For an aluminum plate with porosity: (a) fast fourier transform of front and back surface echoes; (b) attenuation coefficient versus frequency obtained by deconvolving of back surface echo spectrum by front surface (reference) spectrum.

(a)

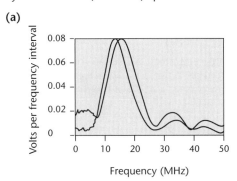

(b)

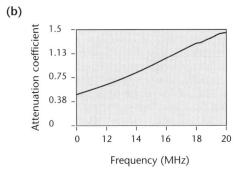

Application of Surface Wave Ultrasound in Aluminum Testing

Surface wave ultrasound is regularly used for tests of aluminum plate surfaces. Cracks and other surface blemishes are likely to occur during the rolling process. These cannot be detected by ultrasonic immersion methods because of the insufficient entry surface resolution inherent in the pulse echo technique.

Surface wave techniques are especially sensitive to these rolling induced discontinuities. A surface wave transducer (contact transducer coupled to an acrylic wedge) is placed on the plate and moved along its edge. The test instrument is calibrated to show a signal from the opposite edge of the plate. The distance between the initial pulse and the edge signal represents the width of the plate. As the transducer is moved along the edge, surface discontinuities can be detected.

Conclusion

Primary metal products such as bar, plate and tubes are manufactured from many metals and metal alloys. The ultrasonic testing technique has proved to be a reliable and efficient means for quality control of these materials in many shapes and many configurations. Ultrasonic tests are also used to detect discontinuities formed during machining, hot working and other finishing processes.

In all primary metal manufacturing, the quality of a finished component directly depends on the quality of the intermediate product. Ultrasonic testing is the most effective method for detecting subsurface discontinuities commonly found in bar, plate and tubes — both forgings and castings. Computers have substantially increased the application and efficiency of ultrasonic tests of primary metal products.

PART 3. Multiple-Transducer Ultrasonic Techniques

General Considerations

Multiple-transducer ultrasonic techniques are used on primary metals (and other materials) to address technical concerns.

An ultrasonic data acquisition system can use more than one transducer. Transducers can be manipulated separately or in an array. Each transducer can use dedicated instrumentation or share instrumentation with other transducers.

The simplest multiple-transducer systems use two-transducer setups. Systems that are more complicated use massive setups of a few transducers, dozens of transducers or hundreds of transducers. Multiple transducers can save time during scanning while using identical transducers and setups. Multiple transducers can also save time during scanning while using dissimilar transducers or setups.

Multiple-transducer setups, even with as few as two or three transducers, can achieve synergism that would be impossible with a single transducer.

Manipulation Separately or as Array

One general consideration for using multiple transducers is whether they are manipulated separately, or manipulated together while embedded in a common housing or jig fixture. The latter approach is generally known as an *array* of transducers.

There are several common designs for arrays.

1. One common design has two or more square or round ultrasonic elements equally spaced along a line, or equally spaced along the circumference of a circle. This is known as a *one-dimensional array* or *linear array*.
2. Another common design has four or more, square or round, ultrasonic elements equally spaced in a two-dimensional grid.

3. An array of transducers with two or more ring shaped ultrasonic elements arranged concentrically is called *annular*. A variation on this design is to break up each full 6.28 rad (360 deg) ring into circumferential sections, such as two 3.14 rad (180 deg) sections, three 2.09 rad (120 deg) sections or four 1.57 rad (90 deg) sections.

Having separate transducers allows maximum flexibility but with two drawbacks:

1. Each transducer requires separate mechanical manipulation hardware, which adds cost.
2. Each transducer must be set up individually, which can be slow.

The alternative of a transducer array inflexibly locks in many ultrasonic characteristics but with two advantages:

1. The cost of mechanical manipulation hardware decreases.
2. An entire group of transducers can quickly be set up together.

Instrumentation for Multiple Transducers

Instrumentation is needed for pulsing and signal processing with multiple transducers. The instrumentation used in multiple-transducer applications is often an engineering compromise between the competing priorities of equipment cost and scanning speed.

At the low cost, low speed end of the spectrum, all transducer signals are processed by a single shared ultrasonic instrument with multiplexed processing. Only one signal can be processed at a time; the processing of any given transducer's signal must be fully completed before the next transducer can be pulsed. So each of the multiple transducers is pulsed in sequence, using a round robin scheme. For any individual transducer, the time between pulses is found by adding together all of the transducers' pulse-to-end-of-signal times. This leads to slow speeds.

At the high cost, high speed end of the spectrum, each transducer signal is parallel processed by its own dedicated ultrasonic instrument. Any number of transducer signals can be processed simultaneously. There is no electronic need to synchronize the pulse rates of any of the transducers. Each transducer can be pulsed as fast as physically practical.

Faster Scanning

Identical Transducers and Setups

Consider the case in which multiple transducers are nominally identical in physical characteristics and in ultrasonic setup. Multiple transducers let signals from multiple surface locations be gathered more quickly than with a single transducer physically scanned from one location to another. Under ideal conditions, if one transducer takes T s to scan a part, then two transducers can scan the part in 0.5 T s, three transducers can scan the part in 0.3 T s and so forth.

If all of a part's scan locations lie on the same test surface, then speed is gained by having multiple transducers divide the task of scanning the single surface (Fig. 19). There are two major variations on single-surface scanning.

1. In the overlapping beams approach, closely packed sensors form a single, wide transducer. The paintbrush transducer array is a classic example, in which the multiple transducers are installed in a common housing. The scan plan can be very simple because it can treat the group of transducers like a single, wide transducer.

2. In the nonoverlapping beams approach, the transducers can either be manipulated as an array (when installed in a common housing or jig fixture), or can be manipulated separately. The scan plan can be somewhat complicated because it must explicitly take into account the spacing between the nonoverlapping beams.

If a part's scan locations lie on two or more test surfaces, then speed can be gained in two ways.

1. Speed can be gained by dedicating at least one transducer to each test surface (Fig. 20). Generally, transducers dedicated to one surface must be manipulated independently of transducers dedicated to another surface, so the scan plan is somewhat complicated.
2. Speed can be gained by treating each test surface as a single test surface, as described above. The task of scanning each surface is divided among multiple transducers.

Dissimilar Transducers or Setups

Multiple transducers save time during scanning when using dissimilar transducers or setups.

1. The transducers can be focused at different depths. This is called the *multizone technique* (Fig. 21).
2. The transducer beams can use different refracted angles or be pointed in different directions relative to the part (Fig. 22).
3. The transducers can use different modes and frequencies (Fig. 22b).

At least one transducer of each dissimilar type or setup must scan an entire test surface.

FIGURE 19. Nonoverlapping beams from multiple transducers.

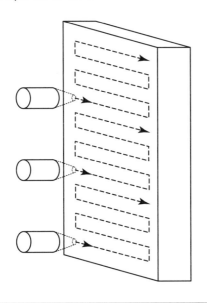

FIGURE 20. If a part's scan locations lie on two or more test surfaces, then speed can be gained by dedicating at least one transducer to each test surface.

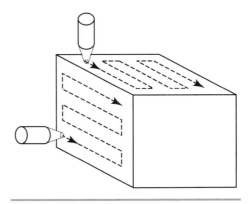

FIGURE 21. Multizone technique divides test object into depth zones and dedicates focused transducer to each.

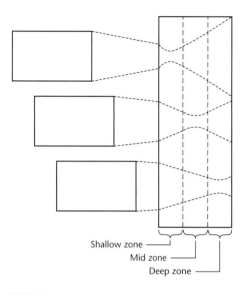

Shallow zone
Mid zone
Deep zone

FIGURE 22. Some parts require dissimilar transducers and/or setups: (a) different refracted angles or directional orientations; (b) different modes or frequencies.

(a)

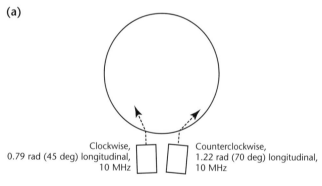

Clockwise, 0.79 rad (45 deg) longitudinal, 10 MHz

Counterclockwise, 1.22 rad (70 deg) longitudinal, 10 MHz

(b)

Axial, 0.79 rad (45 deg) transverse, 2 MHz

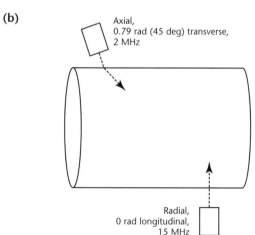

Radial, 0 rad longitudinal, 15 MHz

First, assume the simple situation in which there is only one transducer of each dissimilar type or setup, so each transducer must scan a part's entire test surface. If only one transducer scanned at a time, then the minimum total scan time would be found by adding together all of the individual scan times. (The actual total scan time would also include transducer changeover times.) On the other hand, if all transducers scanned at the same time, then the total scan time would be equal to only a single transducer's scan time (specifically, to whichever transducer's scan time was the longest). This would significantly speed up the scan.

When there is a group of transducers for each dissimilar type and/or setup, then each group of transducers could divide up the task of scanning an test surface, as described in a previous section. This would further speed up the scan.

Synergism Using Multiple Transducers

Pitch Catch Technique in Two-Transducer and Massive Setups

In the classic pitch catch technique, two transducers are used, with each located on a different test surface. One transducer transmits, while the other receives. The receiving transducer monitors decreases in transmitted amplitude. Two transducers allow synergism impossible with a single transducer.

The two transducers can detect discontinuities in the near surface dead zone. For a single transducer, the high amplitude, front surface echo drowns out small amplitude discontinuity signals from immediately below the surface. In pitch catch, however, a discontinuity in the transmitting transducer's dead zone removes some of the transmitted beam's energy and the receiving transducer detects it by a decrease in monitored amplitude.

The two transducers can detect discontinuities that do not reflect ultrasound back to a single transmit/receive transducer. If a rough or abnormally oriented discontinuity removes any of the transmitted beam's energy, then the receiving transducer detects it by a decrease in monitored amplitude.

The classic pitch catch technique is a simple setup for two transducers. However, individual pitch catch transducer pairs can be used as building blocks for a massive setup with four, six, eight or more transducers. (Even for a two-transducer pitch catch setup, the scan plan can be quite complicated if the test specimen surfaces are curved. For a pitch catch setup with a higher number of transducers, the scan plan can be extremely complicated.)

Dual-Element Transducer in Dual-Transducer and Massive Setups

The two elements in the classic dual-element contact transducer make up a short linear array. One element transmits; the other receives. So the dual-element transducer is technically used in pitch catch mode but is treated as if it were a single-element transducer in pulse echo mode. Using two elements allows synergistic effects impossible with a single-element transducer.

The dual-element transducer experiences no near surface dead zone. For a single-element transducer, discontinuity signals of small amplitude from immediately below the surface are drowned out by the high amplitude front surface echo. A dual-element transducer is designed so that the high amplitude, front surface echo is not detected by the receiving element and so cannot interfere with detecting small indications near the surface.

The dual-element transducer does not have to compromise between efficient transmitting and efficient receiving like a single-element transducer. Transmitting and receiving can both be efficient.

The classic dual-element contact transducer is a simple setup with two contact transducers. However, dual-element contact transducers can be used as building blocks for a massive setup with four, six, eight or more transducers.

Automated scanning with contact transducers is uncommon but possible.

Phased Array Technique

The phased array technique can use two transducers, three transducers or a massive number of transducers, depending on the desired effect. The effects depend on one beam interacting with another beam beside it, so the transducers are engineered to have wide beam spreads. The transducers can be arranged in a one-dimensional linear array, a two-dimensional grid array or an annular array. All transducer elements send their beams through a single test surface. All transducer elements can transmit and all transducer elements can receive. The timed pulsing of the transducer elements is coordinated to achieve synergism not possible with a single transducer.

Using two or more transducers in a phased array can result in a combined wave front with a direction different from any of the individual transducers. This technique is known as *beam steering* (Fig. 23). If all transducers were pulsed at once, then the direction of the combined wave front would simply follow the transducers' axis without steering. In beam steering, one transducer pulses; then after a brief delay, a second transducer some distance away pulses; optionally, a third transducer even farther pulses after yet another delay; then a fourth transducer and so on. The combined wave front is steered off axis, in the direction of the delayed transducers.

FIGURE 23. The angle of phased array beam can be directed by changing of pulse delay between transducer elements: (a) upward; (b) no directing; (c) downward.

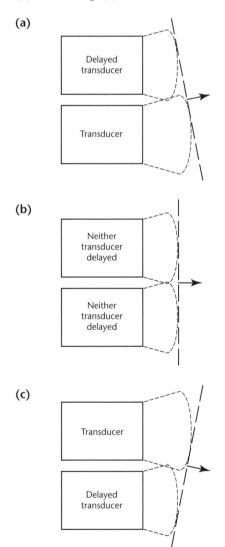

For beam steering, the centers of the transducers must be at different locations. So an annular array with full 6.28 rad (360 deg) rings would not work, but one with two 3.14 rad (180 deg) sections or four 1.57 rad (90 deg) sections would work.

Using three or more transducers a phased array can result in a combined wave front with a focus different from any of the individual transducers. This is known as *dynamic focusing* (Fig. 24). If all transducers were pulsed at once, then the shape of the combined wave front would be flat, with no focusing. In dynamic focusing, there is a central transducer, with a pair of transducers flanking it; optionally, a second pair of transducers could flank the first pair, then a third pair could flank the second pair and so on. The outermost pair is pulsed first; after some delay, the second-to-outermost pair is pulsed; after another delay, the third-to-outermost pair is pulsed; the central transducer is pulsed last. When the array is pulsed with the proper delays, the wave fronts converge at some point under the central transducer. The depth of this convergence point can be changed by varying the delays that are used. (An alternative to pairs of transducers that surround the central transducer is an annular array with full 6.28 rad (360 deg) rings that surround the central transducer.)

On any phased array with at least three elements having centers at different locations, it is possible to perform both beam steering and dynamic focusing at the same time. Without moving the array, it is possible to test the material under the array by using a large number of different beam angles and focal lengths. This virtual manipulation can be faster than a single transducer could be mechanically manipulated for a similar test.

A phased array can be built with a large number of elements having centers at different locations. Within a large array, it is possible to activate a subsidiary array of one or more elements and use it to gather some information, then activate a second subsidiary array and use it to gather some information, then activate a third subsidiary array and so on. Without physically moving the large array, it is possible to test the material under the array using a large number of different beam positions. This virtual scanning can be done much faster than a single transducer could be physically scanned across a test surface.

A subsidiary array with at least two elements can be beam steered as well as virtually scanned. A subsidiary array with at least three elements can be beam steered and dynamically focused, as well as virtually scanned.

Note that each of these capabilities — virtual scanning, beam steering and dynamic focusing — multiplies the ultrasonic data that must be acquired and processed at each array position. Using two or three of these capabilities at once can generate many data and require high end data acquisition and processing.

FIGURE 24. Phased array transducer can be dynamically focused by delayed pulsing of central transducer.

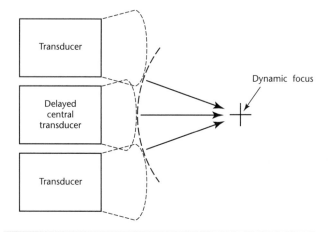

References

1. Ghaziary, H. and T. Kirk. Section 21, "Ultrasonic Testing Applications in Primary Metals." *Nondestructive Testing Handbook,* second edition: Vol. 7, *Ultrasonic Testing.* Columbus, OH: American Society for Nondestructive Testing (1991) p 723-745.
2. ASTM E 317, *Practice for Evaluating Performance Characteristics of Ultrasonic Pulse-Echo Examination Instruments and Systems without the Use of Electronic Measurement Instruments.* West Conshohocken, PA: ASTM International (2001).
3. SAE J 300, *Engine Oil Viscosity Classification.* Warrendale, PA: SAE International (2004).

Bibliography

Brunk, J.A. "The Influence of Ambient Temperature Changes on Angle-Beam Ultrasonic Testing of Steel." *Materials Evaluation.* Vol. 46, No. 9. Columbus, OH: American Society for Nondestructive Testing (August 1988): p 1148-1152.

Hullin, C.G., O.-A. Barbian, G. Haralamb and E. Raeder. "AUGUR — A System Designed for Computer-Aided Evaluation of Ultrasonic Test Data in a Heavy-Plate Mill." *Materials Evaluation.* Vol. 42, No. 12. Columbus, OH: American Society for Nondestructive Testing (November 1984): p 1492-1497.

Howard, Q. and S. Enzukewich. "The Effects of Microstructure on the Ultrasonic Testing of Alloy Steels." *Materials Evaluation.* Vol. 55, No. 12. Columbus, OH: American Society for Nondestructive Testing (December 1997): p 1323-1327.

Lin, L., X.M. Li and J.S. Zhang. "Nondestructive Differentiation of Three Transformation Products in Low Alloy Steel Using Two Ultrasonic Methods." *Materials Evaluation.* Vol. 61, No. 4. Columbus, OH: American Society for Nondestructive Testing (April 2003): p 512-516.

Kumar, A., T. Jayakumar, B. Raj and K.K. Ray. "Ultrasonic Time Domain Technique for Frequency Dependent Attenuation Measurement for Microstructural Characterization of a Titanium Alloy." *Materials Evaluation.* Vol. 61, No. 12. Columbus, OH: American Society for Nondestructive Testing (December 2003): p 1321-1326.

Lebsack, S. and H. Heckhauser. "Immersion Probe Arrays for Rapid Pipeline Weld Inspection." *Materials Evaluation.* Vol. 53, No. 8. Columbus, OH: American Society for Nondestructive Testing (August 1995): p 886-888, 890-891.

Struk, D. *NDT in the Foundry.* Columbus, OH: American Society for Nondestructive Testing (1995).

Aluminum

Debbouz, O. and F. Navai. "Nondestructive Testing of 2017 Aluminum Copper Alloy Diffusion Welded Joints by an Ultrasonic Automatic System." *Materials Evaluation.* Vol. 57, No. 12. Columbus, OH: American Society for Nondestructive Testing (December 1999): p 1263-1269.

Jassby, K. and D. Saltoun. "Use of Ultrasonic Rayleigh Waves for the Measurement of Applied Biaxial Surface Stresses in Aluminum 2024-T351 Alloy." *Materials Evaluation.* Vol. 40, No. 2. Columbus, OH: American Society for Nondestructive Testing (February 1982): p 198-205.

Mansfield, T.L. "Ultrasonic Technology for Measuring Molten Aluminum Quality." *Materials Evaluation.* Vol. 41, No. 6. Columbus, OH: American Society for Nondestructive Testing (May 1983): p 743-747.

Martin, B.G. "The Measurement of Surface and Near-Surface Stress in Aluminum Alloys Using Ultrasonic Rayleigh Waves." *Materials Evaluation.* Vol. 32, No. 11. Columbus, OH: American Society for Nondestructive Testing (November 1974): p 229-234.

Arrays

Beck, K.H. "Ultrasonic Transducer Array Configuration for Interlaced Scanning." *Materials Evaluation.* Vol. 46, No. 6. Columbus, OH: American Society for Nondestructive Testing (May 1988): p 771-778.

Lemon, D.K. and G.J. Posakony. "Linear Array Technology in NDE Applications." *Materials Evaluation.* Vol. 38, No. 7. Columbus, OH: American Society for Nondestructive Testing (July 1980): p 34-37.

McElroy, J.T. and K.F. Briers. "Annular Array Search Units and Their Potential Application in Conventional Ultrasonic Testing Systems." *Materials Evaluation.* Vol. 37, No. 11. Columbus, OH: American Society for Nondestructive Testing (October 1979): p 41-46.

Schwarz, H.-P. "Development of a Divided-Ring Array for Three-Dimensional Beam Steering in Ultrasonic Nondestructive Testing: Theoretical and Experimental Results of a Prototype." *Materials Evaluation.* Vol. 45, No. 8. Columbus, OH: American Society for Nondestructive Testing (August 1987): p 951-957.

Castings

Jiang, G., H. Kato, Y. Yoshida and T. Komai. "Influence of Incident Angle of Ultrasonic Waves on Thickness Measurement of Remelted Zones Formed on Aluminum Alloy Castings." *Materials Evaluation.* Vol. 59, No. 12. Columbus, OH: American Society for Nondestructive Testing (December 2001): p 1421-1425.

Kotval, C. "Ultrasonic Evaluation of Aluminum Master Cylinder Die Castings for Porosity." *Materials Evaluation.* Vol. 38, No. 11. Columbus, OH: American Society for Nondestructive Testing (November 1980): p 23-27.

Palanisamy, S., C.R. Nagarajah and P. Iovenitti. "Effects of Grain Size and Surface Roughness on Ultrasonic Testing of Aluminum Alloy Die Castings." *Materials Evaluation.* Vol. 63, No. 8. Columbus, OH: American Society for Nondestructive Testing (August 2005): p 832-836.

Urich, R.H. and W.H. Sproat. "Ultrasonic Inspection of Gas Turbine Sand Castings." *Materials Evaluation.* Vol. 36, No. 8. Columbus, OH: American Society for Nondestructive Testing (July 1978): p 41-46.

Forgings

Henry, E.B. "The Role of Nondestructive Testing in the Production of Pipe and Tubing." *Materials Evaluation.* Vol. 47, No. 6. Columbus, OH: American Society for Nondestructive Testing (June 1989): p 714-715, 718, 720, 722-724.

Kleven, S. "Ultrasonic Inspection of Commercial Grade Plate and Forgings for Special Applications." *Materials Evaluation.* Vol. 53, No. 9. Columbus, OH: American Society for Nondestructive Testing (September 1995): p 988, 990.

Meyer, P.A. and T.J. Carodiskey. "Ultrasonic Boreside Array for Rapid Heat-Exchanger Tube Inspection." *Materials Evaluation.* Vol. 45, No. 10. Columbus, OH: American Society for Nondestructive Testing (October 1987): p 1190-1194.

Waisman, J.L., L.L. Soffa, P.W. Kloeris and C.S. Yen. "Effect of Internal Flaws on the Fatigue Strength of Aluminum Alloy Rolled Plate and Forgings." *Materials Evaluation.* Vol. 16, No. 6. Columbus, OH: American Society for Nondestructive Testing (November-December 1958): p 477-489.

Wüstenberg, H., B. Rotter, H.P. Klanke and D. Harbecke, "Ultrasonic Phased Arrays for Nondestructive Inspection of Forgings." *Materials Evaluation.* Vol. 51, No. 6. Columbus, OH: American Society for Nondestructive Testing (June 1993): p 669-672. Erratum, Vol. 51, No. 8 (August 1993): p 862.

Standards

Aluminum Standards and Data 2003: Metric SI. Washington, DC: Aluminum Association (2003).

ASTM B 548, *Standard Test Method for Ultrasonic Inspection of Aluminum-Alloy Plate for Pressure Vessels.* West Conshohocken, PA: ASTM International (2003).

ASTM B 594, *Standard Practice for Ultrasonic Inspection of Aluminum-Alloy Wrought Products for Aerospace Applications.* West Conshohocken, PA: ASTM International (2002).

ASTM E 127, *Standard Practice for Fabricating and Checking Aluminum Alloy Ultrasonic Standard Reference Blocks.* West Conshohocken, PA: ASTM International (2005).

ASTM E 428, *Standard Practice for Fabrication and Control of Steel Reference Blocks Used in Ultrasonic Examination.* West Conshohocken, PA: ASTM International (2005).

ASTM E 527, *Standard Practice for Numbering Metals and Alloys (UNS)*. West Conshohocken, PA: ASTM International (2003).

ASTM E 664-93, *Standard Practice for the Measurement of the Apparent Attenuation of Longitudinal Ultrasonic Waves by Immersion Method*. West Conshohocken, PA: ASTM International (2005).

ASTM E 2375, *Standard Practice for Ultrasonic Examination of Wrought Products*. West Conshohocken, PA: ASTM International (2004).

ASTM E 317, *Standard Practice for Evaluating Performance Characteristics of Ultrasonic Pulse-Echo Examination Instruments and Systems without the Use of Electronic Measurement*. West Conshohocken, PA: ASTM International (2001).

AWS D1.1, *Structural Welding Code*. Miami, FL: American Welding Society.

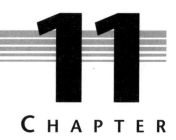

CHAPTER

Chemical and Petroleum Applications of Ultrasonic Testing

David R. Bajula, Acuren Inspection, La Porte, Texas (Parts 1 to 4)

Brozia H. Clark, Jr., Scott Depot, West Virginia (Parts 1 and 2)

Lawrence O. Goldberg, Sea Test Services, Merritt Island, Florida (Part 5)

Gregory A. Hudkins, ExxonMobil Inspection Group, Baytown, Texas (Parts 1 to 4)

D.K. Mak, Nepean, Ontario (Parts 2 and 4)

John Mittleman, United States Navy, Naples, Italy (Part 5)

Roderic K. Stanley, NDE Information Consultants, Houston, Texas (Parts 1, 2 and 4)

PART 1. Chemical and Petroleum Industry

Petroleum Industry

Oil refining began in the early 1850s with the production of kerosene and lamp oil. After 1890, gasoline was needed to fuel the combustion engines in automobiles. Modern refineries and petrochemical plants (Fig. 1) are highly dependent on crude oil and other fossil fuels to produce a wide range of chemicals and products.

Petrochemical plants and refineries are comprised of processing units ranging from simple distillation towers to complex fluid catalytic crackers, hydrotreaters, cokers and other processing units. Process components such as vessels and piping are subject to many forms of service related material degradation. Corrosion and cracking if left unchecked could cause catastrophic failures and loss of life. The history of catastrophic failures in the refining, chemical and other industrial complexes has lead to federal regulation of process safety.[1] Part of the regulatory document covers mechanical integrity. Nondestructive testing is vital in ensuring the mechanical integrity and serviceability of this equipment. Nondestructive testing is important early, during fabrication; later, during maintenance and servicing of vessels and piping; and finally, in on-stream inspection. Owner/user teams and engineering staff use nondestructive test results to plan their maintenance activities, to assess their risks and to implement risk based inspection. Risk based inspection philosophies prioritize inspections, minimize failures and maximize the performance of equipment. Ultrasonic techniques are applied daily to ensure the safety and reliability of vessels, piping and other equipment.

Chemical Industry[2]

The chemical industries use many nondestructive test methods to maintain and ensure safe operation of their production facilities. The goal of such testing programs is to achieve and maintain capacity production. Ultrasonic tests are extensively used by the chemical industries and their material suppliers because of their ease of application, their flexibility and the portability of ultrasonic equipment.

Because ultrasonic testing can be used with either metallic or nonmetallic components, it is the test method most widely used in the chemical industries. Ultrasonic tests are used to ensure structural integrity of construction materials and acceptability of component characteristics before fabrication or machining. Inservice testing is another area of critical application.

In the chemical industries, ultrasonic techniques are typically used in the following sequence: (1) acceptance of base construction materials, (2) acceptance of fabricated materials (tests of the fabrication process) and (3) in-service tests of equipment or material components.

Ultrasonic Test Procedures[2]

When using ultrasonic techniques for inservice inspection, chemical industry inspectors must generally ask the following questions.

1. Has the equipment, component or material had any previous fabrication requirements or nondestructive test requirements? Are there preexisting manufacturer's or purchaser's specifications to a national or local code?
2. What are physical characteristics of the area of interest?
3. What is the surface condition before and after preparation for testing? Will the surface permit adequate sound entry?

FIGURE 1. Photograph of petroleum refinery.

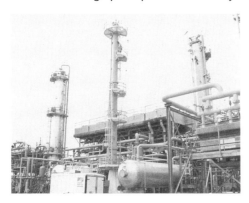

4. Will the test object be subjected to static or dynamic stress?
5. Is the equipment subject to erosion or corrosive service conditions that could cause failure?
6. What temperature is the test object designed to operate in and will it be used within that nominal range?
7. What degree of testing does the test object's use demand?
8. What is the referencing code or standard?

When establishing an ultrasonic procedure, it is frequently difficult to correlate the materials with original procurement specifications. In many cases, the ultrasonic acceptance criteria exceed those originally specified. In the resulting confusion, high quality materials may be rejected and low quality materials could be accepted. The most reliable way to implement accurate ultrasonic procedures is with reference standards. Such standards contain artificial reflectors (discontinuities) such as notches, drilled (horizontal) holes, flat bottom holes or cracks that can be used to set up the discontinuity detector operation. A reference standard helps ensure system sensitivity. System verification, including check of transducer performance characteristics, should also be conducted to ensure test accuracy.

Common Test Techniques

Internal Rotary Ultrasonic Testing

Internal rotary testing is an ultrasonic technique well suited for petrochemical and refinery tube inspections. As shown in Table 1, internal rotary testing is a versatile tube test technique and favored by owners. The technique uses an ultrasonic beam reflected off of a 1.5 rad (90 deg) mirror to scan the tube internal surface in a thread like pattern ensuring that the tube full length is tested (Fig. 2). Scanning or pull speed is critical to establishing 100 percent coverage. The internal rotary system monitors the front

wall and the back wall echoes to precisely measure the tube wall thickness with an accuracy generally within 0.075 to 125 mm (0.003 to 5.00 in.). Essentially, a radial B-scan profiles inside and outside surface pitting and total wall thickness. Newer technology even offers a C-scan presentation, providing a rollout of the tube and global view of the damage (Fig. 3).

One of the drawbacks of internal rotary tests is that the tubes are required to be extremely clean and typically are blasted with water, soda ash or sand. Also,

FIGURE 2. Ultrasonic probe for internal rotary inspection of piping.

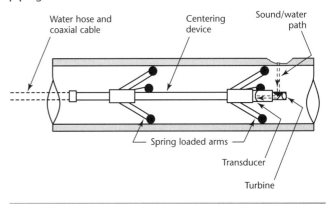

FIGURE 3. Ultrasonic images from internal rotary test of tube: (a) C-scan; (b) B-scan.

(a)

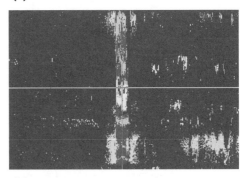

(b)

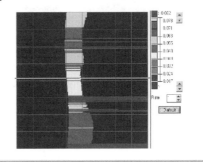

TABLE 1. Applicability of nondestructive tests to ferrous and nonferrous metals.

Technique	Applicability to Metals	
	Ferrous	Nonferrous
Eddy current testing	no	yes
Magnetic flux leakage testing	yes	no
Remote field testing	yes	yes
Laser techniques	yes	yes
Ultrasonic testing	yes	yes

Figure 4. C-scan of pipe at 478 K, or 204 °C (400 °F).

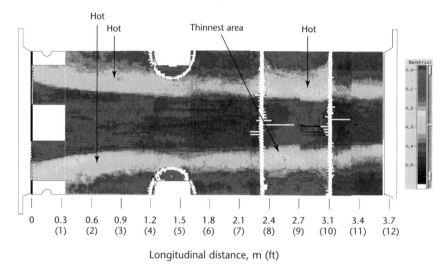

Longitudinal distance, m (ft)

Figure 5. Pipe with hydrogen cracking and stepwise blistering: (a) C-scan, showing side view; (b) volumetric projection, showing blistering with stepwise cracking but not here connecting to inside surface.

(a)

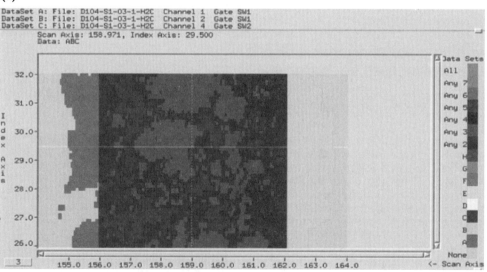

(b)

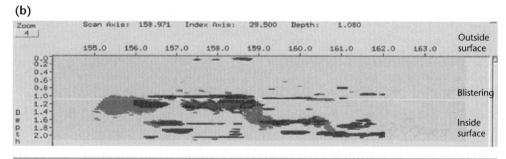

internal rotary testing takes much longer than electromagnetic techniques.

Automated Techniques

Three techniques of automated inspection have important roles in the refinery of the twenty-first century.

C-Scan Corrosion Mapping. Automated ultrasonic tests are vital in the inspection of vessels and piping. One of the most common applications is corrosion mapping. Unlike standard ultrasonic thickness gaging, where typically a single ultrasonic reading is taken, automated ultrasonic C-scan techniques can provide thousands of equivalent ultrasonic readings and cover very large areas in a fraction of the time it would take to gather manual ultrasonic data. Additionally, a C-scan map can provide a valuable global look at corrosion damage and assist in the identification of the lowest or minimum thickness location. Figure 4 shows a C-scan for a section of piping that had major, unexpected corrosion at an injection point.

C-Scan Discontinuity Evaluation. Another common automated ultrasonic test application is C-scan discontinuity evaluation for the detection of cracking and other service related damage. In many refining services, hydrogen sulfide is a byproduct of stripping the sulfur from sour crude or crude having greater than one percent sulfur. Hydrogen sulfide is a deadly gas and, over time, corrodes most carbon steel materials. In addition to corrosion by hydrogen sulfide and other sulfur products, damage to vessels can include hydrogen blistering, hydrogen induced cracking and ultimately stepwise cracking and subsequent failure. Figure 5 shows images of hydrogen blistering and stepwise cracking.

Time-of-Flight Diffraction. Another common automated ultrasonic test application is time-of-flight diffraction (TOFD). Generally the preferred technique for ultrasonic sizing, time-of-flight diffraction quickly and efficiently detects discontinuities. Figure 6 shows a time-of-flight diffraction image of a deep, inside surface crack in a coke drum.

Phased Array Testing. Phased arrays are widely used. This technique is discussed in detail elsewhere in this volume.

FIGURE 6. Deep, inside surface crack in coke drum: (a) photograph of coke drum; (b) time-of-flight diffraction image.

(a)

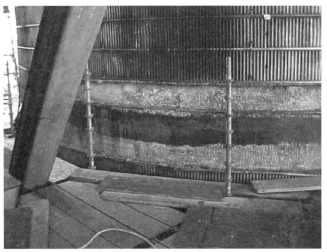

(b)

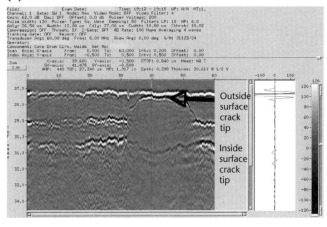

PART 2. Ultrasonic Testing in Processing Plants

Preservice Testing[2]

In the chemical industries, most facilities have a regularly scheduled testing program. Typical chemical production equipment tested by ultrasonic techniques include pressure vessels (Figs. 7 and 8), associated piping, prime movers (pumps and turbines) and other ancillary equipment. Such equipment is typically designed and manufactured in accordance with national standards. Base construction materials for chemical production equipment have specific strength, temperature and stress related characteristics required for safe and effective operation.

In new construction, ultrasonic tests are used to detect many conditions and characteristics critical to the safe and efficient operation of the equipment and to determine if materials and welding adhere to design specifications. In general, ultrasonic techniques are most reliable for tests (1) of weldments joining plate to form a cylindrical shell, cladding and associated bolting (Fig. 9), (2) of nozzle welds, (3) of material grain structure variances in the heat affected zones of welds (Fig. 10), (4) of material work hardening and (5) of effects of heat treatment.

Delamination of Rolled, Clad and Overlaid Material

The detection of delamination in plate materials is a critical chemical industry inspection and is usually considered part of ultrasonic tests of base materials and welds. Cladding interface of composite materials also requires ultrasonic tests for bond integrity. Bond integrity tests are also used to determine the effects of plate rolling because material bending or rolling may cause fractures at the interface of the composite materials. Location of nozzles in new construction could then be a problem.

Locating pinhole leakage through clad material in production vessels is another important application for ultrasonic tests. Such leaks in vessels containing highly corrosive or toxic materials allow corrosion of the backing material, resulting in costly and time consuming repairs. In this application, angle beam scanning at 0.8 to 1.2 rad (45 to 70 deg) depending on the thickness of the backing material plus cladding) may be

FIGURE 7. Ultrasonic testing of high pressure gas cylinders: (a) scanning plan for entire cylinder; (b) detailed cross section scanning plan.

(a)

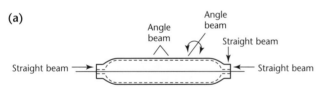

(b)

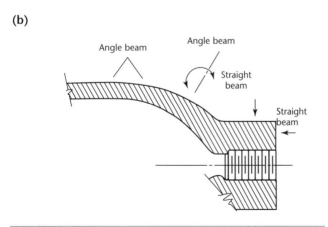

FIGURE 8. Very high pressure columns and cylinders tested with ultrasonic techniques. Arrow indicates field welding region that cannot be radiographically tested.

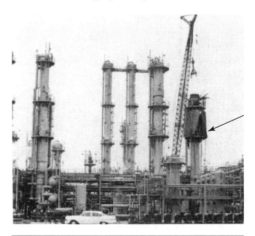

used to locate regions suspected of production clad leakage.

Ultrasonic thickness measurements through the region are used to determine an area's material losses and to indicate if there are other areas of degraded and unacceptable bond integrity through the region.

Another critical ultrasonic application is the test of bond integrity in hard face overlay weld deposits on extruder screw flights. Often, these weld deposits contain severe cracking across the screw flight width and exhibit branch cracks or loops interconnecting to form small isolated pockets. These pockets include the edges of the flight across the crack fissure in the overlay deposit and require ultrasonic testing for bond integrity.

Tube and Pipe Tests

In the chemical industries, welding is widely used for connecting process piping (Fig. 11) and for joint fabrication at plant sites during construction. Ultrasonic testing has proven effective for inspecting welds on heavy wall pipe. Here, ultrasonic tests are used in place of or in addition to radiographic tests.[3] Experience has demonstrated that ultrasonic tests may be more sensitive to critical discontinuities. The ultrasonic procedure used during fabrication is often the same procedure used for inservice tests. The test results during fabrication of such welds often resemble those obtained during inservice tests, except for weld failures or material

FIGURE 9. Ultrasonic scanning plan for heavy walled vessels: (a) thickness scan points; (b) details for unclad (left) and clad welds; (c) anchor bolt scan details.

(a)

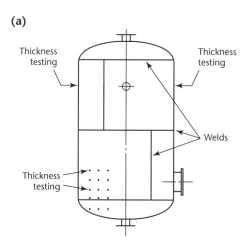

(b)

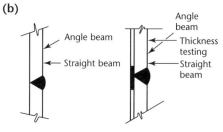

(c)

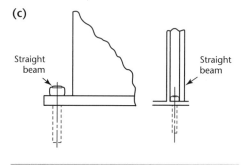

FIGURE 10. Scanning plan for ultrasonic testing of various pipe weld geometries and attendant base materials: (a) groove weld; (b) double-V groove welds; (c) groove weld with backing material.

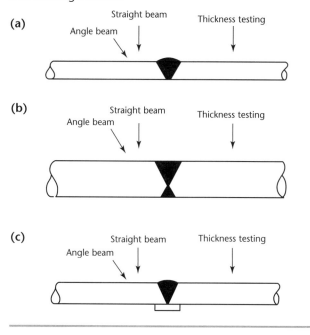

FIGURE 11. Scanning plan for ultrasonic testing of pipe: (a) thin wall; (b) high pressure heavy wall.

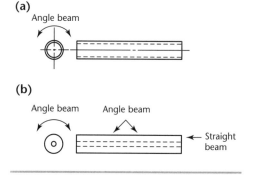

losses upstream or downstream of the process flow and across the root pass of the weld. In such cases, significant differences are expected.

Ultrasonic Tests of Fasteners

Preservice and inservice tests of bolting for discontinuities is widely practiced in the chemical and utility industries. Assemblies (Figs. 12 and 13) must be correctly torqued to ensure proper sealing of mating surfaces. Bolting is exposed to a wide range of dynamic and static conditions. This method of fastening is most frequently used to support process equipment such as tanks and columns and to assemble and seal reactor vessels and pumps. For ultrasonic tests of bolting subject to material fatigue deformation (either tension or compression), the velocity of the ultrasonic wave propagation starts to decrease below an initial value established before deformation. Attenuation increases as deformation continues. This decrease in velocity is characteristic of dislocation

FIGURE 12. Typical scanning plans for fasteners: (a) bolt; (b) stud.

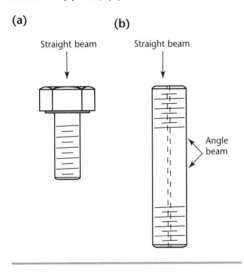

(a)   **(b)**

FIGURE 13. Cracking in bolt threads caused by fatigue loading or intergranular stress corrosion cracking.

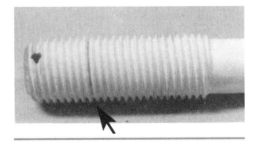

dampening. The change in velocity becomes smaller and attenuation becomes greater as deformation continues. Fatigue deformation of bolts displaying a change in grain structure, including growth in the bolt length, may be the result of abnormally high dislocation density, a result of microcracking.

Bolt stress loading by the so-called *torque measurement technique* depends on friction of the nut and material surfaces and results in inaccurate bolt loading estimates. With ultrasonic techniques this force on the bolt is measured by determining the elongation of the bolt during the torquing procedure. The length of the bolt and the material velocity must first be known. The elongation changes that occur as the bolt is tightened are determined by accurately measuring time of flight as the bolted assembly is torqued to specification requirements. Assuming that the bolting material is in the elastic range, the stress carried by the bolt can then be determined.

Because stress measurements of the bolts can be accurately determined with ultrasonic methods, this technique has proven superior to conventional torque measurements, where uniform stress is required to ensure the integrity of the pressure boundary.

Tests of Forgings

Hot rolled or forged round stock are frequently tested using ultrasonic techniques. Acceptance of raw stock for purposes of machining helps ensure a high quality level for the finished form and has proven to be cost effective by eliminating the costly machining of defective materials. Once the item is machined to the desired geometries, ultrasonic tests are frequently more difficult because of structural reflections and dead zones within the volume of the component. This problem is often experienced with large roller shafts, pump shafts and turbine rotors. Because their surfaces are generally inaccessible after assembly, scanning is a challenge.

The testing of these components before placing them in service is essential. Preservice testing provides a baseline record of discontinuities acceptable for the intended service. Changes in ultrasonic response and patterns (the size of discontinuities observed during inservice testing, for example) must be compared to baseline data to accurately estimate remaining component life.

Ultrasonic tests of rotating components is another excellent application of the technique. Because areas subject to highest stresses are generally inaccessible after assembly, a shaft must be removed from the component if surface tests (magnetic particle or liquid penetrant) are to be effectively used. Because disassembly and removal of shafting is costly or impractical (because of extensive down time), ultrasonic tests are a good choice.

To ensure that materials meet specifications, ultrasonic tests are used before machining and after other processing (heat treating, for example), as shown in Fig. 14. These tests include both angle beam and straight beam tests. Straight beam tests are made from the accessible ends of the shafting to establish a baseline. Fatigue cracking caused by operational loads can be detected soon after initiation and costly down time caused by shaft failures can be avoided (Fig. 15).

Corrosion and Wall Thinning[2]

Many chemical processes are toxic, corrosive and erosive. Equipment to contain such processes is also subject to a range of static and dynamic stress loading, including extreme thermal stresses. Impingement and erosion are directly related to the velocities at which chemicals are conveyed through the system and also contribute to equipment degradation.

Thickness measurements afford one of the best opportunities to demonstrate the versatility and flexibility of ultrasonic testing. Thinning of the walls of process equipment can be caused by chemical and mechanical action. Thinning (material losses) can occur on either the internal or external surfaces of pipe, pressure vessels or fittings (Fig. 16).

The ultrasonic techniques for detecting thinning use one or two transducers. Display of the test results depends on the ultrasonic instrument. Because of its simplicity and reduced dependence on human factors, there are some advantages to using a digital readout. However, test systems with oscilloscope or cathode ray tube presentations provide more meaningful readout data, particularly

FIGURE 14. Ultrasonic scanning plan for shafting: (a) rough round stock; (b) rotating shaft.

(a)

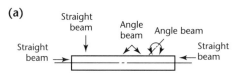

(b)

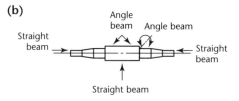

FIGURE 15. Shaft fractured at keyway.

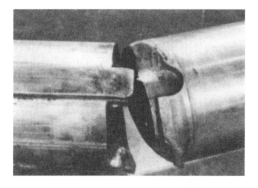

FIGURE 16. Ultrasonic tests in progress on heavy wall vessels: (a) in-service pressure vessel weld test; (b) preservice pressure vessel weld test.

(a)

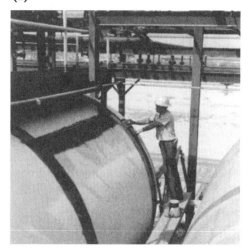

(b)

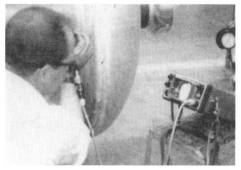

when interpreting the test results, and are frequently preferred over digital readouts. Cathode ray tubes are particularly valuable for determining the difference between thinning losses and material delaminations. Several manufacturers offer equipment with both digital readout and display of ultrasonic response.

Ultrasonic angle beam techniques are used to monitor changes in growth or crack extension, where access to the area by straight beam techniques is impossible. Other techniques have been developed to detect a variety of crack inducing mechanisms, including (1) stress corrosion, (2) thermal fatigue and (3) mechanical fatigue cracking. These conditions are brought on by the environment or process anomalies.

Mechanical equipment subject to fatigue cracking includes compressor connecting rods, crank shafts, turbine blades, rotor shafts in conveyor systems and impeller welds. Ultrasonic testing is also used extensively on heavy lifting equipment.

Piping

In the petrochemical and processing industry, intricate piping systems link process vessels and deliver products to storage tanks for distribution. Many piping systems are broken up into circuits and become systems within systems.

As for vessels, traditional preservice inspections include radiography during fabrication to ensure the quality of the welding. However, enhancements have come through automated imaging and phased arrays.

ASME B31.3, *Process Piping*, includes nondestructive test requirements and acceptance criteria and allow ultrasonic in lieu of radiographic testing.

Once in service, like vessels, the piping relies on ultrasonic techniques for both corrosion and cracking related damage assessments. Inspection for corrosion can range from monitoring the thickness at the same locations to elaborate automated ultrasonic C-scanning to map out and monitor corrosion trends.

Onstream inspections are in many cases performed at high temperatures (Fig. 4). When reciprocal calibrations are not performed at high temperatures, temperature compensation must be performed to ensure accurate readings. A widely used temperature compensation formula is:

$$(1) \quad d_C = d_R \times \left[1.007 - \left(0.0001 \times \theta \right) \right]$$

where d_C is compensated thickness (meter), d_R is the thickness reading (meter) and θ is temperature (celsius).

Heat Exchanger Tubing

Tube testing is vital for the refining and petrochemical industry. Heat exchangers and condensers are designed to sustain 100 percent separation between the products in the tube and products in the vessel. A leaking tube can significantly affect production and also cause catastrophic failure and loss of life. Tube test techniques include internal rotary ultrasonic testing, eddy current testing, remote field eddy current testing, magnetic flux leakage testing and laser profilometry. Electromagnetic and laser techniques complement the ultrasonic method and in many cases are used in parallel.

Tubes may be ferrous or nonferrous. Ferrous materials have magnetic properties and include carbon steel and some stainless steels; nonferrous materials have nonmagnetic properties and include copper, brass, nickel alloys and most stainless steels. Table 2 shows methods for tubes of various materials.

Tube Testing with Two Transducers in Tandem[4]

Trigonometric relationships exist for ultrasonic testing of curved pipe and tube surfaces using a single transducer.[5] Testing using two transducers is also effective and common for measuring the through-wall depth of a discontinuity. The technique is discussed in detail elsewhere.[6]

Pressure Vessels

Pressure vessels are one of the most critical pieces of equipment in a petrochemical plant or refinery and are continually tested. Pressure vessels in service are generally subject to API 510 guidelines and recommended inspections.[7]

Conventional out-of-service tests include visual, manual ultrasonic, magnetic particle, eddy current and alternating current field measurement tests. Traditional preservice inspections include radiographic tests and, more recently, ultrasonic tests in lieu of radiographic tests for weld quality.

Ultrasonic techniques are used for both preservice and in-service inspections. The most common service damage mechanisms for vessels includes corrosion and cracking. Ultrasonic testing offers one of the most reliable techniques for the detection, sizing and evaluation of these damage mechanisms.

Ultrasonic testing can involve simple manual ultrasonic test techniques to advanced, automated ultrasonic testing. Recent advances in automated ultrasonic techniques have allowed on-stream automated ultrasonic testing in lieu of internal inspection.

Establishing manual thickness monitoring locations for condition monitoring is a common practice for ultrasonic testing of both vessels and piping. The thickness monitoring locations are generally tracked in a data base to be compared with future readings and to establish corrosion rates. The practice of collecting thickness monitoring locations varies from company to company. A chart may be used to track thickness monitoring locations.

Although manual ultrasonic testing does well at collecting remaining wall or thickness data, automated ultrasonic techniques are usually required to provide a detailed assessment for large area corrosion concerns. Whereas the thickness monitoring location represents a single-point thickness reading, the automated ultrasonic C-scan data can represent scores of readings per square centimeter (hundreds of readings per square inch).

Equally important is the application of ultrasonic testing for other service related damage such as cracking.

In the petrochemical and refining industry, pressure vessels are subject to degradation due to process variables upsets in normal operation, service life or age. Automated ultrasonic testing is a well established ultrasonic test technique for the detection, sizing, evaluation and monitoring of vessel cracking.

Some of the ultrasonic test techniques include the following.

1. Manual ultrasonic discontinuity detection and sizing use manual ultrasonic discontinuity detection equipment.
2. Automated ultrasonic test equipment uses pulse echo techniques for corrosion mapping, discontinuity detection and sizing using robotic canners at temperatures up to 672 K, that is, 400 °C (750 °F).
3. Automated or semiautomated ultrasonic testing uses time-of-flight diffraction (TOFD) for discontinuity detection and sizing on heavy wall equipment and at temperatures up to 672 K, that is, 400 °C (750 °F).
4. Automated or semiautomated ultrasonic testing uses phased array techniques for discontinuity detection and sizing on all configurations, including complex geometries such as nozzles.

Petroleum Pressure Vessels[4]

Internal damage such as corrosion (pitting, line grooving and galvanic corrosion), erosion, dents, cuts, gouges and other forms of deterioration can be detected with automated ultrasonics if the external surface is accessible and allows the entrance of ultrasound.[8] There are several obvious exceptions, such as the areas directly under plate reinforced nozzles, support pads and other external

TABLE 2. Discontinuity detection by nondestructive tests for ferrous and nonferrous metals in components.

Damage Mechanism	Eddy Current Testing	Magnetic Flux Leakage Testing	Remote Field Testing	Laser Profilometry	Ultrasonic Testing
Nonferrous Materials					
Pitting, inside surface	yes	no	tube and pipe	yes	yes
Pitting, outside surface	yes	no	tube and pipe	no	yes
Stress corrosion cracking, inside surface	yes	no	no	limited	no
Stress corrosion cracking, outside surface	yes	no	no	no	no
Volumetric discontinuities, embedded and other	yes	no	tube and pipe	no	limited
Wall loss, inside surface	yes	no	tube and pipe	limited	yes
Wall loss, outside surface	yes	no	tube and pipe	limited	yes
Ferrous Materials					
Pitting, inside surface	no	yes	tube and pipe	yes	yes
Pitting, outside surface	no	yes	tube and pipe	no	yes
Stress corrosion cracking, inside surface	no	limited	no	limited	no
Stress corrosion cracking, outside surface	no	limited	no	no	no
Volumetric discontinuities, embedded and other	no	limited	no	no	limited
Wall loss, inside surface	no	limited	tube and pipe	limited	yes
Wall loss, outside surface	no	limited	tube and pipe	limited	yes

attachments that prevent sound from entering the shell or head surface.

Hemispherical or torispherical heads of small diameter vessels may not present ideal surfaces for testing with automated robotic scanners. Alternative techniques such as manual ultrasonic testing must then be used.

Large vessels with two or more zones of differing corrosion rates may have each zone independently scheduled for ultrasonic testing.[7] The most active zone of corrosion is the determinant factor in calculating corrosion rate. Ultrasonic tests may be prioritized with emphasis on the active areas or zones of suspected corrosion.[8]

Generally, process equipment is designed for a certain minimum service life under specific operating conditions. On the basis of an annual corrosion rate, a total corrosion allowance is established, which is added to the calculated required thickness.

Different types of petrochemical equipment have typical design lives:[9] (1) twenty years for fractionating towers, catalytic reactors, high pressure heat exchanger shells and other equipment hard to replace; (2) ten to fifteen years for carbon steel drums, removable reactor components and alloy or carbon steel tower internals; and (3) five to ten years for carbon steel piping, heat exchanger tube bundles and various process column internals.

Vessels with expected service lives of twenty years may require many periodic internal and external tests, depending on the testing frequency, and it is essential to maintain accurate and retrievable records. The plan for data retrieval and documentation must be established before periodic testing begins. The automated ultrasonic scanning of a pressure vessel begins with a review of drawings and indicated scan areas. A coordinate system is devised to orient the scanner on the vessel. The reference system is usually governed by the ultrasonic system software.

Robotic scanners are usually servomotor driven magnetic wheeled devices carrying one or more ultrasonic transducers. The scanner can be track mounted or mounted directly on the vessel's surface. For general thickness readings, a free or direct mount has proven effective while maintaining a high degree of positional repeatability, usually within tolerances of ±13 mm (0.5 in.). Paint marking of the vessel surface suffices for indicating scan areas. Outdoor environments may demand a more durable marking medium than those used in protected areas.

Calibration standards used for thickness and corrosion monitoring have proven effective when fabricated (1) with incremental steps for close approximation of vessel thickness and (2) with side drilled or flat bottomed holes for sensitivity calibration. If isolated corrosion pitting is suspected, it is not easily detectable when sensitivity or instrument gain settings are adjusted for thickness readings only.

If erosion is suspected, calibration sensitivity may be adjusted for back wall echoes and thickness readings. However, an inspector may use two or more channels operating multiple-element transducers. This allows simultaneous gathering of thickness data while performing internal surface discontinuity detection in compression and transverse wave modes. Calibration of multiple-element transducers can be time consuming. However, they permit extensive scanning with one pass of the scanner, saving time over the course of the test.

Transducers with up to three pairs of transmitting and receiving elements have been used successfully to scan welds of the vessel shell to internal attachments. With this configuration, suspect areas can be scanned in one pass.

Equipment reliability is essential when operating in a demanding environment, especially when equipment must be operated in remote regions and downtime can mean days without production. Any automated ultrasonic scanning system suitable for use in the field should ideally be repairable in the field with modular components.

In vessels with high concentrations of hydrogen operating at elevated temperatures, laminations or near surface inclusions can contribute to hydrogen blistering. In this case, subsurface discontinuity indications may be relevant. If pitting occurs in service, then hydrogen can lead to embrittlement and blistering. Again, knowing the service or operating conditions of the vessel is vitally important.

PART 3. Storage Tanks

Ultrasonic testing is an important tool for inservice inspection of aboveground storage tanks (Fig. 17), including samples of the walls or shell courses, the roof, pontoons and the floor. In-service inspections may use a tank crawler, capable of collecting data along the walls and the roof, ranging in form from thickness readings at solitary points, to continuous line scans, to full scans in 0.3 m (12 in.) wide strips. Tank crawlers can range from a simple magnetic device attached to a telescope pole that gets pushed up the tank walls to robotic scanners mechanically driven up the tank walls. Ultrasonic instrumentation is interfaced to the crawlers to collect thickness data.

Out-of-service inspections may include detailed ultrasonic thickness surveys of the tank floor. In many cases, ultrasonic tests follow and quantify the results of magnetic flux leakage testing. The magnetic flux techniques for tank floor inspection are detailed elsewhere.[10] Generally, an ultrasonic verification is accomplished by thickness gaging, sometimes by B-scanning with a discontinuity detector or even by automated C-scanning. For stainless steel and other nonferrous tanks, ultrasonic testing is generally preferred.

Standards for Storage Tanks[11]

Several standards are relevant for aboveground storage tanks. In a number of standards and many contracts,

personnel who perform the tests should be qualified and certified by the manufacturer to a program written in conformance to the acceptance guidelines of *ASNT Recommended Practice No. SNT-TC-1A.*[12] In each of the several standards listed below, test requirements may be superseded by the contract or by another standard.

1. API 620, *Design and Construction of Large, Welded, Low-Pressure Storage Tanks,* covers both tanks and liquid spheres containing pressures up to 103.5 kPa (15 lb$_f$·in.$^{-2}$). Test requirements apply to any construction according to the standard's appendices but an appendix may specify a more stringent requirement. Ultrasonic technique requirements of API 620 conform to the *ASME Boiler and Pressure Vessel Code,* Section V, Article 4. The purchaser and manufacturer need to agree to the acceptance criteria for ultrasonic testing.[13]

2. API 650, *Welded Steel Tanks for Oil Storage,* covers certified and noncertified tanks. A section on inspecting joints applies also to tanks built to requirements in any of the appendices to this standard. Ultrasonic technique requirements conform to the *ASME Boiler and Pressure Vessel Code,* Section V, Article 4. The purchaser and manufacturer need to agree to the acceptance criteria for ultrasonic testing.[14]

3. API 653, *Tank Inspection, Repair, Alteration, and Reconstruction,* has requirements that may replace or add to requirements of a standard to which the tested structure was originally built. Ultrasonic testing is required, for example, if the purchaser agreed to acceptance criteria for laminations in plate areas.[15]

FIGURE 17. Aboveground storage tank for petroleum products.

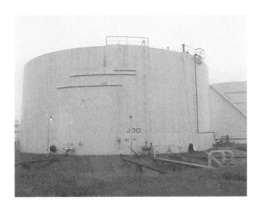

4. In the *ASME Boiler and Pressure Vessel Code,* Section VIII, Division 1 (*Lower Stress Design*) *Requirements*, the ultrasonic test requirements are in Paragraphs UW-11 and UW-53 of "Part UW for Welded Vessels — Technique for Ultrasonic Examination of Welded Joints." Ultrasonic testing is required (1) for 100 percent of electroslag welds in ferritic material after grain refining or after heat treatment following welding and (2) for 100 percent of welds made with the electron beam process. Ultrasonic testing may also be substituted for radiographic testing if construction does not let interpretable radiographic images be made. Lack of suitable radiographic equipment does not justify this substitution.[16]

5. In the *ASME Boiler and Pressure Vessel Code,* Section VIII, Division 2 (*High Stress Design*) *Requirements*, Ultrasonic test requirements can be found in Appendix 9, "Mandatory Nondestructive Examination," Article 9-3, "Ultrasonic Examination of Welds." Ultrasonic testing may be substituted for radiographic testing of some full penetration welds. Ultrasonic testing is required for 100 percent of electroslag welds after grain refining or after heat treatment, (2) for 100 percent of welds made with the electron beam process and (3) for nozzle attachments.[17]

These standards are cited as examples: the list is not exhaustive. Also, some of these examples are more for pressure vessels than storage tanks. Persons planning a testing program need to consult the current versions of all standards that apply to the particular storage tanks to be inspected. Test procedures must conform to other applicable regulations — for example, to other parts of the *ASME Code.*

PART 4. Petroleum Pipes

Pipelines

Pipelines are the arteries between field production (gas and oil extraction) and the refinery and petrochemical plants where gas and crude are processed into useable products. Pipelines are generally made by welding sections of carbon steel line pipe or by laying coiled line pipe from a large drum. Inspection performed during manufacturing of the pipe sections often involves ultrasonic techniques. Because pipelines generally run over several kilometers and across the country and state lines, they are governed by agencies such as the United States Department of Transportation. The construction, maintenance and inspection of these pipelines are critical to the safety of our environment and the general public. Many pipelines are buried and not only have the potential for catastrophic failure but could contaminate lakes, rivers and underground water sources if they leak.

Traditional preservice inspections include radiographic and ultrasonic testing during fabrication to ensure the quality of the welding. Once in service, the pipeline companies depend on inservice testing to assess corrosion and mechanical damage. Inspections before 1970 included leak tests. Since the late 1960s, magnetic flux leakage instruments inserted into the pipelines and propelled by product flow are the main inspection tools.

Quantitative inspections that follow qualitative inspections are commonly called *proveup* inspections. Ultrasonic tests of pipelines or tank floors, for instance, may be used to assess areas of concern highlighted by magnetic flux leakage tests. The proveup test follows up and determines the extent and severity of discontinuities. Many proveup techniques use automated ultrasonic testing and imaging.

Much research has been devoted to ultrasonic testing for stress corrosion cracking and wall thickness measurement in installed pipelines.

A variety of test methods are used before service. For pipes in service, crawlers have been introduced for inspection from the pipe's interior surface. Crawlers are also referred to as *pigs* because of the squealing sound that some models used to make. Smart pigs are inspection vehicles that move inside a pipe line and are pushed along by product flow. At the end of the line or run, the pig is retrieved and the onboard data processing units are analyzed.

Drill Casings[4,18]

Ultrasonic testing on oil field tubular goods has increased with the use of heavy wall casing in oil and gas wells. The techniques generally used before the reintroduction of ultrasonic testing were electromagnetic. The release of API RP5A5, *Recommended Practice for Field Testing of New Casing, Tubing and Plain-End Drill Pipe,* set some basic guidelines for ultrasonic testing, as outlined below.[19]

Equipment

A wide variety of equipment exists as follows.

1. In full body inspection of new tubes, the pipe is rotated under or over a transducer array to ensure full coverage for imperfections and wall thickness. Conventional or phased array techniques are used.
2. In seam weld inspection of new tubes, units are run along the seam weld to inspect it from both sides.
3. For used drill pipe, arrays of transducers fire sound axially, searching for transverse fatigue cracks, often in the presence of pitting.
4. Proveup is generally performed with contact angle beam transverse waves. Note that discontinuity sizing can be quite difficult because of discontinuity orientation. Because many discontinuities are longer than they are deep, the length contributes more to the reflection than the depth does. Further, penetrators in electric resistance welded tubes are virtually impossible to size when they are narrower than the sound beam.
5. Phased array systems have been introduced into several mills and third party inspection companies.

Equipment selection is left to the testing company, with each facility using the equipment that it believes reliably detects all expected discontinuities. These requirements are located in American

Petroleum Institute recommended practices and in other specifications for oil field tubular goods.

Written Procedures

A written practice can refer to ASNT's *Recommended Practice SNT-TC-1A* or specify other personnel qualifying procedures to establish minimum requirements for inspection personnel.[12]

A written procedure outlining all aspects of the company's testing system and personnel is to be available on site. This allows the owner, the oil company, the drilling company or a representative third party to evaluate the procedure for compliance with their requirements. It also allows these parties to determine if the testing company is following its own procedure. The customer representative personnel, an observer, should be qualified and certified to at least the same level as the testing personnel.

Reference Standards

Reference standards for inspections of new material are often full length specimens of the same mass per unit length and attenuation properties as the order, with electrodischarge machine notches eroded into the pipe's inner and outer surfaces. In many cases, it is required to erode these reference indicators before field inspection by a third party, in which case they are made in one of the tubes of the order and then are removed at the conclusion of the inspection. Removal is possible because the notch depths are required to be 5, 10 (for electric resistance welded tubes) or 12.5 percent of the specified wall of the pipe. A minimum wall of 87.5 percent of specified wall permits removal of the reference indicator and of many surface breaking discontinuities found during the testing.

The notches are longitudinal and transverse to the tube axis, although some purchasers require the inspection system to be able to detect notches oriented at angles such as 0.18, 0.38 and 0.79 rad (10, 22 and 45 deg) to the tube axis. The notches are a maximum of 25.4 mm (1.00 in.) long or twice the beam width, 1.0 mm (0.040 in.) wide; in many cases, they must give ultrasonic reflections from both sides that are within 2 dB of each other. If the latter are used, the effective beam width of all transducers must be monitored: if changes are noticed, the transducer may need to be changed.

In the case of electric welded pipe, notches as short as 6.4 mm (0.25 in.) have been used. In the case of used drill stem inspection, transverse inner and outer surface notches are used to simulate fatigue cracks.

For example, with a 180 mm (7 in.), 48 kg·m^{-1} (32 lb$_a$·ft^{-1}) pipe. The specified wall thickness is 11.5 mm (0.453 in.). About 12.5 percent of this is 1.4 mm (0.057 in.) and 5 percent is 0.6 mm (0.023 in.). For this pipe, using the 87.5 percent remaining wall criterion, the specified minimum wall is 157 mm (6.18 in.).

Wall Thickness Eccentricity

Scanning for longitudinal and transverse discontinuities and monitoring the wall thickness are more or less standard ultrasonic test techniques. In the rejection criteria, the 87.5 percent remaining wall creates a potential problem. API Specification 5CT specifies pipe rejection criteria in terms of percentage of wall thickness. Pipe may be repaired or the rejectable part of a pipe may be cut off.[20]

When the material is tested according to API 5CT Supplementary Requirement 2, "Nondestructive Inspection," imperfections between 5 and 12.5 percent must be removed. If an imperfection is on the inside surface and is not removed, the pipe is rejected. If the 87.5 percent remaining wall is the criterion, then a discontinuity larger than 12.5 percent, once removed, can be acceptable and a discontinuity smaller than 5 percent could cause rejection.[20]

The following example uses a 180 mm (7 in.) diameter, 48 kg·m^{-1} (32 lb$_a$·ft^{-1}) casing. The nominal wall is 11.5 mm (0.453 in.). For this demonstration, the inside and outside circumferences are shown as perfect circles (Fig. 18). The pipe is shaped eccentrically, so that the low side wall is 10.0 mm (0.383 in.) thick or 0.25 mm (0.01 in.) greater than the reject level. The high side wall is 13 mm (0.5 in.) or 2.5 mm (0.1 in.) greater than the reject level.

This means that a low side wall discontinuity with a radial depth of 0.4 mm (0.015 in.) should cause rejection because it reduces the wall to 10.0 mm (0.383 in.), 0.13 mm (0.005 in.) less than

FIGURE 18. Cross section of eccentrically shaped pipe.

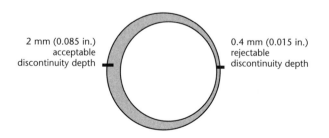

2 mm (0.085 in.) acceptable discontinuity depth

0.4 mm (0.015 in.) rejectable discontinuity depth

the acceptable 87.5 percent remaining wall of 10 mm (0.4 in.). This discontinuity is 35 percent smaller than the 5 percent notch. On the high side wall, a radial discontinuity of 2 mm (0.085 in.) can be accepted if removal is agreed on, as usual. This discontinuity is 50 percent deeper than the 12.5 percent reject level. This example is in strict compliance if 87.5 percent of the remaining wall is the acceptance criterion.

New casing or tubing in the field is inspected according to API RP 5A5 or customer requirements.[19]

PART 5. Inservice Ultrasonic Testing of Offshore Structures[22]

Steel jacketed offshore platforms are distributed throughout the world, supporting oil and gas operations in relatively shallow waters. The steel jacket serves as a template for pilings driven into the sea bed. Additionally, the jacket stiffens the structure and carries a portion of the structural load during the life of the platform. This type of structure is at least as old as 1947, when the first commercially productive offshore unit was placed in the Gulf of Mexico.[23]

Many such platforms have reached and exceeded their original design life. To ensure that the structural integrity of a platform has not been compromised by the loss of material to corrosion, by fatigue or wave, wind and impact forces, divers perform a wide variety of tests on a periodic basis. Visual, ultrasonic and magnetic particle tests are among the methods routinely used to satisfy requirements imposed by regulatory agencies, insurance companies or owners as part of planned maintenance. Tests may also be invoked for specific cause, as when wet weld repair procedures specify underwater testing.

Three major applications of underwater ultrasonic testing are discussed below: (1) thickness gaging for corrosion, (2) weld testing and (3) flooded member detection. Each technique is somewhat unique and although there are topside counterparts to each, there are peculiarities that make underwater ultrasonic testing very challenging. Extensive biofouling, front surface pitting, heavy surge and low visibility are routine impediments facing the diver inspector.[24,25]

Under all but ideal conditions, the diver's tasks should be made as simple as possible. A team — the diver and a topside ultrasonic inspector — is recommended. The diver's responsibilities include locating the proper site, preparing the surface (removal of fouling) and manipulating the transducer to produce the necessary signals. The topside inspector's responsibilities include system calibration, interpretation, guiding the diver's manipulation of the transducer and directing the diver from one location to the next.

While a great deal of excellent ultrasonic information can be obtained underwater, there are also limitations that must be recognized by the supplier and buyer of underwater test services. In this text, each of the three techniques is examined from basic principles through practical implementation.

Steel Jacketed Platforms

Offshore construction is different from that found on shore, with extensive use of tubular products for structural members being an obvious difference. Main platform legs (which also serve to guide the installation of pilings) up to 3 m (10 ft) in diameter and 75 mm (3 in.) wall thickness are locked into a three-dimensional structure by smaller braces typically 0.3 to 1 m (1 to 3 ft) in diameter and up to 25 mm (1 in.) in wall thickness. Most tubular welds are T, K or Y shaped connections, using a variety of joint designs at various points along the welded joint.[26] In some designs, the welded tubular joint has been replaced by a cast node, having stub sleeves for each member.

Offshore platforms are generally welded on land, in a sideways or horizontal position, then towed or carried on a barge to the installation site. There, they are righted and allowed to settle on the sea floor. Even a well constructed fabrication must endure this strenuous installation sequence before its service life begins. The possibility of structural damage during installation cannot be ignored. Once installed, in waters as shallow as 10 m (30 ft) or as deep as 400 m (1300 ft), the structure supports drilling and production operations, hotel services for the operators, berthing of ships and barges and other activities. From the North Sea to the seas of Southeast Asia, platforms endure violent attacks of waves and wind, accidental batterings by ships and the consumption of their materials by corrosion, abrasion and scouring.

Test Requirements

Oil and gas exploration around the United States is subject to many laws. Reasonable test requirements can be demanded as part of the overall design of offshore structures and the periodic fulfillment of testing obligations can be monitored. In the United States, regulatory agencies for oil and gas resources have included the Department of the Interior, the Geological Survey, the Coast Guard and the American Bureau of Shipping. Others around the world include insurance companies.

Owners and operators of offshore structures are motivated to perform tests for reasons more immediate than compliance with regulations: safety, production rates and insurance premiums figure prominently. Testing is a primary means of cost avoidance when it allows rational planning decisions instead of responsive or emergency repairs. Most major operators have testing schedules established for their offshore assets and typically include at least some underwater testing since fixed structures cannot be dry docked. Planned underwater tests are often categorized in three levels: (1) a general visual test for obvious problems such as missing members or collision damage, (2) detailed visual tests requiring surface preparation and (3) other nondestructive tests such as ultrasonic, magnetic particle, eddy current or radiographic tests.

Ultrasonic Thickness Gaging

Both ultrasonic thickness gaging and corrosion testing use the round trip travel time of a compressional wave to calculate the thickness of metal in which the sound traveled. A burst of ultrasound is launched into the water in front of the transducer. After reaching the metal's front surface, a portion of the sound enters the metal and most of it is reflected back to the transducer, producing what is known as the *interface echo*. The sound that enters the metal travels through the metal at longitudinal velocity (about 5.9 km·s^{-1} or 2.3×10^5 in.·s^{-1} in steel) until it arrives at the back surface of the object.

At this point, most of the acoustic energy is reflected back to the front surface. A small amount is transmitted into the medium behind the back surface. Of the sound that reflects back to the front surface, part is transmitted through the front surface and back to the transducer, forming the first back wall echo. Most of the returning sound reflects off the front surface, back to the back wall.

At each interface, there is both reflection and transmission and what arrives at the transducer is a train of pulses from which the metal's thickness can be calculated: travel time divided by sound speed gives distance traveled. If the metal's surfaces are flat, smooth and

parallel, then a very accurate value of thickness is obtained from the difference between successive back wall echo arrival times. If the surfaces are coated, internal reflections from the metal-to-coating interfaces are generally stronger than reflections from the coating-to-water interfaces (the sound path traveled during internal reflections is entirely within the metal and not in the coating). Figure 19 shows the geometry of underwater thickness gaging with a single-transducer pulse echo system.

Ultrasonic Corrosion Testing

Corrosion testing ideally uses the same principle of operation as thickness testing, mapping the thickness of remaining metal and thus revealing thinned and pitted areas. However, the situation is considerably more complicated because, with corroded materials, a series of back wall echoes rarely shows above the system's noise level. Although a thickness measurement taken between the interface echo and the first back wall inherently includes a contribution from any coating, it may be the best signal available.

FIGURE 19. Thickness gaging with ultrasonic testing: (a) test setup; (b) typical oscilloscope display.

(a)

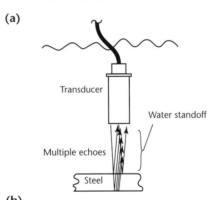

(b)

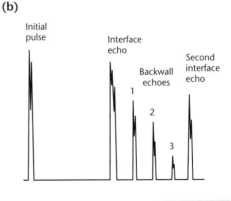

Ultrasonic corrosion testing uses (1) thickness measurement under difficult conditions, (2) deductive information based on the degree of difficulty in making the thickness measurements and (3) information derived from a variety of other sources. For example, the only reliable way to gage the remaining thickness on a heavily pitted surface may be to measure the thickness at a nearby flat spot (uncorroded enough to allow an accurate ultrasonic measurement) and to then subtract from it a direct physical measurement of pit depth.

Differences in Underwater Testing

Underwater thickness gaging and corrosion testing differ from their topside counterparts in three significant respects: front surface roughness, cable length and coordinating the diver's transducer motions with the topside inspector's interpretation of the display.

The problem of surface roughness can be handled by the diver with a heavy hammer because only a small flat area is required for a spot ultrasonic reading. The interior walls of offshore tubular members are expected to be uncorroded and the train of echoes is normally quite clean. When this is not the case, despite a properly flattened front surface, the inspector may presume that internal corrosion has been caused by flooding or water left in the member at the time of fabrication.

Techniques for determining the probable cause of internal corrosion include flooded member detection and comparisons of signal patterns at different depths on the same member. Further testing or mapping of internal corrosion is usually not warranted because repair and maintenance decisions are made on the basis of overall corrosion condition (including the presence or absence of internal corrosion) rather than the details of corrosion at any one location.

The diver's motions must be coordinated with the topside inspector's requirements for producing back wall echoes and this can be approached in several ways. Feedback of signal amplitude to the diver (using an audible signal or a remote video display) is an excellent way to help the diver manipulate the transducer properly. Alternatively, the topside inspector can direct the diver's motions orally, especially if the diver and the inspector have experience together and if the communication system provides clear transmission of both voices. Otherwise, a diver can quickly become frustrated by continual redirection.

Underwater Weld Testing

Weld testing on tubular joints underwater follows standard guidelines[27] for ultrasonic weld testing during fabrication. An angle beam is launched into the steel along a path, insonifying part of the weld length at an angle that causes discontinuities in the weld to reflect sound back to the transducer. If a reflection is received, then the source of the reflection is determined by geometrical calculations and the significance of the discontinuity is evaluated. If no signals are received, the weld is presumed free of internal discontinuities. Figure 20 shows the geometry for a weld test.

Discontinuity Location with Angle Beam Tests

Once smooth surface conditions have been obtained, the key issue for underwater weld testing is the ability to

FIGURE 20. Geometry of ultrasonic testing of weld: (a) skew angle θ; (b) skip distance.

(a)

(b)

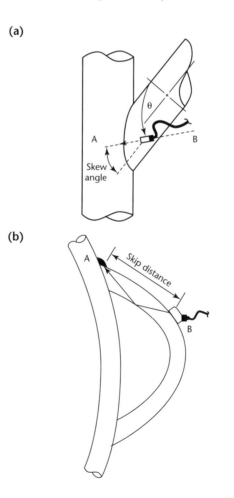

accurately measure the angles and positions required to calculate the location of reflectors within the weld volume. Because of the computational complexity of the tubular joint geometry, this task requires systems that incorporate sophisticated positioning aids. In particular, the unassisted diver is not able to perform underwater transverse wave ultrasonic tests on many tubular joints with a reasonable degree of accuracy.

Consider an angle beam transducer on a tubular member, pointing in a direction parallel to the tube's axis. The geometry of this situation is the same as for a flat plate of the same thickness as the tube, and the curvature of the member is not involved in calculating the sound beam's trajectory. The same transducer turned 1.5 rad (90 deg), however, launches sound into a ring shaped cross section, making the task of ray tracing entirely different. Skip distance is an important parameter and, as shown in Fig. 21, it varies strongly as a function of skew angle.

When the transducer is skewed at an angle between these two perpendicular directions, sound is launched into an elliptical cross section and the skip distance changes continuously around the circumference of the ellipse. To properly calculate the trajectory of the sound beam, the diver must be able to measure both the skew angle (between the transducer's beam axis and the longitudinal axis of the tubular member) and the ellipse defined by the skew angle. Additionally, the diver must (1) measure the distance between the transducer's beam exit point and the weld axis, (2) manipulate the transducer and (3) discriminate between geometric reflectors and discontinuities of concern.

Knowledge of the weld's geometry is essential and successful discontinuity detection in tubular goods is usually

limited to fabrication testing. Without benchmarks to indicate the locations of specific weld details, inservice testing is difficult. For example, an acceptable partial penetration weld may give a signal from the root that could be interpreted as a crack signal.

For these reasons, manual underwater testing of tubular joints is unrealistic but there may arise cases where this difficult task is undertaken. For instance, if visual or magnetic particle testing has revealed a crack in the toe of a weld, ultrasonic testing may be used to determine the depth of the crack and whether it has penetrated through the member.

In the case of very large members or plate-to-tubular joints, curvature related problems may not be significant and transverse wave testing may be desired. Even in these cases, the test system designer must recognize the dexterity problems faced by the diver, the requirement for amplitude feedback to the diver, the need for marking and measuring devices and even provisions for holding all the ancillary items that a topside inspector normally has available in a pocket or tool bag.

Flooded Member Detection

Flooded member detection relies on the same principles as thickness gaging but on a much larger scale. Because the acoustic impedance of steel is vastly different from that of air, virtually all of the sound that arrives at the back surface of an air backed metal plate is reflected. In a flooded member, however, the amount of sound transmitted through the back wall is notable — about 12 percent of the energy is transmitted. With proper instrumentation, it is possible to detect the small amount of ultrasonic energy that penetrates the back surface, travels across the flooded interior of the member, reflects off the opposite inside surface and returns through the original metal thickness to the transducer (Fig. 22). Capturing ultrasonic energy that has traveled this route in air is impossible with conventional instrumentation: a tubular member is almost certainly flooded if the appropriate signal is received.

Sensitivity and Gain

Although flooded member detection can be viewed as a kind of thickness gaging, its implementation stretches the capabilities of conventional ultrasonic systems. The first issue is sensitivity: the ability to transmit energy and receive reflections in water from as much as 3 m

FIGURE 21. Skip distance as function of skew angle. Graph indicates variations in skip distance with transducer position and orientation. Outside diameter of 500 mm (20 in.), thickness $T = 25$ mm (1 in.), skew of $\theta = 0.5$ rad (30 deg) and refracted angle of 1 rad (60 deg).

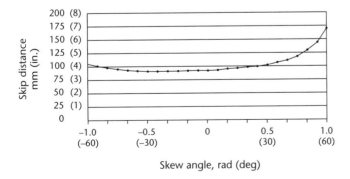

(10 ft) away. Gain is at a premium as square law spreading leads to a 6 dB loss per distance doubling. Large diameter members with legs up to 3 m (10 ft) across require 20 dB gain over that required at 300 mm (12 in.) for through-transmission. An additional 6 dB is required for round trip travel.

Substantial gain is also required to overcome the inefficiencies of energy transmission through the steel-to-water interfaces present in the sound path, if the member is flooded. Traversing the inner surface of the near pipe wall once for the outgoing pulse and again after reflection reduces the signal strength to 1.3 percent of its original strength (12 percent transmission at each boundary plus a reflection of 88 percent), thus requiring an additional 38 dB to maintain the signal. Further losses occur if any surface is rough. In this respect, the entry surface is by far the most important. Experience with typically corroded surfaces suggests that as much as 30 dB may be required to compensate for even mild corrosion and that heavily corroded members might require surface

preparation before any reliability can be expected.

Adequate surface preparation should always be included in planning the diver's workload and associated costs.

Time Constraints

Along with the requirement for adequate sensitivity, the ultrasonic instrument used for flooded member detection must be able to display signals occurring as much as 4 ms after the pulse is launched. This round trip travel time is based on a 3 m (10 ft) diameter flooded member. When compared to tests of steel, the equivalent range requirement is:

$$(2) \quad T_e = T_s + \frac{v_s}{v_w} T_w \cong 4D$$

where D is nominal pipe diameter (millimeter), T_e is equivalent thickness of steel (millimeter), T_s is tube wall thickness (millimeter), T_w is water path length or inside diameter (millimeter), v_s is velocity of sound in steel (5.9 km·s⁻¹) and v_w is velocity of sound in water (1.5 km·s⁻¹). For a tube of moderate size, this range requirement exceeds the capabilities of some instruments.

To attain the best possible penetration, the operating frequency is usually as low as possible. For conventional ultrasonic test systems, the lower limit is about 0.5 MHz because the receiver sections of conventional instruments are optimized for conventional applications. Above 1 MHz, the performance of the system is limited by attenuation and scattering, both of which increase as wavelength decreases. Below 0.5 MHz, performance is limited by the receiver's ability to process low frequency signals. The choice of transducers is made on the basis of its performance with the specific ultrasonic testing instrument, with sensitivity gained at the expense of resolution — for this application, high resolution is not a requirement.

Flooded Member Detection Strategy

The mechanics of flooding dictate the most reasonable strategies for ultrasonic detection. Flooding can result from cracks, corrosion holes, punctures, accidental entrapment of rain water during fabrication, ballasting operations and other causes. Establishing the cause of flooding may be as important as detecting the condition: actions based on flooding differ according to its cause.

Whatever the cause, the final water level should be at least as high as predicted by Boyle's law: for a confined

FIGURE 22. Flooded member detection with ultrasonic testing: (a) sound waves propagate through water, producing back wall reflections; (b) acoustic impedance differences permit no transmission through air filled member.

(a)

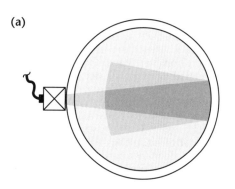

(b)

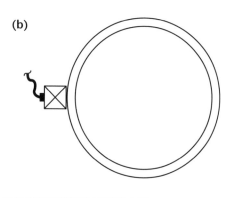

amount of gas, pressure and volume are inversely related ($P \times V$ = constant). When a member floods, the gas that was sealed into it at the time of fabrication is compressed by the entering water. Eventually, the pressure of the compressed gas equals the pressure of the surrounding seawater and flooding stops, there being no further driving force.

However, there are several reasons why the water level might not be near this predicted level. For example, flooding due to water entrapped during fabrication or installation operations is typically far below the predicted level. On the other hand, if flooding is caused by a hole above the predicted level, then gas may bubble out of the member and the final flood level may be well above the predicted level. Finally, after accidental damage results in through-crack flooding, testing after a major storm may fail to detect water at the predicted level.

Underwater Transducers

Single-Element Transducers

For each underwater ultrasonic test, there are several possible transducer types that might be used. Because underwater surfaces are typically coated or pitted, a dual-element transducer is not appropriate. When measuring thickness with a dual-element transducer, a single indication representative of the total time of flight (from the source crystal to the receiving crystal) is measured to calibrate the system — time spent in the transducer's delay lines is subtracted out. On smooth bare metal, the time remaining is related to the travel time of the elastic wave in the metal and so represents the thickness of the material. On a painted or pitted surface, this is not true, because part of the remaining time is spent in the coating layer or in the couplant between the face of the transducer and the bottom of the pit. These conditions must be considered in the calibration of the equipment.

With a single-element transducer, it is often possible to measure the metal's thickness exclusive of time spent in the paint or in a pit. This is done using the difference in arrival time of successive back wall echoes, instead of the difference between the single interface response obtained from the dual transducers.

As explained above, the strongest internal echoes occur at the metal's front and back surfaces, inside any coatings. The difference between successive back walls arises from reflections that exclude coating on either surface. This measurement technique is possible on lightly corroded surfaces but on heavily corroded surfaces it might not be possible to get more than one back wall echo.

Immersion Transducers

Because underwater thickness measurements are taken in an ocean of couplant, there is no compelling reason to use contact transducers. In fact, either contact or immersion transducers work so long as the electrical connector is waterproofed and the transducer's damping allows adequate resolution between closely spaced arrivals that often characterize corroded materials. Because the facing material of an immersion transducer is not designed to resist wear, direct contact with the surface must be avoided.

Because immersion transducers can be obtained in a wide variety of sizes and focal lengths, they are often chosen for underwater thickness gaging. Even the difficulties posed by severe front surface pitting can be tackled successfully by the proper use of a focused immersion transducer.[28] For flooded member detection (where resolution and focus are not critical but penetration is), contact transducers may have an advantage in ruggedness. For weld testing, a conventional angle beam transducer may be fitted with an appropriate wedge or an immersion transducer may be fitted with a properly angled standoff.

Underwater Cabling

Pressure resistant, waterproof instrumentation is not readily available for underwater tests, necessitating transducer cables. These cables are often 300 or 400 m (about 1000 ft) long and are subjected to extremely adverse environmental conditions. Electrical performance and ruggedness are key considerations, particularly when cable failures and poor signal transmission can cause a costly diving operation to be suspended.

Common coaxial cables are available in a variety of wire sizes and characteristic impedances. Waterproof constructions are available to prevent the migration of water into the space between the outer braid and the outer jacket. While vinyl jackets are acceptable for many topside applications, they cut easily and become brittle in low temperatures. Plastic jackets are more suitable for underwater applications.

Electrical problems with long cables can usually be traced to physical damage or improper impedance matching rather than to resistive line losses.[29] The effect of an impedance mismatch can be seen by calculating the approximate travel time of an electrical pulse in a long cable:

$$(3) \quad t = 2\frac{L}{v}$$

where L is cable length (meter), t is the round trip travel time (second) and v is the speed (meter per second) of electromagnetic propagation in the cable.[26] For example, if $L = 100$ m and $v = 2.0 \times 10^8$ m·s⁻¹, then $t = 1$ µs. Consider sound traveling in a 3 mm (0.1 in.) thick steel plate. Using the values for sound in steel, $L = 3.0 \times 10^{-3}$ m, $t = 1$ µs and $v = 6.0 \times 10^3$ m·s⁻¹. If mismatch is present and multiple cable pulses are produced, the two signals can arrive at the same time, resulting in an erroneous thickness reading or an obscured back wall reflection. This case does not have a great deal of field significance because there are very few marine structures made of 3 mm (0.1 in.) thick steel. However, the reflected pulse still interferes with the accurate gaging of much thicker materials because it excites the transducer many times and causes the back wall echo to be less sharp than with a shorter cable.

Figure 23 illustrates the immersion testing of a 19 mm (0.75 in.) thick steel block using a 2 m (6 ft) cable and a 300 m (1000 ft) cable. The spurious signals in Fig. 23b are predictable and can be eliminated by an impedance matching network at the transducer end of the cable.

Another effect of cable length is seen in the hyperbolic forms of transmission line equations, such as the equation relating voltages at the sending and receiving ends of the cable:[30]

$$(4) \quad E_0 = E_L \left[\cos h(GL) + \frac{Z_0}{Z_R} \sin h(GL) \right]$$

where E_0 is the sending end potential (volt), E_L is the receiving end potential (volt), G is the complex constant for phase and cable attenuation, L is the cable length (meter), Z_0 is the cable characteristic impedance (ohm) and Z_R is the receiving end or transducer impedance (ohm).

The complex phase constant G is computed for 50 Ω coaxial cable:[29]

$$(5) \quad G = A + j \times B$$

where B is a phase constant of 9.84 rad ($564 \times F$ deg) per 300 m (1000 ft), F is frequency (megahertz), j is the imaginary number $(-1)^{0.5}$ and A is the attenuation constant:

$$(6) \quad A = \left(4.8\sqrt{F} - 1.4 \right) \text{ dB per 300 m}$$
$$= \frac{\left(4.8\sqrt{F} - 1.4 \right)}{8.68} \text{ Np per 300 m}$$

where 300 m ≅ 1000 ft.

Evaluating the hyperbolic functions for complex arguments leads to periodic functions (sine and cosine) with extreme values at odd and even multiples of one-half the wavelength, respectively. A cable exactly one-half wavelength long performs better than a cable one-quarter wavelength long. For 50 Ω cable carrying 1 MHz signals, one-half wavelength is about 100 m (330 ft). The implication is that even for shallow underwater applications, it is better to use a full 100 m (330 ft) cable for 1 MHz transducers than only half this length. Figure 24 shows the voltage transfer ratio calculated from the previous equations and from Eq. 6, with values appropriate to 50 Ω cable:

FIGURE 23. Effect of cable length on ultrasonic testing: (a) oscillogram from tests of 19 mm (0.75 in.) plate using 2 m (6 ft) cable; (b) degraded performance from 300 m (1000 ft) unmatched cable (note spurious signals at arrows).

(a)

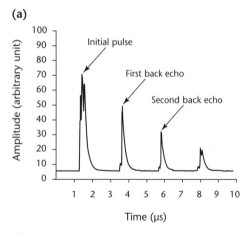

(b)

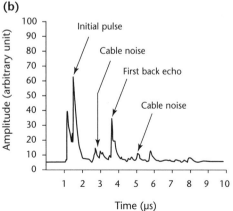

$$(7) \quad V_{TR} \;=\; 20 \log \frac{A}{B}$$

where A is potential (volt) at the transducer end of the cable, B is potential (volt) applied to the instrument end of the cable and V_{TR} is the voltage transfer ratio (decibel).

Clear valleys in this transfer ratio occur at every half wavelength. Peaks in the ratio occur at odd multiples of one-quarter wavelength.

Instrumentation for Underwater Ultrasonic Testing

Effect of Corrosion

For underwater thickness gaging, there is some debate over the choice between a digital thickness gage and an ultrasonic instrument with an A-scan display. On well protected, uncoated surfaces, a digital gage is appropriate for most ultrasonic test procedures, even those made with a dual-transducer setup.

In cases of exceptionally heavy corrosion where the best approach may be a combination of ultrasonic readings on smooth bare areas and direct, physical pit depth measurements, a digital gage may be used. In most cases, where surface corrosion is moderate or where the surface is coated, the A-scan display is preferable. With an A-scan display, an inspector can accurately interpret the screen patterns commonly encountered in underwater tests and can more reliably determine the thickness.

Figure 25 shows three thickness gaging signals. Figure 25a shows a normal screen pattern from uncorroded 13 mm (0.5 in.) steel plate and a series of clean back wall

echoes. The pattern in Fig. 25b shows multiple back wall echoes greatly attenuated by back wall pitting. In Fig. 25c, the front surface pitting shifts the interface echo to the right (showing

FIGURE 25. Effect of surface pitting on ultrasonic test results: (a) normal echoes from specimen 13 mm (0.5 in.) thick; (b) presence of back wall pitting reduces signal strength; (c) effect of front surface pitting.

(a)

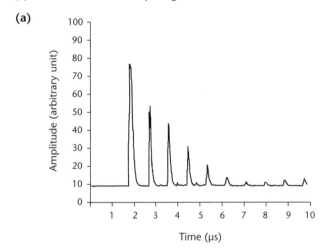

(b)

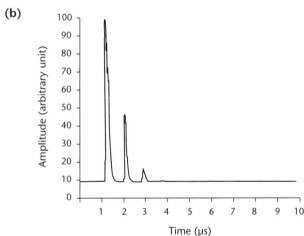

(c)

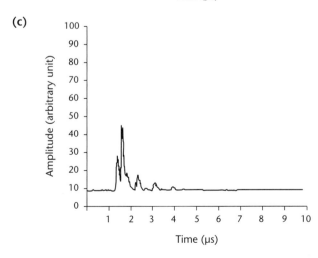

FIGURE 24. Voltage transfer ratio as function of cable length with 1 MHz transducer.

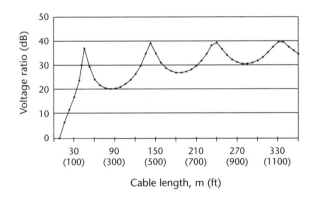

additional time spent in the water between the transducer and the front surface) and reduces the amplitude of back wall echoes.

Pulser Strength

With the difficulties presented by front surface corrosion, several design features of the ultrasonic instrument must be considered. For example, although pulser power varies considerably from instrument to instrument, power itself is not always the most important issue. In a series of experiments characterizing the performance of instruments for flooded member detection, it was found that a very lightweight discontinuity detector with a 200 V pulse can successfully compete with instruments having ten times the pulse strength, provided their receiver noise is low enough to permit use of available gain.

Additionally, for flooded member detection, the total range is very important because it takes about four times as long for sound to travel across a flooded member as it does to travel through the same distance in steel. For corrosion testing, where resolution is the most important parameter, pulser strength means very little but broad band receiving is very important.

System Accuracy

Typical requirements in corrosion testing demand an accuracy on the order of 0.5 mm (0.02 in.), about one-half wavelength when using a 5 MHz transducer. Achieving this level of accuracy in badly corroded material requires that the salient features of the radiofrequency waveform be altered very little in passing to the video display.

If the ultrasonic instrument provides digital readings or an analog thickness signal, it is very important that the gating used to determine thickness be displayed. Without this information, the inspector may have no way of knowing which signals are being interpreted by the digital timing circuits as the front surface and back wall signals.

Ease of Discontinuity Detection

Discontinuity detectors for underwater weld testing must meet the same technical requirements (linearity and calibrated gain) as those used ashore. It should also be remembered that ease of operation translates into reduced time in the water for the diver.

Even the simplest manual skills required for weld testing (marking the transducer location or measuring distances forward of the transducer) may be complicated underwater. It is therefore critically important that fleeting signals be captured quickly and accurately by the topside inspector. Several techniques are available for expediting discontinuity detection. The two most commonly used offshore are automatic distance amplitude compensation (DAC) and direct amplitude feedback to the diver.

1. Distance amplitude compensation is an effective means of preserving signals generated in the weld zone while suppressing entry surface noise. A distance amplitude compensation feature is available on virtually all discontinuity detectors since 1980. While manual distance amplitude compensation procedures give results similar to those of automatic systems (time varying gain), the inspector is alerted to the presence of weld discontinuities more directly when the monitor shows the compensated signal.

2. Direct amplitude feedback to the diver has been accomplished in several ways, dating back to simple tone generators developed in 1978.[31,32] This accessory to the basic discontinuity detector responds to the amplitude of signals in a gate chosen by the topside inspector and produces a whistling tone whose pitch is proportional to the gated signal amplitude. When the tone is fed into the diver's communicator, it allows the diver to produce the discontinuity signal of interest without the need for verbal communication.

Other systems accomplish the same goal in different ways. Perhaps the most sophisticated system uses a television camera aimed at the discontinuity detector. The diver is presented a replica of the monitor signal by means of prisms and a video display mounted in the diving helmet.

Surface Preparation for Underwater Tests

Proper surface preparation is one of the most important factors in successful underwater ultrasonic testing. Topside procedures generally call for surfaces of 250 root mean square (or better) with only a tightly adhering primer allowed. These conditions are rarely possible underwater. Instead, the diver is faced with marine fouling that must be removed from the area of interest. Applied primers or other manufactured coatings, if present, should be preserved.

Hand scrapers, hammers and wire brushes, power brushes, chippers, needle guns and water blasters are all effective for removing marine growth. The scope of the ultrasonic test may determine whether hand or power tools should be used, but it is crucial that the area under the transducer be as smooth as possible to ensure effective coupling throughout the test. For thickness gaging and flooded member detection, a back wall signal always confirms the proper entry of sound into the test object. For weld testing, there is no such confirmation. The surface requirements of conventional topside weld testing documents should be respected.

Diver Location for Underwater Tests

Accurate nomenclature greatly assists the process of locating a diver during underwater testing. Except in rare cases, a platform's nodes (welded intersections of tubular structural members) are not labeled underwater and often visibility is too low to permit the diver to see from one node to the next. The topside inspector must guide the diver from one test area to the next, using engineering drawings or a model of the platform's members.

Nodes are typically designated by their depth and a pair of letters or numbers indicating position in the plan view. Members can be specified by naming the nodes they connect but a description of the member (leg, horizontal, vertical, diagonal) is usually given. All documentary photographs and videotape should include identification of the weld or node in the field of view.

Remote Systems

Remotely operated vehicles can be used to carry ultrasonic transducers, video cameras, water blasters and many other testing tools. For spot readings (thickness gaging or flooded member detection), remotely operated vehicles can effectively reduce the cost of operations in water depths that require saturation diving. For shallower depths, the economic advantage may be lost.

Effective remote system operations depend on the sophistication of their motion control. The unit must be able to find a particular location and remain on site while the transducer is placed and the test signal is received.

Summary

Three areas of underwater ultrasonic testing have been described: thickness gaging, weld testing and flooded member detection. For each application, the use of a diver and topside inspector team is advocated.

1. With specialized training for both the diver and the inspector, the difficult task of corrosion evaluation can be accomplished with a thickness gaging system. On coated or corroded surfaces, an accurate thickness measurement can be obtained using a single-element transducer and measuring travel time between successive back wall echoes. Conventional instrumentation requires little modification before being used offshore. A typical test system consists of an ultrasonic discontinuity detector, an impedance matched cable several hundred meters (about 1000 ft) long, a waterproofed connector, a highly damped transducer (generally 5 MHz) and a transducer housing or standoff.

2. Underwater ultrasonic weld testing on complex tubular joints is discouraged because of the geometrical complexities involved in ray tracing through curved tubular sections. Although the required calculations can be made with a personal computer, the diver must measure the position and angular orientation of the transducer on members having no reference marks. The time and development effort required to train and equip a diver, or provide a transducer tracking unit, have been found economically unacceptable, but without this effort the proper interpretation of ultrasonic signals is impossible. Alternative test methods (visual or magnetic particle testing) are recommended for service induced cracking.

3. Flooded member detection using an extended version of the pulse echo thickness gaging technique provides a global method of determining whether there is water in a member. If there is, then a through-wall crack or penetration due to corrosion is probably present. Although there is a small probability of missing the flooded condition, there is virtually no chance of calling an unflooded member flooded. Proper front surface preparation minimizes the probability of missing the flooded condition.

Under water, ultrasonic testing is an effective method for detecting and quantifying corrosion damage and through-wall cracking. Together with visual and magnetic particle testing, ultrasonic techniques can be effectively used to assess periodically the structural condition of offshore structures.

References

1. CFR 1910.119, *Process Safety Management Regulations.* Washington, DC: Government Printing Office.
2. Clark, B.[H., Jr.] and R.[K.] Stanley. Section 20, "Ultrasonic Testing Applications in the Chemical Industries." *Nondestructive Testing Handbook,* second edition: Vol. 7, *Ultrasonic Testing.* Columbus, OH: American Society for Nondestructive Testing (1991): p 702-721.
3. ASME B31.3, *Process Piping.* New York, NY: ASME International.
4. Engblom, M., D.K. Mak and G. Pont. Section 17, Part 3, "Oil Field Applications of Ultrasonic Testing." *Nondestructive Testing Handbook,* second edition: Vol. 7, *Ultrasonic Testing.* Columbus, OH: American Society for Nondestructive Testing (1991): p 585-591.
5. Johnson, J. "Trigonometric Relations for the Ultrasonic Inspection of Tubular Goods." *Materials Evaluation.* Vol. 43, No. 12. Columbus, OH: American Society for Nondestructive Testing (November 1985): p 1489.
6. Mak, D.K. "Ultrasonic Inspection of Tubular Goods Using Two Probes in Tandem." *Materials Evaluation.* Vol. 45, No. 9. Columbus, OH: American Society for Nondestructive Testing (March 1987): p 396.
7. API 510, *Pressure Vessel Inspection Code: Maintenance Inspection, Rating, Repair and Alteration, Refining Department,* fifth edition. Washington, DC: American Petroleum Institute (December 1987).
8. ANSI/NB-23, *National Board Inspection Code.* Columbus, OH: National Board of Boiler and Pressure Vessel Inspectors (1987).
9. Bednar, H.H. *Pressure Vessel Design Handbook,* second edition. New York, NY: Van Nostrand Reinhold (1986).
10. Amos, D.M. "Magnetic Flux Leakage Testing of Aboveground Storage Tank Floors." *Nondestructive Testing Handbook,* third edition: Vol. 5, *Electromagnetic Testing.* Columbus, OH: American Society for Nondestructive Testing (2004): p 387-389, 399.
11. Sherlock, C.N. "Nondestructive Inspection Requirements for Aboveground Storage Tanks." *Materials Evaluation.* Vol. 54, No. 2. Columbus, OH: American Society for Nondestructive Testing (February 1996): p 145-146, 148-155.
12. *ASNT Recommended Practice No. SNT-TC-1A.* Columbus, OH: American Society for Nondestructive Testing.
13. API 620, *Design and Construction of Large, Welded, Low-Pressure Storage Tanks.* Washington, DC: American Petroleum Institute.
14. API 650, *Welded Steel Tanks for Oil Storage.* Washington, DC: American Petroleum Institute.
15. API 653, *Tank Inspection, Repair, Alteration, and Reconstruction.* Washington, DC: American Petroleum Institute.
16. *ASME Boiler and Pressure Vessel Code,* Section VIII, Division 1 (*Lower Stress Design*) *Requirements* (*Excludes Parts UF, UB, UCI, UCD and ULW*). New York, NY: ASME International.
17. *ASME Boiler and Pressure Vessel Code,* Section VIII, Division 2 (*High Stress Design*) *Requirements* (*Excludes Parts F-7 and F-8*). New York, NY: ASME International.
18. Pont, G.W. "Ultrasonic Inspection of Oil Country Tubular Goods." *Materials Evaluation.* Vol. 46, No. 10. Columbus, OH: American Society for Nondestructive Testing (September 1988): p 1250, 1252-1253.
19. ISO 15463, ANSI/API RP 5A5, *Field Inspection of New Casing, Tubing, and Plain-End Drill Pipe.* Washington, DC: American Petroleum Institute (2005).
20. API SPEC 5CT, *Specification for Casing and Tubing,* eighth edition. Washington, DC: American Petroleum Institute (2006).
21. API RP 5UE, *Recommended Practice for Ultrasonic Evaluation of Pipe Imperfections.* Washington, DC: American Petroleum Institute (2005).
22. Goldberg, L.[O.] and J. Mittleman. Section 19, Part 2, "Ultrasonic Testing of Offshore Structures." *Nondestructive Testing Handbook,* second edition: Vol. 7, *Ultrasonic Testing.* Columbus, OH: American Society for Nondestructive Testing (1991): p 690-702.

23. Traverse, C.A. "Offshore — A New Era." *Petroleum Engineer International*. Vol. 51, No. 10. Houston, TX: Hart Publications (August 1979).
24. Brackett, R.L. "Underwater Inspection of Waterfront Facilities." *Proceedings of the Annual Meeting*. ASME paper 81-WA/OCE-5. New York, NY: American Society of Mechanical Engineers (November 1981).
25. Brackett, R.L., L.E. Tucker and R. Erich. *Pulse Echo Ultrasonic Techniques for Underwater Inspection of Steel Waterfront Structures*. Technical report R-903. Port Hueneme, CA: Naval Civil Engineering Laboratory (June 1983).
26. AWS D1.1-80, *Structural Welding Code: Steel*. Miami, FL: American Welding Society.
27. API RP2X, *Recommended Practice for Ultrasonic Examination of Offshore Structural Fabrication and Guidelines for Qualification of Ultrasonic Technicians*, fourth edition. Washington, DC: American Petroleum Institute (2004).
28. Singh, A. and R. McClintock. "Computer Controlled System for Nondestructive Thickness Measurement of Corroded Steel Structures." *Journal of Energy Resources Technology*. Vol. 105. (December 1983).
29. Mittleman, J. *Impedance Matching for Long Cables Carrying Ultrasonic Signals*. TM 325-81. Panama City, FL: Naval Coastal Systems Center (October 1981).
30. Johnson, W.C. *Transmission Lines and Networks*. New York, NY: McGraw Hill Publishing Company (1950).
31. Mittleman, J. "Underwater Ultrasonic Inspections." *Proceedings of the Twenty-Seventh Defense Conference on Nondestructive Testing* [Yuma, AZ, October 1978].
32. Mittleman, J. and D. Wyman. "Underwater Ship Hull Examination." *Naval Engineer's Journal*. Vol. 92, No. 2. Washington, DC: American Society of Naval Engineers (April 1980).

Bibliography

Alleyne, D.N. and P. Cawley. "Long Range Propagation of Lamb Waves in Chemical Plant Pipework." *Materials Evaluation*. Vol. 55, No. 4. Columbus, OH: American Society for Nondestructive Testing (April 1997): p 504-508.

ANSI/API 573, *Inspection of Fired Boilers and Heaters*. Washington, DC: American Petroleum Institute (2003).

ANSI/ASNT ILI-PQ-2005, *In-Line Inspection Personnel Qualification and Certification*. Columbus, OH: American Society for Nondestructive Testing (2005).

API 570, *Piping Inspection Code: Inspection, Rating, Repair, Alteration, and Rerating of In-Service Piping Systems*. Washington, DC: American Petroleum Institute (2006).

ASME Boiler and Pressure Vessel Code: Section V, *Nondestructive Examination*. New York, NY: ASME International.

Engblom, M. "Considerations for Automated Ultrasonic Inspection of In-Service Pressure Vessels in the Petroleum Industry." *Materials Evaluation*. Vol. 47, No. 12. Columbus, OH: American Society for Nondestructive Testing (December 1989): p 1332, 1334-1336.

Ginzel, E.A. *Automated Ultrasonic Testing for Pipeline Girth Welds: A Handbook*. Waltham, MA: Olympus NDT (2006).

Ginzel, E.A. and G. Legault. "Mechanized Ultrasonic Inspection of Offshore Platform Structures." *Materials Evaluation*. Vol. 56, No. 4. Columbus, OH: American Society for Nondestructive Testing (April 1998): p 511-516.

Harkreader, K. "Effects of Temperature on High Density Polyethylene Piping and Accuracy of Ultrasonic Thickness Gaging." *Materials Evaluation*. Vol. 59, No. 9. Columbus, OH: American Society for Nondestructive Testing (September 2001): p 1033-1036.

Hayden, J.J. and R.W. Pechacek. "Ultrasonic Imaging in the Petroleum Processing Industry." *Materials Evaluation*. Vol. 47, No. 12. Columbus, OH: American Society for Nondestructive Testing (December 1989): p 1372, 1374, 1376.

ISO 11960, *Petroleum and Natural Gas Industries — Steel Pipes for Use as Casing or Tubing for Wells*, third edition. Geneva, Switzerland: International Organization for Standardization (2006).

Joshi, N.R. "Statistical Analysis of UT Corrosion Data from Floor Plates of a Crude Oil Aboveground Storage Tank." *Materials Evaluation*. Vol. 52, No. 7. Columbus, OH: American Society for Nondestructive Testing (July 1994): p 846-849. Erratum, Vol. 52, No. 11 (November 1994): p 1285.

NACE International Publication 8X294, *Review of Published Literature on Wet H_2S Cracking of Steels through 1989*. Item 24185. Katy, TX: NACE International (2003).

Sherlock, C.N. "A Catch-22: Leak Testing of Aboveground Storage Tanks with Double Bottoms." *Materials Evaluation*. Vol. 52, No. 7. Columbus, OH: American Society for Nondestructive Testing (July 1994): p 827-832.

Sherlock, C.N. "A Materials Evaluation Special Issue: Aboveground Storage Tanks." *Materials Evaluation*. Vol. 52, No. 7. Columbus, OH: American Society for Nondestructive Testing (July 1994): p 799.

Stanley, R.K. "Ultrasonic Distances Useful in Oilfield Tubular Inspection." *Materials Evaluation*. Vol. 47, No. 3. Columbus, OH: American Society for Nondestructive Testing (March 1989): p 272, 274-275.

Weisweiler, F.J. and G.N. Sergeev. *Non-Destructive Testing of Large-Diameter Pipe for Oil and Gas Transmission Lines*. Deerfield Beach, FL: VCH (1987).

Proceedings of Chemical and Petroleum Industry Inspection Technology Topical Conferences

Petroleum Industry Inspection Technology [Houston, TX, June 1989]. Columbus, OH: American Society for Nondestructive Testing (1989).

International Petroleum Industry Inspection Technology II Topical Conference [Houston, TX, June 1991]. Columbus, OH: American Society for Nondestructive Testing (1991).

1993 International Chemical and Petroleum Industry Inspection Technology (ICPIIT) III Topical Conference [Houston, TX, June 1993]. Columbus, OH: American Society for Nondestructive Testing (1993).

ASNT's International Chemical and Petroleum Industry Inspection Technology (ICPIIT) IV Topical Conference [Houston, TX, June 1995]. Columbus, OH: American Society for Nondestructive Testing (1995).

ASNT's International Chemical and Petroleum Industry Inspection Technology (ICPIIT) V Topical Conference [Houston, TX, June 1997]. Columbus, OH: American Society for Nondestructive Testing (1997).

ASNT's International Chemical and Petroleum Industry Inspection Technology (ICPIIT) VI Topical Conference: The Challenges to NDT in the New Millennium [Houston, TX, June 1999]. Columbus, OH: American Society for Nondestructive Testing (1999).

Second Pan-American Conference for Nondestructive Testing (PACNDT) and ASNT's International Chemical and Petroleum Industry Inspection Technology (ICPIIT) VII Topical Conference [Houston, TX, June 2001]. Columbus, OH: American Society for Nondestructive Testing (2001).

ASNT's International Chemical and Petroleum Industry Inspection Technology (ICPIIT) VIII Topical Conference [Houston, TX, June 2003]. Columbus, OH: American Society for Nondestructive Testing (2003).

ASNT's International Chemical and Petroleum Industry Inspection Technology (ICPIIT) IX Conference [Houston, TX, June 2005]. Columbus, OH: American Society for Nondestructive Testing (2005).

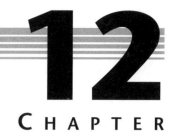

Electric Power Applications of Ultrasonic Testing

Anmol S. Birring, NDE Associates, Webster, Texas

Part 1. Inservice Inspection in Power Plants

Nondestructive testing has been applied with great success to the power generation industry, in both nuclear and fossil plants. Power companies have pooled resources for development of some of the most advanced nondestructive test systems. Basic ultrasonic techniques have been integrated into systems and are routinely applied for inspections.

Nondestructive testing has resulted in safe operation of components, reduced forced outages, extended plant lives and reduced outage periods. Moreover, technologies developed in the power industry have benefited other industries, especially petrochemical.

Components of Power Plant

The power plant can be divided into four basic components: (1) steam generators, (2) steam lines, (3) turbine generators and (4) condensers.

Steam Generation in Nuclear Plants

There are two basic types of nuclear power plants: pressurized water reactor (PWR) and boiling water reactor (BWR). The major difference between them is the means of steam generation. In a pressurized water reactor, steam is generated in a two-step process. In the first step, heat produced by fission of the nuclear fuel is transferred to pressurized water in the reactor pressure vessel. The pressurized water from the reactor pressure vessel is then circulated in the steam generators to produce steam by heat transfer.

The steam generator is basically a large heat exchanger. Typically, a nuclear plant has one reactor pressure vessel and two to four steam generators. The piping system running the pressurized water from the reactor pressure vessel to the steam generator is known as the primary loop. The pressurized water flows through the steam generator tubes and in that process transfers heat to the secondary loop, producing steam. The steam from the steam generators exits to the secondary piping and is sent to the turbines.

The design of the boiling water reactor is different. Unlike the pressurized water reactor, the boiling water reactor has no separate steam generator. Steam is produced in the reactor and is sent directly to the turbines for power generation.

Ultrasonic testing is applied extensively to the reactor pressure vessel, nozzles and the piping systems of nuclear plants.

Steam Generation in Fossil Plant

Steam in a fossil fired power plant is produced in a boiler. Fossil fuel — typically coal, gas or oil — is burned to produce heat. Heat is transferred to the water that flows in the tubes of the boiler wall. The water changes phase and transfers to steam. Steam from the water wall headers is sent into super heater tubes where it picks up additional heat and then cycles to the super heater outlet headers. The main steam lines then carry steam to a high pressure steam turbine. To improve the heat rate, steam from the exhaust of the high pressure steam turbine is returned back to the boiler where it is reheated in tubes known as *reheater tubes*. After reheating, the steam is sent to the low pressure turbines via reheat headers and reheat steam lines. Although the boiler may seem to be a simple component, the high temperatures and pressures encountered in the boiler lead to the use of creep resistant alloy steels in boiler tubes. Other than carbon steel, materials include 1.25 percent chromium, 0.5 percent molybdenum steel; 2.25 percent chromium, 1.0 percent molybdenum steel; and stainless steel. In boiler tubes, the major failure mechanisms are corrosion, erosion, mechanical fatigue, thermal fatigue, creep and oxidation. To avoid such failures, ultrasonic testing is applied extensively in power boilers.

Steam Lines

Steam lines carry high pressure steam from the boiler to the turbine. The line from the superheater headers to the turbine is called the main steam line. When steam is sent back to the boiler, the line is called the *cold reheat line*; after heating, the steam returns to the low pressure turbine in the hot reheat line. The steam lines in a fossil plant are made of 1.25 percent chromium, 0.5 percent molybdenum steel and 2.25 percent chromium, 1.0 percent molybdenum steel. Both magnetic particle testing and ultrasonic testing are used to test steam lines.

Turbines

Turbines convert the energy in the steam to a rotary motion for power generation. There are three types of turbines: high pressure, intermediate pressure and low pressure. Damage mechanisms in turbines differ with operating conditions. High pressure turbines operate at high temperatures in a dry steam environment. Low pressure turbines operate at relatively lower temperatures and in a dry/wet steam environment. Damage mechanisms in turbines include creep, stress corrosion cracking, corrosion fatigue and stress fatigue. Much ultrasonic testing is performed on the steam turbine rotors and disks.

Condensers

Before the steam is sent back to the boiler, it must be condensed. This operation is performed in a condenser, which is basically a large heat exchanger. Water from a lake, sea, river or canal passes through the condenser tubes; steam passes around the tubes and is condensed. Various tube materials are used in condenser tubes. These include copper nickel alloys, brass and titanium. Almost no ultrasonic testing is performed in the condensers.

In addition to these components, nondestructive testing is performed on auxiliary components, including feedwater heaters, boiler feed pump turbines, pumps, valves and pipes.

Inservice Inspection

The driving forces behind the nuclear plant inspections are code requirements, plant life extension and costs. Basic inspections in a nuclear plant are performed in accordance with Section XI of the *ASME Boiler and Pressure Vessel Code*.[1] On the basis of current plant experience and plant life extension, the Nuclear Regulatory Commission mandates additional testing. Furthermore, the move towards deregulation in the United States power industry has reduced outage time for refueling and maintenance. All of these considerations have led to advanced test programs that use the latest technology to minimize inspection time and cost.

The nondestructive testing specified in Section XI is done on a sample of welds. For example, 25 percent of the reactor coolant piping system welds must be examined during each inservice inspection interval. Also, if discontinuities are found, then additional tests are required and components containing discontinuity indications are required to be examined more frequently in the future. Section XI of the *ASME Code* has historically specified nondestructive test requirements on how to perform inspections. The philosophy of the *ASME Code* has gradually changed to specify test criteria, leaving the procedures up to the inspecting organizations. The performance demonstration requirements are intended to verify that nondestructive test systems can detect the minimum discontinuity size identified by acceptance criteria in the *ASME Code*, Section XI.

In addition to the basic inspections as per Section XI, more inspections are required when plants want to extend the license past the normal life of 40 years. Virtually all the major components and structures within a nuclear plant complex must be evaluated in the life extension program.[2] The program therefore triggers inspections in addition to inspections in accordance with Section XI. For the nuclear plants to be economical, the reactor pressure vessel inspections must be conducted in the shortest amount of time. Reactor pressure vessel tests fall on the critical path of a nuclear plant refueling outage.

The philosophy of nondestructive testing in fossil plants differs from nuclear plants. Unlike nuclear plants where inspections are required for regulatory reasons, fossil plants are inspected for reducing forced outages, condition assessment and plant safety. Because of a range of equipment and a number of damage mechanisms, a variety of nondestructive test techniques are applied. These range from simple magnetic particle testing to advanced ultrasonic phased array techniques. Because of minimal regulations, it is easier to implement new nondestructive test technologies in the fossil plants without going through a rigorous administrative and demonstration process. For this reason, some techniques in nondestructive testing are implemented in fossil plants before nuclear plants. However, because of the large resources available for maintenance, the inspection systems in nuclear plants are more sophisticated and advanced.

Another difference between nuclear and fossil inspections are additional requirements because of radiation. Extensive use is made of remote control scanners and robotic devices for areas with hazardous radiation. There is no such requirement for remote inspection in fossil power plants.

Damage is assessed in both nuclear and fossil plants to determine degradation of material properties. Damage assessment tests can include sample removal, hardness testing and in-situ metallographic replication. Proper selection of the nondestructive test is necessary for reliable testing of these components.

Part 2. Nuclear Power Plants

Reactor Pressure Vessels

Pressurized Water Reactors

Ultrasonic testing is performed on nuclear plant components for volumetric inspections. All shell, head, shell-to-flange, head-to-flange and repair welds are subjected to a 100 percent volumetric examination during the first interval.[3] Ensuing test intervals require fewer beltline region, head and repair weld tests. All nozzle-to-safe and butt welds with dissimilar metals (that is, ferritic steel nozzle to stainless steel or to heat resistant nickel chromium alloy) are subjected to volumetric and surface tests at each interval. All studs and threaded stud holes in the closure head studs undergo surface and volumetric tests at each inspection interval. Any integrally welded attachments are required to have surface (or volumetric) tests of welds at each test interval. Ultrasonic testing of the pressurized water reactor is performed after removing the head and internals and placing a tripod device on top of the reactor.

Figure 1 shows a modern ultrasonic test system for pressurized water reactor welds.[4] The system is used for the vessel seam welds, flange-to-shell welds, nozzle-to-shell welds, nozzle-to-piping welds, meridional (lower head) welds, shell-to-lower head welds and nozzle inner radius. The three legs are placed on the vessel flange and can reach approximately 10 m (33 ft) down to the lower head. The reactor is filled with water during the examination. Telescopic devices with transducer heads are then inserted in the nozzles to conduct the tests. The system in Fig. 1 is shown in a compressed position for setup on the vessel. These tests must first be demonstrated on actual mockups of pressurized water reactors to ensure detection of the discontinuities.

Boiling Water Reactors

Boiling water reactor vessels consist of a cylindrical shell and a hemispherical bottom head containing both the control rod penetrations and the in-core instrumentation penetrations. The top head is hemispherical and includes nozzles with bolting flanges attached.

The pressurized water reactor vessel inservice inspection methods and requirements of Section XI of the *Code* are the same for boiling water reactor vessels. However, many older boiling water reactors have very limited accessibility for internal inservice inspection. Typically, 70 to 90 percent of the vessel weld lengths were exempted as inaccessible. The main difficulty in inspection of boiling water reactors is the access to the welds below the top of the core elevation in the boiling water reactor. The inaccessibility results from the narrow clearance between the vessel sidewall and shroud

FIGURE 1. Ultrasonic system for testing of pressurized water reactor welds — welds of vessel seams, of flange to shell, of nozzle to shell, of nozzle to piping, of shell to lower head welds, of meridian (on lower head) and of nozzle inner radius. Unit on left is used to dock the module containing pulser preamps and transducers to change these units quickly without removing device from vessel.

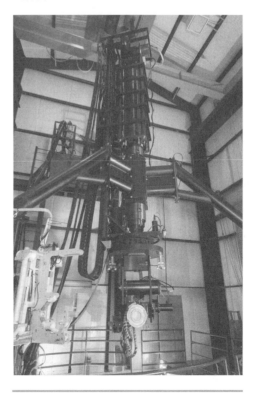

surrounding the core barrel. The clearance is typically in the 150 to 300 mm (6 to 12 in.) range at the top and can be less at the bottom of the vessel. Clearance varies from the top (inlet) to the bottom (outlet) of the jet pumps. For this reason, the boiling water reactor inspections have always been limited to the elevations above the top core level.

The limited examination is however not acceptable for evaluation of aging plants that need license renewal. For this reason, in 1992, the Nuclear Regulatory Commission formally announced that boiling water reactor plants would need to increase the test coverage of welds in boiling water reactors.

To meet the Nuclear Regulatory Commission's requirements, several companies in the nuclear service industry designed robotic tooling to access these welds from the inside surface. Several inspection agencies funded programs to conduct additional inspections required by the Nuclear Regulatory Commission. One such device for conducting inside surface examinations on boiling water reactor shell welds was developed (Fig. 2).

The system combines the mechanical scanner with the advanced ultrasonic data acquisition and analysis system for inspection of vessel welds. Software tools are integrated into these systems for acquisition, for real time data processing and for test tracking. The tracking tool provides a real time display of the surface location of the scan module by using a drawing of the reactor pressure vessel or examination area. The tools are designed to use drawings routinely generated by nondestructive testing companies during planning and scanning. During an examination, these tools are interfaced to the acquisition software to obtain and display the scan module coordinates in real time. Figure 3 displays a rollout drawing of a typical boiling water reactor vessel as well as surface views of the lower and upper head assemblies. For tests, the vessel rollout drawing is used to map a specific examination. During a test, the scan module surface location is recorded on the selected test area drawing (Fig. 3). When the inspection is complete, the user can save the file for subsequent recall and display.

Primary System Piping

Pressurized Water Reactor

The design of coolant piping differs according to the design (Table 1).[5] In many early plants, the main coolant piping is wrought stainless steel.

The type of materials and fabrication results in several ultrasonic procedures for inspection. The two main problems are

FIGURE 3. Circumferential wall of boiling water reactor. Locations of individual measurements are recorded in database to track test progress and examination history.

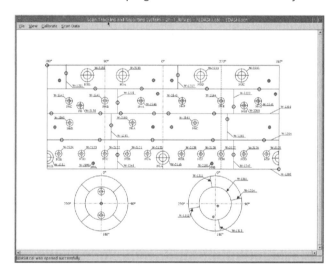

FIGURE 2. Scanner designed to pass through tight spaces in boiling water reactor vessel below top core elevations with gaps of 150 to 300 mm (6 to 12 in.).

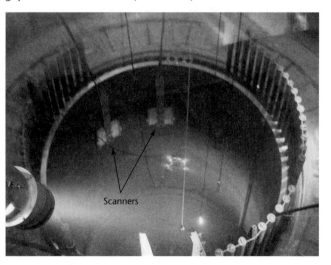

Scanners

TABLE 1. Coolant piping typical in power plants in the United States.

Steel Coolant Piping	Cladding
Centrifugally cast stainless	—
Wrought stainless steel	—
Wrought ferritic	weld deposited stainless
Wrought ferritic	roll bonded stainless

the stainless steel clad and the grain structure of cast stainless piping. The stainless steel clad results in impedance mismatch and multiple signals while performing an ultrasonic test. Anisotropy in the cast stainless steel results in transverse wave velocities that can differ greatly, depending on the direction of sound propagation relative to crystal direction. The velocity of longitudinal waves varies less than that of transverse waves.[6] Angle beam longitudinal waves are therefore used for testing of cast stainless pipes instead of transverse waves. Typically, dual-element refracted longitudinal wave transducers are used to improve sensitivity.

The major locations for pressurized water reactor piping ultrasonic inspections are (1) main coolant pipe nozzles, (2) terminal and dissimilar metal welds and (3) cast stainless steel.

Boiling Water Reactor

Intergranular stress corrosion cracking near weldments in boiling water reactor stainless steel piping has been occurring since the 1980s. Early cases were in relatively small diameter piping. In early 1982, cracking was identified in large-diameter piping in a recirculation system of an operating boiling water reactor plant in this country. Since then, extensive inspection programs have been conducted on boiling water reactor piping systems. These inspections have resulted in the detection of significant numbers of cracked weldments in almost all operating boiling water reactors.[7]

Inservice inspection as required as per Section XI of the *ASME Code* has not always been able to detect cracks that develop during service. Detection of intergranular corrosion is particularly difficult and tests of cast stainless steel is mistrusted. Substantial efforts in research and development have led to the development of test procedures and inspector training for detection and sizing of such cracking. Training programs have been conducted using samples with intergranular stress corrosion cracks. Inspectors are first trained in the ultrasonic techniques and then tested with actual discontinuities. The detection is performed using probes in the frequency range of 1.5 to 2.25 MHz. Although the techniques use conventional pulse echo transverse waves, inspectors are trained to recognize the signals from intergranular stress corrosion cracking.

The sizing of such cracking is more complex. The most accurate technique for measuring the crack depth is tip diffraction. One problem with intergranular stress corrosion cracking is

that, unlike fatigue cracks that have a well defined tip, the crack tips of intergranular cracks are not well defined and blend into the microstructure.

Time-of-flight diffraction in the pitch catch mode is an accurate sizing technique.[8] High attenuation of stainless steels limits the use of higher frequencies such as 10 MHz that are preferred for time-of-flight diffraction. Inspection is done by scanning the probes along the weld length. A set of probes to include pulse echo and time-of-flight diffraction are included in the scanner for ultrasonic inspection. Manual techniques using multiple-beam probes that combine longitudinal and transverse waves are also used for sizing such cracks. These angle beam probes have dual crystals and transmit longitudinal waves at about 1.22 rad (70 deg) and transverse waves at 0.52 rad (30 deg) (Fig. 4). These probes were developed in the mid eighties and are now commercially available. In addition, creeping wave probes that use single element 1.22 rad (70 deg)

FIGURE 4. Multiple-beam approach for ultrasonic sizing of intergranular stress corrosion cracking in stainless steel: (a) cross section; (b) high-frequency waveform.

(a)

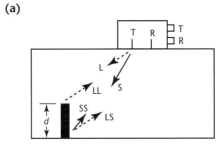

(b)

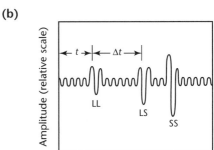

Time (relative scale)

Legend
d = notch depth
L = longitudinal wave
LL = longitudinal wave refracted from longitudinal wave
LS = longitudinal wave reflected from transverse wave
R = receiving element
S = transverse wave
SS = transverse wave reflected from transverse wave
T = transmitting element
t = time interval

longitudinal wave probes are used for crack detection and sizing.

The transition of materials from the reactor body to the piping system is complex and a challenge for ultrasonic testing of nozzles with dissimilar metal welds. Intergranular stress corrosion cracking in dissimilar metal welds has been detected since the 1980s. Cracking initiates in high temperature, nickel chromium alloy welds. The cracking of dissimilar metal welds was addressed first in boiling water reactors and later in pressurized water reactors.

Dissimilar metal welds are between the reactor pressure vessel and the main recirculation piping in the boiling water reactor and between the reactor pressure vessel and the reactor coolant piping in the pressurized water reactor. The reactor pressure vessel nozzles are low alloy carbon steel, and the piping is usually stainless steel. Between the reactor nozzle and the piping is the safe end. A stainless steel or high temperature, nickel chromium alloy weld buffer is deposited on the face of the nozzle weld preparation end. The stainless steel safe end is welded to the reactor nozzle using a stainless steel or high temperature, nickel chromium alloy weld metal. Figure 5 shows a cross section of the dissimilar metal weld. However, the geometries of dissimilar metal welds vary from plant to plant.

In addition to the weld design, the grain growth of the dissimilar metal weld can be quite complex and depends on the weld material, thermal gradient and the welding procedure. Hence, qualification for the ultrasonic method requires tests on mockups that cover the range of dissimilar metal weld designs and welds. In 1990, the United States Nuclear Regulatory Commission issued a notice about weld cracking in boiling water reactors, stating that this application of ultrasonic transverse waves is unreliable.[9] Refracted longitudinal waves must be used to improve the reliability of testing.

Dissimilar metal welds have been tested with 1 to 4 MHz refracted longitudinal waves in the 0.52 to 1.22 rad (30 to 70 deg) range. Both single-crystal and dual-crystal probes are used for this test. Technicians performing such tests are qualified on mockups of dissimilar metal welds with embedded cracks.

Nozzles are another difficult component to test because of their complex geometry. Figure 6 shows a scanner performing a test of a nozzle. The main problem in nozzle testing is to determine the refracted and skew angles of the ultrasonic beam to ensure adequate coverage of the nozzle inner surface. Phased arrays have turned out be a powerful tool for the testing of complex geometries such as nozzles (Fig. 7).[10]

The major locations for boiling water reactor piping ultrasonic tests are (1) furnace sensitized, heat affected zones, (2) high thermal stress regions predicted by stress rule index analysis, (3) austenitic ferritic stainless steel castings with high delta ferrite levels and (4) shaft sleeves and other crevices.

Nuclear Plant Life Extension

Nuclear plants were built with a design life of 40 years. However, as plants approach their end of life, a need arises for plant life extension. Several plant life extension plans were initiated in the mid 1980s. The programs were designed to develop programs for renewing the license of nuclear plants. The Nuclear Regulatory Commission provides significant detail on such inspections.[11,12] Included in these detailed inspections are volumetric (usually ultrasonic) tests for component assessment.

FIGURE 5. Schematic configuration of a typical dissimilar metal weld in a boiling water reactor. The exact geometry and weld configuration will vary from plant to plant.

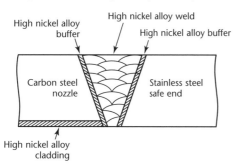

High nickel alloy buffer

High nickel alloy weld

High nickel alloy buffer

Carbon steel nozzle

Stainless steel safe end

High nickel alloy cladding

FIGURE 6. Testing of nozzle in nuclear plant. Scanner using multiple probes operates under remote control.

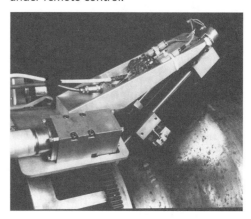

In accordance with the *ASME Code,* the program consists of periodic volumetric, surface and visual tests of reactor vessels, internals and reactor coolant system components and their supports to assess condition, detect degradation and take corrective actions.

This program includes a detailed list of inspections. Some of the inspections include determination of the susceptibility of cast austenitic stainless steel components to thermal aging embrittlement. Loss of material due to general, galvanic, pitting and crevice corrosion could occur in tanks, piping, valve bodies and tubing in the reactor coolant pump oil collection system in fire protection. The fire protection program relies on a combination of visual and volumetric examinations to manage loss of material from corrosion.

Aging is managed through either enhanced volumetric examination or plant specific or component specific discontinuity tolerance evaluation. Inspections require that detection of aging effects should occur before there is a loss of the structure and component intended function(s). The parameters to be monitored or inspected should be appropriate to ensure that the intended functions of the structure and components would be adequately maintained for license renewal under all design conditions. This includes aspects such as method (visual, volumetric or surface testing), frequency, sample size, data collection and timing of new or one-time tests to ensure timely detection of aging effects.

The details of the nuclear plant life extension and license renewal program are discussed elsewhere.[11,12]

FIGURE 7. Phased arrays, beam steering and skewing allow testing of nozzle's complex geometry: (a) cut-away view of nozzle; (b) cross section of nozzle; (c) planar view of water wall tubes.

(a)

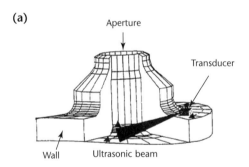

(b)

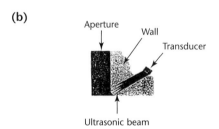

(c)

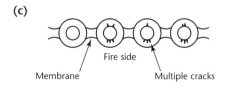

PART 3. Fossil Power Plants

Fossil Plant Boilers

There are 22 failure mechanisms directly responsible for failure of boiler tubes. Table 2 shows test methods used for boiler maintenance. Boiler tubes are usually the number one cause of forced outages in a thermal power plant.

Outside Surface Erosion, Corrosion and Overheating

Erosion, fireside corrosion and short term overheating cause outer diameter wall loss in a boiler. Outside surface erosion is a serious issue in coal fired boilers where high erosion rates require regular inspections. Wall thickness measurements are performed with commercially available ultrasonic digital gages with circuits that detect the signal reflected from the tube's inside surface. The instrument measures the thickness of the wall by converting the signal reflection time into thickness.

The accuracy of digital gages depends on the surface roughness of the component being measured. The gage specifications claim to have an accuracy of 25 µm (0.001 in). However, it is common to find errors as great as 0.25 mm (0.010 in.). These errors are produced by inconsistent procedures. They are not produced because of an instrumentation deficiency. To minimize errors, digital gages with a small A-scan display must be used. The display allows the inspector to validate the signal

TABLE 2. Nondestructive testing of boilers.

Material	Damage Mechanism	Discontinuity	Test Technique
Superheater and reheater tubing			
Chromium molybdenum stainless steel	Long term creep	inside surface oxide scale	high frequency ultrasonic
	creep fatigue in dissimilar metal weld	cracks on ferritic side	transverse wave ultrasonic
	erosion, fire side corrosion	wall loss	longitudinal wave ultrasonic
Waterwall tubing			
Carbon steel	erosion, fire side corrosion, short term overheat	wall loss	longitudinal wave ultrasonic
Carbon molybdenum steel and chromium molybdenum steel	corrosion fatigue, stress corrosion cracking, chemical attack	inside surface cracking	transverse wave ultrasonic
	thermal fatigue, corrosion fatigue	inside/outside surface cracking	visual, transverse wave ultrasonic
	hydrogen damage	inside surface pitting	scanning ultrasonic
	caustic corrosion	inside surface pitting	scanning ultrasonic
	clinker impact	dents, rupture	visual
Waterwall coatings			
—	erosion	loss of coating thickness	electromagnetic thickness gaging, visual
Economizer tubing			
Carbon molybdenum steel	corrosion fatigue	cracking	transverse wave ultrasonic

corresponding to the measurement. Thickness calibration must be performed on a curved calibration block or plate to simulate actual boiler tube geometry. In addition, transducer alignment on both the boiler tube and the calibration block should be identical.

Inside Surface Corrosion

Inside diameter pitting in boiler tubes may be caused by caustic corrosion, hydrogen damage, chemical attack and similar mechanisms. Because this type of pitting is usually isolated, a careful examination of the broiler tube length is required. The process is more difficult than spot thickness measurement of tubes with generalized outside surface wall loss. Digital gages are severely limited when measuring tubes with inside surface pitting. Ultrasonic scattering from inside surface pits produces a noisy reflected signal. This may produce an undefined back surface reflection signal that can create gross errors in measurement.

Digital gages measure the thickness up to the first signal that breaks the threshold. This may be the wrong signal. An error produced by incorrect signal identification may be as high as ±100 percent. For this reason, digital thickness gages without an A-scan display should be used cautiously when measuring thickness of tubes with inside surface pitting. An instrument should be used with an A-scan screen display to identify the back wall reflection. Once the back wall is correctly identified, the thickness can be measured using both screen display and digital readout.

Hydrogen damage is one of the mechanisms that produce inside surface corrosion. This damage is produced in the water wall tubes by imbalance in water chemistry.[12] Tubes experiencing high heat flux (across burners), locations of flow interruptions (tube bends, circumferential welds) are locations most susceptible for such damage. Hydrogen damage is serious because it results not only in inside surface corrosion but also a zone of decarburized material under the corroded area. Ultrasonic thickness scanning is the first step toward detection of corrosion caused by hydrogen damage. Because inside surface corrosion can be caused by other mechanisms, hydrogen damage should be verified by other nondestructive test methods. Decarburization caused by hydrogen damage reduces the ultrasonic velocity. Velocity can therefore be measured to verify such damage.[13]

Cracking

Depending on the damage mechanism, boiler tubes can experience both axial and circumferential cracks on the outside surfaces as well as inside surfaces. Outside surface cracking in a boiler tube can be produced through thermal fatigue, corrosion fatigue and other means. Visual, magnetic particle, liquid penetrant and radiographic testing are commonly applied for detection of cracking on the outside surface. Inside surface cracks with axial orientation may be caused by stress corrosion and corrosion fatigue mechanisms (Fig. 8)

The first step in the inspection process is to determine the optimum refracted angle for the transducer. The maximum refracted angle θ_{max}, which results in a normal incident angle at the inside surface, may be calculated from the incident angle at the outside surface. At this angle, the ultrasonic beam touches the inside surface and is normal to the crack face. Refracted angles higher than θ_{max} cause the ultrasonic beam to not even touch the inside surface and therefore miss small inside surface cracks. A refracted angle that maximizes reflectivity from the crack should be selected.

A 10 mm (0.4 in.) diameter transducer is preferred for 75 mm (3 in.) diameter tubing. Smaller transducers such as 6 mm (0.25 in.) diameter may be used on smaller tubing such as in the super critical units, for example, 40 mm (1.6 in.) diameter tubes. The small diameter transducer is also suited for inspecting the inner radius of tube bends.

Dissimilar metal weld cracking occurs in welds that join the low alloy steels with stainless steel. These welds are present in high temperature sections of the boiler, including the superheater and reheater sections. Dissimilar metal welds crack along or near the fusion line between the low alloy steel tube and the alloy weld. In addition to cracking, an oxide notch is commonly found on the outside surface of the dissimilar metal weld. An oxide notch is initiated because of differences in the creep strength between a weld metal

FIGURE 8. Corrosion fatigue cracking leading to boiler tube failure: (a) side view; (b) end view.

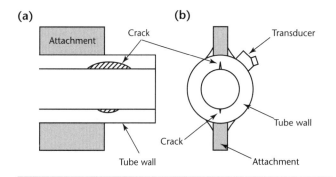

and the low alloy steel heat affected zone. The presence of an oxide notch is not an indication of crack. Ultrasonic testing and radiographic testing are two methods to inspect dissimilar metal welds. When properly applied, these methods can resolve dissimilar metal weld cracking from the oxide notch.

Creep from Inside Surface Oxide Scale

Inside surface oxide scale can be produced when tubes in the reheater and superheater have experienced high temperatures for extended periods of time.[14,15] The formation of inside surface scale reduces heat transfer and results in a further increase of tube metal temperature. The increase in inside surface scale and the associated tube metal temperature promotes creep and reduces tube life. The final outcome of excessive scale is a thick lipped, long term overheat failure (Fig. 9). Scale thickness measurements should be taken just upstream of material upgrade and thickness upgrade locations. A history of prior long term overheat failures should also be used to select tubes for oxide scale testing. The ultrasonic method for measuring scale thickness is based on transmitting a wave through the tube thickness. The thickness is calculated by measuring the time difference between the signals reflected from the interface of steel to scale and the tube inside surface. Because of the extremely small time difference, the application requires high frequency transducers in the range of 15 to 30 MHz. If the scale thickness and the operating hours are known, the remaining life of the tube can be calculated.[14]

Fossil Plant Headers

Circumferential welds in the headers are inspected for cracking in the welds and ligaments (Fig. 10). Testing is done using ultrasonic and wet fluorescent magnetic particle testing. Outside diameter cracking is inspected using magnetic particle testing whereas inside surface or midwall cracks are inspected by ultrasonic testing. Testing is performed with 12 to 19 mm (0.5 to 0.75 in.) diameter transducers producing transverse waves at 2.25 MHz. The test is pulse echo.

A common form of cracking in the headers is called ligament cracking. This cracking is common in the secondary super heater outlet headers with greater wall thickness. There have been several cases at power plants of header leaks because of ligament cracking. Leakage precedes failure in headers. This cracking initiates in the bore holes on the inside surface of the header, grows along the length of the borehole and propagates between the tubes. Historical data reveals that this cracking is generally at the hottest tubes but exceptions can occur. Common to certain designs, the cracking occurs because of cyclic events. These include startups, shutdowns, transients and thermal shocks. There is no correlation of this cracking to the age of the header.

The most common method for inspection of ligament cracking is fluorescent liquid penetrant testing. This test is done after removal of a sample of tubes from the stub tube welds. Ligament cracking can be detected between two adjacent tubes if there is enough space between them for the ultrasonic transducer. However, ultrasonic sizing of

FIGURE 9. Boiler tube failure from creep in reheater tubes. Inside diameter oxide measurements taken using high frequency ultrasonic tests are used to calculate remaining creep life.

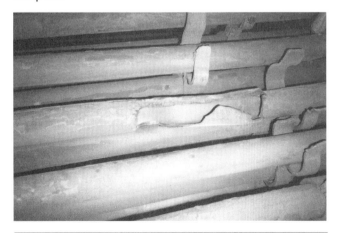

FIGURE 10. Inspection of a header in fossil plant. Ultrasonic testing can be used to detect ligament cracking between tubes if there is enough spacing between tubes for transducer placement.

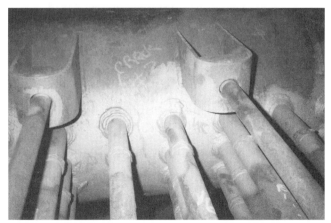

cracks for this inspection is not very reliable. Table 3 lists test methods for headers.

Fossil Plant Steam Lines

There has been significant interest in the inspection of steam lines after some highly publicized failures in the United States. Although cracks in the girth welds produced by fatigue initiate on the outside surface and can be detected by magnetic particle testing, cracking in the seam welded piping can only be detected by ultrasonic testing.

Seam welded pipes can contain a variety of fabrication discontinuities that can act as preferred sites for creep crack initiation and propagation. High temperature creep can cause midwall cracking or inside surface connected cracking in seam welds. Over a long period of time, creep voids can grow to microcracks, interlink and cause failure of a long seam weld.[14,15] The failure of a steam line can either be a *leak before failure* or a rupture. The type of failure depends on the length of the crack. Cracks longer than the critical length can result in rupture. Ultrasonic testing is recommended for such tests.

There are three techniques: pulse echo transverse wave, time-of-flight diffraction and phased arrays. All three are reliable if qualified on representative samples. The techniques have limitations.

1. Manual transverse wave is quite sensitive but full coverage is not guaranteed. There have been cases where inspectors have missed weld areas because of inadequate scanning coverage.
2. Although time-of-flight diffraction is effective, there have been cases where inspectors using low instrument gain have missed relevant discontinuities. Establishing adequate gain is very important for the reliability of time-of-flight diffraction.
3. Phased array ultrasonic testing is effective because it covers a range of angles while conducting the test.

Figure 11 shows ultrasonic scanning performed using a combination of pulse echo and time-of-flight diffraction to improve inspection reliability. Again, the procedure must be qualified on representative discontinuities. The effect of pipe curvature should be accounted for in both the manual transverse wave and phased array techniques. Table 3

TABLE 3. Nondestructive testing of steam lines and headers.

Material	Damage Mechanism	Discontinuity	Test Technique
Hot reheat piping			
Chrome molybdenum stainless steel	creep and fatigue	cracking in girth and long seam welds	transverse wave ultrasonic, magnetic particle, acoustic emission testing
Main stream piping			
Carbon steel	creep and fatigue	cracking in girth welds	transverse wave ultrasonic, magnetic particle, acoustic emission testing
Headers (economizer, hot reheat, superheat outlet)			
carbon, carbon molybdenum, carbon manganese, chromium molybdenum steel	creep and creep fatigue	stub tube and header cracks	magnetic particle testing
		ligament cracking	transverse wave ultrasonic; fiber optic visual testing
		cracks in bore holes	liquid penetrant, eddy current testing
		girth weld cracking, long seam cracking	transverse wave ultrasonic, magnetic particle testing
Drain lines, feedwater recirculation lines			
Carbon steel, chromium molybdenum steel	erosion	wall loss	longitudinal wave ultrasonic
Hangers and supports			
Carbon steel	corrosion, fatigue overload	metal loss, cracking	visual testing; magnetic particle testing

summarizes test methods used for steam lines.

Turbines

Several components are inspected in a turbine: the bore, disk keyway, disk blade attachment area, blades, nozzles, casing and bolts.

Bore

The mechanism of crack growth in a rotor bore is caused by the combined action of creep and fatigue.[14] Creep is more prevalent in high pressure rotors that operate close to 540 °C (1000 °F). Fatigue is more prevalent in low pressure rotors that operate at lower temperatures. Although it is important that the entire length of the bore be inspected for axial cracks, there are certain locations along the bore length that are very critical and require a high sensitivity inspection. Small discontinuities in these locations can grow rapidly and lead to a rotor burst. Critical locations are ones that experience the highest level of hoop stress and temperature. The hoop stress is higher under the disks because of mass loading. The temperature is highest under the control stage. Sensitivity of ultrasonic testing should be highest at the inside bore surface under the high pressure disks.

Three methods are commonly used for bore inspection: magnetic particle, eddy current and ultrasonic testing. The first two methods are limited to surface discontinuities. Magnetic particle testing is performed by applying a circumferential magnetic field at the bore inside surface. The circumferential field detects axial cracks on the bore surface.

Ultrasonic testing is the only method that can perform a complete volumetric examination. A combination of transducer angles is used to perform the inspection, including 0 rad (0 deg), 0.79 rad (45 deg) and 1.05 rad (60 deg), looking in the clockwise and counter clockwise directions. The transducers are installed on a scanner and the data recorded on an ultrasonic imaging system (Fig. 12). Adjusting the step interval between each scan controls the detection sensitivity. In addition to discontinuity detection, damage assessment is done in the bore to determine any loss of fracture toughness. Indirect measurements such as remote replication and small punch test sample removal are performed to assess material degradation.

Solid Rotor

The main advantage of a boreless rotor is its lower level of stresses compared to the bored rotor. The lower level of stress makes the boreless rotor tolerant of larger discontinuities. A solid rotor is tested by using a combination of longitudinal wave and transverse wave transducers. Inspection of boreless rotors requires that the selected angles cover the entire material volume of interest. As an alternative, phased arrays that sweep a range of angles can be used.

Transverse cracking in low pressure rotors initiates from corrosion pits and can grow during service by fatigue corrosion. Transverse cracking is easily detected by application of magnetic particle testing on the rotor outside surface. The depth of the crack can be measured using ultrasonic tip diffraction.

FIGURE 11. Simultaneous application of time-of-flight diffraction and pulse echo techniques to improve discontinuity detection reliability.

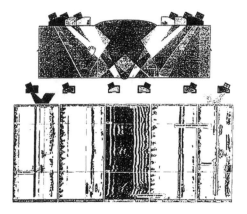

FIGURE 12. Turbine bore is scanned with six ultrasonic probes — 0, 0.75 and 1.0 rad (0, 45 and 60 deg) in clockwise and counterclockwise directions.

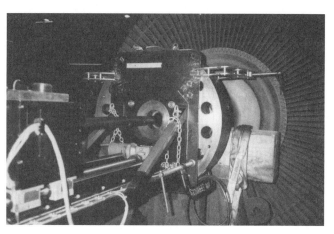

Disk Keyway Cracking

The primary cause of disk keyway cracking is stress corrosion. High stress concentration in the keyway region promotes growth of this cracking. Because of stress corrosion cracking, keyway cracking is mostly observed after steam begins to transform from dry to wet. In some cases, stress corrosion cracking may be found sooner if condensation occurred during standby. Ultrasonic testing of keyway cracking is performed either using multiple refracted angles or using phased array transducers, which can sweep a range of angles electronically.

Both pulse echo and pitch catch modes are used during testing. Alignment of the transducers, in the pitch catch mode, is very important for a reliable inspection.

Attachment of Disk to Blade

The mechanism of crack initiation and growth in the attachment of turbine disk to blade (steeples) depends on three variables: the operating temperature, stresses and environment. Creep is the primary mechanism in high pressure and intermediate pressure rotors, but its mechanism is not discussed here. Stress corrosion cracking, combined with fatigue, is the primary mechanism for low pressure rotors. Initially, cracking in a low pressure rotor grows slowly by stress corrosion. When the stress intensity K_I exceeds K_{th}, crack growth is predominantly due to fatigue. Crack growth rates in this mode are significantly high because of vibratory loads. Generally, failure can be imminent when the threshold for fatigue crack growth K_{th} is reached. Therefore, it is important that nondestructive tests detect cracks before their stress intensity reaches K_{th}.

The test method applied to detect steeple cracking depends on the geometry. Dovetail shaped turbine blades are inspected only by ultrasonic testing.[16] Phased array or multiple single-element transducers are used for inspection. Side entry steeples allow access for surface inspection.

Figure 13 shows ultrasonic inspection of the blade attachment areas. The ultrasonic probes are placed on a stationary arm and the turbine is placed on turning rolls. Data are taken as the turbine rotates slowly, once or twice per minute. In addition to ultrasonic testing, these disks can be inspected by eddy current testing and magnetic particle testing. However, ultrasonic testing is the only method that can inspect the entire length of the side entry steeple under the blade.

Once the blades are removed, wet fluorescent magnetic particle testing is preferred for testing steeples. The slow process results in a highly sensitive inspection.

Blades

The failure mechanism of turbine blades depends on their temperature, environment and stress state. Corrosion fatigue is the major failure mechanism of blades in the next-to-last stage of the low pressure turbine. Creep blade failures are limited to high pressure turbines. Cracking of blades occurs at the following three locations: blade attachments, airfoil and tenon. Eddy current and magnetic particle testing are the two methods used to inspect the blade attachment areas of side entry blades.

Blade tenons are located at the tip of the blades and hold the shroud. Cracking and failure of the tenons may release the shroud and cause mechanical damage to other blades. The only method available to inspect blade tenons is ultrasonics. An ultrasonic transducer is placed on a flat surface of the tenon so that a contact with a transducer can be achieved. Tenons without a flat face cannot be inspected unless they are ground flat.

High Temperature Bolts

Creep rupture and brittle fracture are two primary reasons for bolt failures. The low toughness that leads to brittle fracture is due to the inherent high strength of bolts. The failures are usually initiation controlled. Hence, the failure time is very short after the crack initiation.

Cracking in bolts occurs only in the threads next to the joint. These threads experience the highest level of stress. The stress on the last thread at the end of the bolt is almost zero. Therefore, the

FIGURE 13. Inspection turbine disk blade attachment areas. Turbine placed on rollers rotates while test data are acquired.

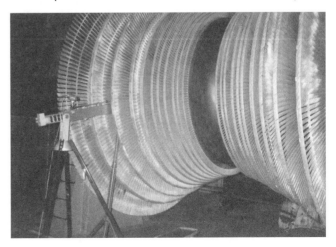

inspector should carefully investigate threads right next to the joint.

Ultrasonic testing is the only method that can inspect bolts without removing them from the casing. One of two ultrasonic approaches is used for this inspection. A zero degree examination is performed when the top surface of the bolt is flat because it allows placement of a normal beam transducer. But when the top face of the bolt is not flat, an angle beam test is performed through the heater holes in the bolt.

Retaining Rings

The susceptibility of 18 percent manganese, 5 percent chromium steels to stress corrosion cracking produces cracking in retaining rings when moisture enters and settles on the inner surface. The initiation time of the cracks is long but, once the crack has begun, crack growth can be rapid. The high crack growth rate limits nondestructive testing for crack detection. No effort is made to size the cracks once they are detected. Repair or replacement actions are initiated once a crack is positively detected.

Four methods are generally used when inspecting the retaining rings: (1) visual, (2) fluorescent liquid penetrant, (3) eddy current and (4) ultrasonic testing. Visual, eddy current and fluorescent methods can be applied only after ring removal. Visual testing is accomplished using borescopes that detect moisture in accessible areas of the inside surface. Evidence of moisture is an indication of possible crack initiation. The penetrant examinations are performed using the fluorescent penetrant method. High sensitivity lipophilic emulsifiers are used for these inspections. Ultrasonic testing is the only method that may be applied without removal of the retaining ring, however its detection sensitivity is limited. A combination of adverse factors, such as high ultrasonic attenuation and spurious geometrical reflections, results in the low ultrasonic detection sensitivity.

Condensers

The testing of condensers is normally limited to a 2 to 5 percent random sample of tubes. The information from the test can then be used to make decisions on replacement of all the tubes.

Conventional eddy current testing is applied for inspection of condenser tubing. Because of the long length of the tubing, inspection of condenser tubing is done at high speed manually or using pusher/pullers.

Feedwater Heaters

Tube failures in feedwater heaters are a major cause of forced outages in a fossil power plant. Inspection of high pressure feedwater heaters produces one of the highest cost benefits of any nondestructive test in a power plant. Conventional eddy current is applied for nonferromagnetic materials. Remote field eddy current is quite effective for testing of carbon steel tubing. Ultrasonic internal rotary testing is typically not used for feedwater tube inspections because it is slow.

Closing

Nondestructive testing has been developing in terms of damage assessment, data acquisition, analysis and reliability. Methods to detect and characterize incipient or early stages of damage will be applied on a wider scale. More sophisticated systems will be introduced for inspection using faster, smaller and economical computer hardware. There will be more emphasis on improving the reliability of nondestructive test methods, especially characterization of discontinuities. This may include upgrading personnel qualification to improve inspection reliability.

In summary, ultrasonic tests for power plants include (1) thickness measurements, (2) thickness scanning, (3) high frequency testing for scale measurements, (4) transverse wave testing for crack detection and sizing, (5) longitudinal wave testing for crack detection, (6) multimode testing for crack detection and sizing, (7) automated testing for corrosion mapping, (8) automated testing for crack detection and sizing, (9) time-of-flight diffraction for crack detection and sizing, (10) phased arrays for crack detection and sizing and (11) phased arrays for complex geometries, such as nozzles.

In addition to the above list, nuclear plant inspections include (1) inspection of cast stainless steels, (2) detection and sizing of intergranular stress corrosion cracking, (3) detection and sizing of underclad cracking, (4) inspection of nozzles from inside surface and outside surface, (5) inspection of dissimilar metal welds, (6) detection of radiation embrittlement and other aging mechanisms that cause embrittlement and decrease fracture toughness, (7) detection of cladding disbond, (8) remote inspections and (9) inspections in areas with limited accessibility.

References

1. *ASME Boiler and Pressure Vessel Code:* Section XI, *Rules for Inservice Inspection of Nuclear Power Components.* New York, NY: ASME International (2001).
2. Shah, V.N. and P.E. McDonald, eds. NUREG/CR-4731, *Residual Life Assessment of Major Light Water Reactor Components.* Washington, DC: United States Nuclear Regulatory Commission (Vol. 1, June 1987; Vol. 2, November 1989).
3. Server, W.L., G.R. Odette and R.O. Ritchie. "Pressurized Water Reactor Pressure Vessels." NUREG/CR-4731, *Residual Life Assessment of Major Light Water Reactor Components.* Vol. 1. Washington, DC: United States Nuclear Regulatory Commission (June 1987): p 12-31.
4. Hamlin, D.R., J.L. Fisher and J.F. Crane. "Acquisition and Analysis System for Rapid Inspection of Large Structures." *Proceedings of the 2nd EPRI Conference on NDE in Relation to Structural Integrity for Nuclear Pressurized Components* [Charlotte, NC, 2000]. Palo Alto, CA: Electric Power Research Institute (2000).
5. Cloud, R.L. and W.L. Server. "Pressurized Water Reactor Coolant Piping." NUREG/CR-4731, *Residual Life Assessment of Major Light Water Reactor Components.* Washington, DC: United States Nuclear Regulatory Commission (June 1987): p 55-65.
6. Singh, A. "Flaw Location Errors in Extruded Stainless Steel Pipes." *Ultrasonics.* Vol. 21, No. 6. Surrey, United Kingdom: Elsevier (November 1983): p 270-274.
7. Mantle, H. "Boiling Water Reactor Recirculation Piping." NUREG/CR-4731, *Residual Life Assessment of Major Light Water Reactor Components.* Washington, DC: United States Nuclear Regulatory Commission (June 1987): p 108-113.
8. Charlesworth, J.P. and J.A.G. Temple. *Engineering Applications of Time-of-Flight Diffraction.* Taunton, Somerset, United Kingdom: Research Studies Press (1989).
9. NRC Information Notice 90-30, *Ultrasonic Inspection Techniques for Dissimilar Metal Welds.* Washington, DC: United States Nuclear Regulatory Commission (1990).
10. Dube, N. *Introduction to Phased Array Ultrasonic Technology Applications.* Quebec, Canada: RD Tech (2004).
11. NUREG-1800, *Standard Review Plan for Review of License Renewal Applications for Nuclear Power Plants.* Washington, DC: United States Nuclear Regulatory Commission (July 2001).
12. NUREG-1801, *Generic Aging Lessons Learned (GALL) Report.* Vol. 1, Rev. 1. Washington, DC: United States Nuclear Regulatory Commission (September 2005).
13. French, D.N. *Metallurgical Failures in Fossil Fired Boilers.* New York, NY: Wiley (1993).
14. Birring, A.S., D.G. Alcazar, J.J. Hanley and S. Gehl. "Ultrasonic Detection of Hydrogen Damage." *Materials Evaluation.* Vol. 47, No. 3. Columbus, OH: American Society for Nondestructive Testing (March 1989): p 345-350, 369.
15. Viswanathan, R. *Damage Mechanisms and Life Assessment of High-Temperature Components.* Materials Park, OH: ASM International (1989).
16. Viswanathan, R., S.R. Paterson, H. Grunloh and S. Gehl. "Life Assessment of Superheater/Reheater Tubes in Fossil Boilers." *ASME Journal of Pressure Vessel Technology.* Vol. 116, No. 1. New York, NY: ASME International (February 1994).
17. Ciorau, P. and D. MacGillivray. "In Situ Examination of Low Pressure Steam Turbine Components Using Phased Array Technology." *Proceedings 2nd International Conference on NDE.* [New Orleans, LA, 2000]. Palo Alto, CA: Electric Power Research Council (2000).

Bibliography

Avioli, M., Jr., M. Behravesh, M. Engblom, D. Kupperman, D.K. Mak and G. Pont. Section 17, "Ultrasonic Testing Applications in Utilities." *Nondestructive Testing Handbook,* second edition: Vol. 7, *Ultrasonic Testing.* Columbus, OH: American Society for Nondestructive Testing (1991): p 569-591.

Birring, A.S. "Selection of NDT Techniques for Heat Exchanger Tubing." *Materials Evaluation.* Vol. 59, No. 3. Columbus, OH: American Society for Nondestructive Testing (March 2001): p 382-391.

Birring, A.S., M. Riethmuller and K. Kawano. "Ultrasonic Techniques for Detection of High Temperature Hydrogen Attack." *Materials Evaluation.* Vol. 63, No. 2. Columbus, OH: American Society for Nondestructive Testing (February 2005): p 110-115.

Birring, A.S. and B.K. Nidathavolu. "Ultrasonic Testing of Welds by Time of Flight Diffraction: Codes, Guidelines and Standards." *Materials Evaluation.* Vol. 63, No. 9. Columbus, OH: American Society for Nondestructive Testing (September 2005): p 910-914.

Light, G.M., N.R. Joshi and S.-N. Liu. "Cylindrically Guided Wave Technique for Inspection of Studs in Power Plants." *Materials Evaluation.* Vol. 44, No. 5. Columbus, OH: American Society for Nondestructive Testing (April 1986): p 494.

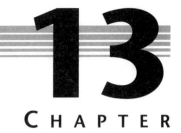

CHAPTER

Infrastructure Applications of Ultrasonic Testing

Amos E. Holt, Southwest Research Institute, San Antonio, Texas (Part 1)

John S. Popovics, University of Illinois, Urbana, Illinois (Part 2)

PART 1. Ultrasonic Testing of Wood and Structural Steel[1]

Need for Ultrasonic Testing of Structures

Nondestructive testing of buildings and highway bridges is variously performed as maintenance, performance demonstration, degradation studies, load verification or quality assurance inspection — depending on the location or technical discipline. Such testing functions are carried out periodically to meet a variety of local, state and federal regulations. For bridges, the testing criteria can depend on many factors, including increased or altered operating conditions, system problems, transient events and aging. The purpose of the nondestructive test is to ensure the continued safe operation of the structure by detecting or verifying a condition that makes the structure incapable of performing its design function and so makes it a threat to safety.

As population density and technology accelerate, the need for nondestructive testing is increasingly evident. In heavily populated areas, for example, bridges are now used as pathways over large masses of the population. Consequently, there is a need to improve the nondestructive tests used to detect degradation in bridge structures. In addition, bridges are now being built with inexpensive, lighter weight materials, again necessitating improved nondestructive test methods.

Typically, bridges are visually tested. If an anomaly is detected visually, then other test methods are used. Ultrasonic testing is done to evaluate the material rather than to diagnose problem areas.

Highway Bridges

Some bridge types in highway systems around the world are shown in Fig. 1.[2] A typical bridge consists of a substructure, a superstructure and a deck.

The substructure includes (1) abutments, supporting the end of a single span or the extreme end of a multispan superstructure, (2) piers, transmitting the load of the superstructure to the foundation and providing intermediate support between abutments, (3) bearings, transmitting the superstructure load to substructure and providing for longitudinal movement caused by expansion, contraction and rotation from deflection and (4) piles, transmitting the bridge loads to the foundation. Concrete, stone masonry, steel and wood are typical materials for the substructure.

The superstructure is typically built with (1) reinforced concrete beams, (2) rolled steel beams (I beam or channel) for short spans, (3) steel plate girders (made by riveting or welding a web plate to the top and bottom flanges) for intermediate span lengths and (4) steel trusses or arches for spans requiring lengths longer than girders.

The deck includes (1) the structural slab (the load carrying capacity of the deck system), (2) a wearing course (traffic surface) placed on top of the slab, (3) sidewalks, (4) curbs and (5) railings. Typical materials used for the deck elements (excluding the wearing course) are steel plates and beams, prestressed concrete box beams, reinforced concrete and timber.

FIGURE 1. Typical bridge types:
(a) continuous girder; (b) through arch truss;
(c) suspension; (d) cable stayed.

(a)

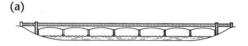

(b)

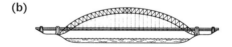

(c)

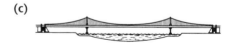

(d)

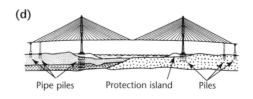

Pipe piles　　Protection island　　Piles

Four construction materials — concrete, steel, wood and fiberglass reinforced plastic — are typically used in bridges and buildings. Many nondestructive testing methods have been developed for these materials. The application of ultrasonic techniques is detailed below.

Ultrasonic Testing of Steel Structures

Steel is an important material in bridges and other civil structures. The two major mechanisms that reduce strength in steel structures are cracking and corrosion. Cracking is usually produced under dynamic loading or fatigue. Corrosion is produced by the environment or deicing chemicals, particularly on steel structures in coastal regions. Corrosion reduces the steel thickness, causing a loss of structural strength.

In significant contrast to concrete testing, ultrasonic frequencies used for testing steel are quite high: 2 to 10 MHz. Both longitudinal and transverse waves are used for steel testing. The speed of longitudinal waves in carbon steel is 5.9 km·s^{-1} and the speed of transverse waves is 3.2 km·s^{-1}.

Thickness measurement is always taken with longitudinal waves and crack detection is usually performed with transverse waves. Corrosion assessment is done with ultrasonic thickness measurements. Digital thickness gages can be used if the corrosion produces a smooth surface. Such gages are not recommended for measurements on rough, corroded or pitted surfaces (error in thickness measurements with digital gages can be as high as 100 percent on rough surfaces). When making thickness measurements on corroded surfaces, a water delay line (bubbler) may be used to couple the ultrasound.

Crack detection in steel frames can be performed using conventional ultrasonic techniques, including angle beam transverse or longitudinal waves.[3]

Many infrastructural fabrications are welded in compliance with the American Welding Society's *Structural Welding Code*.[4] Bridges in particular are welded in compliance with the *Bridge Welding Code*.[5]

Ultrasonic Testing of Wooden Structures

Loss of strength in wood primarily results from decay, infestation (fungi and borers) and mechanical damage. Various fungi attack wood at the surface while borers typically burrow into underwater structures, creating large voids inside the volume of the material. Because of their small entrance holes on the surface, borer damage is very difficult to detect visually.

The most influential factor affecting wave propagation in wood is anisotropy produced by grain structure. The ultrasonic speed along the grains is about three times the speed across the grain (velocity along the grains is about 4.5 km·s^{-1}). Frequencies used for wood testing are the same as those for concrete, ranging from 50 to 150 kHz. Higher frequencies can be used on wood with fine grain or smooth machined surfaces.

Several ultrasonic techniques can be used to detect damage in wood poles.[6] One approach is to measure the travel time in through-transmission mode across the grain. In one application, travel time across the diameter of a pole was measured[7] and an empirical formula was derived to relate this value to the diameter of the decay pocket in the wood. Another detailed study correlates the ultrasonic wave speed with the compression strength of wood exposed to brown rot fungi.[8] A similar approach has been devised for lumber discontinuity detection, where a decrease in wave speed is used to indicate discontinuities.[9]

The wave speed technique has been integrated into a lumber testing system that scans a wooden board, acquires ultrasonic data and processes it to display the location of discontinuities. The technique is limited to a minimum thickness of 50 mm (2 in.). This limit is determined by the rated frequency (0.25 MHz) of the transducers.

Internal damage in wood pilings under water can be detected if the sound propagates in the axial direction (propagation speed is about three times that in water). Ultrasonic testing of piles cannot be performed across the grain because the values of speed and impedance for cross grain wood and water are similar. Marine borer damage can be detected by propagating ultrasound along the wood grain.

Attenuation measurement of ultrasonic waves in the pulse echo mode has also been done.[10] An assessment of the degradation of wood can be made by measuring the attenuation of sound waves. A system based on this technique has been used in commercial applications in Canada. The system uses two magnetostrictive transducers separated by a distance of 1.1 m (42 in.). The transducers generate sound waves at 30 kHz. An electronic instrument measures the attenuation of the signal against a predetermined value and presents it as a reading on water content, a direct indication of the loss of material.

Resonance Test

Resonance and pulse echo tests are based on propagation of compressional waves and can be used along the length of a wooden component.[6] These techniques require access to one end of a wooden pole to transmit and receive the wave. When the end of the pole is not available, a hole can be drilled to position a transducer for transmission and reception of sound waves.

Standing waves are generated with a frequency f that depends on pole length:

$$(1) \quad f = \frac{v}{2\ell}$$

where ℓ is the length (meter) of the pole and v is the speed (meter per second), or velocity, of compressional waves.

Damage in a certain area affects the attenuation of waves and broadens the resonance peaks. The width of the resonance peaks can be correlated to damage in the poles. In place of the resonance technique, the pulse echo technique also can be used. The sound is transmitted along the length of the wood pole, and the durations and intervals of the reflected signal are measured. In cases of internal damage, time measurements of ultrasonic signals can be used to infer the discontinuity location.

Field Testing of Bridges

Bridges are susceptible to environmental stresses, corrosion, earthquake damage, wind damage and fatigue from cyclic traffic loads. Because bridges are more vulnerable to damage or deterioration in service than buildings, bridges require more monitoring of their structural integrity and serviceability. Buildings also tend to be hyperengineered, that is, designed to bear stress greater than that encountered in service. For these reasons, ultrasonic testing is used more often on bridges than on buildings.

Bridge Materials

Reinforced concrete is common in short spans, expressway overpasses and abutments to long span bridges. Steel is the material most used in bridges where tensile strength is needed to support spans and cantilevers. The types of discontinuities found in steel bridge members are different from those found in concrete structures. Some typical forms of degradation common to steel structures include corrosion, fatigue cracking and weld discontinuities.

There are many advantages to ultrasonic testing for inspecting and monitoring bridge structures.[11] For example, ultrasonic testing is less expensive, less hazardous and less cumbersome than radiographic testing.

Ultrasonic instruments with angle beam transducers provide excellent results for detecting cracks, lack of fusion, incomplete penetration and slag in welds. Furthermore, the location and the depth of discontinuities are easily determined with ultrasonic tests. Although size discrimination is a problem and surface finish must be taken into account, the training and experience of the operator compensate for these difficulties.

Ultrasonic test procedures have been performed on a variety of bridge materials, including stone masonry.[12] Knowing the thickness of the materials, time measurements are taken to calculate the speed. From the speed measurements obtained at several points, it is possible to determine the basic internal construction of the bridge, including areas of rubble, fill, solid stone and the lime mortar/masonry hybrid. Speed data reflect also the quality of the bridge construction at different locations on the structure.

Bridge Weld Tests

Ultrasonic discontinuity testing in support of quality standards for welds in bridge construction has been developed at British Rail, addressing weld discontinuities no deeper than 3 mm (0.1 in.). With glass models of weld discontinuities, the procedure for sizing discontinuities was developed by using a distance amplitude correction curve. Weld discontinuities in steel test objects were used to transfer the relation of reflector area to reflected signal amplitude for use in the field.

Steel reference standards were made with 2, 4 and 6 mm (0.08, 0.16 and 0.24 in.) lack of fusion in 35 mm (1.4 in.) thick plate. Except for the 6 mm (0.24 in.) discontinuity, the ultrasonic response correlated with the results on flat bottom hole tests and the glass discontinuity models. The deviation of the 6 mm (0.24 in.) discontinuity occurred because the reflector was larger in area than the ultrasonic transducer.

Two, fixed angle, 1 rad (60 deg) transverse wave transducers and a variable angle transducer set to the optimum angle for maximum reflection from the discontinuity were used in the distance amplitude curve development. Table 1 shows the test results for sidewall lack of fusion. This work, along with preliminary tests on reference standards with flat bottom holes for calibration, established a standard procedure for weld discontinuity detection by ultrasonic techniques in steel bridge structures.

Pin Assemblies[13]

In June 1983 in Connecticut, three people were killed and three more injured when a pin and hanger bridge carrying three eastbound lanes of an interstate highway collapsed and fell 20 m (70 ft) into the Mianus River. In March 1987, a contractor's employee noticed that one span of a highway bridge in Saint Louis, Missouri, had dropped about 45 mm (1.75 in.) at its expansion device. At the end of the investigation, it was found that four of the bridge's twelve pins had failed. In December 1988, the Arkansas River Bridge in Kansas was closed after federally mandated inspections showed it to be in need of repair. Eight of the bridge's ten pins and hangers had failed.

The critical member in each of these incidents is the pin and hanger assembly shown in Fig. 2. The assembly comprises two pins and two hanger plates. The top pin is in a cantilever girder and the other pin is in a suspended girder connected by the two hanger plates.

TABLE 1. Ultrasonic tests of welds containing lack of sidewall fusion.

Actual Area (mm²)	Ultrasonic Signal[a] (dB)	Discontinuity Area Measured Ultrasonically (mm²)
14	6	17
31	14	36
47	14	36

a. Ultrasonic signal with respect to 3 mm (0.12 in.) distance amplitude correction curve.

FIGURE 2. Cantilevered and suspended girder hanger plate and pin assembly.

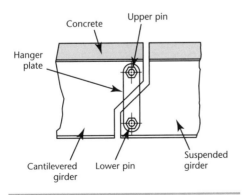

Figure 3 shows a cross section of the pin and hanger assembly. This configuration was designed to allow rotation of the pin in response to temperature induced expansion and contraction. Complications occur when the pin becomes corroded and can no longer move within the assembly. This seizure may result in pin wear and cracking at the hanger locations, potentially causing the pin to fail.

To detect a fracture before total failure, the Federal Highway Administration's National Bridge Inspection Standard mandates that all fracture critical members be tested ultrasonically. The standard includes a brief description of an ultrasonic field demonstration originated to familiarize state Department of Transportation personnel with various bridge inspection techniques, including the ultrasonic testing of bridge pins.[14]

The discontinuity detector used in these demonstrations was chosen for two reasons. First, the unit can be programmed, making each calibration repeatable, accurate and quick. Second, an A-scan presentation or menu screen may be stored and later printed out. Because the Federal Highway Administration requires a copy of all test results, this printout feature is important to most bridge inspection teams.

Straight and angle beam tests are performed to detect a crack, warranting the replacement of a fracture critical member. The straight beam test transmits ultrasound from one end of the pin to the opposite end, to detect fractures that occur where the hanger plates are seated. The test needs to be performed from both ends of the pin to inspect the critical locations on both hanger plates (Fig. 4a).

The angle beam test (Fig. 4b) is used to enhance the reflection of outside diameter cracks and to avoid obstacles or acceptable discontinuities such as cotter pin holes. The beam is directed at a slight angle past the cotter pin hole and strikes

FIGURE 3. Cross section of pin and hanger assembly.

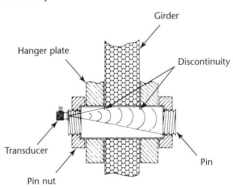

the side wall of the bridge pin. Angle beam testing can reveal cracking or deterioration from corrosion.

The equipment needed to complete such a test includes a contact transducer, an angle beam wedge and transducer and a discontinuity detector. The test procedure is specific to the pin and hanger design. Other bridge testing problems are being solved by transducers and fixtures specifically designed for the variety of bridge pins in use. Sealed transducers are used for underwater tests of bridge components.

Closing

Phased arrays are an important technique in the ultrasonic testing of steel bridge components.[15] This application and others are discussed at length in studies by the United States Federal Highway Administration.[16,17]

Ultrasonic testing has become widely applied for the inspection of concrete, wood and steel structural members. Ultrasonic methods are frequently found to provide more detection sensitivity and discontinuity sizing accuracy than radiographic testing. Additionally, the ultrasonic method is more portable and flexible than radiography and testing can be performed without clearing the area for safety. Despite these advantages, the size and complexity of some bridges make it impractical to perform more than sampling tests of high stress or high fatigue areas.

Continued development of ultrasonic techniques and automated scanners may be necessary as building materials change.

FIGURE 4. Setups for ultrasonic testing of bridge pins: (a) straight beam; (b) angle beam.

(a)

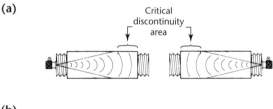

Critical discontinuity area

(b)

Critical discontinuity area

0.09 rad (5 deg)   0.09 rad (5 deg)

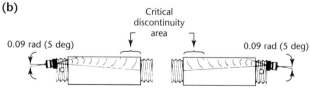

PART 2. Ultrasonic Testing of Structural Concrete[18]

Although conventional ultrasonic techniques are limited by the nature of concrete, modified ultrasonic techniques have been applied to detect internal cracking and other discontinuities, to monitor changes such as deterioration in aggressive environments, to estimate in-place strength and to monitor material strength and stiffness over time. The following discussion reviews the application of selected ultrasonic nondestructive test techniques to concrete structures. The theory and application of through-thickness wave speed testing, ultrasonic imaging and high frequency ultrasonic interface reflection measurements are described.

Introduction

Structural concrete constitutes a significant part of the total infrastructure in the United States. Much of this concrete infrastructure has passed its original design life.[19] Before appropriate rehabilitation can be prescribed, the condition of the structures must be assessed. Nondestructive tests that can detect, localize and characterize damage, deterioration and discontinuities in concrete are of great interest to infrastructure management agencies. Nondestructive testing is important for concrete structures because internal discontinuities may remain hidden from view yet significantly compromise the overall integrity of the structure.

Early detection of discontinuities is the most effective way to reduce maintenance and rehabilitation costs, thereby improving public safety. The deterioration and damage of concrete structures can be described by a variety of physical and environmental damage modes. Common discontinuity modes include delamination, spalling, cracks and voids. In other cases, the geometry or size of a concrete element should be verified by nondestructive means: for example, verifying the thickness of pavement slabs or the depth and shape of poured concrete shafts that act as the supporting foundations for tall buildings. Finally, the strength and stiffness development of concrete over time may be needed.

Concrete structures present specific challenges before nondestructive testing

can be applied effectively. The structures are usually large, and much time is needed to adequately test the entire structure and deep material penetration is often difficult. In addition, concrete naturally exhibits large scale heterogeneous material structure and a variability in local material property. Portland cement as opposed to bituminous asphaltic concrete can have a wide range of mechanical properties. Structural concrete is composed of graded mineral aggregates, up to 30 mm (1.2 in.) in size, bound by an inorganic cement matrix. In addition, most structural concrete contains a grid of reinforcing steel bars or cables. For these reasons, many conventional nondestructive test techniques that work well for steel and other homogeneous materials cannot be applied to concrete. Concrete is unable to transmit high frequencies, as the heterogeneity of the concrete causes signals of smaller wavelengths or wavelengths equal to the nominal aggregate size to be highly scattered and attenuated. For example, high frequency pulse echo A-scans or C-scans cannot be performed directly on concrete because of the intensive backscatter caused by the aggregates.

Nevertheless, some forms of ultrasonic tests have found application in concrete structures. In the present discussion, ultrasonic tests are defined as dynamic measurements using wave frequencies of 20 kHz and greater, where the waves are generated by an electromechanical transducer. Nondestructive testing that makes use of waves generated by an impact event, or sonic tests, will not be discussed here. The development of through thickness ultrasonic wave speed measurement, sometimes referred to as the ultrasonic *pulse velocity* technique, began in Canada and the United Kingdom in the 1940s. Since then, many nations have adopted standardized procedures to measure wave speed in concrete. In the 1960s, one-sided pulse echo systems were developed for concrete.[20] Over the next several decades, additional advances in ultrasonic testing of concrete have been introduced, both for field applications and for laboratory research.[21-25] Nevertheless, through-thickness wave speed tests have remained the most common ultrasonic tests and the only ones standardized for concrete. Below, three types of ultrasonic tests for concrete structures are described: (1) the through-thickness wave speed test, (2) ultrasonic imaging and (3) high frequency ultrasound interface reflection measurements.

Ultrasonic Wave Speed

Background

The ultrasonic wave speed test uses two ultrasonic transducers to measure the travel time of pulses of ultrasonic longitudinal waves (also called *compressional waves*) over a known path length. To measure the ultrasonic wave speed, the sending transducer, driven by a generator, transmits a wave pulse into the concrete. The receiving transducer, separated from the sender by the distance L, receives the pulse through the concrete at another point. The wave pulse transmitted to the concrete undergoes scattering at various boundaries binding aggregate to cement. By the time the pulse reaches the receiving transducer, it gets transformed into a complicated form, which contains multiple reflected longitudinal waves and mode converted transverse waves. However, longitudinal waves travel the fastest and thereby arrive first at the receiver. The wave speed instrument then measures this time of flight T for the first arriving longitudinal wave pulse to travel through the concrete. Alternatively, T can be determined by direct testing of the received wave signal with respect to the known start time of the signal if the equipment is connected to an oscilloscope, or other display device, to observe the nature of the received wave signals. The longitudinal wave speed, or pulse velocity V, is then given by:

$$(2) \quad V = \frac{L}{T}$$

The speed of a wave depends on the elastic properties and density of the medium. For elastic, homogeneous solid media, the longitudinal wave speed is given by the following:[26]

$$(3) \quad V = \sqrt{\frac{KE}{\rho}}$$

where E is the modulus of elasticity, μ is Poisson's ratio, ρ is density and K is defined:

$$(4) \quad K = \frac{1 - \mu}{(1 + \mu)(1 - 2\mu)}$$

The value of K varies within a fairly narrow range. For example, as μ increases from 0.15 to 0.25 (67 percent increase), K increases from 1.06 to 1.20 (12 percent increase). Variations in E and ρ have more significant effects on V than variations in μ has. For concrete, V typically ranges from 3000 to 5000 m·s⁻¹ (9840 to 16 400 ft·s⁻¹), depending on concrete strength, age, moisture content, type and amount of aggregate and proximity to steel reinforcing bars.[27]

Portable ultrasonic wave speed testing units have become available worldwide. Transducers with frequencies of 25 to 100 kHz are usually used for testing concrete, but transducer sets having different resonant frequencies are available for special applications. For concrete, the upper limit of usable frequency is about 500 kHz because the associated wavelength is in tens of millimeters, the size of coarse aggregate particles. As a result, the path length that can be effectively traversed at this upper limit of frequency before the wave pulse becomes completely scattered is only several centimeters. Greater path lengths can be traversed using lower frequencies (and thus larger wavelengths); a frequency of 20 kHz can usually traverse up to 10 m (32.8 ft) of concrete.[28]

To transmit and receive the wave pulse, the transducers must be well coupled to the concrete; otherwise, an air pocket between the transducer and test medium may introduce an error in the indicated transit time. Petroleum jelly has proven to be a good couplant for many cases. If the concrete surface is very rough, thick grease should be used as a couplant. In some cases, the rough surface may have to be ground smooth or a smooth surface may have to be established with plaster of paris, quick setting cement paste or quick setting epoxy mortar.

There are three possible configurations in which the transducers may be arranged (Fig. 5). These are (1) direct transmission (through-thickness transmission), (2) semidirect transmission and (3) indirect or surface transmission. The direct transmission method is the most desirable and satisfactory arrangement because, with this arrangement, maximum energy of the pulse is transmitted and received. The semidirect transmission configuration can also be used quite satisfactorily. However, care should be exercised that the transducers are not too far apart, otherwise the transmitted pulse might attenuate and thus not be detected. The indirect or surface transmission configuration is least satisfactory because the amplitude of the received signal is significantly lower. This technique is also more susceptible to errors and may necessitate a special procedure for determining the wave speed.[29,30]

Wave Speed in Concrete

Aggregate Size, Grading, Type and Content

Wave speed is affected significantly by the type and amount of mineral aggregate in the concrete.[31-35] In general, the longitudinal wave speed of the cement binder is lower than that of aggregate. For the same concrete mixture at the same compressive strength level, concrete with rounded gravel had the lowest wave speed, crushed limestone resulted in the highest wave speed and crushed granite had a speed between these two. Research findings indicate that, at the same strength level, the concrete having the higher aggregate content gives a higher wave speed. The effects of varying the proportion of coarse aggregate in a concrete mixture on the wave speed versus compressive strength relationship

FIGURE 5. Testing configurations for ultrasonic wave speed test: (a) direct; (b) semidirect; (c) indirect.

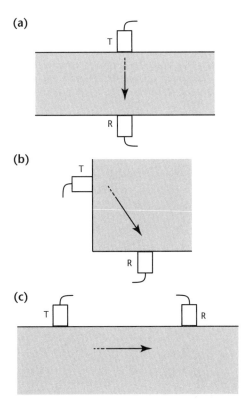

(a)

(b)

(c)

Legend
R = receiving transducer
T = transmitting transducer

are shown in Fig. 6. The figure shows that, for a given value of wave speed, the higher ratio of aggregate to cement, the lower the compressive strength.[36]

Moisture and Curing Condition of Concrete

Concrete is porous and will absorb externally supplied water into its internal pore structure. The wave speed for saturated concrete is higher than for dry concrete. A 4 to 5 percent increase in wave speed can be expected when dry concrete is saturated.[28] It was found that the pulse velocities for laboratory cured specimens were higher than for the site cured specimens.[37] Wave speed in columns cast from the same concrete were lower than in the site cured and laboratory cured specimens.

Presence of Reinforcing Steel

A significant factor that influences the wave speed of concrete is steel reinforcement. The longitudinal wave speed in steel is 1.4 to 1.7 times that in plain concrete. Therefore, wave speed readings in the vicinity of reinforcing steel are usually higher than those in plain concrete. Whenever possible, test readings should be taken such that the reinforcement is avoided in the wave path. If reinforcements cross the wave path, correction factors should be used.

FIGURE 6. Effect of proportions of cement to fine aggregate to coarse aggregate on the relationship between wave speed and compressive strength.[33]

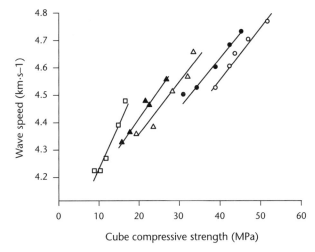

Legend
o = 1:1:2 aggregate ratio
● = 1:1.5:3 aggregate ratio
△ = 1:2:4 aggregate ratio
▲ = 1:2.5:5 aggregate ratio
□ = 1:3:6 aggregate ratio

The importance of including bar diameters as a basic parameter in the correction factors has been demonstrated.[38,39] It should be emphasized, however, that in heavily reinforced sections it might not be possible to measurements the concrete wave speed accurately.

Concrete Compressive Strength and Young's Modulus

The in-place compressive strength of concrete is an important design factor for structural engineers. Concrete gains strength over the first several months after casting as a result of a chemical reaction (the hydration reaction) between the inorganic cement binder and water. The strength of concrete is generally controlled by the relative amount of water to cement binder (the ratio of water to cement by mass) in the concrete mixture and also the age of the concrete. As the ratio of water to cement increases, the compressive and flexural strengths and the corresponding wave speed decrease, assuming no other changes in the composition of the concrete.[37]

The effect of concrete age on the wave speed is similar to the effect upon the strength development of concrete. The speed increases very rapidly initially but soon flattens out.[28] This trend is similar to the curve of strength versus age for a particular type of concrete but wave speed flattens sooner than strength. Once the wave speed curve flattens out, experimental errors make it impossible to estimate the strength with accuracy. Nevertheless, wave speed provides a means of estimating the strength of both in-situ and precast concrete, although there is no physically based relation between the strength and speed.

The strength can be estimated from the wave speed by a preestablished graphical correlation between the two parameters, an example of which is shown in Fig. 7.[36] The relationship between strength and wave speed is not unique: it is affected by other factors such as moisture content and aggregate size, type and content, as described above. No attempts should be made to estimate compressive strength of concrete from wave speed values unless similar correlations have been previously established for the type of concrete under investigation. The American Concrete Institute provides recommended practices to develop the relationship between wave speed and compressive strength, which can be later used for estimating the in-situ strength based on wave speed.[40]

The speed of a longitudinal wave traveling through an elastic material is uniquely defined by the elastic constants and density of the material by wave propagation theory (Eq. 3). Therefore, it is possible to compute the modulus of elasticity of a material if the ultrasonic wave speed is measured where the values of Poisson's ratio and density are known or assumed. This approach has an advantage over another standardized technique, which uses of vibration frequencies, in that the testing is not restricted to specially shaped laboratory specimens. Nevertheless, the estimation of the dynamic modulus of elasticity in concrete from ultrasonic wave speed measurements is not normally recommended for two reasons.

1. The error resulting from inaccurate estimation of Poisson's ratio is significant.
2. Equation 3 is appropriate only for homogeneous materials leaving the validity for heterogeneous composite materials, such as concrete, in doubt.

Usually, the dynamic modulus of elasticity estimated from wave speed measurements is higher than that obtained from vibration measurements, even when the value of Poisson's ratio is known.[41]

Internal Discontinuities

Cracks, voids and other internal discontinuities in concrete will cause variations in the measured wave speed. For example, the diffraction of a wave pulse around an internal air void will cause an increase in the time of propagation with respect to a path through the void center. The measured apparent speed decreases because mechanical waves in solids are not readily transmitted across air or water interfaces.

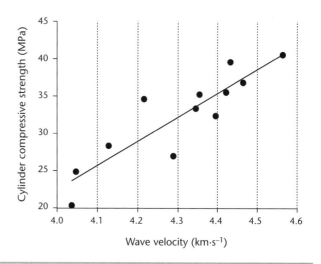

FIGURE 7. Example of relationship of strength versus wave speed for estimation of concrete strength, with an estimated standard error of 2.89 MPa.[33]

However, only large cracks and voids, generally larger than the transducer contact face, will cause measurable reduction in speed.[28] In this regard, the wave speed technique is effective in establishing comparative data for qualitative testing of concrete and is suitable for the study of concrete's heterogeneity.

Here, heterogeneity is defined as interior cracking, deterioration, honeycombing and variations in mixture proportions. For obtaining these qualitative data, a system of measuring points — for example, a grid pattern — should be established. Depending upon the quantity of the concrete to be tested, the size of the structure, the variability expected and the accuracy required, a grid of 300 mm (11.8 in.) spacing, or greater, should be established. Generally about 1 m (39.4 in.) of spacing is adequate.[26]

Other applications of this qualitative comparison of in-situ or test specimen concrete are (1) to check the variation of concrete density to test the effectiveness of consolidation, (2) locating areas of honeycombed concrete and (3) localizing internal cracks and voids.

Several researchers have applied ultrasonic wave speed to measure the depth of surface breaking cracks in concrete using the indirect testing configuration.[42,43] If a pulse traveling through the concrete comes upon an air filled crack or a void whose projected area perpendicular to the path length is larger than the area of the transmitting transducer, the pulse will diffract around the discontinuity (Fig. 8).[36]

For this reason, the pulse travel time will be greater than that through similar concrete without any discontinuity. This technique has serious limitations in locating discontinuities. For example, if cracks and other discontinuities are small, if they are filled with water or other debris (thus allowing the wave to propagate through the discontinuity) or if the crack tip is not well defined, the wave speed will not significantly decrease, implying that no discontinuity exists.[27]

Ultrasonic Imaging

Individual wave data characterize the material along a given wave path. Because the presence of discontinuities and variation in the internal material properties affect the travel time and amplitude of ultrasonic waves along each path, multiple exterior ultrasonic data projections may be assembled to build up a three-dimensional image of the interior of the test object. Tomographic approaches and the synthetic aperture focusing technique enable the assembly of large amounts of data to form such images and have been applied to concrete structures.[44] Both the tomographic and the synthetic aperture focusing technique require collection of many data to reconstruct adequate images, which is computationally and labor intensive.

Tomography

The tomographic technique combines large amounts of physical data, most often ultrasonic speed values, taken from many different intersecting ray paths through the material. The projections are then used to reconstruct a cross sectional view or a three-dimensional property map (for example, a velocity map) of the structure within a specific region. Tomographic imaging software must be used to reconstruct the data collected along ray paths at varying angles; the reconstruction process can be computationally intensive. Several different reconstruction algorithms may be applied, but sufficient data are needed to ensure convergence to the correct solution.[45] Greater numbers of measurements and intersecting ray paths result in more accurate tomograms.[46] In a tomographic reconstruction of speed data collected from a concrete beam. voids and poor concrete regions are indicated by regions of low apparent speed.

Synthetic Aperture Focusing

The synthetic aperture focusing technique numerically superimposes many ultrasonic pulse echo time signals, measured at several positions, to create a high resolution image. The signals are assembled and integrated, or focused, with respect to the time-of-flight surface in volume and time space for each voxel of material. Thus, structural noise is suppressed by spatial superposition[47]

FIGURE 8. Scheme for measurement of surface breaking crack depth h.[33]

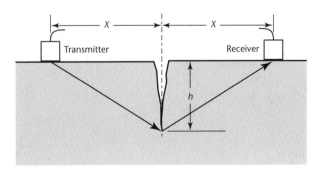

Legend
X = distance from transducer to crack
h = crack depth

Limitations to conventional ultrasonic A-scan testing — limitations due to the high heterogeneity of concrete — are thereby overcome. The synthetic aperture focusing technique provides a three-dimensional map of the backscatter intensity from inside the structure, which may then be interpreted in area (C-scan) or depth (B-scan) slices.[48] Indications of significant backscatter indicate locations of interior air filled voids and cracks.

Reconstruction algorithms for one-dimensional, two-dimensional and three-dimensional synthetic aperture focusing from contact pulse echo measurements have been used to identify and locate indications of significant backscatter from backwall echoes, tendon ducts, voiding and steel reinforcement inside concrete.[44] Transducer arrays are usually used in the measurement. The synthetic aperture focusing technique requires good coupling between transducers and the test surface, which is often difficult to apply to practical testing of concrete because of its inherently rough surface. In addition, only larger discontinuities (greater than 200 mm [7.9 in.] in size) can be detected reliably.[49]

Interfacial Wave Reflection

As cement sets, its stiffness changes because of the hydration of the cement binder. Monitoring the setting and hardening of concrete is often important for economy and structural safety. For example, the efficiency of precast concrete element production can be raised or the timing of concrete form removal can be optimized. Investigators have reported nondestructive monitoring of the hydration process of cement, including several that use ultrasound for this purpose. Early efforts applied ultrasonic through-transmission measurements to characterize the development of the mechanical properties of concrete.[50,51] Since then, it has been shown that the interfacial wave reflection technique has significant advantages over the through-transmission technique. The test can be applied to structures allowing limited access. Data collection can be started immediately after mixing and continue indefinitely. Several researchers have shown that these wave reflection data are directly connected to the mechanical properties of the stiffening concrete, including its strength development.[52-54]

In the technique, an ultrasonic wave pulse (usually 1 to 5 MHz) is launched in a steel plate in contact with the concrete and reflections from the steel-to-concrete interface are monitored. The wave reflection technique monitors the development of the reflection coefficient at the interface between steel and concrete over time, thus the stiffness change (the setting) of the concrete is inferred. When a wave encounters the steel-to-concrete interface, part of the wave energy is transmitted into the concrete and part is reflected back to the transducer. Some of this wave energy is then again reflected from the transducer-to-steel interface into the steel and is again partially reflected when it again hits the steel-to-concrete boundary. The process is illustrated in Fig. 9 where S_T is the transducer signal transmitted into the steel, R_1 and R_2 are the first and second reflections captured by the transducer and T_1 and T_2 are the first and second pulses into the concrete. When a longitudinal wave or transverse wave is reflected at a boundary between two different materials, the reflection coefficient r can be calculated:

$$(5) \quad r = \frac{\rho_2 v_2 - \rho_1 v_1}{\rho_2 v_2 + \rho_1 v_1}$$

where v_1 is the wave speed in material 1, v_2 is the wave speed in material 2, ρ_1 is the density of material 1 and ρ_2 is the density of material 2.

The development of concrete's shear modulus in particular is related to how the microstructure of hydrating cement binder evolves as a result of curing, indicating the development of compressive strength. Thus, transverse waves are often used because the reflection coefficient so determined is

FIGURE 9. Schematic representation of reflection and transmission at interface of steel to concrete.[51]

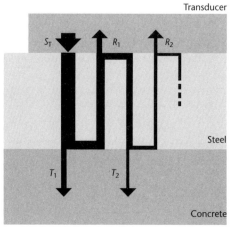

Legend
R_1 = first reflected signal
R_2 = second reflected signal
S_T = signal from transducer
T_1 = first signal transmitted into concrete
T_2 = second signal transmitted into concrete

governed by the development of the concrete shear modulus. A transverse wave traveling through metal and incident upon a steel-to-fluid interface is entirely reflected. Thus, at early ages most of the transverse wave energy is reflected and the amplitude of the received wave is large. As the concrete stiffens, more of the wave energy is transmitted through the concrete and less is reflected at the interface. The magnitude wave reflection can be quantified by using a wave reflection factor, which defines the ratio of the amount of incident wave energy reflected from an interface between two materials[52] or the same ratio expressed in decibels, called *reflection loss*.[54]

Experimental test results show that certain features in the reflection coefficient development curves of concrete correlate well to pin penetration tests and concrete temperature measurements. Plots of typical transverse wave reflection loss (expressed in decibels) as a function of time are shown in Fig. 10. The reflection is measured continuously after casting up to 72 h. Significant changes in the early response of the reflection factor coincide with distinctive stages of hydration. In the initial stage, the temperature inside the concrete decreases followed by a dormant period of thermal inactivity. The reflection loss during this stage remains constant near zero. During this dormant period, the concrete mixture maintains considerable plasticity for several hours, allowing mixing, casting and finishing operations to be carried out. At the beginning of the acceleration period, the temperature inside the specimen increases due to the exothermal reaction of the cement coinciding with initial stiffening and setting. After 5 h, the concrete begins to stiffen noticeably, corresponding with the end of the induction period. At this time,

there is a noticeable increase in the reflection loss response away from zero. This point has been shown to correlate well with the time of initial setting. Afterwards, there is a steady, almost linear increase in the reflection loss, indicating that the observed trends are owing to the change in the mechanical properties of concrete. Inferences about concrete strength development are made during this stage.

Closing

Despite the limitations imposed by the material character, ultrasonic tests have been applied successfully to concrete structures. The ultrasonic wave speed measurement is an effective and practical technique for investigating the uniformity of concrete and, with imaging procedures, provides an effective means to locate interior discontinuities within concrete. The technique can also be used to estimate the strength of concrete in place; however, many variables affect the relations between the strength parameters of concrete and its wave speed. The use of ultrasonic wave speed to estimate the compressive or flexural strengths of concrete is not recommended unless previous correlation testing has been performed. The ultrasonic interfacial wave reflection technique is effective in monitoring the stiffening and hardening process of early age concrete.

FIGURE 10. Transverse wave reflection loss development for three different concrete batches.[51]

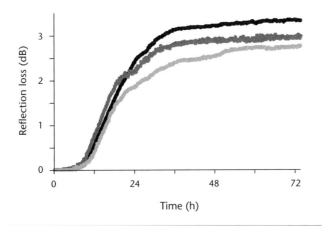

References

1. Holt, A.[E.] and M.[J.] McCurdy. Section 19, Part 1. "Ultrasonic Testing of Bridges and Buildings." *Nondestructive Testing Handbook,* second edition: Vol. 7, *Ultrasonic Testing.* Columbus, OH: American Society for Nondestructive Testing (1991): p 680-689, 701-702.
2. *Manual for Bridge Maintenance.* Washington, DC: American Association of State Highways and Transportation Officials (1976).
3. Krautkrämer, J. and H. Krautkrämer. *Ultrasonic Testing of Materials,* fourth edition. New York, NY: Springer (1990).
4. AWS D1.1/D1.1M, *Structural Welding Code Steel,* Rev. 06. Miami, FL: American Welding Society (2006).
5. AASHTO/AWS D1.5M/D1.5, *Bridge Welding Code.* Washington, DC: American Association of State Highway and Transportation Officials. Miami, FL: American Welding Society (2002).
6. Singh, A., W.D. Jolly, K.J. Krzywosz, E. Reuscher and C.A. Keeney. "Investigation of Inspection Techniques for Timber Waterfront Structures." *Proceedings of the Fourteenth Symposium on Nondestructive Evaluation.* San Antonio, TX: Nondestructive Testing Information Analysis Center (1983): p 513-519.
7. Breeze, J.E. and R.H. Nilberg. "Predicting by Sonic Measurements the Strength of Logs and Poles Having Internal Decay." *Forest Products Journal.* Vol. 21, No. 5. Madison, WI: Forest Products Society (1971): p 39-43.
8. Pellerin, R.F., R.C. DeGroot and G.R. Esenther. "Nondestructive Stress Wave Measurements of Decay and Termite Attack in Experimental Wood Units." *Proceedings of the Fifth Nondestructive Testing of Wood Symposium.* Madison, WI: United States Department of Agriculture, Forest Products Laboratory (1969).
9. McDonald, K.A., R.G. Cox and E.H. Bulgrin. FPL-120, *Locating Lumber Defects by Ultrasonics.* Madison, WI: United States Department of Agriculture, Forest Products Laboratory (1969).
10. Okyere, J.G. and A.J. Cousin. "On Flaw Detection in Live Wood." *Materials Evaluation.* Vol. 38, No. 3. Columbus, OH: American Society for Nondestructive Testing (March 1980): p 43-47.
11. Schaeffer, G.M. "Today's Level of Achievement in NDE in the Bridge Fabrication Industry." Fall Conference [Pittsburgh, PA, October 1982]. *1982 Paper Summaries.* Columbus, OH: American Society for Nondestructive Testing (1982): p 297-301.
12. Whittington, H.W. "Sonic Testing of Civil Engineering Sub and Super Structures." *Proceedings of the Ultrasonics Symposium.* Vol. 2. New York, NY: Institute of Electrical and Electronics Engineers (1984): p 869-876.
13. McCurdy, M.[J.] "Ultrasonic Inspection of Pin Assemblies in Bridges." *Materials Evaluation.* Vol. 47, No. 12. Columbus, OH: American Society for Nondestructive Testing (December 1989): p 1340-1341.
14. 23 CFR 650, *Code of Federal Regulations:* Title 23, *Highways:* Part 650, *Bridges, Structures, and Hydraulics.* Subpart C, "National Bridge Inspection Standards": Paragraph 650.303, "Inspection Procedures." Washington, DC: United States Department of Transportation, Federal Highway Administration; Government Printing Office (2002).
15. *Introduction to Phased Array Ultrasonic Technology Applications.* Waltham, MA: R/D Tech [Olympus NDT Canada] (2004).
16. Moore, M., B.M. Phares and G.A. Washer. FHWA-HRT-04-042, *Guidelines for Ultrasonic Inspection of Hanger Pins.* McLean, VA: Federal Highway Administration (July 2004).
17. Rezai, A., M. Moore, T. Green and G.[A.] Washer. FHWA-HRT-04-124, *Laboratory and Field Testing of Automated Ultrasonic Testing (AUT) Systems for Steel Highway Bridges.* McLean, VA: Federal Highway Administration (April 2005).
18. Popovics, J.S. "Ultrasonic Testing of Concrete Structures." *Materials Evaluation.* Vol. 63, No. 1. Columbus, OH: American Society for Nondestructive Testing (January 2005): p 50-55.

19. *Report Card for America's Infrastructure.* Reston, VA, American Society of Civil Engineers (2003).
20. Bradfield, G. and E.P.H. Woodroffe. "Determining the Thickness of Concrete Pavements by Mechanical Waves: Diverging Beam Method." *Magazine of Concrete Research.* Vol. 16. London, United Kingdom: Thomas Telford (1964): p 45-63.
21. Suaris, W. and V. Fernando. "Ultrasonic Pulse Attenuation As a Measure of Damage Growth during Cyclic Loading of Concrete." *ACI Materials Journal.* Vol. 84. Farmington Hills, MI: American Concrete Institute (1987): p 185-193.
22. Jacobs, L.J. and R.W. Whitcomb. "Laser Generation and Detection of Ultrasound in Concrete." *Journal of Nondestructive Evaluation.* Vol. 16. New York, NY: Plenum (1997): p 57-65.
23. Selleck, S.F., E.N. Landis, M.L. Peterson, S.P. Shah and J.D. Achenbach. "Ultrasonic Investigation of Concrete with Distributed Damage." *ACI Materials Journal.* Vol. 95. Farmington Hills, MI: American Concrete Institute (1998): p 27.
24. Popovics, S., N.M. Bilgutay, M. Karaoguz and T. Akgul. "High-Frequency Ultrasound Technique for Testing Concrete." *ACI Materials Journal.* Vol. 97. Farmington Hills, MI: American Concrete Institute (2000): p 58-65.
25. Purnell, P., T.H. Gan, D.A. Hutchins and J. Berriman. "Noncontact Ultrasonic Diagnostics in Concrete: A Preliminary Investigation." *Cement and Concrete Research.* Vol. 34. Amsterdam, Netherlands: Elsevier (2004): p 1185-1188.
26. ACI 228.2R-98, *Nondestructive Test Methods for Evaluation of Concrete in Structures.* Farmington Hills, MI: American Concrete Institute (1998).
27. *CRC Handbook for Nondestructive Testing of Concrete,* second edition. Boca Raton, FL: CRC Press (2004).
28. Jones, R. *Non-Destructive Testing of Concrete.* London, United Kingdom: Cambridge University Press (1962).
29. Qixian, L. and J.H. Bungey. "Using Compression Wave Ultrasonic Transducers to Measure the Velocity of Surface Waves and Hence Determine Dynamic Modulus of Elasticity for Concrete." *Construction and Building Materials.* Vol. 10. Amsterdam, Netherlands: Elsevier (1996): p 237.
30. Benedetti, A. "On the Ultrasonic Pulse Propagation into Fire Damaged Concrete." *ACI Structural Journal.* Vol. 95. Farmington Hills, MI: American Concrete Institute (1998): p 259.
31. Kaplan, M.F. "The Effects of Age and Water to Cement Ratio upon the Relation between Ultrasonic Pulse Velocity and Compressive Strength of Concrete." *Magazine of Concrete Research.* Vol. 11. London, United Kingdom: Thomas Telford (1959): p 85.
32. Anderson, D.A. and R.K. Seals. "Pulse Velocity as a Predictor of 28 and 90 Day Strength." *ACI Journal.* Vol. 78. Farmington Hills, MI: American Concrete Institute (1981): p 116.
33. Sturrup, V.R., F.J. Vecchio and H. Caratin. "Pulse Velocity as a Measure of Concrete Compressive Strength." ACI SP-82, *In Situ/Nondestructive Testing of Concrete.* Farmington Hills, MI: American Concrete Institute (1984): p 201-227.
34. Swamy, N.R. and A.H. Al-Hamed. ACI SP 82, *The Use of Pulse Velocity Measurements to Estimate Strength of Air-Dried Cubes and Hence In Situ Strength of Concrete.* Farmington Hills, MI: American Concrete Institute (1984): p 247.
35. Popovics, S., J.L. Rose and J.S. Popovics. "The Behavior of Ultrasonic Pulses in Concrete." *Cement and Concrete Research.* Vol. 20, No. 2. Amsterdam, Netherlands: Elsevier (1990): p 259-270.
36. Naik, T.R. and V.M. Malhotra. "The Ultrasonic Pulse Velocity Method." *CRC Handbook on Nondestructive Testing of Concrete,* first edition. Baton Rouge, LA: CRC Press (1991): p 169-188.
37. Kaplan, M.F. "Compressive Strength and Ultrasonic Pulse Velocity Relationships for Concrete in Columns." *ACI Journal.* Vol. 29. Farmington Hills, MI: American Concrete Institute (1958): p 675.
38. Chung, H.W. "Effect of Embedded Steel Bar upon Ultrasonic Testing of Concrete." *Magazine of Concrete Research.* Vol. 30. London, United Kingdom: Thomas Telford (1978): p 19.
39. Bungey, J.H. ACI SP 82, *The Influence of Reinforcement on Ultrasonic Pulse Velocity Testing.* Farmington Hills, MI: American Concrete Institute (1984): p 229.
40. ACI 228.1R-03, *In-Place Methods to Estimate Concrete Strength.* Farmington Hills, MI: American Concrete Institute (2003).
41. Philleo, R.E. "Comparison of Results of Three Methods for Determining Young's Modulus of Elasticity of Concrete." *ACI Journal.* Vol. 26. Farmington Hills, MI: American Concrete Institute (1955): p 461.

42. Knab, L.J., G.V. Blessing and J.R. Clifton. "Laboratory Evaluation of Ultrasonics for Crack Detection in Concrete." *ACI Journal*. Vol. 80. Farmington Hills, MI: American Concrete Institute (January-February 1983): p 17-27.

43. Rebic, M.P. "The Distribution of Critical and Rupture Loads and Determination of the Factor of Crackability." ACI SP 82, *In Situ/Nondestructive Testing of Concrete*. Farmington Hills, MI: American Concrete Institute (1984): p 721-730.

44. Rhazi, J., Y. Kharrat, G. Ballivy and M. Rivest. ACI SP 168, *Application of Acoustical Imaging to the Evaluation of Concrete in Operating Structures*. Farmington Hills, MI: American Concrete Institute (1997): p 221.

45. Gomm, T.J. and J.A. Mauseth. "State of the Technology: Ultrasonic Tomography." *Materials Evaluation*. Vol. 57, No. 7. Columbus, OH: American Society for Nondestructive Testing (July 1999): p 747-752.

46. Martin, J., K.J. Broughton, A. Giannopolous, M.S.A. Hardy and M.C. Forde. "Ultrasonic Tomography of Grouted Duct Post-Tensioned Reinforced Concrete Bridge Beams." *NDT&E International*. Vol. 34, No. 2. Amsterdam, Netherlands: Elsevier (March 2001): p 107-113.

47. Schickert, M., M. Krause and W. Muller. "Ultrasonic Imaging of Concrete Elements Using Reconstruction by Synthetic Aperture Focusing Technique." *ASCE Journal of Materials in Civil Engineering*. Vol. 15. Reston, VA, American Society of Civil Engineers (2003): p 235-246.

48. Krause, M., F. Mielentz, B. Milman, W. Muller, V. Schmitz and H. Wiggenhauser. "Ultrasonic Imaging of Concrete Members Using an Array System." *NDT&E International*. Vol. 34. Amsterdam, Netherlands: Elsevier (2001): p 403-408.

49. Popovics, J.S. "NDE Techniques for Concrete and Masonry Structures." *Progress in Structural Engineering and Materials*. Vol. 5. New York, NY: Wiley (2003): p 49-59.

50. Boumiz, A., C. Vernet and F. Cohen Tenoudji. "Mechanical Properties of Cement Pastes and Mortars at Early Ages." *Journal of Advanced Cement-Based Materials*. Vol. 3, No. 3-4. New York, NY: Elsevier Science (1996): p 94-106.

51. Arnaud, L. "Rheological Characterization of Heterogeneous Materials with Evolving Properties." *ASCE Journal of Materials in Civil Engineering*. Vol. 15, No. 3. Reston, VA, American Society of Civil Engineers (June 2003): p 255-265.

52. Öztürk, T., J. Rappaport, J.S. Popovics and S.P. Shah. "Monitoring the Setting and Hardening of Cement-Based Materials with Ultrasound." *Concrete Science and Engineering*. Vol. 1, No. 2. Bagneux, France: RILEM Publications (1999): p 83-91.

53. Valic, M.I. "Hydration of Cementitious Materials by Pulse Echo USWR Method, Apparatus and Application Examples." *Cement and Concrete Research*. Vol. 30. Amsterdam, Netherlands: Elsevier (2000): p 1633-1640.

54. Voigt, T., Y. Akkaya and S.P. Shah. "Determination of Early-Age Mortar and Concrete Strength by Ultrasonic Wave Reflections." *ASCE Journal of Materials in Civil Engineering*. Vol. 15. Reston, VA: American Society of Civil Engineers (2003): p 247-254.

Bibliography

Achenbach, J.D., I.N. Komsky and P.J. Stolarski. "A Self-Compensating Ultrasonic System for Flaw Characterization in Steel Bridge Structures." *Structural Materials Technology: An NDT Conference* [Atlantic City, NJ, February 1994]. Lancaster PA: Technomic Publishing (1994): p 26-30.

Finch, K.J., M.P. Freeman and S. Snyder. "NDT (UT) Inspection and Data Management for Bridge Pins and Trunnions." *Structural Materials Technology: An NDT Conference* [Atlantic City, NJ, February 1994]. Lancaster PA: Technomic Publishing (1994): p 257-260.

Gessel, R.D. and R.A. Walther. "Ultrasonic Inspection of Bridge Pin and Hanger Assemblies." *Structural Materials Technology: An NDT Conference* [San Diego, CA, February 1996]. Lancaster PA: Technomic Publishing (1996): p 28-33.

Harland, J.W., R.L. Purvis, D.R. Graber, P. Albrecht and T.S. Flournoy. *Inspection of Fracture Critical Bridge Members*. McLean, VA: Federal Highway Administration (September 1986).

Harm, E.E. and G.A. Washer. Problem Statement 95-D-33, "Improving the Correlation of Ultrasonic Testing Results to the In Place Condition of Bridge Suspension Pins." Springfield, IL: Illinois Department of Transportation (1993).

Hosseini, Z., M. Momayez and F. Hassani. "Application of SAFT for Inspection of Cracks in Concrete." *NDE Conference on Civil Engineering: A Joint Conference of the 7th Structural Materials Technology: NDE/NDT for Highways and Bridges and the 6th International Symposium on NDT in Civil Engineering* [Saint Louis, Missouri, August 2006]. Columbus, OH: American Society for Nondestructive Testing (2006): p 438.

Komsky, I.N. and J.D. Achenbach. "A Computerized Imaging System for Ultrasonic Inspection of Steel Bridge Structures." *Structural Materials Technology: An NDT Conference* [San Diego, CA, February 1996]. Lancaster PA: Technomic Publishing (February 1996): p 40-45.

Miller, W.J. and M.K. Chaney. "NDT of Bridge Pins on PennDOT Structures." *Structural Materials Technology: An NDT Conference* [Atlantic City, NJ, February 1994]. Lancaster PA: Technomic Publishing (1994): p 252-256.

Prine, D.W. et al. FHWA/RD-83-006, *Improved Fabrication and Inspection of Welded Connections in Bridge Structures.* Springfield, VA: National Technical Information Service for the United States Department of Transportation, Federal Highway Administration (1984).

Thomas, G., S. Benson, P. Durbin, N. Del Grande, J. Haskins, A. Brown and D. Schneberk. "Nondestructive Evaluation Techniques for Enhanced Bridge Inspection." *Review of Progress in Quantitative Nondestructive Evaluation* [Brunswick, ME, August 1993]. Vol. 13. New York, NY: Plenum (1994): p 2083-2090.

Woodward, C., G. Reyes and B. Stone. "Guided Wave Evaluation of Steel Bridge Beams." *Topics on Nondestructive Evaluation [TONE]:* Vol. 2, *Nondestructive Testing and Evaluation of Infrastructure.* Columbus, OH: American Society for Nondestructive Testing (1998): p 25-36.

Structural Materials Technology Proceedings

Proceedings: Nondestructive Evaluation of Civil Structures and Materials [Boulder, CO, May 1992]. Boulder, CO: Atkinson-Noland and Associates (1992).

Structural Materials Technology: An NDT Conference [Atlantic City, NJ, February 1994]. Lancaster PA: Technomic Publishing (1994).

Structural Materials Technology II: An NDT Conference [San Diego, CA, February 1996]. Lancaster PA: Technomic Publishing (1996).

Structural Materials Technology III: An NDT Conference [San Antonio, TX, September 1998]. Bellingham, Washington: Society of Photographic Instrumentation Engineers [International Society for Optical Engineering] (1998).

Structural Materials Technology IV: An NDT Conference [Atlantic City, NJ, February-March 2000]. Lancaster PA: Technomic Publishing (2000).

Structural Materials Technology V: An NDT Conference [Cincinnati, OH, September 2002]. Columbus, OH: American Society for Nondestructive Testing (2002).

Structural Materials Technology VI: An NDT Conference [Buffalo, NY, September 2004]. Columbus, OH: American Society for Nondestructive Testing (2004).

NDE Conference on Civil Engineering: A Joint Conference of the 7th Structural Materials Technology: NDE/NDT for Highways and Bridges and the 6th International Symposium on NDT in Civil Engineering [Saint Louis, Missouri, August 2006]. Columbus, OH: American Society for Nondestructive Testing (2006).

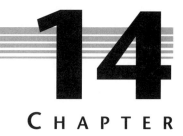

CHAPTER

Aerospace Applications of Ultrasonic Testing

Richard H. Bossi, Boeing Aerospace, Seattle, Washington (Parts 1 to 3)

Laura M. Harmon Cosgriff, National Aeronautics and Space Administration, Langley Research Center, Hampton, Virginia (Part 4)

Andrew L. Gyekenyesi, National Aeronautics and Space Administration, Glenn Research Center, Cleveland, Ohio (Part 4)

Donald J. Hagemaier, Huntington Beach, California (Parts 1 to 3)

Eric I. Madaras, National Aeronautics and Space Administration, Langley Research Center, Hampton, Virginia (Part 4)

Richard E. Martin, National Aeronautics and Space Administration, Glenn Research Center, Cleveland, Ohio; Cleveland State University, Cleveland, Ohio (Part 4)

William H. Prosser, National Aeronautics and Space Administration, Langley Research Center, Hampton, Virginia (Part 4)

Gary L. Workman, University of Alabama, Huntsville, Alabama (Part 4)

PART 1. Overview of Aerospace Applications of Ultrasonic Testing

Ultrasonics plays a critical role in the production and inservice testing of aerospace structures. It is applied to metallic and composite parts using a wide range of techniques, frequencies and waveform types. The applications can be routine or unique. The ultrasonic techniques check for discontinuities such as cracks, delaminations, porosity and inclusions. Ultrasonics may also be used to measure dimensions and material properties. Table 1 lists aerospace materials that are ultrasonically tested. Eddy current, radiographic, liquid penetrant, magnetic particle and other nondestructive test methods may be more appropriate for particular types of quality issues. Table 2 lists the advantages and limitations of ultrasound as a function of test issues. For the most part, ultrasound is best when inspecting for planar discontinuities lying parallel to the test surface. If the back surface of the object is also parallel, it simplifies the test.

Figure 1 shows basic configurations used in aerospace ultrasonic testing. Through-thickness ultrasonic testing uses two probes placed on each size of the object. The alignment for through-thickness testing may be by robotics, magnetic coupling or simply hand held. For hand held through-thickness testing, one transducer is usually held at a fixed position while the other is moved to obtain the peak signal. The pulse echo technique is simple to use and is the most common hand held test.

The reflector plate pulse echo technique can also be very useful. It has the advantage of being sensitive to changes in material properties because the sound passes through the sample twice. It is also very useful for parts that have surfaces slightly nonparallel by several dozen millirad (a few degrees) because the reflector plate can be aligned normal to the beam.

The through-thickness or pulse echo technique with longitudinal waves is used at frequencies appropriate for the thickness and attenuation characteristics of the materials. The sensitivity to fine detail is a function of wavelength and active beam size. At long wavelengths and large beams, details are lost but attenuation is less, so penetration is greater. Short wavelengths and small beams have greater detail resolution on thinner structures. Table 3 lists several aerospace materials with their wave speeds and the wavelengths as a function of frequency. For composite materials with layers typically around 0.2 mm (0.008 in.) thickness, the ability to count individual plies is lost below 5 MHz frequency or about 0.6 mm wavelength.

Sizing of discontinuities is a function of orientation and beam size. When the beam is normal to the discontinuity and the beam is smaller than the discontinuity, the size can be estimated on the basis of signal loss as the beam is scanned over the discontinuity zone. When the beam is larger than the discontinuity, the sizing is based on the amplitude of the signal. The amplitude based sizing must be calibrated against a standard. When using angle beams and corner trap detection for discontinuity detection, sizing is based on the signal amplitude compared to a standard. Discontinuities whose reflection intensity is different from the standard may not be sized precisely. However, accept/reject criteria for discontinuities are normally based on the reflection amplitude in the standard, usually a notch machined and set to be a conservative signal. Cracks in thick metal structure may be sized by crack tip diffraction. Crack tip diffraction can be more accurate than amplitude sizing for uneven crack discontinuities but is rarely used on aerospace structures.

The ability of ultrasound to detect features during testing is a function of the changes in acoustic impedance at interfaces. The transmission and reflection

FIGURE 1. Basic ultrasonic test techniques.

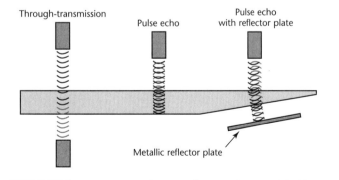

Through-transmission

Pulse echo

Pulse echo with reflector plate

Metallic reflector plate

TABLE 1. Aerospace material test issues.

Material	Inspection Issues	Ultrasonic Testing
All types	curved surfaces, radii, discontinuity orientation, noodles	Ultrasonic testing requires precise beam alignment, either normal to test surface or at precise angles. Normality is found by peaking signal response for entry surface, simulated discontinuity or alignment of through-transmission transducers. Curved surfaces require surface following so beam can be oriented normal to surface. Radii require special orientation of probes to remain normal in radius.
Fiber reinforced polymer composite laminate/glass epoxy	consolidation, porosity, inclusions, fiber-to-resin ratio, delaminations, wrinkles, surface layers, curved surfaces, radii, noodles	Through-transmission or pulse echo testing are main techniques for acceptance of composite laminates, using automated scanning with water coupled piezoelectric transducers. Test variations depend on material, configuration, thickness and sensitivity requirements and include handheld, resonance, laser coupled, air coupled, lamb wave, spectroscopic and roller probe techniques. All testing requires correlation with acceptance standards. Generally, consolidation and porosity are monitored by acoustic attenuation using through-transmission or pulse echo testing with reflector plate. Delaminations, voids and some inclusions are detectable with through-transmission testing but pulse echo reflection may be more sensitive to inclusions in some materials. Wrinkles are detectable with pulse echo B-scanning at high frequency (>3 MHz). Surface coatings are monitored with high frequency (such as 20 MHz) pulse echo or resonance testing. In some cases, pitch catch configuration may be used across radii to check for quality of noodles in root of T and I shaped structure.
Foam core composite	cracking, voids, density, bonding to skin, inclusions, fluid ingress, skin quality, skin porosity	Through-transmission technique is common. Water squirter systems at 1 MHz look for wide range of discontinuities. Air coupling may be acceptable.
Honeycomb core structure	bonding of core to skin, crushed/damaged core, filled core, inclusions, skin quality, skin porosity	Through-transmission technique is common with standard water squirter systems at 1 MHz, looking for delaminations and porosity. Air coupling may be acceptable.
Carbon-to-carbon	consolidation, dry ply, porosity, delamination, inclusions, wrinkles	Ultrasonic testing detects delaminations and porosity. Concerns exist with means of coupling to carbon-to-carbon surface.
Castings	cracks, voids/porosity, inclusions, shrinkage, weld repairs, dimensional tolerances	Pulse echo angle beams, normal beams and phased arrays are used to detect and locate discontinuities. Grain size noise affects sensitivity.
Forgings	cracks, inclusions, grain size, residual stress	Pulse echo testing of billets for inclusions, porosity and voids. Angle beams look for cracks.
Machined parts	cracks, residual stress, dimensional tolerance, repairs	Pulse echo angle beams and phased arrays are used to detect cracks. Internal dimensional checks can sometimes be performed at high frequency.
Fastened structure	cracks, corrosion, alloy type	Pulse echo ultrasonic testing with angle beams is used for cracks around fasteners. Normal beam ultrasonic testing is used for corrosion detection, loss of material in top layer.
Welded joints	voids, porosity, lack of fusion, lack of penetration, undercut, shrinkage, cracks, slag, inclusions, residual stress	Normal or angle beam ultrasonic testing is used for cracks, voids, inclusions, lack of fusion and lack of penetration in welds. Phased arrays can be used for beam steering in both pulse echo and pitch catch modes along welds.
Bonded joint assemblies	surface wetting, bond strength, voids, disbonds, degradation	Ultrasonic testing normal to bond interface detects disbonds and voids. Spectroscopy can be sensitive to interface that correlates to bond quality. Under special conditions, changes in acoustic attenuation or wave speed can indicate adhesive degradation.
Coatings	paint thickness, conductive layers, thermal coatings, insulation, low observable coatings	High frequency pulse echo technique can gage paint thickness. Thermal coatings, insulation and low observables may need low frequency in through-transmission or resonance mode.
Subsystems	cracks, residual stress, surface condition	Pulse echo angle and normal ultrasonic testing are useful for crack detection.
Inservice or damaged structure	impact damage, heat damage, moisture ingress, fatigue cracks, corrosion, lightning strike, disbonds, delaminations	Ultrasonic testing is useful for composite impact damage, disbonds and delaminations with normal beams. Moisture ingress can be detected through changes in wave speeds and attenuation. Fatigue cracks in top layers are detectable with normal or angle beams. Thickness changes in accessible layers indicate corrosion.

of ultrasound pressure across interfaces is given by:

(1) $\quad T = \dfrac{2Z_2}{Z_2 + Z_1}$

and:

(2) $\quad R = \dfrac{Z_2 - Z_1}{Z_2 + Z_1}$

where R is the reflection coefficient, T is the transmission coefficient and Z_1 and Z_2 are the acoustic impedances of material 1 and material 2 of an interface. Table 4 lists interface transmission and reflection coefficients and their corresponding amplitudes for some possible aerospace test interfaces.

Because of the large change in acoustic impedance at an air interface, it is difficult to couple sound into air. Cracks are an interface between the material and air that do not transmit and thus provide a large amplitude reflection. Inclusions are interfaces between the base material and the inclusion material and may not have sufficient reflection for detection, depending on the relative impedances. Table 4 points out the difficulty of air coupled ultrasound because of the low transmission of ultrasound from a lead zirconate titanate transducer into air compared to the transmission from the transducer into water. The same applies for coupling through material samples. Air coupled ultrasound suffers from the decibel insertion losses and thus loses sensitivity relative to immersion or

TABLE 2. Advantages and limitations of ultrasonic testing.

Material	Inspection Issues	Ultrasonic Testing
Planar discontinuities such as delaminations and disbonds	Ultrasonic testing is well suited to planar discontinuities.	Ultrasonic testing does not see behind one discontinuity to detect another. Inspection from both sides of object may be required to verify. Ultrasonic testing is applicable to top layer of fastened structure.
Cracks detection	Ultrasonic testing is sensitive to very small cracks.	Beam must be oriented to intersect crack so that sound wave is returned to transmitter/receiver or separate receiving probe.
Crack sizing	Amplitude from well oriented cracks can be calibrated for sizing. Crack tip echoes and timing are used for sizing.	Cracks that do not grow planar and smooth will not be accurately sized by ultrasonic testing. Crack tip detection requires materials with little internal scatter.
Thickness measurement	Ultrasound can be very accurate if material is uniform with known wave speed.	Must be able to sense back echo. Wave speeds must be known.
Porosity	Ultrasonic signal is scattered by porosity and can be detected by signal loss from back of part.	Porosity can be difficult to calibrate. Usually, acoustic attenuation is a criterion, but calibration standards must match test object.
Thin material	Ultrasonic testing can be performed at high frequencies such that the wavelength is much shorter than thickness.	Near surface detection of features is subject to quality of signal insertion. Delay lines may be used to avoid having ringdown of pulse. Near field transducer effects limit near surface sensitivity.
Thick materials	Ultrasonic testing can be performed at low frequencies to obtain penetration through thick material.	As frequency is decreased, sensitivity to fine detail is lost with ultrasonic testing, and some discontinuities can be missed.
Inclusions	Ultrasonic testing can detect inclusions by either reflected echo or an attenuation effect on transmitted beam.	To detect inclusions, difference between material and inclusion must be enough to generate echo or reduce transmission. Inclusion must be oriented for beam detection.
Multilayer structure	Ultrasonic testing can be transmitted through layered structures bonded or in intimate contact. It is useful to detect delaminations between layers. Resonance testing is useful for in-service testing of multilayer structures such as honeycomb.	Ultrasonic testing is limited to top layer of fastened multilayer structure.
Complex structure	Beams can be oriented to inspect zones in complex structures by adjusting beam angles with specially oriented shoes, computer control immersion systems or phased arrays.	Highly complex structures may not be inspectable with ultrasound because beams may not reach critical zones or orientation of beam relative to discontinuity may not be sufficiently normal to provide sensitivity.

TABLE 3. Wavelength in common materials.

Material	Density (g·cm⁻³)	Acoustic Impedance (kg·cm⁻²·s)	Wave Type	Speed (km·s⁻¹)	Wavelength 0.5 MHz (mm)	1 MHz (mm)	2.25 MHz (mm)	3.5 MHz (mm)	5 MHz (mm)	10 MHz (mm)	15 MHz (mm)	20 MHz (mm)
Air	0.0012	0.04	longitudinal	0.33	0.66	0.33	0.15	0.094	0.066	0.033	0.022	0.017
Water	1.00	148	longitudinal	1.48	2.96	1.48	0.66	0.423	0.296	0.148	0.099	0.074
Acrylic	1.15	310	longitudinal	2.70	5.40	2.70	1.20	0.771	0.540	0.270	0.180	0.135
			transverse	1.10	2.20	1.10	0.49	0.314	0.220	0.110	0.073	0.055
Graphite epoxy	1.55	465	longitudinal	3.00	6.00	3.00	1.33	0.857	0.600	0.300	0.200	0.150
Aluminum	2.71	1710	longitudinal	6.30	12.60	6.30	2.80	1.800	1.260	0.630	0.420	0.315
			transverse	2.50	5.00	2.50	1.11	0.714	0.500	0.250	0.167	0.125
Magnesium	1.72	1000	longitudinal	5.80	11.60	5.80	2.58	1.657	1.160	0.580	0.387	0.290
			transverse	2.30	4.60	2.30	1.02	0.657	0.460	0.230	0.153	0.115
Titanium	4.50	2730	longitudinal	6.07	12.14	6.07	2.70	1.734	1.214	0.607	0.405	0.304
			transverse	2.40	4.80	2.40	1.07	0.686	0.480	0.240	0.160	0.120
Steel, mild	7.80	4600	longitudinal	5.90	11.80	5.90	2.62	1.686	1.180	0.590	0.393	0.295
			transverse	2.30	4.60	2.30	1.02	0.657	0.460	0.230	0.153	0.115
Steel stainless	7.83	4540	longitudinal	5.80	11.60	5.80	2.58	1.657	1.160	0.580	0.387	0.290
			transverse	2.30	4.60	2.30	1.02	0.657	0.460	0.230	0.153	0.115
Nickel	8.88	5000	longitudinal	5.63	11.26	5.63	2.50	1.609	1.126	0.563	0.375	0.282
			transverse	2.96	5.92	2.96	1.32	0.846	0.592	0.296	0.197	0.148
Steel, nickel chromium	8.59	5000	longitudinal	5.82	11.64	5.82	2.59	1.663	1.164	0.582	0.388	0.291
			transverse	3.02	6.04	3.02	1.34	0.863	0.604	0.302	0.201	0.151

TABLE 4. Interface transmission and reflection coefficients.

Interface	Transmission Coefficient $2Z_2 \cdot (Z_2+Z_1)^{-1}$	Reflection Coefficient $(Z_2-Z_1) \cdot (Z_2+Z_1)^{-1}$	Transmission Amplitude (dB)	Reflection Amplitude (dB)
Lead zirconate titanate to air	0.00002	−0.99998	−92.69	−0.0002
Air to lead zirconate titanate	1.99998	0.99998	6.02	−0.0002
Lead zirconate titanate to water	0.08227	−0.91773	−21.70	−0.75
Water to lead zirconate titanate	1.91773	0.91773	5.66	−0.75
Graphite epoxy to air	0.00017	−0.99983	−75.29	−0.0015
Air to graphite epoxy	1.99983	0.99983	6.02	−0.0015
Water to graphite epoxy	1.51713	0.51713	3.62	−5.73
Graphite epoxy to water	0.48287	−0.51713	−6.32	−5.73
Acrylic to graphite epoxy	1.20000	0.20000	1.58	−13.98
Graphite epoxy to acrylic	0.80000	−0.20000	−1.94	−13.98
Aluminum to air	0.00005	−0.99995	−86.58	−0.00041
Air to aluminum	1.99995	0.99995	6.02	−0.00041
Water to aluminum	1.84046	0.84046	5.30	−1.51
Aluminum to water	0.15954	−0.84046	−15.94	−1.51
Water to titanium	1.89715	0.89715	5.56	−0.94
Titanium to water	0.10285	−0.89715	−19.76	−0.94
Water to steel	1.93766	0.93766	5.75	−0.56
Steel to water	0.06234	−0.93766	−24.10	−0.56

FIGURE 2. Simulated 5 MHz signals as function of interface materials in acrylic sample for water immersion test: (a) setup; (b) A-scan of crack; (c) A-scan away from discontinuity; (d) A-scan of steel inclusion.

(a)

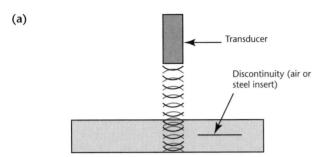

(b)

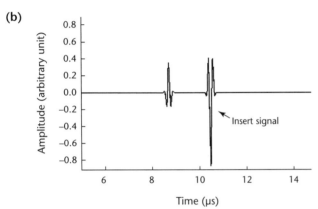

(c)

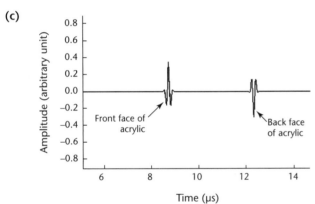

(d)

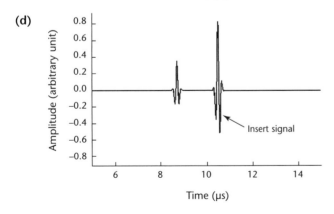

contact ultrasonic testing. Alternative transducers with better acoustic matching to air are needed to improve the air coupled test sensitivity. The equation for the reflection coefficient can result in a negative number: the wave form is phase reversed at the interface. This effect can be seen in the acoustic waveform and can be useful for the interpretation of interfaces. Figure 2, using simulation software shows the change in waveform for different interfaces for an acrylic block scanned in water at 5 MHz. It can be seen that an insert of air (crack) versus an inclusion of steel changes the phase of the reflected waveform.

PART 2. Aerospace Material Production Inspection[1]

Aircraft production uses a wide range of materials. The following discussion expands on Table 1 for some ultrasonic test applications.

Care must be taken to prepare and use reference standards in production ultrasonic testing. Table 5 lists types of ultrasonic reference standards for aerospace materials and issues with ultrasonic reference standards.

Fiber Reinforced Polymer Composite Laminate Glass Epoxy

Composite materials are a matrix material reinforced with another material, often a fiber. Carbon fiber reinforced polymer composite materials are attractive for advanced structural applications because of their excellent strength-to-weight ratios, high toughness, controlled anisotropy and ability to be fabricated in any desired shape. Composite materials are widely used in aircraft and spacecraft and are the largest area of ultrasonic testing requirements for aircraft. Figure 3 shows the growth in the use of

composites for aircraft. Primary structural composites must be 100 percent inspected by ultrasound to verify that the laminate is properly consolidated and is clear of porosity and of foreign materials.

Carbon fiber reinforced plastics are anisotropic media: acoustic plane waves moving through the material are often only quasi longitudinal or quasi transverse (containing both longitudinal and transverse characteristics). Because of the layered structure, the ultrasonic waves interact at the ply layer interfaces. Ultrasound can travel along fibers and therefore certain ultrasonic test techniques can be highly sensitive to the fiber orientation in the structure. For the general testing of carbon fiber reinforced plastic, however, ultrasonic beams oriented perpendicular to the ply layers are used. As the ultrasonic beam passes through the composite material, it will be attenuated by scattering and absorption. Features in the composite larger than about 0.1× the wavelength will contribute to the scatter. As shown in Table 3, wavelengths between 0.3 and 0.03 mm (0.012 and 0.0012 in.) represent 1 and 10 MHz respectively. The attenuation due to scatter and absorption of the sound

TABLE 5. Ultrasonic testing reference standards.

Material	Type	Comments
General	all	Construct standards using material like that being tested. Include discontinuity simulation sizes above and below critical discontinuity sizes specified by engineering. Include material thickness ranges in standard that bound materials being tested. Includes steps reasonably close (for example, within 10 percent acoustic signal) of material under test.
Composite laminates	step wedge, porosity, inclusions, delaminations and voids, flat bottom holes	Inserts represent factory foreign materials that could be left in laminate. Simulated delaminations may be made with nonbonding materials such as fluorocarbon resin, release coated brass shims and release ply materials. Flat bottom holes may be used to simulate delaminations or voids for one sided tests but not for through-transmission testing unless backside is potted. Locations of inserts include near surface, middle and far surface.
Honeycomb and foam	step wedges, voids, flat bottom holes	Step configuration with sufficient range to cover thickness of structure. Plug backside drilled holes.
Metallics	International Institute of Welding blocks, step wedges, custom configurations	Step wedge for thickness gaging. Custom configuration to match structure and discontinuity type.
Bonds	voids, unbonds	Create joint configuration. Create disbond inserts using release ply material on each interface side of bond.

pressure of a plane wave can be represented by:

$$(3) \quad p = p_0 e^{-\alpha d [\text{Np}]}$$

$$= p_0 10^{-\frac{\alpha d [\text{dB}]}{20}}$$

where d is the distance traveled (meter), p is the end pressure (pascal), p_0 is the initial pressure (pascal) and α is the attenuation coefficient. The attenuation coefficient (decibel per meter) is obtained from by rearranging and taking the log of the above equation:

$$(4) \quad \alpha d = 20 \log \frac{p_0}{p}$$

where $20 \log (p_0 \cdot p^{-1})$ is the ratio of the initial to final pressure in decibels. Figure 4 shows generic plots of attenuation of a composite material as a function of thickness at 1 and 5 MHz. In this example, the attenuation coefficient is in range of 0.5 and 1 dB·mm^{-1} at 1 and 5 MHz respectively. The attenuation can be highly variable among different composite materials. The higher testing frequency will be more sensitive to material changes. However, as the sample becomes thicker, the dynamic range of the ultrasonic test system limits the testing and needs lower frequencies.

Most composite material tests are specified to be through-thickness or pulse echo. The coupling of the ultrasound to the composite is usually through water in immersion tanks, bubbler/dribbler or squirter systems. For bubbler and squirter systems, the surface must be wettable for adequate coupling. Surfactants are often added to the water systems to ensure coupling. In immersion systems, air bubbles or entrapped air on the part can cause significant signal variations and must be removed for proper testing. Table 6 compares the common scanner types. Figure 5 shows an automated ultrasonic system with motion control squirters programmed for contour following that can perform through-thickness and pulse echo scanning simultaneously. Laser ultrasonic

FIGURE 4. Graph of sample composite attenuation at 1 and 5 MHz.

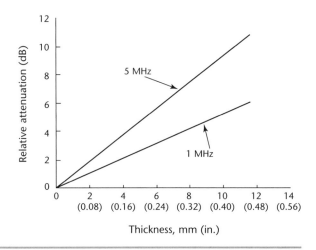

FIGURE 3. The use of composites in aircraft has increased with time.

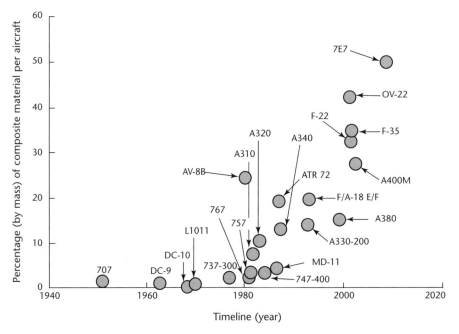

test systems exist but have been relatively uncommon in the first decade of the twenty-first century. Air coupled ultrasound is used for low sensitivity applications, typically of noncritical, structural aerospace materials.

For through-thickness tests, the pulser can use a tone burst (several cycles of the waveform) to increase the acoustic power. Through-thickness systems can have a wide dynamic range (>100 dB on some systems) and easily detect problems in multiple-layered structures. By comparing through-thickness signal attenuation between a standard and the material under test, porosity, inclusions, unbonds, wrinkles or delaminations can all be detected. For example, porosity in the 1 to 2 percent range corresponds to a change of 4 to 8 dB in signal level for approximately 6 mm (0.25 in.) of material at 2.25 MHz and 10 to 20 dB at 5 MHz. Through-thickness ultrasonic techniques do not determine the depth of detected discontinuities. Depth is determined by pulse echo time-of-flight (TOF) scanning.

The horizontal spatial resolution for the data must allow for an adequate number of test points over the smallest discontinuity of interest, normally 2 to 3 points in each direction. For 6 mm (0.25 in.) resolution, data spacing of 2 to 3 mm (0.08 to 0.12 in.) would be used. For pulse echo testing, a spike or square wave pulse is desired for a broad bandwidth and depth resolution. In pulse echo testing, the sound is reflected from the front and back surfaces of the composite material as well as from internal discontinuities. Figure 6 shows a 5 MHz

TABLE 6. Advantages and limitations of automated scanning system.

Method	Advantage	Limitation
Water squirter	Handling of large parts, fast scanning of up to 1 m·s⁻¹ (40 in.·s⁻¹), contour following, through-transmission or pulse echo modes.Resolution and power of sound can be tailored (spike or tone burst).	Complex manipulators. Alignment of through-transmission mode transducers to each other. Alignment of pulse echo mode to surface. Water splash. Cannot use focused transducers effectively.
Bubbler or dribbler	Low implementation cost; surface following; transducer arrays often used for high rate.	Edge or cutout test limitations. Speeds may be limited (< 0.5 m·s⁻¹). Pulse echo mode (through-transmission testing can be performed with magnetic coupling).
Immersion	Excellent signal quality; good spatial resolution; ability to use focused transducers, arrays, angle beams and either through-transmission or pulse echo.	Part size, buoyancy, tank depth, scanning speed limitations.
Laser ultrasonic testing	Easy to scan contoured parts, noncontact.	Surface must be suitable to generate ultrasound without damage. Broadband signal, signal quality may be degraded relative to standard transducers. Can be large, expensive and require laser safe room.
Air coupled ultrasonic testing	Noncontact, low frequency penetration for attenuative materials.	Lower sensitivity than water coupled. Lower frequency applications (<1 MHz). Edge effects.

FIGURE 5. Example of overhead gantry water squirter through-transmission and pulse echo system for large composite objects.

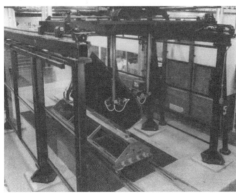

FIGURE 6. Pulse echo data trace of composite with internal feature.

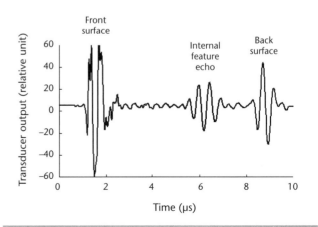

test of composite structure. The first pulse is the front surface echo of the part (the interface between the coupling media and the part). The third pulse is the back surface echo of the part. Any laminar discontinuities (inclusions or delaminations) appear as echoes between the front and back surfaces (second pulse). The amplitude of the echo correlates to the acoustic impedance mismatch of the discontinuity to the composite. If the discontinuity is longer than the beam size and the impedance mismatch is significant, then the back surface echo will be lost or significantly reduced. The depth of the discontinuity is obtained by knowing the wave speed in the material and the time of the reflection from the waveform. Carbon-to-epoxy composite materials have a characteristic wave speed around 3 mm·µs⁻¹, ±5 percent.

Automated pulse echo examinations generally create both amplitude and time-of-flight C-scan images for interpretation. The amplitude images may be gated for the full thickness of the part or gated in regions of the part, such as at particular zones or just the back wall. Time-of-flight images may use the time of either the peak signal or the first signal in the gate. The imaging possibilities allow important differences in the interpretation of discontinuities in samples or the detection of subtle features. For example, some inclusions may be difficult to detect with a back wall echo gate but can be detected by an internal time-of-flight gate in the material. Wrinkles are generally below the threshold commonly applied for porosity testing but can be found by B-scan data sets. Figure 7 shows the scan of a composite test sample containing flat bottom holes. The amplitude and time-of-flight C-scans show the features. Different colors or gray scales indicate the echo amplitude or, in the case of time of flight, the part thickness or depth. In Fig. 7, the amplitude of the echoes from the holes are close to the amplitude signal from the back of the part, so the holes are detected by the presence of the edges. In the time-of-flight image, the holes have different gray scale levels due to the time of the signal. The B-scan of a line trace across the time-of-flight image shows the difference in time location of the signal between the front surface and the back of the part. Care must be taken in evaluating pulse echo amplitude images as discontinuity reflections or multiple indications of the discontinuity can be in the amplitude gate. Porosity detection with pulse echo amplitude is usually more sensitive than through-thickness testing because the back wall or reflector plate technique of Fig. 1 makes the signal pass through the part twice. For comparison of

signals for internal features, *distance amplitude correction* (also called *time corrected gain*) should be used to keep the discontinuity sensitivity constant throughout the composite thickness. Discontinuities near the back wall of the composite are electronically enhanced to bring amplitude up to about the same level as a front surface discontinuity.

Composite structure can be made in many shapes that complicate ultrasonic tests. Figure 8 shows a picture of a T section and some options for testing. Radius testing can be performed with a special shoe for a hand-held transducer, with a special array of transducers or with contour following automated scanning systems. Laser ultrasonic testing is suited for radius testing because it can be easy to set up. Figure 9 shows radius testing using miniature squirters and an automated

FIGURE 7. Pulse echo data on composite test sample with flat bottom holes: (a) amplitude display; (b) time-of-flight display; (c) B-scan.

(a)

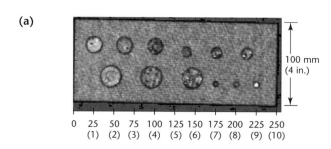

```
0   25   50   75  100  125 150  175 200  225 250
(1)  (2)  (3)  (4)  (5)  (6)  (7)  (8)  (9) (10)
```

Distance, mm (in.)

(b)

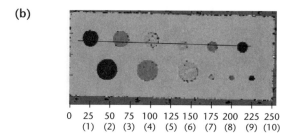

```
0   25   50   75  100  125 150  175 200  225 250
(1)  (2)  (3)  (4)  (5)  (6)  (7)  (8)  (9) (10)
```

Distance, mm (in.)

(c)

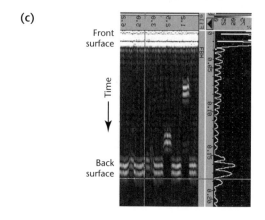

scanner. When angle beams are used in composites for access to particular locations, care must be taken as to where the beam is transmitted. As noted above, the multiple layers in a composite result in multiple mode conversions. The layered structure and strong anisotropy can have significant effects on the beam performance. Figure 10 shows an experimental setup where the angle of a composite part in a through-thickness system was changed. The plot is a notional extraction of the data from multiple tests showing how the ultrasound signal varies significantly in amplitude as a function of the orientation. This demonstrates that care must be taken to maintain normality to the surface of composites and that an angle beam test can be highly variable.

FIGURE 8. Options for ultrasonic testing of T section: (a) T section; (b) pulse echo test of radius; (c) pitch catch test of noodle; (d) pulse echo test of noodle.

(a)

(b)

(c)

(d)

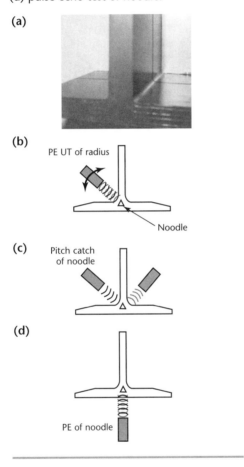

FIGURE 9. Miniature water squirter radius inspection.

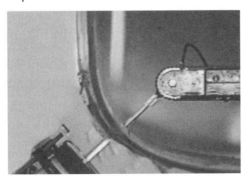

Honeycomb and Foam Core Laminates

Honeycomb and foam core laminate structures are inspected primarily with through-thickness testing for production. A lower frequency, around 1 MHz, is used compared to the higher frequencies used for solid laminate. Internal delaminations, nonbonded inclusions and core damage will be detected. Figure 11 is a photograph

FIGURE 10. Effect of angle on transmission of ultrasound in composites: (a) scan diagram; (b) results.

(a)

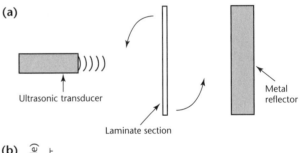

(b)

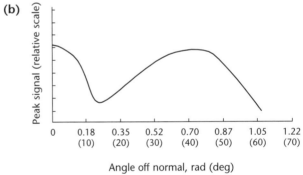

FIGURE 11. Honeycomb core sample.

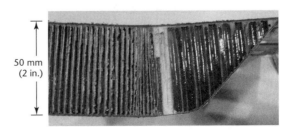

of a sectioned honeycomb sample having a thin skin, two sizes of honeycomb and a taper. Figure 12 shows a system for inspecting large aerospace structures. Calibration with a standard helps establish sensitivity to the features of interest. The bonding of the skin to the honeycomb core should have proper adhesive fillets. Lower frequencies and the signal variations inherent in many core structures prevent the detection of low levels of porosity (less than 4 percent) in the laminate skins. In most cases, the application for the honeycomb and foam core structure and the thin (three-ply to ten-ply) skins do not require an ultrasonic test for porosity. When porosity testing may be desired, a high frequency pulse echo scan may be performed. Over foam core, the back echo from the skin is likely to be lost at the interface. High frequencies (above 10 MHz) and high scanning spatial resolution may be used to look in the surface layers and detect porosity. Full waveform data are taken and then analyzed ply by ply.

Carbon-to-Carbon

Carbon-to-carbon structures are used in aerospace for their strength at high temperature and for their light weight. Ultrasound is typically performed at 1 MHz because the material is relatively attenuative. At 1 MHz, thickness up to around 20 mm can be inspected. Care must be taken with coupling to the carbon-to-carbon because water should be avoided. Moisture content in carbon-to-carbon is unacceptable. Alcohol, or alcohol in a 50 percent mix with deionized water, is acceptable. With carbon-to-carbon structure, the amount of couplant can affect the signal levels and therefore needs to be applied consistently. Contact pressure can also be an issue. An elastomeric material is recommended

FIGURE 12. Large aerospace structure inspection system.

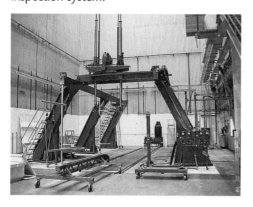

between the transducer and the carbon-to-carbon surface. The transducer near field and ringdown characteristics need to be carefully selected to allow near-surface testing. The back face reflection was used to detect porosity or unconsolidated structure. Delaminations, dry ply and inclusions are detectable by internal reflection. Wrinkles will have a weak change in the back reflected signal and may have a weak internal reflection but be detectable because of the linear indication in scanned image. Carbon-to-carbon standards can be difficult to work with because the repeated application of couplant changes the response. An alternate material, such as phenolic, matched to the appropriate attenuation can be used to calibrate the transducer and receiver setup.

Castings, Forgings and Machined Parts

Ultrasonic testing is not the main method for inspection of aerospace castings, forgings and machine parts. The shape and locations of the discontinuities are better inspected in most cases with other nondestructive test methods. However occasions exist, particularly with cracking where ultrasound may be used as a backup test and sometimes as a primary test.

Castings can be difficult for ultrasonic testing because of the surface conditions, grain size and complex structures. Crack detection at specific locations where the beam can be suitably oriented may be performed using standard angle beam ultrasonic test techniques. Phase array ultrasonic testing can be useful for these applications and has been applied to complex titanium aerospace castings. The phased array allows the beam to be scanned for internal coverage without moving the probe. This is particularly useful for locations that may not be accessible by a standard probe.

Aerospace forgings may be inspected in the billet stage with ultrasonic testing. Titanium billets are an example for engine applications. Focused ultrasonic testing is performed on the billets by using a range of transducers to focus the beam at appropriate depths to achieve required detection sensitivity.

Welded Joints

Aerospace welds are usually thin and typically are tested radiographically, as are other industrial welded joints. Calibration for ultrasonic testing is performed with standard International Institute of

Welding blocks. For aerospace structures, a particular weld routinely inspected with ultrasonic testing is the friction stir weld. Figure 13a shows the weld scheme. This type of weld is subject to curved discontinuities in the vertical plane of the weld. The weld discontinuity does not lend itself to common corner trap ultrasound detection. Phased array ultrasonic testing has been found to be an excellent technique to test the weld. The basic phased array technique is shown in Fig. 13b.

Bonded Joints

Bonded structures offer significant advantages in aircraft design, manufacture and performance over traditional fastened structures. Bond quality is often assessed looking for nonbonded regions with ultrasonic and other techniques.

1. Shearography, an optical rather than an acoustic technique, can be used as an alternative on bonds with thin skin, <2.5 mm (<0.1 in.), depending on the materials and structures.

FIGURE 13. Friction stir weld: (a) welding scheme; (b) phased array testing.

(a)

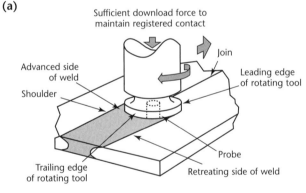

(b)

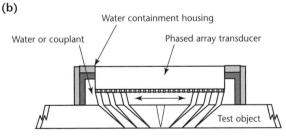

2. Tap testing with a coin or computerized tap testing is perhaps the most common bond test. The signal's frequency is in the sonic rather than the ultrasonic range. It is most useful on thin structures. In the case of composites, it should not be considered reliable on structures with top skins of more than three to five plies. The tap test should be performed in a consistent grid pattern on the structure. The sound should be clear over good structure and change to a dull or muffled sound over poor bonds.

3. Specially dedicated acoustic devices commonly called *bond testers* use low frequency vibration schemes, often in a pitch catch mode, to excite the structure and sense a difference between good and bad bonds. Such bond testing is similar to the ultrasonic technique called *resonance mode testing,* using a transducer with continuous or wave train frequencies of hundreds of kilohertz. These techniques can be scanned over a part to extract image data from the sensor. Typically, sensing is based on a comparison of the input waveform to the received waveform.

4. In pulse echo mode, ultrasonic waveforms are used to measure bond line thickness and interface echo signals. B-scans are often studied to assess the reflection intensity and uniformity of bond quality. Film adhesives will be relatively thin, usually less than 0.25 mm (0.01 in.). Paste adhesive bonds tend to be thicker, from 0.25 mm (0.01 in.) to over 2 mm (0.08 in.). The attenuation characteristics of the adhesive can indicate the adhesive condition in some bonds.

5. Ultrasonic spectroscopy has been used on bonded interfaces and is sensitive to variations in bond quality beyond the sensitivity of standard ultrasound. For critical primary structure applications, the bond quality assessment procedure may include a verification of bond strength. Nondestructive techniques have not been successful in determining bond strength because the strength parameter is measured only at failure. Proof testing of a joint is required to ensure adequate strength. It is possible to perform localized proof testing using laser generated shock waves. This technique makes a dynamic strength assessment as a very localized proof test of the bond.

6. Controlled, localized stress waves in materials and bonded joints offer opportunities for the characterization of structures, in particular the strength monitoring of bonded joints. Stress waves of intensity sufficient to evaluate bonding can be generated by electron beam, mechanical impact or laser pulse. The laser beam shape results in controlled, very localized testing of internal strength. The technique is sensitive to weak bonds created by poor adhesive mixing, improper surface preparation or contamination.

PART 3. Inservice Inspection of Aircraft

Aircraft structures may develop cracks during service because of stresses experienced during flight and landing. Composite structures are subject to impact damage from birds, hail, service vehicles and other sources. Therefore, airline operators require that the aircraft manufacturer provide a nondestructive testing manual with information and procedures for determining the condition of these structures. The manual supplies information about the possible locations of cracks and other service induced conditions and recommends applicable techniques for detecting them. If the anticipated crack is on an accessible surface, test methods such as visual, liquid penetrant, magnetic particle or eddy current testing may be selected for detection. However, numerous locations throughout the structure are made up of multiple layers of detail components joined together by rivets or bolt fasteners. At these locations, it is possible for cracks to be generated in a subsurface member and go undetected until they propagate to a surface. Early detection of subsurface cracks is possible with ultrasonic and radiographic testing. Composite assessment is based on visual detection of damage followed by ultrasonic testing. Composite structures are designed to tolerate barely visible impact damage. Damage that does not cause a visible indication can be tolerated in the structure.

Reference Standards for Tests of Aircraft

The purpose of an ultrasonic reference standard (or calibration standard) is to provide a test specimen that simulates as nearly as possible discontinuities that may be encountered in actual tests. Reference standards help establish instrument calibration and are used to ensure that particular discontinuities are detected with a predetermined sensitivity. Reference standards are used not only to facilitate initial adjustment but also to check periodically on the reproducibility of the measurement.

Preparation of Reference Standards

The first step in creating a reference standard is to select sound material of convenient size to eliminate edge effects in the area of interest. The material should be as free from natural imperfections as possible and should be similar to the test object in chemical composition, heat treatment, attenuation, velocity and shape (geometry). Next, artificial discontinuities, representative of those to be detected, are created with saw cuts, drilling, fatigue cracks or electric discharge machining. These manufactured discontinuities are used to generate a response equivalent to that expected in actual tests, allowing the instrumentation to be set at a specific sensitivity level and to indicate discontinuity resolution for various techniques. The proper selection and use of reference standards is the key to successful ultrasonic testing of aircraft components and permits the use of terms and values that have significant meaning for describing test results. Without proper use of reference standards, test results have little or possibly no significant value. Usually, the type and orientation of discontinuities are known in advance. By using reference standards with calibrated reflectors similar to the discontinuities of interest, proper testing procedure can be established and validated. If the testing procedure can clearly indicate artificial discontinuities in a reference standard, then there is a high probability that it can also indicate natural discontinuities in actual test objects. If the sensitivity level is too low, harmful discontinuities may not be detected. Conversely, if the level is too high, natural material characteristics may be mistaken for discontinuities.

Testing Procedure

For a typical ultrasonic test, the following steps are performed.

1. A reference standard is prepared for calibration.
2. The component is prepared for testing by removing loose paint and dirt.
3. The ultrasonic test instrument is set up, and the calibration standard is used to adjust controls and get a discontinuity pattern on the A-scan.

4. An appropriate couplant is selected and applied to the area of interest.
5. The test object is scanned according to detailed instructions specific to the component.
6. All indications of discontinuities are located and identified.
7. After testing, the ultrasonic equipment is withdrawn and the couplant is removed from the test surface.

Figures 14 and 15 show an example of a landing gear inspection. Figure 14 shows a standard created for the test. Figure 15 shows the ultrasonic waveforms at several locations along the standard and for a crack in the part (Fig. 15).

Cracks

Ultrasonic testing is often used on aircraft structure to detect discontinuities radiating from attachment holes in fatigue sensitive areas. Anticipated crack areas can be tested using one or more wave modes. Holes with access limited to a curved surface may require only a refracted longitudinal wave technique. An example of this application is the detection of cracks radiating from attachment holes in the curved attached fittings on the horizontal stabilizer, elevator, rudder, flap and aileron in Fig. 16. Several techniques may be used to establish the proper angle of the transducer. The mathematics of these techniques are discussed in detail elsewhere.[1]

One of these techniques allows testing holes of different diameters with the same apparatus. The incident beam needs to be perpendicular to the axis of the hole and allow lateral movement of the transducer to achieve a refracted longitudinal wave tangential to the inner curved surface. Figure 17 shows this configuration. A clear plastic shoe must be fabricated to fit the outer radius of the test object and to allow the transducer to move laterally in the shoe on a plane perpendicular to the center line of the shoe. The lateral motion of the transducer d within the plastic shoe effectively changes the angle of incidence and thus the angle of refraction at the curved interface. By adjusting the lateral position of the transducer in the shoe, the

FIGURE 14. Crack testing of landing gear: (a) landing gear; (b) enlarged area of interest; (c) reference standard.

(a)

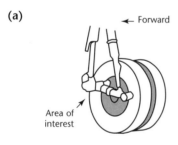

Forward

Area of interest

(b)

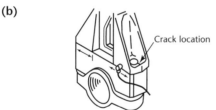

Crack location

(c)

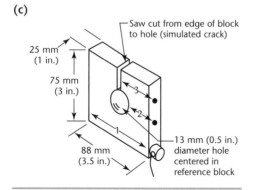

Saw cut from edge of block to hole (simulated crack)

25 mm (1 in.)

75 mm (3 in.)

88 mm (3.5 in.)

13 mm (0.5 in.) diameter hole centered in reference block

FIGURE 15. Display patterns for ultrasonic testing of landing gear: (a) signal at location 1 of Fig. 14c; (b) signal at location 2 of Fig. 14c; (c) signal at location 3 of Fig. 14c; (d) small crack signal in landing gear.

(a)

(b)

(c)

(d)

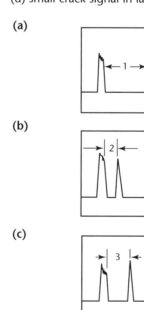

longitudinal wave may be refracted tangentially to the circumference of any size hole (Fig. 17):

(5) $\quad d = r_0 \dfrac{V_1}{V_m} \sin \theta_r$

and:

(6) $\quad \sin \theta_r = \dfrac{r_i}{r_0}$

and:

(7) $\quad d = r_i \dfrac{V_1}{V_m}$

where d is the transducer offset (meter) from the centerline of the tube or shoe, r_i is the inner radius (meter) of the tube or hinge, r_0 is the outer radius of the tube or hinge, V_1 is the velocity (meter per second) of the sound beam in the plastic offset shoe (meter per second), V_m is the velocity (meter per second) of the sound beam in the tube or hinge depending on critical angle, θ_1 is the incident angle (degree) of the beam in plastic and θ_r is the desired refracted angle of the test beam for beam tangency at the inside diameter surface (degree).

FIGURE 16. Ultrasonic detection of cracks in hinge fittings: (a) test of assembly with eyebolt in place; (b) test from above; (c) test from below.

(a)

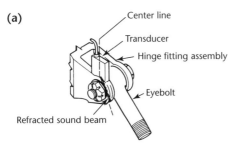

(b)

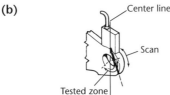

(c)

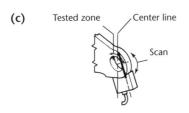

The technique requires only one shoe fabricated to fit the outer radius, regardless of the hole diameter. The test object, unlike the reference standard, may have only a semicircular surface on which scanning can be accomplished. Therefore, to obtain maximum coverage around the hole, the transducer and shoe are moved around the entire curved surface in one direction and are then rotated 3.14 rad (180 deg), and the scan is completed in the opposite direction. Figure 18 shows an example of piston cylinder lug inspection.

Such techniques use fundamental ultrasonic principles programmed into codes for modeling tests with a computer. Fig. 19 shows an example using computer graphics to model the optimum angles. Once the geometry of the object is input into the program, the orientation of the transducer can be adjusted to peak the reflected signal. In Fig. 19, the signal is peaked for either a longitudinal wave or a transverse wave test of the object. The angles of refraction where the signals are peaked are found by changing the parameters in the model. The model also provides estimates of the timing of the reflection which are useful to aid in interpretation. In some cases, echoes may be obtained by both the longitudinal and transverse waves. The model will help determine the source and timing of these signals.

FIGURE 17. Transducer offset for longitudinal ultrasonic tests.

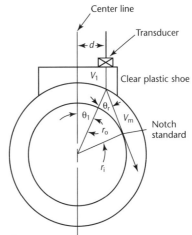

Legend
r_i = inner radius of tube or hinge (meter)
d = transducer offset from the centerline of tube or shoe (meter)
r_0 = outer radius of tube or hinge (meter)
θ_1 = incident angle of beam in plastic (degree)
θ_r = desired refracted angle of the test beam (transverse θ_3 or longitudinal θ_2) for beam tangency at inside diameter surface (degree)
V_1 = velocity of sound beam in plastic offset shoe (meter per second)
V_m = velocity of sound beam in the tube or hinge (shear V_3 or longitudinal V_2) depending on critical angle (meter per second)

Tests for Cracked Structures

An example of ultrasonic testing as applied to aircraft structures is shown in Fig. 18. An angle beam technique is used to detect fatigue cracks at the inside diameter of the attachment lug holes without removing the bushings or disassembly from the aircraft. Cracks as small as 0.25 mm (0.01 in.) deep can be detected with a transverse wave incident to the inner surface at an angle of 0.8 or 1 rad (45 or 60 deg) rather than at a tangent to it. Acrylic (methyl methacrylate) shoes and transducers are used. Reference standards are made of Unified Numbering System H41300 chromium molybdenum steel, with a reference notch 0.25 mm (0.01 in.) deep.[1]

The D_0 and D_i dimensions are used to make the reference standard. Figures 20 and 21 show a transverse wave check of a wing spar splice. Transducer location, reference standard dimensions and typical scope presentations are illustrated. The reference standard design is obtained from data in the engineering drawings. The

FIGURE 18. Ultrasonic testing of piston cylinder lugs: (a) from side and above; (b) looking inboard; (c) from below.

(a)

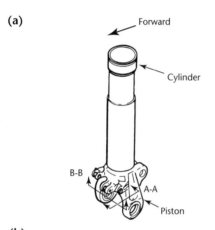

(b)

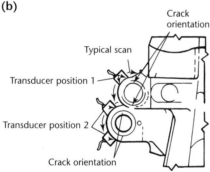

View A-A (looking inboard)

(c)

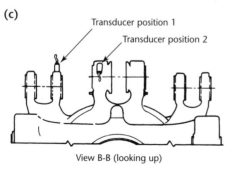

View B-B (looking up)

FIGURE 19. Computer model of ultrasonic testing: (a) 0.5 rad (30 deg) for longitudinal wave test; (b) longitudinal peak signal; (c) 1 rad (60 deg) for transverse wave test; (d) transverse peak signal.

(a)

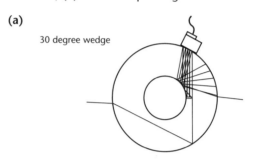

(b)

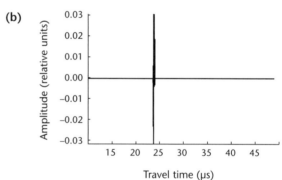

(c)

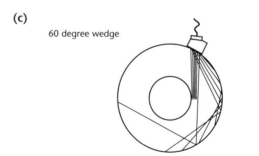

(d)

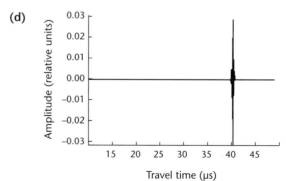

transverse wave test is used to locate fatigue cracks in the horizontal and vertical legs of the lower spar cap. The high stresses associated with these positions usually generate cracks adjacent to the outer two rows of fasteners (as denoted by the darkened fastener pattern). The cracks are oriented parallel to the forward and aft direction so the transverse wave testing is done normal to the crack direction. The cracks in the spar cap are covered by the doubler and the ultrasonic beam is directed under the doublers to detect cracks in the caps.

Unified Numbering System A97075 and A97079 wrought aluminum alloys are highly susceptible to stress corrosion cracking when in the temper 6 (solution heat treatment and aged) condition, especially in the short transverse grain direction. Unfortunately, these alloys, when in temper 6, are used for many primary structural applications because of their high yield and tensile strength properties. For stress corrosion cracking to occur, the object must be exposed to the corrosive environment and subjected to a sustained tensile stress for an undetermined period of time. The time required for the object to crack is directly related to the stress intensity and the type and quantity of corrosive products in the environment. The variability of the time to crack is a major concern because a repetitive testing interval is difficult to establish. In some cases, components have been found cracked by high residual stresses before installation on the aircraft. Similar cracks have occurred in the A97075, temper 6, overwing frame forgings, as illustrated in Fig. 22. Testing these forgings requires removal of cabin seats and interior side panels. Visual testing may be difficult to perform or may not be effective for detecting small cracks.

FIGURE 20. Ultrasonic tests of center wing front spar splice: (a) diagram of component; (b) diagram of wrought aluminum alloy reference standard.

(a)

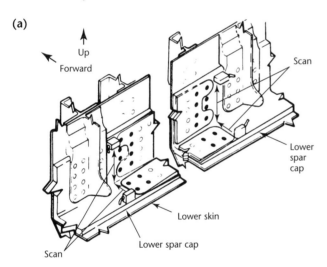

(b)

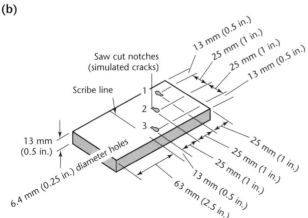

FIGURE 21. A scan display from ultrasonic test of center wing front spar splice: (a) reflection from center hole 1; (b) crack extending from edge of hole 1; (c) crack extending from edge of hole 3; (d) no cracks. Dashed lines represent positions of holes 1, 2 and 3 of Fig. 20.

(a)

(b)

(c)

(d)

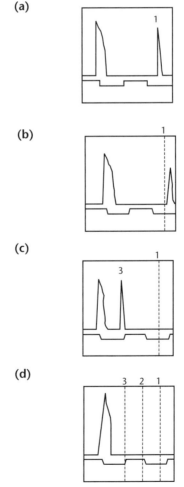

When visual testing is impractical, ultrasonic longitudinal wave (straight beam) techniques may be used as shown in Figs. 23 and 24. In this example, the transducer is placed at the edge of the forging so that the ultrasonic beam is normal to the crack plane for maximum reflection.

Figure 25 shows an example of cracks in the horizontal stabilizer constant section integral machined skin panels (planks) made from Unified Numbering System 97075 wrought aluminum alloy, temper 6. The cracks typically run forward and aft between the bolt holes common to the operating bulkhead. Extensive cracks of this type are possible in the panels and could reduce the strength of the horizontal stabilizer. Ultrasonic testing of the skin panels can detect cracks and

determine their length. A decision to either repetitively test panels with cracks within flyable limits or replace panels with cracks beyond flyable limits can be reached to maintain the structural integrity of the horizontal stabilizer.

Corrosion

Although contact between two galvanically dissimilar metals such as steel and aluminum is a known cause of galvanic exfoliation corrosion, the design of aircraft structures occasionally requires that such metals be joined. When joining them is unavoidable, it is a design requirement that contacting surfaces be electrically insulated with organic paint or that one of the surfaces be coated with a metallic coating galvanically similar to the other surface. For example, on many types of aircraft, cadmium plated steel bolts are used. The cadmium plating not only protects the steel bolts from corrosion but also provides a surface galvanically similar to aluminum so that the possibility of corrosion is greatly reduced. However, if the cadmium is depleted or if a crevice where moisture can collect exists between the fastener head and the aluminum skin, pitting and intergranular corrosion may occur (Fig. 26).

FIGURE 22. Stress corrosion cracking of frame forging of Unified Numbering System A97075 wrought aluminum alloy, temper 6.

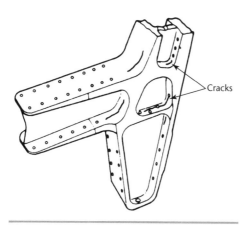

Cracks

FIGURE 23. Ultrasonic testing of frame forging for stress corrosion cracks: (a) from above; (b) cross section.

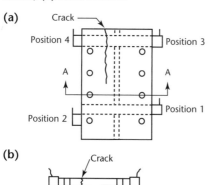

(a)

Crack

Position 4

Position 3

A   A

Position 2

Position 1

(b)

Crack

Transducer positions

Section A-A

FIGURE 24. A scan display of ultrasonic test of frame forging for stress corrosion cracks: (a) position 1 back reflection; (b) position 2 reflection from fastener hole; (c) position 3 crack reflection, far flange; (d) position 4 crack reflection, near flange.

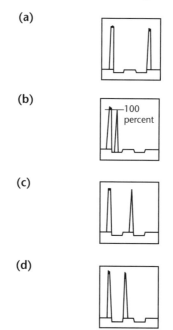

(a)

(b)

100 percent

(c)

(d)

Intergranular corrosion occurs along aluminum grain boundaries which in sheet and plate are oriented parallel to the surface of the material because of the rolling process. Intergranular corrosion in its more severe form is called *exfoliation corrosion* — an intergranular delamination of thin layers of aluminum parallel to the surface, with white corrosion products between the layers. Where fasteners are involved, the corrosion extends outward from the fastener, either from the entire circumference of the hole or in one direction from a segment of the hole. In advanced cases, the surface bulges upward; in milder cases, there may be no bulging and the corrosion can be detected only by eddy current or ultrasonic testing. The ultrasonic testing may be performed as shown in Figs. 27 and 28.

FIGURE 25. Stress corrosion cracks in integrally machined skin panels of horizontal stabilizer constant section: (a) side view; (b) upper skin panel; (c) lower skin panel.

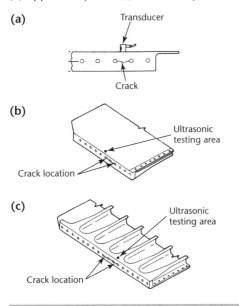

FIGURE 26. Galvanic aspects of corrosion in aluminum cladding.

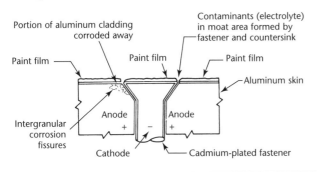

FIGURE 27. Detection of intergranular corrosion with ultrasonic tests: (a) response from unpainted or normal paint thickness with no corrosion; (b) response from paint buildup area with no corrosion; (c) response from corroded area with loss of back reflection.

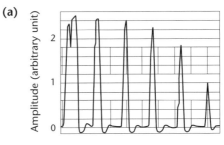

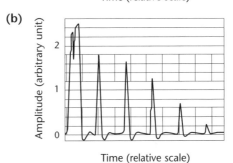

FIGURE 28. Typical exfoliation corrosion in spar cap of extruded Unified Numbering System A97075 wrought aluminum alloy, temper 6: (a) cap; (b) cross section.

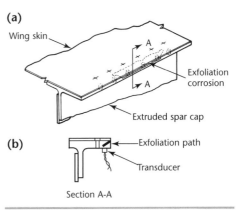

Composite Damage

Composites are nondestructively tested in service to determine the extent of damage and to evaluate repairs. Damage may occur from impact, lightning, erosion, stress or fatigue. Discontinuities include holes, cracks, delaminations, distortion, erosion, water entrapment in honeycomb and burned or overheated surfaces. Ultrasonic testing is used to detect interply delaminations in laminates and skin-to-core disbonds in honeycomb. For honeycomb inspection with access to both sides, through-transmission techniques are preferred using a water coupled test yoke. Transducer frequency is 1 to 2.25 MHz.

Pulse echo techniques are preferred for inspecting a laminate composite structure for interply delamination from one side. Contact probes with soft tip (dry coupled) and conventional contact with appropriate couplants may be used. The most common frequency range is then 2.25 to 5 MHz. Higher frequencies can be used for thin samples, such as less than 2.5 mm (0.1 in.) thick. The transducer should be highly damped and delay lines used to resolve discontinuities near the surface.

Figure 29 shows an ultrasonic C-scan of a damaged composite. The time-of-flight display shows how in composites the damage takes on different shapes with depth in the laminate. In a color version, the near surface appears dark blue. Light blue, green and yellow are deeper and orange is the back surface. It is common in composite damage for ply damage to be larger below the surface. The overall shape of the damage is a function of ply layup. Damage must be mapped for structural repair.

FIGURE 29. Ultrasonic time-of-flight C-scan of damaged region in composite sample.

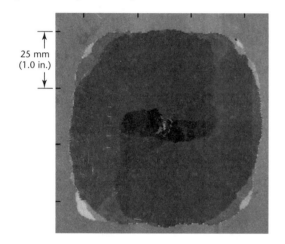

25 mm
(1.0 in.)

Bond Testing[2]

Bond testing is performed on both aluminum bonded and honeycomb composite structures. The common techniques are listed in Table 7 with comments on their application. Bond testing using continuous waves is discussed elsewhere in this volume, in connection with instrumentation.

Bond Testing Instrumentation

An effective tool for bond testing has a combined phase and amplitude detection circuit for detecting and quantifying certain disbond conditions and marginal adhesive strength.

TABLE 7. Bond testing technique.

Technique	Methodology	Comments
Tap testing	Coin tapping or mechanical tap hammer.	Useful on thin structure (three-ply to four-ply composite). Coin test requires operator to listen for dull sound. Tap hammer provides numerical output.
Ultrasonic resonance testing	Ultrasonic transducer is driven at resonance frequency. The electrical impedance of transducer is monitored to detect changes as function of changes in test object.	Reference null is used to set signal and then look for changes as transducer is scanned. Self nulling is also possible. Resonance test can see significant changes, >12 mm (> 0.5 in.) in composite and honeycomb.
Pitch catch	Generation and detection of plate waves affected by poor bonding. Transducer frequency may be swept or constant. Detection may test for time, amplitude or phase effects.	For low frequencies, contact may be made without couplant by using transducers with tips.
Mechanical impedance analysis	Low frequency (audible range) single-contact probe. Loading, like resonance ultrasonic testing, affects amplitude and phase.	Proper test frequency is needed for sensitivity. Setup uses frequency sweep for operator to choose best frequency on test standard. Single-point contact is good for uneven structure. Sensitive to honeycomb far side discontinuities.

The bond tester operates by exciting the test material with a series of pulses from a transmitting transducer. Adhesive bond discontinuities are detected by comparing the wave train from the test object to the wave train received during calibration from a reference standard of known bond integrity.

Pulse transmission is predominantly by lamb waves, because the test object thickness in this application is only a fraction of the wavelength. Transmitted pulses are detected by the receiving transducer and electronically compared to those received from the reference bond. Phase and amplitude change because the pulse travels along a layer of unbonded material. The unbonded layer is more free to vibrate at higher amplitude, with less energy dissipation and lower wave velocity than a bonded reference standard.

Bond Testing System Modes

Alarm Mode. To make a valid comparison of pulses from test objects of unknown integrity, the bond tester is first calibrated to a standard. Amplitude and phase are adjusted to prescribed values while the reference standard is monitored. Then the alarm mode is selected, and its level is set. There are two choices for discontinuity detection in the alarm mode: (1) sensing deviations of the phase from its reference value; (2) sensing the combined deviations of the phase and amplitude. Sensing the combined deviations is recommended. After the amplitude and phase levels are adjusted, the alarm's activation level determines the increase in amplitude and shift in phase required for discontinuity indication by alarm. When testing bond joints in alarm mode, the activation level, amplitude and phase adjustments remain set after calibration. The alarm activation level can be used as a quantitative indicator of bond joint integrity under known conditions.

Metering Mode. In addition to the alarm mode for which the bond tester was designed, a test procedure can be verified by reading the instrument response to the ultrasonic properties of the local bond region. This attempt to quantify bond tester response allows correlation of responses with bond strength, at least for certain failure modes. The bond tester alarm circuit is altered so that the potential difference between the base of transducer and the ground could be measured with a digital volt meter. Voltage readings are recorded as bond integrity measurements for each bond locale.

Bond Reference Standards

The proper preparation and selection of a bond reference standard is a prerequisite to obtaining meaningful and consistent results from ultrasonic tests of bond joints. A reference standard compares the ultrasonic characteristics of test objects with those of a reference standard with known bond integrity. It is essential that the reference standard resemble the test object in material composition and bond joint geometry. It should also possess a level of bond integrity equal to or slightly better than that required in the final product.

A reference standard is required for each material type and for geometry and composition corresponding to the test object. Each reference standard must be prepared under adhesive bonding conditions that closely simulate accepted and expected production practice. The reference standards contain no adhesive discontinuities.

PART 4. Ultrasonic Testing for Space Systems and Aeronautics

Introduction

Ultrasonic nondestructive testing plays a major role in the manufacturing and operations of both space systems and aeronautics. The National Aeronautics and Space Administration has research programs at field centers to develop nondestructive test techniques for assessment of critical structures in manufacturing and in operation. These programs comprise basic and applied research in a broad spectrum of aerospace related sciences and technologies. Many of the nondestructive test activities are also included in programs for the National Aeronautics and Space Administration to transfer its technological expertise to other users — interacting with universities, industry and other government agencies to enhance its research.

Ultrasonic tests and characterizations of advanced material systems play a large role in the agency nondestructive test programs, with a major emphasis on aerospace propulsion systems and space structures. Feasibility of testing is included in every phase of the design and development activities leading to the deployment of critical space hardware. In addition, the National Aeronautics and Space Administration also has a mission objective in aeronautics to develop an understanding of aircraft materials and structures. Typical material systems include composite structures, monolithic ceramics, superalloys and materials for operations at extreme temperature.

Applications covered below include (1) assessment of fatigue and thermal damage in composites using lamb waves, (2) assessment of aging wire insulation, (3) studying fatigue of complex composites and flywheel rotors composed of carbon fiber reinforced polymer matrix composites for energy storage on the *International Space Station,* (4) reinforced carbon-carbon materials for the space shuttle and (5) creep damage in superalloys with acoustoultrasonics.

Lamb Wave Assessment of Fatigue and Thermal Damage in Composites

Composite materials are being used more widely today by both aeronautics and space systems. In addition other industry applications are increasing, including automotive, sports equipment and many others. These increased usages are due to the high strength-to-weight ratio and versatility in design. Composites also provide weight savings over traditional metals without sacrificing strength.[3]

It is important to understand fatigue and thermal damage in composites and how that will affect critical applications.[3] Various techniques have been tested in the past, in particular in ultrasonic testing and characterization. Ultrasonic lamb waves provide a convenient means of evaluating material changes in composites. As a composite material is damaged, the elastic parameters of the structure change and in turn change the lamb wave velocity. This characteristic provides an effective tool to determine damage in composites by monitoring the wave velocity changes. Lamb wave measurements are better than through-thickness ultrasonic measurements because they are sensitive to in-plane elastic properties and can propagate over long distances.[3] It is important to recognize also that thermal degradation as well as mechanical fatigue damage may occur under general thermal mechanical loading.

The correlation between lamb wave velocity and stiffness was measured with strain gages and by correlating lamb wave velocity and crack density for mechanically fatigued composite samples.[3] The fatigue damage experiments were performed using both strain gage and lamb wave velocities. The composite samples were AS4/35001-6 graphite epoxy with a stacking sequence of $[0/90_3]_S$. Two 305×381 mm (12×15 in.) plates were fabricated and C-scanned before being cut into small test samples to check for abnormalities. The scans revealed a porosity level of 5 to 7 percent by volume. The plates were then cut into 280×38 mm (11×1.5 in.) coupons with an average thickness of 1.2 mm (0.05 in.). Two 6.35 mm (0.25 in.) strain gages were attached to each sample: one axial and one transverse. Young's modulus and Poisson's ratio were then obtained from the measurements of the stress, axial strain and transverse strain. Loading to ultimate strength was determined by loading to failure.

The coupons were subjected to tension-tension fatigue in a 380 MPa (55 000 lb$_f$·in.$^{-2}$) capacity load frame at 10 Hz and at an R (ratio of minimum load to maximum load) value of 0.3. The upper load was set to 160 MPa (23 000 lb$_f$·in.$^{-2}$) — 33 percent of ultimate strength. Higher fatigue cycle values were successively applied to the specimens. In this region, only the S_0 and A_0 modes allow for the leading part of the wave to be identified as the lowest order nondispersive symmetric wave. The distances were measured at a precision of 1 mm (0.04 in.), and a least squares fit of the time and distance gave the velocity of the S_0 mode. The velocity of the lowest order symmetric lamb mode was measured and the modulus was obtained from the strain gage measurements both before and after each cyclic loading. The samples were then removed from the load frame at intermediate values of the fatigue cycles to make the contact measurements.

For both fatigued and unfatigued samples, an immersion measurement was also performed to obtain dispersion curves to compare with earlier reported results (Fig. 30).[3] The immersion measurement results agreed with previous tests in a similar arrangement.[4] The results showed that the contact results gave roughly a 7 percent difference in velocity for the symmetric mode when fatigued.[3]

In similar experiments, a correlation with crack density was obtained when performed with the loading raised up to 45 percent ultimate failure at 200 MPa using pin transducers placed on the coupon to obtain lamb wave signals. Crack density measurements within the same 25 × 25 mm (1 × 1 in.) area on the coupon were made optically by counting through a microscope. As expected, the crack density increased with increasing cycles and the velocity squared decreased with increasing cycles, as before. The decrease in modulus was estimated from the crack density measurements using the expression reported by Caslini.[5] For a $[0_m/90_n]_S$ laminate, the stiffness loss was calculated:

$$(8) \quad \frac{E}{E_0} = \frac{1}{1 + \left(\dfrac{nE_2}{mE_1} \dfrac{\tanh \dfrac{\lambda}{2D}}{\dfrac{\lambda}{2D}} \right)}$$

where D is crack density (1 meter), E is modulus for the damaged state, E_0 is modulus for undamaged state, E_1 is longitudinal modulus, E_2 is transverse modulus, G_{12} is shear modulus, h is lamina thickness (meter), m is number of 0 deg layers in the half thickness of the plate, n is number of 90 deg layers in the half thickness of the plate and λ is defined by Eq. 9:

$$(9) \quad \lambda^2 = \frac{3G_{12}E_0}{h^2 E_1 E_2} \frac{n+m}{n^2 m}$$

The results gave a normalized modulus as a function of crack density (Fig. 31).[3]

Thermal experiments were performed using heat damaged samples of 16-ply, uniaxial plates of woven carbon epoxy prepreg with an average thickness of 3.05 mm (0.12 in.). As in the fatigue study above, the lowest order symmetric mode was used for the measurement. The results show a dramatic decrease in velocity with thermal damage along the fiber direction.

Follow-up studies were performed by Seale and Madaras[6] to measure the lamb

FIGURE 30. Plot of lower modes of experimental dispersion curves for one undamaged specimen and one fatigued for 1000 h.[3]

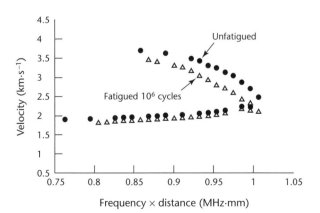

FIGURE 31. Calculated normalized modulus (solid line) as function of normalized velocity squared as function of crack density for all samples.[3]

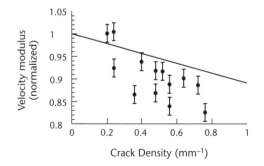

wave velocity over a wide frequency range while subjecting two different composite specimens to thermal mechanical cycling. The composite materials were graphite fiber reinforced amorphous thermoplastic polyimide laminates and high performance graphite fiber reinforced bismaleimide thermoset composite.[6] The 1.22 m by 305 mm samples were manufactured with 16 and 32 plies with stacking sequences of $[45/0/-45/90]_{2S}$ and $[45/0/-45/90]_{4S}$. Thermal mechanical cycling of the samples was performed with either 151 MPa (22 000 $lb_f \cdot in.^{-2}$) or 345 MPa (50 000 $lb_f \cdot in.^{-2}$) capacity load frames equipped with environmental chambers with a thermal control range of –54 °C to 344 °C (–65 °F to 651 °F). The chamber dimensions were 400 mm (16 in.) wide by 686 mm (27 in.) tall by 400 mm (16 in.) deep. The upper and lower sections of the samples remained outside the chamber and only the middle 670 mm (27 in.) section was subjected to thermal extremes.

For all the samples, the load was applied along the length of the samples in the 0 rad (0 deg) direction. Both high and low strain profiles as well as high and low temperature profiles were used. The low strain profiles had strain levels that ranged from 0 to 2000 microstrain with a sustained strain at or above 1040 microstrain for 10 800 s (180 min). The high strain profiles had strain levels ranging from 0 to 3000 microstrain with a sustained strain at or above 1560 microstrain for 10 800 s (180 min). The temperature extremes for the high temperature cycling was –18 °C to 177 °C with a sustained temperature of 177 °C for 10 800 s (180 min) whereas the low temperature cycling was –18 °C and 135 °C with a sustained temperature of 135 °C for 10 800 s mm (180 min). Each

loading cycle lasted for a total of 15 300 s (255 min).

The temperature and strain axes are normalized to sustained levels in the thermal mechanical loading profile (Fig. 32).[6] The graphite fiber reinforced amorphous thermoplastic polyimide laminate samples were subjected to high temperature profiles and both high and low temperature profiles. The 32-ply samples were exposed to low temperature and high strain profiles only.

A digital lamb wave imaging device (Fig. 33)[6] was used in this set of measurements. A unique feature of this system is bicycle tire patch material as couplant between the test sample and the transducers (Fig. 33).

The elastic bending stiffness and out-of-plane stiffness of the sample materials were computed from a reconstruction of the flexural plate mode dispersion curves according to laminated plate theory.[6] For propagation in the 0 rad (0 deg) direction, the only stiffness constants significantly affecting the curve are bending stiffness constant D_{11} and the out-of-plane stiffness constant A_{55}. Consequently, curve fitting of the experimental data was restricted to these two parameters. Figure 34 shows the effect of bending and out-of-plane stiffness constants by reducing the lamb wave velocity.[7] The dispersion curve for propagation in the 1.57 rad (90 deg) direction has similar trends except that D_{22} and A_{44} become the controlling stiffness coefficients for curve fitting of the experimental data.

A reduction in composite stiffness due to matrix cracking was observed. Typical results are shown in Fig. 35 and Table 8. More results are given elsewhere.[6,7] A much larger difference in stiffness loss for the samples loaded at high temperatures as compared to low temperatures was observed, with the graphite fiber reinforced bismaleimide thermoset composite not performing well at high temperatures. The results also indicated

FIGURE 32. Thermal-versus-mechanical profile.[6]

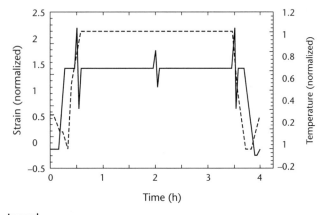

Legend
——— = Strain
- - - - = Temperature

FIGURE 33. Image of scanner, showing frame, bridge and head.[6]

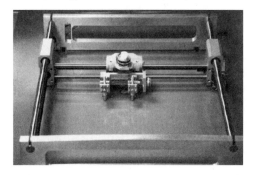

that the out-of-plane shear load carrying capabilities are matrix dominated and that matrix cracking due to mechanical fatigue damage in composites leads to a decrease in elastic moduli. Bending stiffness showed few effects of the thermal mechanical loading: the matrix was insensitive to matrix cracking as well as the large standard deviations in the frequency range used.[8]

Assessment of Aging of Wiring Insulation

Environmental aging of wiring insulation in critical systems because of the onset of brittleness and cracking in both insulation and conductor materials has become an important issue to government agencies such as the Department of Defense, the National Aeronautics and Space Administration and the Federal Aviation Administration and to the industry that manufactures and maintains these critical systems. With this broad interest, a number of different test techniques have been tried, including the development of

an ultrasonic test technique for the aging effects.[9-11] Experiments were performed with military specification wire samples normally used in aircraft: wiring specimens were heat damaged in an oven over a range of heating conditions while measuring axisymmetric mode phase velocities. Samples include a range of types and gages.

FIGURE 35. Mapping of A_{55} stiffness coefficient for composite samples when unaged and when aged for 10 000 h at indicated strain level: (a) 16-ply thermoplastic; (b) 16-ply thermoset; (c) 32-ply thermoset.

(a)

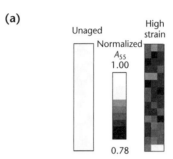

(b)

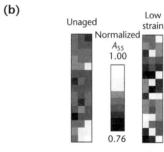

(c)

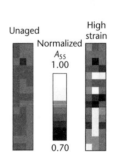

FIGURE 34. Flexural dispersion curves comparing velocities with 25 percent reduction from full values for D_{11} and A_{55} stiffness constants.[7]

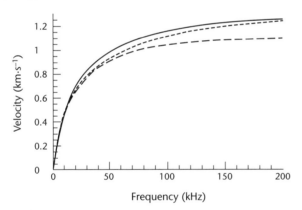

Legend

—— = full stiffness values

- - - - = D_{11} reduced by 25 percent

— — — = A_{55} reduced by 25 percent

TABLE 8. Normalized values for time of flight in aged samples. Time measurements are in seconds.

Direction of Time of Flight	16-Ply Thermoplastic				16 Ply-Thermoset				32-Ply Thermoset			
	Unaged		High Strain		Unaged		High Strain		Unaged		High Strain	
	Time of Flight	Standard Deviation	Time of Flight	Standard Deviation	Time of Flight	Standard Deviation	Time of Flight	Standard Deviation	Time of Flight	Standard Deviation	Time of Flight	Standard Deviation
0 rad (0 deg)	1.03	0.01	1.07	0.02	1.11	0.01	1.09	0.03	1.08	0.01	1.07	0.02
1.57 rad (90 deg)	1.05	0.01	1.07	0.02	1.07	0.01	1.08	0.03	1.06	0.01	1.05	0.02

Development of an applicable model was simplified by the fact that a number of researchers have studied acoustic guided wave propagation in cylinders. In these models, a number of axisymmetric modes propagate in an isotropic cylinder as a function of material properties, geometry, frequency, propagation order and circumferential order. The axisymmetric mode was investigated to determine its ability to detect and quantify degradation in electrical wire insulation because of its nondispersiveness at the low frequencies. The initial experiments measured the dispersion curves on a simple model consisting of a solid cylinder and a solid cylinder with a polymer coating. The lowest order axisymmetric mode was sensitive to stiffness changes in the wire insulation.[9]

Two ultrasonic transducers are used in a pitch catch configuration to generate and receive an ultrasonic guided wave in the wire (Fig. 36).[10] The wave will propagate in both the wire and the insulation, with the amplitude and overall wave speed being affected by the condition and stiffness of the wire

insulation. Experimental details are found elsewhere.[9-11]

The angular dependence of the wave amplitude was examined by holding the transmitting transducer while rotating the receiving transducer in a fixed location in increments of 0.18 rad (10 deg). Axisymmetric modes exhibit no angular dependence, making identification straightforward (Fig. 37).[10]

As an example, the effect of heat damage is shown in Figs. 38 and 39 for MIL-W-22759/34 wire samples of each

FIGURE 38. Images of MIL-W-22759/34 16 gage wire as exposed to room temperature: (a) virgin wire; (b) 349 °C (660 °F) for 1 h; (c) 399 °C (750 °F) for 1 h.[10]

(a)

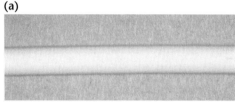

(b)

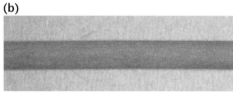

(c)

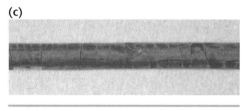

FIGURE 36. Attachment of transducers to insulated wire.[10]

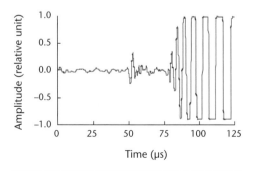

FIGURE 39. Bar chart showing phase velocity for each gage family and each heat damage condition in insulated wire (sheathed in polymer of tetrafluoroethylene and ethylene) using MIL-W-22759/34.[9]

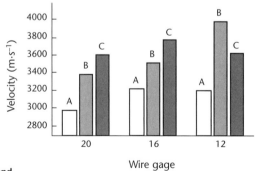

Legend
A. Baseline.
B. Aged 1 h at 349 °C (660 °F).
C. Aged 1 h at 399 °C (750 °F).

FIGURE 37. Typical ultrasonic signals from a polymer coated aluminum rod, showing axisymmetric wave and first flexural wave.[10]

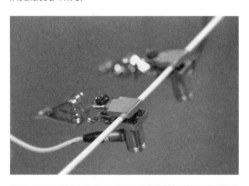

gage to 270 °C (518 °F) for up to 200 h.[9-13] Ultrasonic measurements were taken on samples removed from the oven every 3 h for 15 h and then every 20 h. The results are shown in Fig. 39.[9] The data for each gage show a rapidly increasing phase velocity at short oven exposure times and a slower increasing phase velocity at longer oven exposure times. The measurements of the condition of the insulation appeared to approach a limiting phase velocity value. The damaged wire insulation also became darker and more brittle as the tests continued (Fig. 38).[10]

Similar experiments with the use of lamb waves on composite materials to determine fiber volume fractions in composites showed further applications of lamb waves and provided useful information on composite characteristics.[14]

Ultrasonic Resonance Spectroscopy Applied to Composite Flywheel Rotors

Flywheel energy storage devices comprising multilayered composite rotor systems are being studied extensively for the *International Space Station*. A flywheel system includes the components necessary to store and discharge energy in a rotating mass. The rotor is the complete rotating assembly portion of the flywheel, composed primarily of a metallic hub and a composite rim. The rim may contain several concentric composite rings (Fig. 40).[15] Advances in current ultrasonic spectroscopy research were used to inspect such composite rings and rims and a flat coupon manufactured to mimic the manufacturing of the rings.

Ultrasonic spectroscopy can be a useful nondestructive test technique for material characterization and discontinuity detection.[16,17] Other approaches have used a wide bandwidth frequency spectrum created from a narrow ultrasonic signal and analyzed for amplitude and frequency changes. An ultrasonic resonance spectroscopic system[18] has been developed that uses a continuous swept sine waveform in a pitch catch or through-transmission mode and performs a fast fourier transform on the frequency

FIGURE 40. Simple rotor is metallic hub with rim of eight concentric rings.[15]

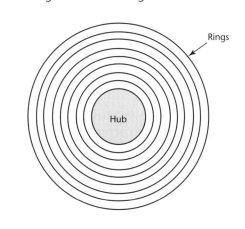

FIGURE 41. Through-transmission ultrasonic spectroscopy on acrylic sample: (left) digital input waveform in time domain; (center) digital output waveform in time domain; (right) typical output display of spectrum and spectrum resonance spacing domains.[15]

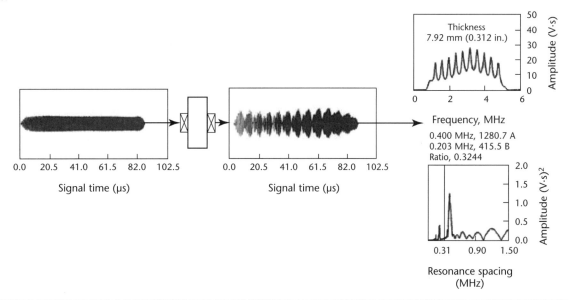

spectrum to create the spectrum resonance spacing domain, or fundamental resonant frequency. Ultrasonic responses from composite flywheel components have been analyzed to assess this nondestructive test technique for the quality assurance of flywheel applications. The objectives of this study were to determine the effects of the constituents of single and multilayer composite material systems and interfacial bond properties within those systems on the frequency responses and the effects of intentionally seeded and naturally occurring discontinuities on the resonant frequencies in the various structures to assess the technique for certifying composite flywheels in the *International Space Station.*

All specimens were measured in the through-transmission, pitch catch configuration using liquid or gel couplant (Fig. 41). Coaxial cables and medium damped transducers were used to maximize energy and bandwidth. The transducer frequency depended on the upper limit of the frequency sweep for the 5 MHz and 10 MHz transducers.

Amplitude and frequency changes in the spectrum and spectrum resonance spacing domains were evaluated from the ultrasonic responses of a flat composite coupon, thin and thick composite rings and a multiple-ring composite rim.[15] Full thickness resonance was produced in discontinuity-free composite rings. Foreign materials and delaminations in composite rings were detected as amplitude reductions in the spectrum domain and changes in fundamental resonant frequency. Manufacturing

variations between the flat composite coupon and composite rings were detected as major differences in the response signals (Fig. 42). The presence of discrete and clustered voids with widths greater than 1.7 mm (0.07 in.) was detected in thick composite rings as an amplitude reduction in the spectrum and spectrum resonance spacing.

A unique detection of kissing disbonds requires further investigation, as their existence in composite rings was not confirmed destructively or corroborated with other nondestructive techniques. Voids with a width of 1.5 mm (0.06 in.) or smaller were not detected in the multiple-ring composite rim. The ultrasonic responses before and after proof spin testing contained the same resonances for the four outer rings, suggesting that damage was not introduced to the rim. As a result, the signals from the multiple-ring composite rim are baseline signatures to be compared after fatigue testing. On the basis of these findings, ultrasonic spectroscopy is a potential nondestructive test tool for flight certification of flywheel rotors for the *International Space Station.*

Impact Damage in Reinforced Carbon-Carbon on Space Shuttle Thermal Protection

Following the space shuttle *Columbia* accident in 2003, an extensive investigation was conducted to determine the physical cause of the orbiter failure and to prevent future mishaps. Analysis of debris, flight data and video revealed the loss of *Columbia* and its crew was caused by a breach of the thermal protection system on the leading edge of the shuttle's left wing. The breach was initiated by insulating foam shedding off of the external tank and striking the reinforced carbon-carbon leading edge structure on ascent. Upon orbiter re-entry, the breach allowed superheated gasses to enter the interior of the wing and melt support structures. Based on these findings, the Columbia Accident Investigation Board made recommendations to develop and validate a physics based model to estimate the severity of damage to the thermal protection system for any future debris impact. The investigators further recommended establishing damage thresholds that would trigger corrective action such as on-orbit inspection or repair. Nondestructive test methods, mainly ultrasonic and thermal, played a key role in both of these efforts.

FIGURE 42. Response from flat composite coupon compared with response from composite ring: (a) spectrum; (b) spectrum resonance spacing.[15]

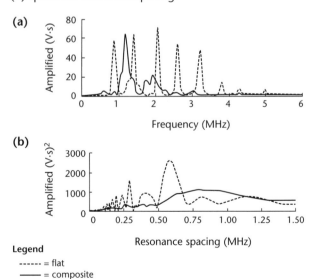

Legend

------ = flat

—— = composite

To achieve the goals requested by the Columbia Accident Investigation Board, researchers at the National Aeronautics and Space Administration first developed a dynamic finite element analysis model to predict the amount of damage resulting from a debris impact with reinforced carbon-carbon. The two main debris types considered were external tank foam insulation and ice. To validate this analytical model, a series of ballistic impact tests were conducted on 150×150×6 mm (6 × 6 in. × 0.25 in.) thick reinforced carbon-carbon panels using projectiles made from representative debris types as shown in Fig. 43.[19] Impacts were conducted over speeds from 91 to 732 m·s⁻¹ (300 to 2400 ft·s⁻¹), and test results were used to validate finite element analysis predictions, to refine the model and to determine the threshold of damage. Results from ultrasonic and thermographic tests were used to measure the damage in the panel because visual testing alone was insufficient.

Each reinforced carbon-carbon panel used in the validation study was inspected before and after ballistic impact using both through-transmission ultrasonic C-scan and pulsed thermography. Ultrasonic tests were conducted using water immersion and 1 MHz transducers for sending and receiving the ultrasonic signal. Because of scattering and attenuation in the woven reinforced carbon-carbon, higher frequencies were found to be ineffective. Nondestructive testing before and after impact was conducted to provide baseline images for comparison and to identify material anomalies in the as received state. Thermographic testing of the panels used xenon flash lamp excitation and a focal plane array infrared camera for image acquisition. Through-transmission ultrasonic testing and thermography turned out to be complementary methods in terms of the types of discontinuities they are most sensitive to (perpendicular to the excitation direction) and were used together extensively to validate findings.

Figure 44 shows images of the baseline and postimpact ultrasonic results for a reinforced carbon-carbon panel subjected to foam impact at 643 m·s⁻¹ (2109 ft·s⁻¹).[19] In addition, postimpact thermography results are also shown for comparison. The ultrasonic images shown represent the peak amplitude of the through-transmission ultrasonic signal received during the tests. It should be noted that the dark, damaged region in the image cannot be identified visually but is easily seen by using ultrasound and thermography together

This project provided the National Aeronautics and Space Administration some very useful data for the Columbia Accident Investigation Board and the Shuttle Program. Ultrasonic imaging, coupled with pulsed thermography, enabled researchers to determine impact energies above which damage was noticeable and below which no detectable change resulted in the nondestructive testing signals. Measurement of this threshold velocity and feedback into the impact model were a vital part of the effort to return the space shuttle to flight.

FIGURE 43. Optical image of reinforced carbon-carbon panels following ballistic impact: (a) impacted with ice projectile at 91 m·s⁻¹ (300 ft·s⁻¹) with no apparent visible damage; (b) impacted with foam at 732 m·s⁻¹ (2400 ft·s⁻¹), with visible damage on both the front and rear of the panel.[19]

(a)

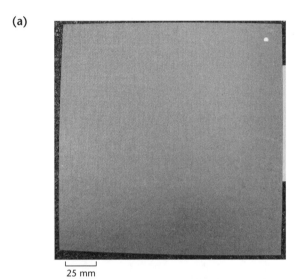

25 mm
(1 in.)

(b)

25 mm
(1 in.)

Acoustoultrasonic Assessment of Creep Damage in Nickel Alloy

Metallic turbine components in operation for long periods of time may experience creep behavior due to elevated temperatures and excessive stresses. As a

FIGURE 44. Nondestructive test results for reinforced carbon-carbon panel subjected to ballistic foam impact: (a) baseline through-transmission ultrasound; (b) postimpact ultrasonic results revealing damage zones; (c) pulsed thermography to confirm ultrasonic results.[19]

(a)

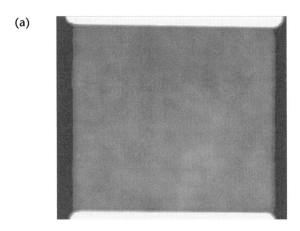

(b)

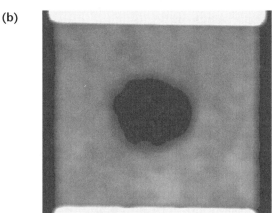

(c)

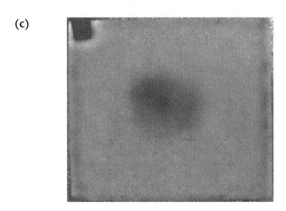

result, it is desirable to monitor and assess the current condition of these components, particularly for early damage detection as well as to prevent failure during operation. Acoustoultrasonics was used to monitor the state of the material at various percentages of creep life in a precipitation hardenable, nickel based alloy.[20] For polycrystalline metals, the permanent deformations associated with creep are due to various stress assisted, thermally activated micromechanisms. These include the generation and mobilizations of dislocations, escape of dislocations from their glide planes, grain boundary sliding and diffusion of atoms and point discontinuities.[19] These mechanisms characterize the majority of the creep life as defined by the primary and secondary portions of a typical strain versus time creep curve. As failure approaches, an increase in strain rate is noticed and is identified as the tertiary portion of the creep curve. The increase in the strain rate is assumed to occur because of additional mechanisms such as the growth and accumulation of cavities along grain boundaries. The growing cavities reduce the effective area of the material with the final result being creep rupture.[21,22]

Acoustoultrasonic testing was used as a nondestructive testing technique for disclosing distributed material changes that occur before the local damage detected by other means of testing. A dual-element (25 MHz broad band, 50 MHz acquisition rate, 10 μs window), contact ultrasonic transducer, in a send/receive arrangement, was used for investigating a region of interest. The intent of the technique was to correlate certain parameters in the detected waveform to characteristics of the material being interrogated. In these experiments, the parameter of interest was the attenuation due to internal damping. The parameters used to indirectly quantify the attenuation were the ultrasonic decay rate as well as various moments of the frequency power spectrum.[23,24]

Creep rupture tests were conducted on specimens of Unified Numbering System N07520, a precipitation hardenable, nickel base alloy. The specimens were designed with a multiple-step gage region to simulate areas of different remaining life, as shown in Fig. 45c.

The overall specimen length was 150 mm (6 in.) — each step, including the grip region, having a length of 25 mm (1 in.). The thickness was 4 mm (0.16 in.). The four gage widths were designed to correspond to 12.5, 25, 50 and 100 percent of used life with fracture in the cross section of smallest area. Hence, the four gage widths ranged from 22.9 to 30 mm (0.9 to 1.2 in.). Additional specimens were stressed at various levels at 732 °C (1350 °F) and at 816 °C (1500 °F). Specimens were also thermally aged without load to compare acoustoultrasonic results of creep tested versus thermally aged conditioning. Figure 45 shows the obtained acoustoultrasonic results as a function of position (that is, used up creep life) compared to an image of the failed specimen.

The first waveform parameter used was the diffuse decay rate, which quantifies the internal damping of the vibration. Damping was measured through determination of the volume averaged decay rate as function of frequency and time. Then the mean square value of the power spectral density M_0 measured the overall energy of the received waveform. Lastly, the shape parameters f_c, f_0 and f_p represented centroid of power spectrum, f_0 the frequency of mean crossings with positive slopes and f_p the frequency of maxima in the time domain.

The data (Fig. 45) show that there was an overall increase in the attenuation. This increase was indicated by the increase in the diffuse field decay rate and the decrease in the ultrasonic wave energy M_0 as the failure region (100 percent of life used) was approached from the right. Another observed effect was the preferential attenuation of the low frequency signal components, which caused the shape parameters f_c, f_0 and f_p to increase with damage. A comparison of the aged specimens (that is, elevated temperatures but no stress) to the creep tested specimens (that is, stress as well as elevated temperatures) showed that the large majority of the changes in the acoustoultrasonic parameters were driven by the creep mechanisms. As a final note, the acoustoultrasonic approach was also applied to characterize the above discussed flywheel materials and showed success in monitoring degradation due to spin testing.

FIGURE 45. Acoustoultrasonic parameters as functions of used up creep life, concerning specimen B2 tested at 732 °C (1350 °F): (a) M_0 and decay rate; (b) f_c, f_0 and f_p; (c) photograph of fractured specimen. Four gage areas on test object represent (from left) 100, 50, 25 and 12.5 percent used up creep life. Scale above specimen shows position: specimen photo is approximately aligned with positions in graphs.[20]

(a)

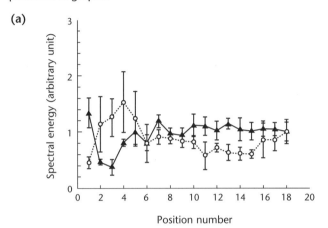

(b)

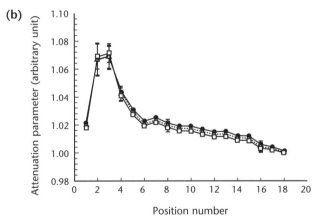

(c)

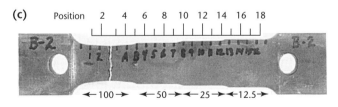

Used up life (percent)

Legend

▲ = M_0
○ = decay rate
● = f_c
△ = f_0
□ = f_p

References

1. Hagemaier, D.J. "Ultrasonic Maintenance Testing of Aircraft Structures." *Nondestructive Testing Handbook,* second edition. Columbus, OH: American Society for Nondestructive Testing (1991): p 635-648.
2. Chapman, G. "Ultrasonic Testing of Automotive Composites." *Nondestructive Testing Handbook,* second edition. Columbus, OH: American Society for Nondestructive Testing (1991): p 649-667.
3. Seale, M.D., B.T. Smith and W.H. Prosser. "Lamb Wave Assessment of Fatigue and Thermal Damage in Composites." *Journal of the Acoustical Society of America.* Vol. 103, No. 55. Melville, NY: American Institute of Physics, for the Acoustical Society of America (May 1998): p 2416-2424.
4. Balasubramaniam, K. and J.L. Rose. "Physically Based Dispersion Curve Feature Analysis in the NDE of Composites." *Research in Nondestructive Evaluation.* Vol. 3. Columbus, OH: American Society for Nondestructive Testing (1991): p 41-67.
5. Caslini, M., C. Zanotti and T.K. O'Brien. "Fracture Mechanics of Matrix Cracking and Delamination in Glass/Epoxy Laminates." *Journal of Composites Technology and Research.* Vol. 9. Amsterdam, Netherlands: Elsevier (Winter 1987): p 121-130.
6. Seale, M.D. and E.I. Madaras. NASA/TM-2000-210628, *Use of Guided Acoustic Waves to Assess the Effects of Thermal Mechanical Cycling on Composite Stiffness.* Washington, DC: National Aeronautics and Space Administration (2000).
7. Seale, M.D. and E.I. Madaras. "Lamb Wave Stiffness Characterization of Composites Undergoing Thermal-Mechanical Aging." *NASA 1998 Technical Documentation CD.* New Port Richey, FL: Integrated Publishing (1998).
8. Seale, M.D. and E.I. Madaras. "Lamb Wave Characterization of the Effects of Long Term Thermal-Mechanical Cycling on Composite Stiffness." *Journal of the Acoustical Society of America.* Vol. 106, No. 3. Melville, NY: American Institute of Physics, for the Acoustical Society of America (September 1999): p 1346-1352.
9. Anastasi, R.F. and E.I. Madaras. "Investigating the Use of Ultrasonic Guided Waves for Aging Wire Insulation." *Fifth Joint NASA/FAA/DoD Conference on Aging Aircraft* [Orlando, FL, September 2001]. NASA Langley, VA: National Aeronautics and Space Administration (2001).
10. Anastasi, R.F. and E.I. Madaras. "Application of Ultrasonic Guided Waves for Aging Wire Insulation Assessment." *Material Evaluation.* Vol. 63, No. 2. Columbus, OH: American Society for Nondestructive Testing (February 2005): p 143-147.
11. Madaras, E.I., T.W. Kohl and W.P. Rogers. "Measurement and Modeling of Dispersive Pulse Propagation in Drawn Wire Waveguides." *Journal of the Acoustical Society of America.* Vol. 97, No. 1. Melville, NY: American Institute of Physics, for the Acoustical Society of America (January 1995): p 252-261.
12. MIL-W-22759/87, *Wire, Electrical, Polytetrafluoroethylene/Polymide Insulated, Normal Weight, Nickel Coated Copper Conductor, 200 Degrees, 600-Volts, for Crimp Applications.* Arlington, VA: Defense Information Systems Agency (1994).
13. MIL-W-22759/34, *Wire, Electrical, Fluoropolymer-Insulated, Crosslinked Modified ETFE, Normal Weight, Tin-Coated Copper, 150 Deg. C, 600 Volt.* Arlington, VA: Defense Information Systems Agency (1994).
14. Seale, M.D., B.T. Smith, W.H. Prosser and J.N. Zalameda. "Lamb Wave Assessment of Fiber Volume Fraction in Composites." *Journal of the Acoustical Society of America.* Vol. 104, No. 3. Melville, NY: American Institute of Physics, for the Acoustical Society of America (1998): p 1399-1403.
15. Harmon, L.M. and G.Y. Baaklini. "Ultrasonic Resonance Spectroscopy of Composite Rings for Flywheel Rotors." *Nondestructive Evaluation of Materials and Composites V. SPIE Proceedings,* Vol. 4336. Bellingham, WA: SPIE — International Society for Optical Engineering (2001): p 24-35.
16. Fitting, D.W. and L. Adler. *Ultrasonic Spectral Analysis for Nondestructive Evaluation.* New York, NY: Plenum (1981).

17. Krautkrämer, J. and H. Krautkrämer. *Ultrasonic Testing of Materials,* fourth edition. New York, NY: Springer (1990).

18. Tucker, J.R. United States Patent 5 591 913, *Apparatus and Method for Ultrasonic Spectroscopy Testing of Materials* (January 1997).

19. *Columbia Accident Investigation Board (CAIB) Mishap Report.* Vol. 1. Washington, DC: United States Government Printing Office, for the National Aeronautics and Space Administration (August 2003).

20. Gyekenyesi, A.L., H.E. Kautz and W. Cao. NASA/TM-2001-210988, *Damage Assessment of Creep Tested and Thermally Aged Udimet 520 Using Acousto-Ultrasonics.* Washington, DC: National Aeronautics and Space Administration (2001).

21. Shames, I.H. and F.A. Cozzarelli. *Elastic and Inelastic Stress Analysis,* revised printing. Philadelphia, PA: Taylor and Francis (1997).

22. Gittus, J.H. *Creep, Viscoelasticity, and Creep Fracture in Solids.* London, United Kingdom: Applied Science Publishers (1975).

23. Tiwari, A. NASA CRT-198374, *Real Time Acousto-Ultrasonics NDE Technique Monitoring Damage in Ceramic Composites under Dynamic Loads.* Washington, DC: National Aeronautics and Space Administration (1995).

24. Lot, L.A. and D.C. Kunerth. "NDE of Fiber-Matrix Interface Bonds and Material Damage in Ceramic/Ceramic Composites." *Conference on Nondestructive Evaluation of Modern Ceramics* [Columbus, OH, July 1990]. Columbus, OH: American Society for Nondestructive Testing (1990): p 135-139.

Bibliography: Ultrasonic Testing of Jet Engines

"NDT of Jet Engines: An Industry Survey." *Materials Evaluation.* Columbus, OH: American Society for Nondestructive Testing. Part One, Vol. 44, No. 13 (December 1986): p 1477-1478, 1480-1482, 1484-1485. Part Two, Vol. 45, No. 1 (January-February 1987): p 26, 28, 30-34.

Bossi, R.H., K.R. Housen and W.B. Shepherd. "Using Shock Loads to Measure Bonded Strength." *Materials Evaluation.* Vol. 60, No. 11. Columbus, OH: American Society for Nondestructive Testing (November 2002): p 1333-1338.

Bossi, R.H., K.R. Housen and W.B. Shepherd. "Application of Stress Waves to Bond Inspection." *SAMPE 2004* [Long Beach, CA, May 2004]. Covina, CA: Society for the Advancement of Materials and Process Engineering (2004).

Brasche, L. "The Use of Nondestructive Inspection in Jet Engine Applications." *Materials Evaluation.* Vol. 60, No. 7. Columbus, OH: American Society for Nondestructive Testing (July 2002): p 853-856.

Bratt, M.J. and V.I.E. Wiegand. "Detection of Flaws in Jet Engine Parts by Ultrasonics." *Nondestructive Testing.* Vol. 13, No. 5. Columbus, OH: American Society for Nondestructive Testing (September-October 1955): p 45-47, 59.

Davis [Witmann], R.S. "Nondestructive Inspection of Jet Engine Assemblies and Components." *Materials Evaluation.* Vol. 48, No. 12. Columbus, OH: American Society for Nondestructive Testing (December 1990): p 1485-1486, 1488-1490.

Ortolano, R.J., B. Kotteakos and M.L. Luttrell. "Automated Ultrasonic Inspection of Turbine Blade Tenons." *Materials Evaluation.* Vol. 51, No. 5. Columbus, OH: American Society for Nondestructive Testing (May 1993): p 568-571.

Papadakis, E.P. "Justification for Engine Parts Testing in Manufacture." *Materials Evaluation.* Columbus, OH: American Society for Nondestructive Testing (December 2002): p 1399-1400.

Vaerman, J. and H. Forsans. AD0196517, *Ultrasonic Testing of Ball Bearings.* Fort Belvoir, VA: Defense Technical Information Center (1971).

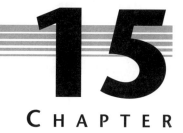

15
CHAPTER

Special Applications of Ultrasonic Testing

David S. Forsyth, Texas Research Institute, Austin, Texas (Part 1)

Lawrence W. Kessler, Sonoscan, Elk Grove Village, Illinois (Part 4)

Francesco Lanza di Scalea, University of California — San Diego, La Jolla, California (Part 2)

Roger D. Wallace (Part 3)

PART 1. Reliability of Nondestructive Testing

Nondestructive testing has critical roles in process control and in inspection of safety critical physical assets such as aircraft, pressure vessels, nuclear reactor components and pipelines, so the measurement of the performance of nondestructive testing has become important. It is no longer sufficient in many cases simply to assume that an inspection is a perfect process of unbounded capability; rather, it is imperative to know the probability of finding discontinuities of interest. This is usually called the *probability of detection.* Probability of detection is described below in terms of cracks but has been applied to other discontinuities such as corrosion loss, impact damage or delamination. Figure 1 shows a representative curve used for analysis of probability of detection for a given application.

The most commonly used measure of nondestructive testing performance is probability of detection. Other measures of nondestructive test performance are considered below. The exact definition of probability of detection, and statistical methods used to calculate probability of detection, have evolved over time. In the 1970s, some probability of detection

curves were constructed by using moving averages, or averaging the response of all cracks in an interval and manually fitting a curve through these points.[1,2] The probability of detection for each interval on the moving average was used to calculate confidence intervals.

Early work was sponsored by the National Aeronautics and Space Administration, and the United States Air Force was moving along a similar path. In both cases, the motivation was the use of damage tolerance philosophies in design and maintenance: it would be assumed that parts contained discontinuities when they left manufacturing, and these discontinuities would grow as cracks under the expected operation of the part. The other technology advance that enabled this approach was the maturing of fracture mechanics models for crack growth in metals.

The National Aeronautics and Space Administration would adopt a damage tolerance approach for the space shuttle program. The United States Air Force adopted fracture mechanics and damage tolerance in response to structural failures in jet aircraft that were virtually new.[3] The Air Force released MIL-STD-1530 in 1972

FIGURE 1. Probability of detection curve from transverse ultrasonic testing of welds for longitudinal cracks in flush grounded, gas tungsten arc welds made of Unified Numbering System A92219, heat treatable, wrought aluminum alloy. Three operators detected 291 indications in 345 opportunities for a combined probability of detection of 90 percent at 7.54 mm (0.030 in.).[6]

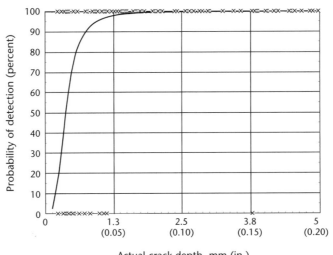

to revise their Aircraft Structural Integrity Program to include damage tolerance.[4] In 1974, MIL-A-83444 detailed the damage tolerance requirements for airplane safety of flight structure.[5] The essence of these approaches is illustrated in Fig. 1: the time for a severe initial cracklike discontinuity a_0 (often called the *rogue discontinuity*) to grow a crack until failure is estimated.[6] Inspections are scheduled to have one or more opportunities in this time to detect the crack and to repair or replace the part before failure.

The approach to damage tolerance illustrated in Fig. 2 shows a single crack size a_{NDT}, defining a threshold above which all cracks would be found. Given a probability of detection curve, the simple answer for picking this size for nondestructive testing would be at the point where probability of detection is 100 percent. However, the binomial statistics used to estimate probability of detection and confidence bounds in the early works required very large numbers of trials to obtain high values of probability of detection and high statistical confidence. In the mid 1970s, the threshold for probability of detection was chosen to be the 95 percent lower confidence bound at the probability of detection of 90 percent. This is often referred to as $a_{90/95}$ or simply the *90/95 value*. The acceptance of the 90/95 criterion as a threshold for inspection capability was due to four factors.

1. A threshold was needed for deterministic fracture mechanics. Damage tolerance approaches of the United States Air Force and the National Aeronautics and Space Administration were such that a crack growth analysis was started from a rogue discontinuity, and the time to crack instability was calculated from this starting point. Inspections are used to detect the crack before instability. To reduce risk, one would prefer 100 percent probability of detection at crack sizes greater than the rogue size. Because 100 percent probability of detection is not likely at any size of crack, a lesser threshold had to be chosen.

2. Binomial statistics were in use to calculate probability of detection and confidence bounds.

3. Using binomial statistics to demonstrate high probability of detection numbers requires many tests: 29 successes out of 29 trials is required for 95 percent confidence that probability of detection is 90 percent. Many more trials are required to increase this confidence.

4. A confidence level of 90/95 percent was consistent with the USAF MIL-HDBK-5 B basis materials allowables, and thus familiar to the people working with the damage tolerance approaches.[7,8]

A published standard or guideline on how to perform an experiment to estimate a probability of detection curve was not available immediately. Within the American Society for Nondestructive Testing, an effort was initiated by W.H. Lewis to develop a recommended practice document. Although the final version was finished in 1976, publication did not occur until 1982.[9,10] This recommended practice was based on binomial methods. In the meantime, the *ASM Handbook* included a section describing possible binomial techniques for estimating the probability of detection. It was acknowledged that the ASM document was developed in concert with the ASNT authors.[11]

The most common technique of estimating probability of detection curves from inspection data are based on USAF MIL-HDBK-1823, released in 1992 as a document of the North Atlantic Treaty Organization.[12,13] The Federal Aviation Administration has also published ways to conduct a probability of detection study, based on the statistical methods described in MIL-HDBK-1823.[14] These statistical methods were developed by Berens and Hovey at the University of Dayton in the 1980s.[15,16] Two principles underpin the approach.

FIGURE 2. Damage tolerance approach to structural integrity used by United States Air Force and National Aeronautics and Space Administration.

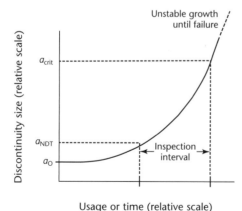

Legend
a_{crit} = discontinuity of critical size
a_{NDT} = discontinuity at moment of test
a_0 = discontinuity before propagation

1. Different cracks of the same size will not be detected with the same probability of detection.
2. In many cases the relationship between the signal from the nondestructive testing system and the size of the crack are linearly related if plotted on a logarithmic chart.

These principles (Fig. 3) give rise to the use of the log normal equation to fit the relationship of crack size and probability of detection.[12]

Nondestructive Test Measures in Practice

The techniques of probability of detection have been continually refined to reduce unpredicted variations in reliability.[12,17-25]

Estimation of Probability of Detection

Both the United States Air Force and the Federal Aviation Administration have published guidelines that describe in detail the experiments required to estimate the probability of detection of an inspection system. These documents are in the public domain and can be obtained for free from the government agencies as well as the Department of Defense's Advanced Materials, Manufacturing, and Testing Information Analysis Center. The United States Air Force and National Aeronautics and Space Administration have updated key handbooks and guidelines.[12,17-19] Requirements for other industries appear in their standards, such as the *ASME Boiler and Pressure Vessel Code*.[26] The reference to be used in a particular application should be based on the regulating body that requires the assessment.

There are a number of useful general statements that can be made.

1. The process of probability of detection estimation requires a number of inspections to be performed.
2. The predefined inspection system being assessed should be complete, including representative equipment, procedures, inspectors and target parts.
3. Parts used should have discontinuities that represent the discontinuities of interest, or a means to assess the difference between the two: for example, using machined notches or flat bottomed holes can provide a useful measure of capability but should not be assumed to represent cracks or other natural discontinuities.
4. The inspection procedure and environment should be typical of the deployed environment. Human factors studies have shown that the relationship of factors — such as environment (such as lighting and temperature), training, experience, motivation and others — to inspection performance is not simple and often not intuitive.

To estimate the probability of detection, it is key to understand the physical parameters that may affect the response to a discontinuity. Parts with discontinuities arising from actual service are optimal but often not available. Therefore every reasonable effort should be made either to replicate the service discontinuities as closely as possible or to carefully define the difference between the probability of detection experiment and inservice conditions.

False Call Rates

The number of false positives or false calls made during inspections is very important in practical applications because of the cost implication and the trust in the nondestructive test procedure. The detection threshold is often lowered to reduce the quantity of dangerous false negatives. However, lowering the detection threshold to capture smaller discontinuities increases false calls. The appropriate level will depend on individual situations. Key factors to consider include the cost of false calls and the cost of passed discontinuities, that is, false calls.

The tradeoff between false calls and the detection of discontinuities of a single size can be visualized using the receiver operating characteristic curve.

Receiver Operating Characteristic

The receiver operating characteristic is a measure in a system of the separation of the noise signals from the signals due to

FIGURE 3. Log linear relationship observed between test signal magnitude and crack size.

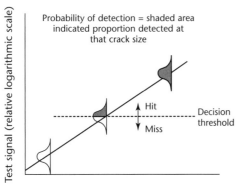

the item of interest (for example, cracks). This measure originated in the evaluation of radar signals in World War Two. It shows how the decision threshold affects the tradeoff between false calls and detection of discontinuities at a single size (Fig. 4).

To plot the receiver operating characteristic curve requires making measurements of the signal distributions from noise and from discontinuities, as shown in Fig. 4. The receiver operating characteristic curve is then plotted by changing the decision threshold and plotting the fraction of detected discontinuities as a function of the fraction of false calls. Starting with a decision threshold at positive infinity, one would find zero discontinuities and have zero false calls. As the decision threshold goes lower, the detection rate goes up with few false calls. As you continue to lower the threshold, the detection rate will increase slowly and the false call rate will increase rapidly.

A set of receiver operating characteristic curves is shown below. The perfect curve is one where the noise signal and discontinuity signal distributions do not overlap, as shown in Fig. 4a. This makes a receiver operating characteristic curve as shown in Fig. 5a. A more realistic curve is the one shown in Fig. 5b, corresponding to Fig. 4b. The worst possible receiver operating characteristic curve is when the noise and discontinuity signal distributions are identical and completely overlap: the inspection cannot

distinguish between the two. This line is at a 0.79 rad (45 deg) angle on the receiver operating characteristic plot (Fig. 5a).

It must be noted that the receiver operating characteristic curve plot applies only to a single discontinuity size and thus provides less information than the probability of detection curve.

Common Mistakes in Estimation of Nondestructive Test Reliability

The means used to assess nondestructive testing reliability have evolved significantly since 1970 and the statistical basis of assessment is often at a level beyond the statistical knowledge of most nondestructive test practitioners. A few errors in the estimation of nondestructive testing reliability are common and must be avoided.

FIGURE 5. Various receiver operating characteristic curves for tests of different capability: (a) best and worst case; (b) realistic case.

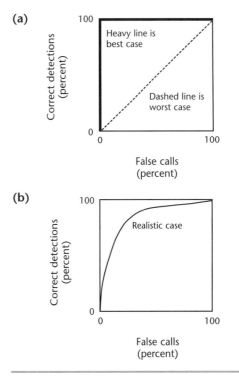

FIGURE 4. Distributions of signals from noise and discontinuities: (a) ideal case of perfect detection, with zero false calls; (b) realistic distribution, in which a higher detection rate also gives higher rate of false calls. Distance between distributions is measure of capability of test and can be represented in receiver operating characteristic curve.

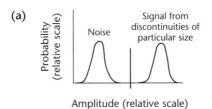

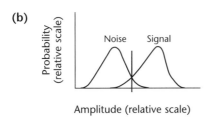

1. Often the customer for nondestructive testing reliability information is the design engineer, who may have very little knowledge of nondestructive testing. It is crucial to know what the end use of the information will be, in order to provide the best estimate of reliability. Often designers will ask for the *smallest discontinuity that can be found.* The nondestructive test practitioner is cautioned to avoid simply replying *the smallest discontinuity ever found.* Rather, the question needs to be clarified so that the designer understands the statistical nature of nondestructive testing. This understanding will help meet the customer's needs and provide the inspector with reasonable expectations.

2. The most common mistake in nondestructive test reliability is the use of pre-existing probability of detection information beyond its scope of applicability. The cost and time required to do a study as described in the USAF MIL-HDBK-1823 may be prohibitive, and the temptation to apply data from previous studies strong. However, old data can be used only with careful engineering judgment and an understanding of all the factors that affect nondestructive test capability in a particular situation. Residual stresses are only one example of factors that are often undocumented but can have an enormous impact on the detectability of cracks.

3. Another common mistake is to assume that repeated inspections will increase probability of detection. Recognizing the statistical nature of the inspection process, many people have then assumed that inspections are independent and therefore repeating the inspections will improve the probability of detection. It must be understood that the concept of statistical independence applies to random events like a coin toss, and an inspection is not a random event.

4. Finally, the use of proper technique documentation, calibration procedures and training are essential to ensure that the carefully controlled data acquired in a probability of detection study can be reproduced in service.

application. The most common technique for assessing nondestructive testing performance is the probability of detection curve. MIL-HDBK-1823 provides detailed information on the experiments required to estimate the probability of detection for a specific inspection technique and application.[12]

Summary

The measurement of the performance of nondestructive testing is important for maintaining safety, for scheduling inspections and maintenance and for technique selection for a particular

Part 2. Ultrasonic Testing in the Railroad Industry

Introduction

Railroad components such as tracks, axles and wheels are usually designed for an infinite life performance based on the fatigue endurance limit of the material. The need to design for infinite life arises from the fact that these components far exceed the 10^6 to 10^7 cycles generated in a common fatigue test, which measures the stress versus the number of cycles to failure. For example, for a typical service duty of 400 000 km per year for high speed railroad systems, the number of cycles that axles and wheels experience is on the order of 2×10^8.[27] Unfortunately, there is no deterministic guarantee that the goal of *infinite life* will be met, for two reasons.

1. Loads experienced in practice differ from hypothetical loads considered in the design phases.
2. Discontinuities can be originated in the manufacturing process or generated by unexpected service events, such as debris impact.

Thus railroad components are maintained with a damage tolerance concept.[28]

According to this philosophy, it is accepted that cracks grow in tracks, axles and wheels provided that these cracks do not reach their critical size during the component's life. Nondestructive testing becomes a critical link of the damage tolerant philosophy. Nondestructive testing allows engineers to make decisions on remaining useful life as well as schedule the frequency of subsequent inspections. Without nondestructive testing, structural failures caused by growing discontinuities may have catastrophic consequences with potential for loss of human life and large direct cost associated to repairs and indirect cost associated to traffic disruptions.

Ultrasonic testing is routinely used for the nondestructive testing of tracks, axles and wheels.[29] Ultrasonic testing is often used with other nondestructive test methods, such as magnetic induction testing in tracks and magnetic particle testing in axles.

Ultrasonic Testing of Rail Track

Motivation

Rail track failures are a cause of great concern to railroad operators and owners. The United States Federal Railroad Administration maintains updated safety statistics on train accidents and associated causes. According to these records, in the decade from 1992 to 2002, track discontinuities causing accidents in the United States were responsible for 2600 derailments and 441 000 000 dollars in reportable damage cost. Unfortunately, these numbers get worse with aging infrastructure and heavier tonnages.

Rail Track Discontinuities

Discontinuities in rail tracks are classified according to their orientation with respect to the major geometrical planes of the track (Fig. 6). The major distinction is between longitudinal discontinuities preferentially oriented in the horizontal plane or in the vertical plane of Fig. 6, and transverse discontinuities (the most severe ones) preferentially oriented in the transverse plane of Fig. 6.[30] Figure 7 schematizes the most typical track discontinuities, including longitudinal discontinuities (horizontal split heads, vertical split heads and vertical split webs), transverse discontinuities

FIGURE 6. Geometrical planes of railroad track.

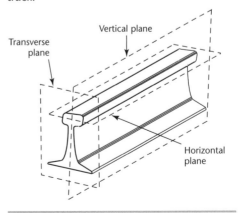

(transverse fissures, detail fractures and compound fractures) and other types of discontinuities internal to the track (weld discontinuities, head web separation, split webs, bolt hole cracks and broken bases). Discontinuities at the surface of the track include shelling, head checks, head squats, engine burn fractures and corrugated track.

Some of these discontinuities originate during manufacturing, such as the transverse fissure from hydrogen nuclei. Others originate in service because of the wheel-to-rail fatigue. Rolling contact fatigue discontinuities initiate at the surface of the rail head as horizontal head checks or squats. A few millimeters from the surface, they can turn to a transverse crack and develop a detail fracture. Because rolling contact fatigue discontinuities tend to form almost continuously in a given track, they are of greater concern than other track discontinuities.

Practice of Rail Track Ultrasonic Testing

In addition to electromagnetic tests, ultrasonic testing has been widely used for discontinuity detection in rail tracks since the 1960s. Normally, the ultrasonic test is targeted to detecting discontinuities in the track head and web, with only limited coverage of the track base.

The frequency of rail track inspection varies from country to country. In the United States, the Federal Railroad Administration mandates that inspections for track discontinuities be made at least once every 40.6×10^9 kg (40×10^6 long tons) or once a year, whichever interval is shorter, for tracks over which passenger trains operate. For tracks over which passenger trains do not operate, the inspection must be carried out every 30.5×10^9 kg (30×10^6 long tons) or once a year, whichever interval is longer.

Tracks testing are tested ultrasonically with longitudinal or transverse transducers in a pulse echo mode or a pitch catch mode. The transducers are in wheels filled with water or a water solution that runs over the surface of the track. Sleds, rather than wheels, can also be used to host several transducers in a smaller area. Specialized test cars typically perform the inspection. Details on common transducer configurations can be found in various references.[31-33] The most common configuration (Fig. 8a) uses transducer orientations to generate ultrasonic beams propagating at normal incidence (0 rad, 0 deg) and at 1.22 rad (70 deg) from the normal to the rail surface. The 0 rad (0 deg) probe targets horizontal cracks while the 1.22 rad (70 deg) probe targets the transverse cracks that tend to grow in a 0.35 rad (20 deg) direction from the transverse plane. A 0.65 rad (37 deg) or 0.79 rad (45 deg) probe is also often used in addition to the previous two orientations to target other discontinuities, including bolt hole cracks and weld discontinuities (Fig. 8a). To target vertical discontinuities, complete search units also host *side looking* transducers, generating beams in the transverse plane, rather than in the vertical plane of the track, typically at 0.79 rad (45 deg) orientations (Fig. 8b).

Wheels or sleds are often used in tandem to provide complete coverage. Using tandem configurations also allows adding pitch catch testing capability to the pulse echo capability of a single wheel.

The standard transducer of a rail track ultrasonic test unit operates at 2.25 MHz; 3 MHz transducers can also be used.

The test car inspections of rail tracks are followed by manual scanning to confirm the presence of a discontinuity and to size it. Generally, both normal beam transducers and angle beam transducers (with conventional acrylic wedges) can be used in manual scanning. As mentioned above, normal beam transducers target horizontal discontinuities whereas angle beam transducers target transverse

FIGURE 7. Typical discontinuities in rail: (a) in the vertical plane; (b) in the transverse plane.

(a)

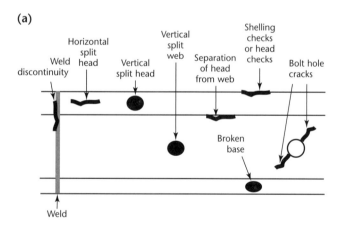

(b)

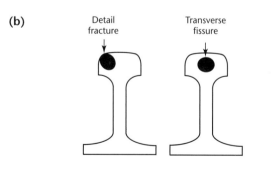

discontinuities. Discontinuities are sized by simply scanning the normal beam transducer for horizontal discontinuities and by using a conventional technique while scanning the angle beam transducers. In addition to conventional normal beam or angle beam configurations, more complex transducer arrangements can be used in manual scanning. Skewed transducer orientations can be used, for example, for the detection of detail fractures.[31] In skewed arrangements, the ultrasonic wave propagates along planes inclined with respect to both the vertical and the transverse plane to enhance the interaction with certain types of discontinuities.

Manual ultrasonic testing is required in the United States to verify any discontinuity indication from the test car search units — the *stop and confirm* test mode. Europe operates, instead, in a nonstop test mode, whereby indications are verified by manual ultrasonic testing only days or weeks after the test car has passed.[34] Modern test cars can operate fast, over 64 km·h⁻¹ (40 mi·h⁻¹), although stopping and confirming in the United States limits the effective testing speed to as slow as 15 km·h⁻¹ (10 mi·h⁻¹).

One serious drawback of current wheel or sled transducer arrangements is the fact that internal transverse discontinuities in the track may be missed by the inspection in the presence of shallow horizontal cracks, such as head checks and shelling. Another drawback is that the high probing frequency (2.25 MHz to 3 MHz) of the transducers is sometimes not effective in penetrating aluminothermic welds due to their grain structure, coarser than that of the surrounding steel.[34,35]

Other Techniques of Rail Track Ultrasonic Testing

To avoid the drawbacks of contact between the test probes and the test rail, noncontact techniques for ultrasonic testing of rail tracks also exist. These include techniques based on electromagnetic acoustic transducers,[36] air coupled transducers,[37,38] and combinations of lasers and air coupled transducers.[39-41] These noncontact approaches are particularly effective when generating ultrasonic guided waves along the rail running direction. Ultrasonic guided waves have been used to inspect rails at probing frequencies ranging from a few tens of kilohertz to a few megahertz (rayleigh waves). Besides providing large inspection ranges, guided waves are particularly sensitive to transverse discontinuities, the most critical in rails. More importantly, they do not suffer from the masking effects of horizontal head checks or shells that instead affect bulk waves excited by wheel or sled transducer configurations as mentioned above.[35,38,39,42,43] Discontinuities are generally detected and sized by measuring reflection or transmission coefficients of the guided waves. A rayleigh wave arrangement (laser or air coupled) that works on a transmission discontinuity detection mode is shown in Fig. 9. In this system, discontinuities in the rail head between the two sensors are detected and sized by monitoring changes in the ratio between the strengths of the two sensor readings.

FIGURE 8. Common transducer arrangements for rail track tests: (a) vertical plane; (b) transverse plane.

(a)

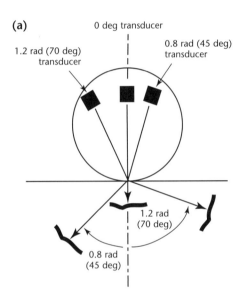

(b)

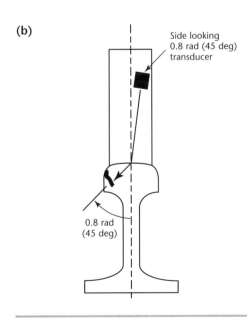

Automatic discontinuity classification capabilities have also been added to guided wave ultrasonic testing of rail tracks through pattern recognition algorithms.[41,44]

Measurement of Residual Stress in Rail Tracks by Ultrasonic Testing

Another successful application of ultrasonic testing of rail tracks is the measurement of longitudinal stresses that develop from temperature gradients and can lead to buckling of the track. Acoustoelastic ultrasonic tests, based on the measurement of ultrasonic velocity, can be used for this purpose.[45-47] Acoustoelastic techniques have proven effective to nondestructively measure stress levels once the effects of material texture and temperature are removed.

Ultrasonic Testing of Axles

Motivation

Train accidents due to axle failures occur worldwide. In the three years from 2002 to 2004, for example, axle failures were the eighth largest cause of accidents having electrical and mechanical causes, with almost 16 000 000 dollars in reportable damage. In the same category of primary cause and during the same period, the journal overheating was the first cause of accidents, associated to reportable damage of 35 000 000 dollars. Reported axle failures in the United Kingdom amount to one or two per year.[48] In Japan, the number of axle failures was greatly reduced with the introduction of ultrasonic testing in 1957 and, subsequently, of angle ultrasonic testing in 1963. After 1963, nevertheless, yearly axle failures were still reported at

0.5 percent, and yearly axle replacement rates were up to 10 percent.[49]

Axle Discontinuities

The causes of failures and methods of inspection in railway components, including axles, has been summarized in the literature.[28] Figure 10 shows the most typical discontinuities found in train axles. These include radial fatigue cracks from fretting at the fitted parts (that is, at the wheel seats), at the brake disk seats (for trailing axles) and at the gear seats (for driving axles); radial fatigue cracks in the transition regions between two principal diameters; radial fatigue cracks at the journal fillet; radial fatigue cracks in the free region of the axle (less frequent); and discontinuities caused by corrosion, for example, when protective coatings are removed accidentally (less frequent).

Fretting remains the most common cause of fatigue cracks in axles, despite measures in various countries to increase fretting fatigue strength.

Practice of Axle Ultrasonic Testing

Railroad axles have been tested by nondestructive testing since the 1950s. Ultrasonic testing is also often combined with magnetic particle testing to probe specific critical surfaces of the axle. As for rail track inspections, the frequency of axle inspections varies from country to country. In the United Kingdom, axles are subjected to ultrasonic testing every 200 days of service or 240 000 km (150 000 mi).[27] Japanese high speed rail axles are inspected for cracks every 30 000 km (19 000 mi) regularly, every 450 000 km (280 000 mi) in inspection of

FIGURE 10. Common discontinuities in train axles.

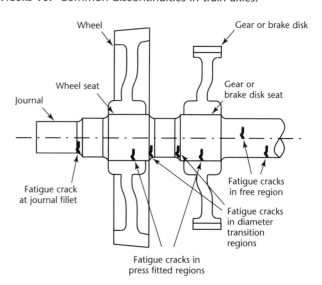

FIGURE 9. Noncontact laser and air coupled arrangement for rail track tests in transmission mode for discontinuity detection.

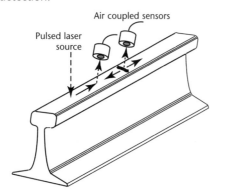

bogies (speed reducing axle components) and every 900 000 km (560 000 mi) in a general inspection.[28]

Most commonly, ultrasonic testing of axles is performed by longitudinal transducers positioned at the axle free ends and operated in either a pulse echo or a pitch catch mode (Fig. 11a). Generally the inspections are performed from both ends of the axle and a discontinuity echo is only flagged as such if it is measured in the same axial position of the axle when testing from either end. The transducers operate in the 1 to 3 MHz frequency range and can be arranged to generate beams in a given direction between 0 rad (0 deg) normal incidence and 0.28 rad (16 deg) angled incidence. The normal incidence is effective for detecting internal cracks whereas the angled incidence configurations are used to probe surface cracks in specific regions of the axle. Although manual scanning of the ultrasonic transducer is most common for the free end inspections, more sophisticated systems can be used. These include either arrays of up to ten transducers, opportunely multiplexed, that can substantially increase the coverage of the axle cross section, or motorized systems that provide automatic scanning of the transducer while maintaining it in constant contact with the axle surface through liquid couplant or dry pressure.

One problem of free end tests is the fact that ultrasonic echoes from the diameter fillets must be distinguished from discontinuity echoes. Ultrasonic angle probes positioned at critical positions along the axle length, developed in the 1960s, have improved the coverage of press fitted areas in axles. The conventional ultrasonic angle probes require manual scanning of the ultrasonic beam to cover the entire cross section of the axle (Fig. 11b). Recently, ultrasonic phased arrays have been proposed to detect radial cracks in the press fitted areas of axles without requiring manual scanning (Fig. 11c). The phased array technique consists of a set of several normal ultrasonic transducers driven at slightly different times, so that they interfere constructively and destructively into an angled wave. Typical ultrasonic operating frequencies for phased array transducers are 3 MHz. The ultrasonic beam is swept electronically with typical steering angles covering a span as large as 0.3 to 1.3 rad (20 to 80 deg).

The phased array technique for axle inspection can be computerized and synchronized with the rotation of the axle to provide full coverage of the axle cross section. The section is covered by mounting phased array probes on manipulators put in contact with the surface of the axle through a water gap while the axle is being rotated. Results are displayed in terms of ultrasonic amplitude versus axle rotational position in cascading charts. Ultrasonic indications (reflections) from variations in diameters, that are circular and symmetric, appear as vertical straight lines; ultrasonic indications from discontinuities, instead, appear as isolated events because most discontinuities do not extend to the entire circumference of the axle. One such computerized phased array system for axle inspection has been used by German Railways.[50]

FIGURE 11. Transducer arrangements for axle tests: (a) longitudinal transducer at axle free end; (b) angle beam transducers; (c) phased array transducers.

(a)

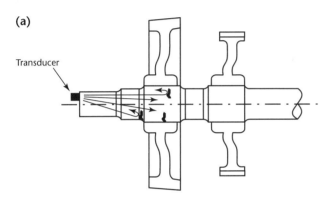

Transducer

(b)

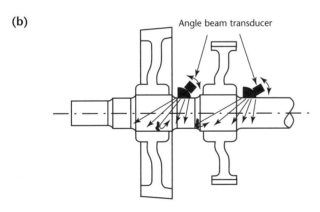

Angle beam transducer

(c)

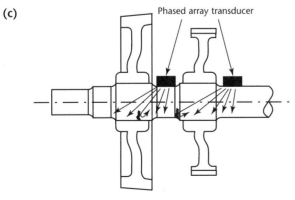

Phased array transducer

A different version of an ultrasonic scanning system is used for the inspection of hollow axles found in urban transit systems. In this case, transverse rather than longitudinal transducers (about 3 MHz frequency) are hosted in a piglike probe inserted into the hollow of the axle. Angle beam testing, typically at 0.79 rad (45 deg) and 1.13 rad (65 deg), is used to detect the cracks. Three-dimensional coverage is provided by rotating the pig and then translating it to a new axial position.

One challenge associated with any ultrasonic technique of axle inspection is that results vary because of inconsistent coupling between the ultrasonic probes and the axle surface. This problem is particularly critical in automated scanning systems where data are acquired in real time while the axle rotates.

Ultrasonic Testing of Wheels

Motivation

Failure of the wheels is another problem of railroad systems, flanges being the top wheel problem. For example, anomalous flanges caused about 360 of the total 680 derailments attributed to wheel failures from 1992 to 2002 in the United States, corresponding to about 30 000 000 dollars in reportable damage.

Wheel Discontinuities

Discontinuities found in train wheels include broken and worn flanges, broken rims and thermal cracks formed by heat generated friction and quenching.

Practice of Wheel Ultrasonic Testing

Most commonly, ultrasonic wheel inspection is performed using surface waves on the wheel tread and flange (Fig. 12).[51] For complete coverage, scanning can be done in both the axial direction (across the rim section) and the radial direction (from the tread surface).[52] Both reflection and transmission measurements can be used for detecting discontinuities. Phased arrays can also be used to relax the requirements for scanning. Both stationary and in-motion tests are possible. In-motion tests use either dry coupling, water immersion or noncontact electromagnetic acoustic transducers. Full inspection is accomplished by a single 6.3 rad (360 deg) rotation of the wheel.

Ultrasonic Measurement of Residual Stress in Wheels

Circumferential tensile stresses can build up in wheels because of heat input from braking. As for rail tracks, residual stresses in wheels can be measured with acoustoelastic ultrasonic tests.[53]

FIGURE 12. Transducer arrangements for wheel tests.

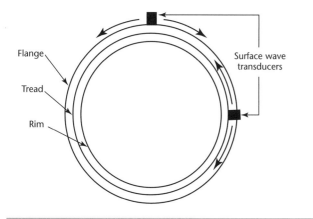

PART 3. Ultrasonic Testing in Marine Industry[54]

Ultrasonic testing is an important tool in the marine industry, in new construction and in ship repairs. Its primary purpose is to ensure that materials and components in a ship's construction or repair meet prescribed quality levels such that the vessel meets its performance requirements as designed. Ultrasonic testing is used in naval and commercial shipbuilding. Although governed by different specifications and codes, the ultrasonic tests are very similar.

Applications of ultrasonic testing in the marine industry vary widely depending on the type of vessel, its operating environment and its use. The materials and components to be tested, the extent of the testing and the criteria used for the tests are specified by the vessel's designer or owner. In general, there are three major testing categories: (1) material testing, (2) fabrication testing and (3) inservice testing. Some common techniques are briefly described below.

Ultrasonic Material Tests

Tests of Plate

During the plate rolling process, impurities or voids present in the ingot become compressed into laminar discontinuities in the finished plate. A compressional wave test from one major surface is used to detect and evaluate this condition. Calibration may be based on the response from flat bottomed holes drilled to mid thickness but is most often based on the back surface reflection height.

Such tests may involve 100 percent scanning of one major surface, scanning along grid lines or static tests at criticality of a grid, depending on the effect of laminations on the intended use of the plate.

Small laminar discontinuities are usually not considered critical to a plate's serviceability: they are judged by size and proximity to each other. However, plates in applications where stress loads are perpendicular to their planar surfaces may be required to be free of laminar discontinuities.

Tests of Pipe

The extrusion and drawing processes used to manufacture pipe tend to elongate discontinuities in a direction parallel to the pipe axis. The most common pipe discontinuities are laps, seams and cracks. These are easily detected using transverse wave ultrasonic tests around the circumference of the pipe.

Such techniques involve 100 percent scanning and may be in only one or in two opposite circumferential directions, some specifications also requiring an axial scan. Calibration is based on inside and outside diameter notches, with depths typically equal to 3 or 5 percent of the wall thickness. Acceptance is based on amplitude comparison.

Tests of Bar Stock

The rolling or forging processes used to manufacture bar stock also tend to elongate discontinuities in an axial direction. The discontinuities are usually toward the center of the bar and are best detected by compression wave testing transverse to the axis.

The test typically involves scanning at least half the circumference of round stock and one of each pair of parallel sides for multisided bar. Calibration is based on drilled flat bottomed holes. Bars may also be tested in the axial direction by inducing sound through one end and monitoring the back reflection.

Tests of Forgings

Forging discontinuities are usually oriented in the direction of the forging flow lines. However, in complex shapes, discontinuities may lie in more than one direction and are often difficult to predict. Consequently, a combination of transverse and compression waves is often used to ensure adequate coverage of the forging in two or three directions.

The number and type of scans depend on the type of forging (hollow, rectangular, round, multisided or disk). Calibration is based on flat bottomed holes for compression wave testing and 3 or 5 percent notches for transverse wave tests. Size and amplitude are the deciding factors.

Tests of Castings

The most common discontinuities found in castings are porosity, slag inclusions, shrinkage, cold shuts, hot tears and cracks. Most of these discontinuities are oriented completely at random. Consequently, compression wave ultrasonic tests in three directions 1.5 rad (90 deg) to each other are recommended when possible.

Calibration is usually based on the response from drilled flat bottomed holes of varying depths but also may be based on the back reflection height. Amplitude and size are used to determine acceptability.

Thickness Tests

With the exception of some cast materials, ultrasonic testing often can be used to measure material thicknesses. Accurate ultrasonic thickness measurement is not possible for stainless steel castings and some nonferrous castings because of variations in sound wave velocity through the cast structure.

Thickness testing involves a basic compression wave test from one surface. Calibration is based on known thicknesses of acoustically similar materials. In addition to a single thickness at a given point, scans may be performed over large areas so that minimum or maximum thicknesses are obtained. Static readings on a grid pattern can also be taken for specific thickness plots.

Fabrication Tests

In the shipbuilding industry, most ultrasonic tests are made on welds. Welding is the primary joining process for marine vessels and the most common discontinuities found in welds are cracks, incomplete fusion, incomplete penetration, slag and porosity.

The extent of testing is governed by the design of the structure and the materials used in construction. Depending on the intended service and requirements of the designers, testing may cover a small sampled area or a percentage, up to 100 percent coverage. Ultrasonics may be used with radiography for greater assurance. Ultrasonics is used to identify the planar discontinuities (such as lack of fusion and cracking) and radiography is used to identify nonplanar discontinuities (such as slag and porosity).

Volumetric Tests of Butt and Corner Welds

Contact transverse wave techniques are primarily used with beam directions perpendicular to the weld in opposite directions and also parallel to the weld. The refracted angle of 0.8, 1.0 or 1.2 rad (45, 60 or 70 deg) depends on the thickness of the weld being tested. Welds may be scanned in the as welded condition or in the flush (ground) condition for butt and corner welds.

Calibration is based on the reflections from side drilled holes in a reference standard. Acceptance criteria are usually based on length of discontinuity and height of reflected signal.

Discontinuities in T Welds

If a T weld requires 100 percent joint efficiency, it may be ultrasonically tested to ensure second side welding. The test is performed using a compressional wave technique from the through-member side. The calibration standard may be a through member (back reflection technique) adjacent to the weld area, or a manufactured piece of similar material and thickness with a specific size machined square notch. Acceptance is usually based on length and height of the reflected signal.

Full and partial penetration T welds are tested for underbead discontinuities that extend into the through-member attachment. A transverse wave technique is used, with the beam directed beneath the weld. The refracted angle, 0.8 or 1 rad (45 or 60 deg), depends on the through-member thickness. Calibration is based on side drilled holes. Acceptance is usually judged on length, height of signal and vertical height (distance of propagation into the through member) for all recordable discontinuities detected in the area of interest.

Bonding Tests

Ultrasonic techniques are used to determine the degree of bonding in such items as silver brazed pipe fittings, lead or babbitt bearings and overlay cladding. Bonding is determined by comparing the ultrasonic test response to the signal patterns obtained from areas of bond and unbond in a reference standard. Areas of unbond produce reflections from the interface. Bonded areas permit ultrasound to pass through the interface and produce reflections from the composite thickness.

Inservice Tests

Weld Tests

Throughout the life of a pressure vessel, surveillance testing is performed at specific intervals to monitor known discontinuities for changes and to detect service induced cracks. The technique is similar to the technique used for the original weld testing.

Thickness Measurement

Ultrasonic thickness measurement is used extensively in the marine industry to monitor changes in thickness caused by corrosion and steam or water erosion or for any reason that thickness monitoring becomes necessary.

The most common uses for thickness surveillance are (1) to monitor the hull thickness for corrosion caused by exposure to sea water and (2) to monitor piping systems for both corrosion and erosion.

Water Level Determination

The level of water in a tank or piping system can often be determined with ultrasonic techniques. If the tank or pipe is vertical, the presence of water is indicated by the ability to transmit sound through the diameter and obtain reflections from the opposite wall. If a tank is lying horizontally, the sound can be transmitted from places on the bottom of the tank and reflected off the surface of the water, so the actual height of the water can be measured.

PART 4. Acoustic Microscopy[55]

Acoustic microscopy is a general term applied to high resolution, high frequency ultrasonic test techniques that produce images of features beneath the surface of a test object. Because ultrasonic energy requires continuity to propagate, discontinuities such as voids, inclusions, delaminations and cracks can interfere with the transmission or reflection of ultrasonic signals.

Conventional ultrasound techniques operate between 1 and 10 MHz. Acoustic microscopes operate up to and beyond 1 GHz, where the wavelength is very short and the resolution correspondingly high. In the early years of acoustic microscopy, it was thought that the highest frequencies would dominate applications. However, because of high attenuation, the frequency range from 10 to 100 MHz is used most extensively.

Acoustic microscopy comprises three distinct techniques: (1) scanning laser acoustic microscopy (SLAM), introduced in the literature in 1970 (Fig. 13),[56,57] (2) C-mode scanning acoustic microscopy, a variation of familiar C-scan instrumentation and (3) scanning acoustic microscopy (SAM).[57,58]

These techniques are complementary to each other. Often, only one technique is suited to a particular application. Acoustic microscopes have been especially useful in solving problems with new materials and components not previously available. The three types of acoustic microscopes are very different from each other and this discussion should provide the potential user with an awareness of their distinctions to maximize opportunities for successful acoustic microscopy.

Fundamentals of Acoustic Microscopy Techniques

For the purposes of comparison, the scanning laser acoustic microscope is primarily considered a transmission mode instrument that creates true real time images of a test object throughout its entire thickness. (The reflection mode is sometimes used.) In operation, ultrasound is introduced to the bottom surface of the test object by a piezoelectric transducer and the transmitted wave is detected on the top by a rapidly scanning laser beam.

The other two systems are primarily reflection mode instruments that use transducers with an acoustic lens to focus the wave at or below the test object

FIGURE 13. Principle components of scanning laser acoustic microscope.

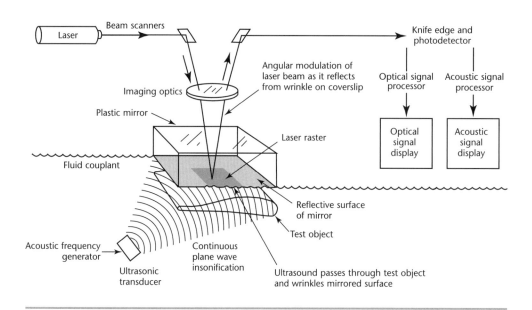

surface. The transducer is mechanically translated (scanned) across the test object in a raster fashion to create the image. The C-scan acoustic microscope system can image several millimeters or more into most test objects and is ideal for analyzing at a specific depth. Because of a very large top surface reflection from the test object, this type of microscope is not effective in the zone immediately below the surface unless rayleigh waves are used with wide aperture transducers.

The scanning acoustic microscope uses rayleigh waves for very high resolution images of the surface and near surface of a test object. Penetration depth is limited to one wavelength of sound because of the geometry of the lens. For example, at 1 GHz, the penetration limit is about 1 µm (4×10^{-5} in.). The C-scan acoustic microscope is designed for moderate penetration into a test object, and transmission mode imaging is sometimes used. This instrument uses a pulse echo transducer, and the specific depth of view can be electronically gated.

Scanning Laser Acoustic Microscopy Operating Principles

A collimated plane wave of continuous wave ultrasound at frequencies up to several hundred megahertz is produced by a piezoelectric transducer beneath the test object (Fig. 13). Because this ultrasound cannot travel through air (making it an excellent tool for crack, void and disbond detection), a fluid couplant is used to bring the ultrasound to the test object. Distilled water, spectrophotometric grade alcohol or other more inert fluids can be used, depending on user concerns for test object contamination.

When the ultrasound travels through the test object, the wave is affected by the homogeneity of the material. Wherever there are anomalies, the ultrasound is differentially attenuated and the resulting image reveals characteristic light and dark features, corresponding to the localized acoustic properties of the test object. Multiple views can be made to determine the specific depth of a discontinuity — such viewing is performed by stereoscopy.[59]

A laser beam is used as an ultrasound detector by sensing the infinitesimal displacements at the surface of the test object — that is, the rippling from the ultrasound. In typical test objects that do not have polished, optically reflective surfaces, a mirrored plastic block, or cover slip, is placed close to the surface and is acoustically coupled with fluid. The laser is focused onto the bottom surface of the cover slip, which has an acoustic pattern that corresponds to the test object surface. By rapid sweeping of the laser beam,

images are produced in real time (30 images per second) and are displayed on a high resolution monitor. In contrast to less accurate uses of the term *real time*, the scanning laser acoustic microscope can be used to observe events as they occur — for example, a crack propagating under an applied load.

The images produced by scanning laser acoustic microscopy are shadowgraphs of structure throughout the thickness of the test object. This provides the distinct advantage of simultaneous viewing of the entire test object thickness, as occurs in X-radiography. In situations where it is necessary to focus on one specific plane, holographic reconstruction of the scanning laser acoustic microscopic data can be used.[60,61]

In a scanning laser acoustic microscope, in addition to an acoustic image on the display, an optical image is produced by means of the direct scanned laser illumination of the test object surface. For this mode, the reflective coating on the cover slip is made semitransparent. The optical image serves as a reference view of the test object that the operator consults for landmark information, artifacts and positioning of the test object to known areas.

These acoustic images also provide useful and easily interpreted quantitative data about the test object.[62] For example, the brightness of the image corresponds to the acoustic transmission level. Precise insertion loss data can be obtained by removing the test object and restoring the image brightness level with a calibrated electrical attenuator placed between the transducer and its electrical driver. With the acoustic interference mode, the velocity of sound can be measured in each area of the test object.[63] When these data are used to determine regionally localized acoustic attenuation loss, modulus of elasticity and so on, the elastic microstructure can be well characterized.

The simplest geometries for scanning laser acoustic microscopic imaging are flat plates or disks. However, with proper fixturing, complex shapes and large test objects can also be accommodated. For example, tiny hybrid electronic components, large metal plates (250×250 mm or 10×10 in.), aircraft turbine blades and ceramic engine cylinder liner tubes have been tested with scanning laser acoustic microscopy.

C-Scanning Acoustic Microscopy Operating Principles

The C-scanning acoustic microscope is primarily a pulse echo (reflection) microscope that generates images by mechanically scanning a transducer in a raster pattern over the test object. A focused spot of ultrasound is generated by an acoustic lens assembly at frequencies from 10 to 100 MHz.

The ultrasound is brought to the test object by a coupling medium, usually water or an inert fluid. The angle of the rays from the lens is generally kept small so that the incident ultrasound does not exceed the critical angle of reflection between the fluid coupling and the solid test object. The focal distance into the test object is shortened considerably by the liquid-to-solid refraction. The transducer alternately acts as sender and receiver, being electronically switched between the transmit and receive modes. A very short acoustic pulse enters the test object and return echoes are produced at the object surface and at specific interfaces within the test material.

Pulse return times are a function of the distance from the interface to the transducer. An oscilloscope display of the echo pattern (an A-scan) clearly shows these levels and their time-versus-distance relationships from the test object surface. This response provides a basis for investigating anomalies at specific levels within a test object. An electronic gate selects information from a specified level while it excludes all other echoes. The gated echo brightens a spot on a display showing the C-scan. The image follows the transducer position and is brightened by signals in the gate.

Older, conventional C-scan instruments produce monoamplitude output on thermal paper when a signal exceeds an operator selected threshold. By comparison, the output of the C-scanning acoustic microscope is displayed in full gray scale, the gray level being proportional to the amplitude of the interface signal. The gray scale can be converted into false color and the images can be color coded with echo polarity information.[64]

In such displays, positive echoes arise from reflections off lower impedance interfaces and are displayed in a different color. This allows quantitative determination of the nature of the interface within the test object. For example, the echo amplitude from a plastic ceramic boundary is very similar to that from a plastic air gap boundary, except that the echoes are 3.14 rad (180 deg) out of phase. To determine whether or not an epoxy is bonded to a ceramic, echo amplitude analysis alone is not sufficient.

The color coded enhanced microscope is further differentiated from conventional C-scan equipment by the speed of the scan. Here, the transducer is positioned by a very fast mechanical scanner that produces images in tens of seconds for typical scan areas the size of an integrated circuit.

It is well known that the large echo from a liquid-to-solid interface (the top surface of the test object) masks the small echoes that may occur near the surface within the solid. This characteristic is known as the *dead zone* and its size is usually on the order of a few wavelengths of sound. Below the surface, the maximum depth of penetration is determined by the attenuation losses in the test object and by the geometric refraction of the acoustic rays, which shorten the lens focus by the solid material. Appropriate transducers and lenses must be used for optimum test results, depending on the depth of interest.

Scanning Acoustic Microscopy Operating Principles

The scanning acoustic microscope is primarily a reflection microscope that generates very high resolution images of surface and near surface features by mechanically scanning a transducer in a raster pattern over the test surface. In the normal mode, an image is generated from echo amplitude data over an X,Y scanned field of view. As with scanning laser acoustic microscopy, a transmission interference mode can be configured for velocity of sound measurements. In contrast to C-scan acoustic microscopy, a more highly focused spot of ultrasound is generated by a very wide angle acoustic lens assembly at frequencies typically ranging from 100 to 2000 MHz. The angle of the sound rays is well beyond the critical cutoff angle, so that there is essentially no wave propagation into the material.

There is a rayleigh (surface) wave at the interface and an evanescent wave reaches to about one wavelength below the surface. As in the other techniques, the ultrasound is brought to the test object by a coupling medium, usually water or an inert fluid. The transducer alternately acts as sender and receiver, being electronically switched between the transmit and receive modes. However, instead of a short pulse of acoustic energy, a long pulse of gated radiofrequency energy is used. No range gating is possible, as in C-scan acoustic microscopy, because of the design of the scanning acoustic microscope. The returned acoustic signal level is determined by the elastic properties of the material at the near surface zone. The returned signal level modulates a cathode ray tube synchronized with the transducer position. In this way, images are produced in a raster scan on the cathode ray tube. As with C-scan acoustic microscopy, complete images are produced in about 10 s.

With the scanning acoustic microscope operating at very high frequencies, it is possible to achieve resolution approaching that of a conventional optical microscope. This technique is used in much the same way as an optical microscope, with the important exception that the information relates to the elastic properties of the material. Even higher resolution than an optical microscope can be obtained by lowering the temperature of operation near absolute zero and using liquid helium as a coupling fluid. The wavelength in the liquid helium is very short compared to that of water, and submicron resolution can be obtained.[65]

The scanning acoustic microscope has been found useful for characterizing the elastic properties of a test object over a microscopic area determined by the transducer's focal spot size. In this technique, the reflected signal level is plotted as a function of the distance between the test object and the lens. Leaky surface waves are generated by mode conversion at the liquid-to-solid interface as the test object is defocused toward the lens. For this reason, an interference signal is produced between the mode converted waves and the direct interface reflection.

The curve obtained is known as the *V(z) curve*. By analyzing its periodicity, the surface wave velocity can be determined. Furthermore, defocusing the lens enhances the contrast of surface features that do not otherwise appear in the acoustic image.[66,67] In addition, by using a cylindrical lens instead of a spherical lens, the anisotropy of materials can be uniquely characterized.[68]

Acoustic Microscopy Applications

Acoustic microscopy is compatible with most metals, ceramics, glasses or polymers and composites made from combinations of the above materials. The compatibility of a material is limited by ultrasound attenuation from scattering, absorption or internal reflection.

In metals, the grain structure causes scattering losses. In ceramics, porosity may cause losses. The magnitude of these effects generally increases with ultrasonic frequency and the dependence is monotonic. The quantitative aspects of this phenomenon have not yet found widespread industrial acceptance although they provide a basis for materials characterization. The techniques of scanning laser acoustic microscopy, C-mode scanning acoustic microscopy

and scanning acoustic microscopy all produce quantitative data in addition to images.

The most popular application of scanning laser acoustic microscopy and C-scanning acoustic microscopy is for nondestructive tests of bonding, delamination and cracks in materials. These instruments are often used for process and quality control although a significant percentage of the devices are placed in analytical and failure analysis laboratories. The most popular application of scanning acoustic microscopy uses its very high magnification mode as a counterpart to conventional optical and electron microscopy, to see fine detail at or near surfaces. The scanning acoustic microscope, like the other acoustic microscopy methods, produces image contrast that is a function of the elastic properties of the test material (nonacoustic techniques may not).

Acoustic Microscopy Tests of Composite Materials

With a combination of materials having different properties and manufactured anisotropy, acoustic microscopy can clearly define the relevant property distribution at the microscopic level. In general, composites contain interfaces that cause scattering of ultrasound and differential attenuation within the field of view. This can be important in determining the population density shifts of fibers within a test object.

Acoustic microscopy can be used to differentiate fibers bonded to the matrix from fibers that are separated from the matrix. Excessive stress, for example, causes a separation. Scanning laser acoustic microscopy can be used to image complex shapes even though the curvature may cause some restriction of the field of view because of critical angle effects and lenslike actions by the test object.

In C-scan acoustic microscopy, the acoustic lens is focused within the material near the top surface of the test object and the electronic gate is set to receive the backscattered signal. Where the test object is made with fibers distributed throughout its volume, acoustic energy is scattered from all depths, and distinct, time separated echoes are not generated. When the transducer is focused deep into the test object, there is less definition of the fibers in the acoustic image, similar to that seen in the scanning laser acoustic microscope image.

Acoustic Microscopy Tests of Ceramic Materials

Ceramic materials are used in many ways and in many industries, including electronics where they serve as substrates for delicate hybrid circuits. In structural applications, ceramics are used where high temperature and light weight are important. Silicon nitride, silicon carbide and zirconia are being studied for combustion engine applications.

Because of the inherent brittleness of ceramic materials, small discontinuities which may contribute to localized stress concentrations are very critical to structural integrity. The successful use of these materials necessitates careful nondestructive testing.

Attenuation changes in ceramics correlate well with variations in strength.[69]

Acoustic microscopy is a powerful tool for nondestructively testing ceramic materials and displaying internal discontinuities and density gradients such as porosity.

References

1. Pettit, D.E. and D.W. Hoeppner. Contract Report NAS 9-11722 LR 25387, *Fatigue Flaw Growth and NDI Evaluation for Preventing Through Cracks in Spacecraft Tankage Structures.* Washington, DC: National Aeronautics and Space Administration (September 1972).
2. Rummel, W.D., P.H. Todd, Jr., R.A. Rathke and W.L. Castner. "Detection of Fatigue Cracks by Nondestructive Evaluation Methods." *Materials Evaluation.* Vol. 32, No. 10. Columbus, OH: American Society for Nondestructive Testing (October 1974): p 205-212.
3. Haviland, G.P. and C. Tiffany. AIAA Paper No. 73-18, "The USAF Aircraft Structural Integrity Program (ASIP)." *Proceedings of the American Institute of Aeronautics and Astronautics 9th Annual Meeting and Technical Display* [Washington, DC, January 1973]. Reston, VA: American Institute of Aeronautics and Astronautics (1973).
4. MIL-A-83444, *Airplane Damage Tolerance Requirements (for Future Procurements)* [superseded by MIL-A-87221]. Philadelphia, PA: Document Automation and Production Service, for the Aeronautical Systems Center of the United States Air Force (1987).
5. MIL-STD-1530, *Aircraft Structural Integrity Program (ASIP).* Philadelphia, PA: Document Automation and Production Service, for the Aeronautical Systems Center of the United States Air Force (2005).
6. Rummel, W.D. and G.A. Matzkanin. *Nondestructive Evaluation (NDE) Capabilities Data Book*, third edition. Austin, TX: Nondestructive Testing Information and Analysis Center (1997).
7. USAF MIL-HDBK-5, *Metallic Materials and Elements for Flight Vehicle Structure*, Part B [superseded by *Metallic Material Properties Development and Standardization* (MMPDS)]. Washington, DC: United States Department of Defense.
8. DOT/FAA/AR-MMPDS, *Metallic Material Properties Development and Standardization.* Washington, DC: United States Department of Transportation (2003).
9. Lewis, W.H., B.D. Dodd, W.H. Sproat and J.M. Hamilton. USAF SA-ALC/MEE 76-6-38-1, *Reliability of Nondestructive Inspections — Final Report (Have Cracks, Will Travel)* (1978).
10. Rummel, W.D. "Recommended Practice for a Demonstration of Nondestructive Evaluation (NDE) Reliability on Aircraft Production Parts." *Materials Evaluation.* Vol. 40, No. 9. Columbus, OH: American Society for Nondestructive Testing (August 1982): p 922-932.
11. Packman, P.F., S.J. Klima, R.L. Davies, J. Malpani, J. Moyzis, W. Walker, B.G.W. Yee and D.P. Johnson. "Reliability of Flaw Detection by Nondestructive Inspection." *Metals Handbook*, Vol. 11: *Nondestructive Inspection and Quality Control*, eighth edition. Materials Park, OH: ASM International (1976): p 414-419.
12. USAF MIL-HDBK-1823, *Nondestructive Evaluation System, Reliability Assessment.* Philadelphia, PA: Document Automation and Production Service, for the Aeronautical Systems Center of the United States Air Force (1999).
13. Anderson, R.T., T.J. DeLacy and R.C. Stewart. NASA CR-128946, *Detection of Fatigue Cracks by Nondestructive Testing Methods.* Washington, DC: National Aeronautics and Space Administration (March 1973).
14. Spencer, F.W., G. Borgonovi, D. Roach, D. Schurman and R. Smith. DOT/FAA/CT-92/12, II, *Reliability Assessment at Airline Inspection Facilities*: Vol. 2, *Protocol for an Eddy Current Inspection Reliability Experiment.* (1993).
15. Berens, A.P. "NDE Reliability Data Analysis." *Metals Handbook:* Vol. 17, *Nondestructive Evaluation and Quality Control*, ninth edition. Materials Park, OH: ASM International (1988): p 659-701.
16. Berens, A.P. and P.W. Hovey. "Statistical Methods for Estimating Crack Detection Probabilities." *Probabilistic Fracture Mechanics and Fatigue Methods: Applications for Structural Design and Maintenance.* Special Technical Publication 798. West Conshohocken, PA: ASTM International (1983): p 79-94.

17. NASA-STD-5009, *Nondestructive Evaluation Requirements for Fracture Control Programs* [draft]. Washington, DC: National Aeronautics and Space Administration (2005).

18. NASA-STD-5013, *Nondestructive Evaluation Requirements for the Durability and Damage Tolerance of Composites*. Washington, DC: National Aeronautics and Space Administration (2000).

19. NASA-STD-5014, *Nondestructive Evaluation (NDE) Implementation Handbook for Fracture Control Programs* [draft]. Washington, DC: National Aeronautics and Space Administration (2003).

20. Forsyth, D.S., A.P. Berens and W.D. Rummel. "Nondestructive Inspection Reliability and Risk in the Field and Depot." *USAF Aircraft Structural Integrity Program* [San Antonio, TX, November 2006]. Dayton, OH: Universal Technology Corporation, for the United States Air Force Research Laboratory (2006).

21. Singh, R. Report Karta-3510-99-01 (AF Contract F41608-99-C-0404), *Three Decades of NDI Reliability Assessment*. San Antonio, TX: Karta Technology (2000).

22. Hyatt, R.W., G.E. Kechter and R.G. Menton. "Probability of Detection Estimation for Data Sets with Rogue Points." *Materials Evaluation*. Vol. 49, No. 11. Columbus, OH: American Society for Nondestructive Testing (November 1991): p 1402-1408.

23. Fahr, A., D.S. Forsyth and M. Bullock. Report LTR-SMPL-1993-0102, *A Comparison of Probability of Detection Data Determined Using Different Statistical Methods*. Ottawa, Ontario, Canada: National Research Council Canada (December 1993).

24. Fahr, A., D.S. Forsyth, M. Bullock and W. Wallace. NRCC-LTR-ST-1961, *NDT Techniques for Damage Tolerance–Based Life Prediction of Aero-Engine Turbine Disks*. Ottawa, Ontario, Canada: National Research Council Canada (February 1994).

25. Spencer, F.W. "Identifying Sources of Variation for Reliability Analysis of Field Inspections." RTO-MP-10, AC/323 (AVT) TP/2, *RTO Meetings Proceedings 10: Airframe Inspection Reliability under Field/Depot Conditions* [Brussels, Belgium]. Neuily-sur-Seine, France: Research and Technology Organization (1998): p 11·1–11·8.

26. *ASME Boiler and Pressure Vessel Code*. New York, NY: ASME International.

27. Smith, A. "Fatigue of Railway Axles: A Classical Problem Revisited." *Thirteenth European Conference on Fracture (ECF)* [San Sebastian, Spain, October 2000]. Amsterdam, Netherlands: Elsevier (2000): p 173-181.

28. Zerbst, U., K. Mädler and H. Hintze. "Fracture Mechanics in Railway Applications — An Overview." *Engineering Fracture Mechanics*. Vol. 72, No. 2. London, United Kingdom: Elsevier (2005): p 163-194.

29. Bray, D.[E.] and G. Vezina. "Ultrasonic Applications in the Railroad Industry." *Nondestructive Testing Handbook*, second edition: Vol. 7, *Ultrasonic Testing*. Columbus, OH: American Society for Nondestructive Testing (1991): p 594-634.

30. *Rail Defect Manual*. Danbury, Connecticut: Sperry Rail Service (1989).

31. Report FRA/ORD-88-39. Washington, DC: Federal Railroad Administration (1988).

32. Anon, F. "Rail-Flaw Detection: A Science That Works." *Railway Track and Structures*. Vol. 86, No. 5. New York, NY: Simmons-Boardman (1990): p 30-32.

33. Grewal, D.S. "Improved Ultrasonic Testing of Railroad Rail for Transverse Discontinuities in the Rail Head Using Higher Order Rayleigh (M_{21}) Waves." *Materials Evaluation*. Vol. 54, No. 9. Columbus, OH: American Society for Nondestructive Testing (September 1996): p 983-986.

34. Clark, R. and S. Singh. "The Inspection of Thermite Welds in Railroad Rail — A Perennial Problem." *Insight*. Vol. 45, No. 6. Northampton, United Kingdom: British Institute of Non-Destructive Testing (June 2003): p 387-393.

35. Wilcox, P., M. Evans, B. Pavlakovic, D. Alleyne, K. Vine, P. Cawley and M. Lowe. "Guided Wave Testing of Rail." *Insight*. Vol. 45, No. 6. Northampton, United Kingdom: British Institute of Non-Destructive Testing (June 2003): p 413-420.

36. Alers, G.A. Report DOT/FRA/ORD-88/09, *Railroad Rail Flaw Detection System Based on Electromagnetic Acoustic Transducers*. Washington, DC: United States Department of Transportation (1988).

37. Wooh, S.C. "Doppler-Based Airborne Ultrasound for Detecting Surface Discontinuities on a Moving Target." *Research in Nondestructive Evaluation*. Vol. 12, No. 3. Columbus, OH: American Society for Nondestructive Testing (2000): p 145-166.

38. Rose, J.L., M.J. Avioli, P. Mudge and R. Sanderson. "Guided Wave Inspection Potential of Defects in Rail." *NDT&E International.* Vol. 37, No. 2. London, United Kingdom: Elsevier (March 2004): p 153-161.

39. Lanza di Scalea, F., I. Bartoli, P. Rizzo and J. McNamara. Report DOT/FRA/ORD-04/16, *On-Line High-Speed Rail Defect Detection.* Washington, DC: United States Department of Transportation (2004).

40. Lanza di Scalea, F., I. Bartoli, P. Rizzo and M. Fateh. "High-Speed Defect Detection in Rails by Noncontact Guided Ultrasonic Testing." *Journal of the Transportation Research Board.* Vol. 1916. Washington, DC: Transportation Research Board (2005): p 66-77.

41. Lanza di Scalea, F., P. Rizzo, S. Coccia, I. Bartoli, M. Fateh, E. Viola and G. Pascale. "Non-Contact Ultrasonic Inspection of Rails and Signal Processing for Automatic Defect Detection and Classification." *Insight.* Vol. 47, No. 6. Northampton, United Kingdom: British Institute of Non-Destructive Testing (June 2005): p 346-353.

42. Rose, J.L., M.J. Avioli and W.-J. Song. "Application and Potential of Guided Wave Rail Inspection." *Insight.* Vol. 44, No. 6. Northampton, United Kingdom: British Institute of Non-Destructive Testing (June 2002): p 353-358.

43. Cawley, P., M.J.S. Lowe, D.N. Alleyne, B. Pavlakovic and P. Wilcox. "Practical Long Range Guided Wave Testing: Applications to Pipes and Rail." *Materials Evaluation.* Vol. 61, No. 1. Columbus, OH: American Society for Nondestructive Testing (January 2003): p 66-74.

44. McNamara, J., F. Lanza di Scalea and M. Fateh. "Automatic Defect Classification in Long-Range Ultrasonic Rail Inspection Using a Support Vector Machine-Based 'Smart System.'" *Insight.* Vol. 46, No. 6. Northampton, United Kingdom: British Institute of Non-Destructive Testing (June 2004): p 331-337.

45. Egle, D.M. and D.E. Bray. Report DOT/FRA/ORD-77/341, *Nondestructive Measurement of Longitudinal Rail Stresses: Application of the Acousto-Elastic Effect to Rail Stress Measurement.* Washington, DC: United States Department of Transportation (1977).

46. Egle, D.M. and D.E. Bray. "Application of the Acoustoelastic Effect to Rail Stress Measurement." *Materials Evaluation.* Vol. 37, No. 4. Columbus, OH: American Society for Nondestructive Testing (March 1979): p 41-46, 55.

47. Bray, D.E. and D.M. Egle. "Ultrasonic Studies of Anisotropy in Cold-Worked Layer of Used Rail." *Metal Science.* Vol. 15, No. 11-12. London, United Kingdom: Institute of Metals (1981): p 574-582.

48. Benyon, J.A. and A.S. Watson. "The Use of Monte Carlo Analysis to Increase Axle Inspection Interval." *Proceedings of the 13th International Wheelset Congress* [Rome, Italy, September 2001]. Brussels, Belgium: Union of European Railway Industries, for the European Railway Wheels Association (2001).

49. Hirakawa, K., K. Toyama and M. Kubota. "The Analysis and Prevention of Failure in Railway Axles." *International Journal of Fatigue.* Vol. 20, No. 2. London, United Kingdom: Elsevier (February 1998): p 135-144.

50. Hansen, W. and H. Hintze. "Ultrasonic Testing of Railway Axles with the Phased Array Technique: Experience during Operation." *Insight.* Vol. 47, No. 6. Northampton, United Kingdom: British Institute of Non-Destructive Testing (June 2005): p 358-360.

51. Bray, D.E., N.G. Dalvi and R.D. Finch. "Ultrasonic Flaw Detection in Model Railway Wheels." *Ultrasonics.* Vol. 11, No. 2. Guildford, United Kingdom: Butterworth Scientific (1973): p 66-73.

52. *Manual of Standards and Recommendation Practices — Wheel and Axle Manual — Section G.* Washington, DC: Association of American Railroads (1998).

53. Fukuoka, H., H. Toda, K. Hirakawa, H. Sakamoto and Y. Toya. "Acoustoelastic Measurements of Residual Stresses in the Rim of Railroad Wheels." *Wave Propagation in Inhomogeneous Media and Ultrasonic Nondestructive Evaluation.* AMD, Vol. 62. New York, NY: ASME International (1984): p 185-193.

54. Wallace, R.[D.] "Ultrasonic Testing in the Marine Industry." *Nondestructive Testing Handbook,* second edition: Vol. 7, *Ultrasonic Testing.* Columbus, OH: American Society for Nondestructive Testing (1991): p 668-669.

55. Kessler, L.W. "Acoustic Microscopy: Industrial and Electronics Applications." *Nondestructive Testing Handbook,* second edition: Vol. 7, *Ultrasonic Testing.* Columbus, OH: American Society for Nondestructive Testing (1991): p 797-817, 826-827.

56. Korpel, A., L.W. Kessler and P.R. Palermo. "Acoustic Microscope Operating at 100 MHz." *Nature.* Vol. 232, No. 5306. Hampshire, United Kingdom: Macmillan (9 July 1971): p 110-111.

57. Kessler, L.W. "Acoustic Microscopy Commentary: SLAM and SAM." *1985 IEEE Transactions on Sonics and Ultrasonics.* Vol. SU-32, No. 2. New York, NY: Institute of Electrical and Electronics Engineers (1985): p 136-138.

58. Lemons, R.A. and C.F. Quate. "Acoustic Microscope — Scanning Version." *Applied Physics Letters.* Vol. 24, No. 4. Melville, NY: American Institute of Physics (1974): p 163-165.

59. Kessler, L.W. and D.E. Yuhas. "Acoustic Microscopy." *Proceedings of IEEE.* Vol. 67, No. 4. New York, NY: Institute of Electrical and Electronics Engineers (April 1979): p 526-536.

60. Lin, Z.C., H. Lee, G. Wade, M.G. Oravecz and L.W. Kessler. "Holographic Image Reconstruction in Scanning Laser Acoustic Microscopy." *Transactions on Ultrasonics, Ferroelectrics and Frequency Control.* Vol. UFFC-34, No. 3. New York, NY: Institute of Electrical and Electronics Engineers (May 1987) p 293-300.

61. Yu, B.Y., M.G. Oravecz and L.W Kessler. "Multimedia Holographic Image Reconstruction in a Scanning Laser Acoustic Microscope." *Acoustical Imaging.* Vol. 16. New York, NY: Plenum (1988): p 535-542.

62. Yuhas, D.E., M.G. Oravecz and L.W. Kessler. "Quantitative Flaw Characterization by Means of the Scanning Laser Acoustic Microscope (SLAM)." *Proceedings of IEEE.* Vol. 67, No. 4. New York, NY: Institute of Electrical and Electronics Engineers (April 1979): p 526-536.

63. Oravecz, M.G. and S. Lees. "Acoustic Spectral Interferometry: A New Method for Sonic Velocity Determination." *Acoustical Imaging.* Vol. 13. New York, NY: Plenum (1984): p 397-408.

64. Cichanski, F.J. United States Patent 4 866 986, *Method and System for Dual Phase Scanning Acoustic Microscopy* (September 1989).

65. Foster, J.S. and D. Rugar. "Low-Temperature Acoustic Microscopy." *Transactions on Sonics and Ultrasonics.* Vol. SU-32. New York, NY: Institute of Electrical and Electronics Engineers (1985): p 139-151.

66. Liang, K.K., G.S. Kino and B.T. Khuri-Yakub. "Material Characterization by the Inversion of V(z)." *Transactions on Sonics and Ultrasonics.* Vol. SU-32. New York, NY: Institute of Electrical and Electronics Engineers (1985): p 213-224.

67. Weglein, R.D. "Acoustic Micro-Metrology." *Transactions on Sonics and Ultrasonics.* Vol. SU-32. New York, NY: Institute of Electrical and Electronics Engineers (1985): p 225-234.

68. Kushibiki, J. and N. Chubachi. "Material Characterization by Line-Focus-Beam Acoustic Microscope. *Transactions on Sonics and Ultrasonics.* Vol. SU-32. New York, NY: Institute of Electrical and Electronics Engineers (1985): p 189-212.

69. Oishi, M. "Nondestructive Evaluation of Materials with the Scanning Laser Acoustic Microscope." *IEEE Electrical Insulation Magazine.* Vol. 7, No. 3. New York, NY: Institute of Electrical and Electronics Engineers, Dielectrics and Electrical Insulation Society (May-June 1991).

Additional Resources on Probability of Detection

Anderson, R.T., T.J. DeLacy and R.C. Stewart. NSAS CR-128946, *Detection of Fatigue Cracks by Nondestructive Testing Methods* (March 1973).Berens, A.P. and P.W. Hovey, AFWAL-TR-81-4160, *Evaluation of NDE Reliability Characterization.* Wright Patterson Air Force Base, OH: United States Air Force (1981).

Forsyth, D.S. and M. Bullock. NRCC-LTR-ST-1947, *A Comparison of Probability of Detection Data Determined Using Different Statistical Methods.* Boucherville, Quebec, Canada: National Research Council Canada (December 1993).

Haviland, G.P. and C. Tiffany. "The USAF Aircraft Structural Integrity Program (ASIP)." *Proceedings of the American Institute of Aeronautics and Astronautics Ninth Annual Meeting and Technical Display* [Washington, DC, January 1973]. Reston, VA: American Institute of Aeronautics and Astronautics (1973).

Packman, P.F., H.S. Pearson, J.S. Owens and G.B. Marchese. AFML-TR-68-32, *The Applicability of a Fracture Mechanics–Nondestructive Testing Design Criterion* (May 1968).

Pettit, D.E. and D.W. Hoeppner. NASA Contract Report CR NAS 9-11722 LR 25387, *Fatigue Flaw Growth and NDT Evaluation for Preventing Through Cracks in Spacecraft Tankage Structures*. Washington, DC: National Aeronautics and Space Administration (September 1972).

Rummel, W.D., P.H. Todd, Jr., R.A. Rathke and W.L. Castner. "Detection of Fatigue Cracks by Nondestructive Evaluation Methods." *Materials Evaluation*. Vol. 32, No. 10. Columbus, OH: American Society for Nondestructive Testing (October 1974): p 205-212.

Rummel, W.D., P.H. Todd, Jr., S.A. Frecska and R.A. Rathke. NASA CR-2369, *The Detection of Fatigue Cracks by Nondestructive Testing Methods* (February 1974).

Rummel, W.D., R.A. Rathke, P.H. Todd, Jr. and S.J. Mullen. MCR-75-212, NASA Contract Report NASA-CR-144639, *The Detection of Tightly Closed Flaws by Nondestructive Testing Methods*. Washington, DC: National Aeronautics and Space Administration (October 1975).

Spencer, F. and D. Schurman. DOT/FAA/CT-92/12, III, *Reliability Assessment at Airline Inspection Facilities: Vol. 3, Results of an Eddy Current Inspection Reliability Experiment*. Washington, DC: United States Department of Transportation (May 1995).

Yee, B.G.W., F.H. Chang, J.C. Couchman and G.H. Lemon. NASA CR-134991, *Assessment of NDE Reliability Data*. Washington, DC: National Aeronautics and Space Administration (1975).

16

Ultrasonic Testing Glossary

Stephen D. Hart, Alexandria, Virginia

PART 1. Terms

Introduction

Many of the definitions in this glossary are adapted from the second and third edition of the *Nondestructive Testing Handbook*.[1-16] The definitions have been modified to satisfy peer review and editorial style. For this reason, references at the end of this glossary should be considered not attributions but acknowledgments and suggestions for further reading.

The definitions in this *Nondestructive Testing Handbook* volume should not be referenced for tests performed according to standards, specifications or contracts. Written procedures should refer to definitions in standards.

This glossary is provided for instructional purposes. No other use is intended.

A

acceptance standard: Document defining acceptable discontinuity size limits.[7] See also *standard*.

acoustic emission: Transient elastic waves resulting from local internal microdisplacements in a material. By extension, the term also describes the technical discipline and measurement technique relating to this phenomenon.[16]

acoustic impedance: Material property defined as the product of sound velocity and density of the material. The relative transmission and reflection at an interface are governed in part by the acoustic impedances of the materials on each side of the interface.[7,22] See also *characteristic acoustic impedance; specific acoustic impedance*.

acoustic microscopy: General term referring to the use of high resolution, high frequency ultrasonic techniques to produce images of features beneath the surface of a test object.[7]

AE: *Acoustic emission* method of nondestructive testing.

amplitude linearity: See *linearity, amplitude*.

amplitude, echo: Vertical height of a received signal on an A-scan, measured from base to peak for a video presentation or from peak to peak for a radio frequency presentation.[7]

analog-to-digital converter: Circuit whose input is analog and whose output is digital.[16]

angle beam: Ultrasound beam traveling at an acute angle into a medium. The angle of incidence or angle of refraction is measured from the normal to the entry surface.[7,22]

angle of incidence: Included angle between the beam axis of the incident wave and the normal to the surface at the point of incidence.[7,21]

angle of reflection: Included angle between the beam axis of the reflected wave and the normal to the reflecting surface at the point of reflection.[7,21]

angle of refraction: Angle between the beam axis of a refracted wave and the normal to the refracting interface.[7,21]

angle beam testing: Technique of ultrasonic testing in which transmission of ultrasound is at an acute angle to the entry surface.[7,21]

angle beam transducer: Transducer that transmits or receives ultrasonic energy at an acute angle to the surface. This may be done to achieve special effects such as setting up transverse or surface waves by mode conversion at an interface.[7,21]

anisotropy: Condition in which properties of a medium (velocity, for example) depend on direction in the medium.

anomaly: Variation from normal material or product quality.[10]

antinode: Point in a standing wave where certain characteristics of the wave field have maximum amplitude.[7,21]

area linearity: See *linearity, area*.

array: Group of transducers used for source location.[16]

array transducer: Transducer made up of several piezoelectric elements individually connected so that the signals they transmit or receive may be treated separately or combined as desired.[7] See also *phased array*.

artificial discontinuity standard: See *acceptance standard*.

A-scan: One-dimensional display of ultrasonic signal amplitude as function of time or depth in test object.

ASNT *Recommended Practice No. SNT-TC-1A*: See *Recommended Practice No. SNT-TC-1A.*

ASNT: American Society for Nondestructive Testing.

attenuation coefficient: Factor determined by the degree of diminution in sound wave energy per unit distance traveled. It is composed of two parts, one (absorption) proportional to frequency, the other (scattering) dependent on the ratio of grain size or particle size to wavelength.[7,23] See also *ultrasonic absorption.*

attenuation: (1) Decrease in acoustic energy over distance. This loss may be caused by absorption, leakage, reflection, scattering or other material characteristics. (2) Decrease in signal amplitude caused by acoustic energy loss or by an electronic device such as an attenuator.[10,16,21]

attenuator: Device for varying the signal amplitude on an ultrasonic instrument. Usually calibrated in decibels.[7,21]

B

back reflection: Signal received from the far boundary or back surface of a test object.[7,21]

background noise: Extraneous signals caused by random signal sources within or exterior to the ultrasonic testing system, including the test material.[7,21] It has electrical, mechanical or chemical origins.[16] Sometimes called *grass* or *hash.*

baseline: Horizontal trace across the A-scan display. It represents time and is generally related to material distance or thickness.[7]

beam exit point: See *probe index.*

beam spread: Widening of the sound beam as it travels through a medium.[21] Specifically, the solid angle that contains the main lobe of the beam in the far field.[7]

bel (B): See *decibel.*

boundary echo: Reflection of an ultrasonic wave from an interface.[7,22]

brittleness: Material characteristic that leads to crack propagation without appreciable plastic deformation.[10]

broad band: Having a relatively wide frequency bandwidth. Used to describe pulses that display a wide frequency spectrum and receivers capable of amplifying them.[7]

B-scan: Data presentation technique typically applied to pulse echo techniques. It produces a two-dimensional view of a cross sectional plane through the test object. The horizontal sweep is proportional to the distance along the test object and the vertical sweep is proportional to depth, showing the front and back surfaces and discontinuities between.[7,22]

bubbler: See *water column.*

burst, forging: See *crack, forging.*

C

calibration, basic: Procedure of standardizing an instrument by using a reference standard.

calibration reflector: Reflector with a known dimensioned surface in a specified material, established to provide an accurately reproducible reference level.[7] See also *reference standard.*

cathode ray: Stream of electrons emitted by a heated filament and projected in a more or less confined beam under the influence of a magnetic or electric field.[7,22]

cathode ray tube: Vacuum tube containing a screen on which ultrasonic scans may be displayed. Used for A-scans or B-scans in the twentieth century.[7]

certification: With respect to nondestructive test personnel, the process of providing written testimony that an individual has met the requirements of a specific practice or standard. See also *certified* and *qualified.*

certified: With respect to nondestructive test personnel, having written testimony of qualification. See also *certification* and *qualification.*

characteristic acoustic impedance: Acoustic impedance typical or *characteristic* of a particular material. See *acoustic impedance; specific acoustic impedance.*

compensator: Electrical matching network to compensate for electrical impedance differences.[7,22]

compressional wave: Wave in which particle motion in the material is parallel to the wave propagation direction. Also called *longitudinal wave.*[7]

contact technique: Testing technique in which the transducer face makes direct contact with the test object through a thin film of couplant.[7,22]

contact transducer: Transducer used in the contact technique.[7]

continuous wave: Wave of constant amplitude and frequency.

contracted sweep: Misnomer that refers to extending the duration of the sweep to permit viewing discontinuities or back reflections from deeper in the test object. The sweep appears to be compressed.[7]

corner effect: Strong reflection obtained when an ultrasonic beam is directed toward the intersection of two or three intersecting surfaces.[7,22]

couplant: Substance used between the transducer and the contacting surface to permit or improve transmission of ultrasonic energy into or from the test object.[7,22]

crack: (1) Break, fissure or rupture, sometimes V shaped in cross section and relatively narrow. By convention, a discontinuity is called a *crack* if it is at least three times longer than it is wide. (2) Propagating discontinuity caused by fatigue, corrosion or stresses such as heat treating or grinding. May be difficult to detect unaided because of fineness of line and pattern (may have a radial or latticed appearance).[10]

crack, cold: Crack that occurs after solidification, because of high stresses from nonuniform cooling.[10]

crack, cooling: Crack resulting from uneven cooling after heating or hot rolling. Cooling cracks are usually deep and lie in a longitudinal direction but are usually not straight.[10]

crack, fatigue: Progressive growth of a crack that usually develops on the surface and is caused by the repeated loading and unloading of the object.[10]

crack, forging: Crack developed by forging at too low a temperature, resulting in rupturing of the material.[10] Also called *burst*.

crack, hot: Crack that develops before the material has completely cooled, as contrasted with cold cracks that develop after solidification.[10]

crack, quenching: During quenching of hot metal, rupture produced by more rapid cooling and contraction of one portion of a test object than occur in adjacent portions.[10]

critical angle: Incident angle of the ultrasound beam where the refracted beam is parallel to the surface and above which a specific mode of refracted energy no longer exists.[7,21]

cross coupling: *Cross talk.*

cross noise: *Cross talk.*

cross talk: Unwanted signal leakage (acoustical or electrical) across an intended barrier, such as leakage between the transmitting and receiving elements of a dual transducer.[7,22] Also called *cross noise* and *cross coupling*.

CRT: See *cathode ray tube*.

crystal: See *transducer element*.

crystal, X-cut: Cut with face perpendicular to the X-dirction of the piezoelectric crystal.[7] In a quartz slice so cut, a thickness mode of vibration occurs when the slice is electrically stimulated in the X direction.[7,22]

crystal, Y-cut: Piezoelectric crystal whose cut face is perpendicular to the Y direction. In quartz, a transverse mode of vibration is obtained when the slice is electrically stimulated in the Y direction.[7,22]

crystal mosaic: Multiple crystals mounted in the same surface on one holder and connected so as to cause all to vibrate as one unit.[7,22]

C-scan: Presentation technique applied to acoustic data and displaying an image of two-dimensional test object with scaled grays or colors representing the ultrasonic signals. The amplitude represented in each pixel may be a pulse echo, through-transmission or pitch catch value calculated from each A-scan datum.

cutoff frequency: Upper or lower spectral response of a filter or amplifier, at which the response is a specified amount less (usually 3 or 6 dB) than the maximum response.

D

damping: (1) Limiting the duration or decreasing the amplitude of vibrations, as when damping a transducer element.[22] (2) Deliberate introduction of energy absorbers to reduce vibrations.[7]

damping capacity: Measure of the ability of a material to dissipate mechanical energy.[7,23]

damping material: Highly absorbent material used to cause rapid decay of vibration.[7]

damping, transducer: Material bonded to the back of the piezoelectric element of a transducer to limit the duration of vibrations.[7,21]

damping, ultrasonic: Decrease or decay of ultrasonic wave amplitude controlled by the instrument or transducer.

dead zone: Interval following the initial pulse at the surface of a test object to the nearest inspectable depth.[21] Any interval following a reflected signal where additional signals cannot be detected.[7]

decibel (dB): Logarithmic unit for expressing relative signal power, such as the loudness of a sound, in proportion to the intensity of a reference signal. One tenth of a *bel*. Decibel in signal amplitude is twice that in signal power.[16] One decibel equals ten times the base ten logarithm of the ratio of two powers.

defect: Discontinuity whose size, shape, orientation or location (1) makes it detrimental to the useful service of its host object or (2) exceeds an accept/reject criterion of an applicable specification.[10,18] Some discontinuities do not exceed an accept/reject criterion and are therefore not defects. Compare *crack; discontinuity; indication*.[10]

delamination: Laminar discontinuity, generally an area of unbonded materials.[7]

delay line: Material (liquid or solid) placed in front of a transducer to cause a time delay between the initial pulse and the front surface reflection.[7,22]

delayed sweep: See *sweep delay*.

delayed time base: See *delayed sweep*.

delta effect: Reradiation or diffraction of energy from a discontinuity.[22] The reradiated energy may include waves of both the incident mode and converted modes (longitudinal and transverse).[7]

delta *t* (Δ*t*): Duration measured between two points in time. Also called *time differential*.

depth compensation: See *distance amplitude correction*.

depth of field: *Focal zone*.

depth of focus: *Focal zone*.

detectability: A measure of the ability to detect signals from small reflectors. Limited by the signal-to-noise ratio.

diffraction: Deflection of a wavefront when passing the edge of an ultrasonically opaque object.[7,22]

diffuse reflection: Scattered, incoherent reflections from rough surfaces.[7,21]

discontinuity: Interruption in the physical structure or configuration of a test object. After nondestructive testing, a discontinuity indication can be interpreted to be a *flaw* or a *defect*.[10] Compare *defect; indication*.

dispersion: In acoustics, variation of wave phase with frequency.[7]

dispersive medium: Medium in which the propagation velocity depends on the wave frequency.[7]

distance amplitude correction: Compensation of gain as a function of time for difference in amplitude of reflections from equal reflectors at different sound travel distances.[7] Refers also to compensation by electronic means such as swept gain, time corrected gain, time variable gain and sensitivity time control.[7,22]

divergence: Term sometimes used to describe the spreading of ultrasonic waves beyond the near field. It is a function of transducer diameter and wavelength in the medium.[7] See *beam spread*.

double-crystal technique: See *pitch catch technique*.

dual transducer: See *send/receive transducer*.

dynamic range: Ratio of maximum to minimum reflective areas that can be distinguished on the display at a constant gain setting.[7,19]

E

echo: Reflected acoustic energy or signal indicating such energy.[7]

effective penetration: In a material, the maximum depth at which a test signal can reveal discontinuities.

electrical noise: Extraneous signals caused by external sources or electrical interferences within an ultrasonic instrument.[21] A component of *background noise*.[7]

electromagnetic acoustic transducer: Transmitting transducer based on the force exerted on a current flowing in a magnetic field. A receiving transducer that detects the current produced by moving a conductor in a magnetic field.[7]

EMAT: See *electromagnetic acoustic transducer*.

evaluation: Process of deciding the severity of a condition after an indication has been interpreted. Evaluation determines if the test object should be rejected or accepted.[7] See also *indication* and *interpretation*.

expanded sweep: Short duration horizontal sweep positioned to allow close examination of a signal.[7]

F

false indication: See *indication, false.*

far field: Zone beyond the near field in front of a plane transducer in which signal amplitude decreases monotonically in proportion to distance from the transducer.[7] Also called the *fraunhofer zone.*

filter: (1) Electrical circuit that leaves a signal unaffected over a prescribed range of frequencies and attenuates signal components at all other frequencies.[10,20] (2) Data analysis process for treating data files.

flat bottom hole: Type of reflector commonly used in reference standards. The end (bottom) surface of the hole is the reflector.[7]

flaw location scale: Specially graduated ruler that can be attached to an angle beam transducer to relate the position of an indication on the display to the actual location of a discontinuity within the test object.[7]

flaw: Unintentional anomaly or imperfection. See also *defect* and *discontinuity.*[10]

focal zone: Distance before and after the focal point in which the intensity differs a specified amount (usually 6 dB) from the focal intensity.[7] Also called *depth of field* or *depth of focus.*

focused beam: Sound beam that converges to a cross section smaller than that of the element.

focused transducer: Transducer that produces a focused sound beam.[7]

fraunhofer zone: See *far field.*

frequency, fundamental: In resonance testing, the frequency at which the wavelength is twice the thickness of the test material.[7,22]

frequency, pulse repetition: Number of pulses per second.[7]

frequency, test: Nominal ultrasonic wave frequency used.[7,22]

frequency: Number of complete wave cycles passing a given point per second or the number of vibrations per second.[7]

fresnel field: See *near field.*

fresnel zone: See *near field.*

front surface: First surface of the test object encountered by an ultrasonic beam.[7]

G

gate: (1) Electronic device for selecting signals in a segment of the trace on an A-scan display. (2) The interval along the baseline that is monitored.[7]

general examination: In personnel qualification, a test or examination of a person's knowledge, typically (in the case of nondestructive test personnel qualification) a written test on the basic principles of a nondestructive test method and general knowledge of basic equipment used in that method. (According to ASNT's guidelines, the general examination should not address knowledge of specific equipment, codes, standards and procedures pertaining to a particular application.)[10]

ghost: Aliasing indication arising from certain combinations of pulse repetition frequency and time base frequency.[7,23] See also *wrap around.*

grass: See *background noise.*

grinding crack: Shallow crack formed in the surface of relatively hard materials because of grinding heat. Grinding cracks typically are 90 degrees to the direction of grinding.[10]

group velocity: Speed at which the envelope of an ultrasonic pulse (many frequencies) propagates through the medium.[7]

H

hardness: Resistance of metal to denting, to plastic deformation by bending or to mechanical deformation by scratching, abrasion or cutting. Typically measured by indentation.

harmonic: Vibration frequency that is an integral multiple of the fundamental frequency.[7,21]

hash: See *background noise.*

heat affected zone: Base metal that was not melted during brazing, cutting or welding but whose microstructure and physical properties were altered by the heat.[10]

hertz (Hz): Measurement unit of frequency, equivalent to one cycle per second.[10,17]

horizontal linearity: Measure of proportionality between positions of indications on the horizontal trace and the positions of their corresponding reflectors.

I

immersion technique: Test technique in which the test object and the transducer are submerged in a liquid (usually water) that acts as the coupling medium.[22] The transducer is not usually in contact with the test object.[7]

impedance, acoustic: See *acoustic impedance.*

indication: Nondestructive test equipment response to a reflector, requiring interpretation to determine its relevance. Compare *crack; defect; discontinuity; indication, false.*[10]

indication, discontinuity: Visible evidence of a material discontinuity. Subsequent interpretation is required to determine the indication's significance.[10]

indication, false: Test indication that originates where no discontinuity exists in the test object. Compare *defect; indication, nonrelevant.*[10]

indication, nonrelevant: Indication possibly caused by an actual discontinuity that does not affect the usability of the test object (a change of section, for instance) or that is smaller than a relevant indication. Compare *indication, false* and *indication, relevant.*[10]

indication, relevant: Indication from a discontinuity (as opposed to a nonrelevant indication) requiring evaluation by a qualified inspector, typically with reference to an acceptance standard, by virtue of the discontinuity's size, shape, orientation or location. Compare *indication, nonrelevant.*[10,19]

initial pulse: Pulse applied to excite the transducer. It is the first indication on the screen if the sweep is undelayed. Also called the *main bang.* May refer to an electrical pulse or an acoustic pulse.[7]

insonification: Irradiation with sound.[7]

interface: Physical boundary between two adjacent media.[7,21]

interface synchronization: See *interface triggering.*

interface triggering: Triggering the sweep and auxiliary functions from an interface echo occurring after the initial pulse.[7] Also called *interface synchronization.*

interpretation: Determination of the source, significance and relevance of test indications.[10]

isotropy: Condition in which significant medium properties (sound speed, for example) are the same in all directions.[7]

L

lamb wave: Type of ultrasonic wave propagation in which the wave is guided between two parallel surfaces of the test object. Mode and velocity depend on the product of the test frequency and the thickness. Plate wave.[7]

linearity, amplitude: Constant proportionality between the signal input to the receiver and the amplitude of the signal appearing on the display of the ultrasonic instrument or on an auxiliary display.[7,19] Also called *vertical linearity.*

linearity, area: Constant proportionality between the signal amplitude and the areas of equal discontinuities located at the same depth in the far field. Necessarily limited by the size of the ultrasonic beam and configuration of the reflector.[7]

logarithmic decrement: Natural logarithm of the ratio of the amplitudes of two successive cycles in a damped wave train.[7]

longitudinal wave: Wave in which points of same phase lie on parallel plane surfaces.[7,23]

loss of back reflection: Absence or significant reduction of an indication from the back surface of the test object.[7,21]

M

main bang: See *initial pulse.*

manipulator: In immersion testing, a device for angular orientation of the transducer[7,24] and for scanning motion in three axes.

markers: Series of indications on the horizontal trace of the display screen to show increments of time or distance.[7,21]

material noise: Random signals caused by the material structure of the test object.[7,21] A component of *background noise.*

mechanical properties: Measurable properties of a material related to its behavior, such as toughness, hardness and elasticity. Compare *physical properties.*

mode conversion: Change of ultrasonic wave propagation mode upon reflection or refraction at an interface.[7]

mode converted signal: Unintended signal from mode conversion of primary test angle, due to interaction with component geometry such as the signals after back wall signal when testing a long narrow bar.

mode of vibration: Manner in which an acoustic wave is propagated, as characterized by the particle motion in the wave[21] (transverse, lamb, surface or longitudinal).[7]

model, analytical: Mathematical representation of a process or phenomenon.

multiple back reflections: Repetitive echoes from the far boundary of the test object.[7,21]

multiple-echo technique: Technique where thickness is measured between multiple back reflections, minimizing error from coatings or from changes in temperature or contact pressure.

N

narrow band: Relative term denoting a restricted range of frequency response.[7,22]

NDC: Nondestructive characterization.

NDE: (1) *Nondestructive evaluation.* (2) *Nondestructive examination.*

NDI: *Nondestructive inspection.*

NDT: *Nondestructive testing.*

near field: Distance immediately in front of a plane transducer in which the ultrasonic beam exhibits complex and changing wavefronts. Also called the *fresnel field* or *fresnel zone.*[21]

neper: Natural logarithm of a ratio of two amplitudes (equal to 8.686 dB) used as a measure of attenuation. Power ratios are expressed as half the natural logarithm.[7]

nodal points: In angle beam testing, the location of reflections at opposite surfaces as a wave progresses along a test object.[7]

noise: Undesired or unintended signals that tend to interfere with normal reception or processing of a desired signal. The origin may be an electric or acoustic source, small discontinuities or abrupt changes in the acoustic properties of the test material.[7,22] See also *signal-to-noise.*

noncontact transducer: In ultrasonic testing, a sensor designed for wave propagation through gas.

nondestructive characterization (NDC): Branch of nondestructive testing concerned with the description and prediction of material properties and behavior of components and systems.

nondestructive evaluation (NDE): Another term for nondestructive testing. In research and academic communities, the word *evaluation* is sometimes preferred because it implies interpretation by knowledgeable personnel or systems.[10]

nondestructive examination (NDE): Another term for nondestructive testing. In the utilities and nuclear industry, the word *examination* is sometimes preferred because *testing* can imply performance trials of pressure containment or power generation systems.[10]

nondestructive inspection (NDI): Another term for nondestructive testing. In some industries (utilities, aviation), the word *inspection* often implies maintenance for a component that has been in service.[10]

nondestructive testing (NDT): Determination of the physical condition of an object without affecting that object's ability to fulfill its intended function. Nondestructive test methods typically use an appropriate form of energy to determine material properties or to indicate the presence of material discontinuities (surface, internal or concealed).[10]

nonrelevant indication: See *indication, nonrelevant.*

normal incidence: (1) Condition in which the axis of the ultrasonic beam is perpendicular to the entry surface of the test object. (2) Condition where the angle of incidence is zero.[7]

O

optimum frequency: Probe frequency that provides the highest signal-to-noise ratio compatible with the detection of a specific discontinuity. Each combination of discontinuity type and material may have a different optimum frequency.[7,22]

orientation: Angular relationship of a surface, plane, discontinuity or axis to a reference plane or surface.[7,21]

oscillogram: Common term for a record or photograph of data displayed on screen.[7,22]

P

parasitic echo: See *spurious echo.*

particle motion: Movement of particles of material during wave propagation.[7]

penetration, ultrasonic: Propagation of ultrasonic energy into a material.[7] See also *effective penetration.*

period: Value of the minimum duration after which the same characteristics of a periodic waveform or a periodic feature repeat.[10]

phantom: Reference standard used to verify the performance of diagnostic ultrasound systems.[7]

phase velocity: Velocity of a single frequency continuous wave.[7]

phased array: Mosaic of transducer elements in which the timing of the elements' excitation can be individually controlled to produce certain desired effects, such as steering or focusing the beam.

physical properties: Nonmechanical properties such as density, electrical conductivity, heat conductivity and thermal expansion.[10] Compare *mechanical properties*.

piezoelectric effect: Ability of certain materials to convert electrical energy (voltage) into mechanical energy (stress) and vice versa.[7,22]

pitch catch technique: Ultrasonic test technique that uses two transducers, one transmitting and the other receiving on the same or opposite surface.[7,21,22] Also called *double-crystal technique* or *two-transducer technique*.

plane wave: See *longitudinal wave*.

plate wave: See *lamb wave*.

point of incidence: Point at which the axis of the sound beam leaves the wedge of an angle beam transducer and enters the test object.[7,22] See also *probe index*.

poling: Process of reorienting crystal domains in certain materials by applying a strong electric field at elevated temperatures, inducing macroscopic polarization and piezoelectric behavior.[7]

presentation: Technique used to show ultrasonic information. This may include A-scans, B-scans or C-scans, displayed on various types of recorders or display instruments.[7,21]

primary reference response level: Ultrasonic response from the basic reference reflector at the specified sound path distance, electronically adjusted to a specified percentage of full screen height.[7]

probe: See *sensor; transducer*.

probe index: Point on a transverse wave or surface wave transducer through which the emergent beam axis passes.[7,23] See also *point of incidence*.

propagation: Movement of a wave through a medium.[7,21]

pulse: Transient electrical or ultrasonic signal that has a rapid increase in amplitude to its maximum value, followed by an immediate return.[16]

pulse echo technique: Ultrasonic test technique in which discontinuities are detected by return echoes from the transmitted pulses.[7]

pulse length: Measure of pulse duration expressed in time or number of cycles.[7,22]

pulse repetition frequency: See *repetition rate*.

pulse tuning: Control of pulse frequency to optimize system response.[7]

Q

qualification: Process of demonstrating that an individual has the required amount and the required type of training, experience, knowledge and abilities.[10] See also *certification* and *qualified*.

qualified: Having demonstrated the required amount and the required type of training, experience, knowledge and abilities.[10] See also *certified* and *qualification*.

quality: Ability of a process or product to meet specifications or to meet the expectations of its users in terms of efficiency, appearance, reliability and ergonomics.[10]

quality assurance: Administrative actions that specify, enforce and verify quality.[10]

quality control: Physical and administrative actions required to ensure compliance with a quality assurance program. Quality control may include nondestructive testing in the manufacturing cycle.[10]

R

radian (rad): Measurement unit of plane angle subtending, in a circle, an arc equal in length to the radius.

radio frequency display: Presentation of unrectified signals.[7,22] See also *video presentation*.

range: Maximum ultrasonic path length that is displayed.[7] See also *sweep length*.[22]

rarefaction: Thinning or separation of particles in a propagating medium due to the decompression phase of an ultrasonic cycle. Opposite of compression. A compressional wave is composed of alternating compressions and rarefactions.[7,21]

rayleigh wave: Ultrasonic wave that propagates along the surface of a test object. The particle motion is elliptical in a plane perpendicular to the surface, decreasing rapidly with depth below the surface. The effective depth of penetration is considered to be about one wavelength.[7] Also called *surface wave*.

receiver: (1) Section of the ultrasonic instrument that amplifies echoes returning from the test object. (2) Transducer that picks up the echoes.[7]

recommended practice: Set of guidelines or recommendations.[10]

Recommended Practice No. SNT-TC-1A: Set of guidelines published by the American Society for Nondestructive Testing, for employers to establish and conduct a qualification and certification program for nondestructive testing personnel.[10]

reference standard: (1) Test object containing known reflectors representing accept or reject criteria. (2) Sample test object selected for reference.

refracted beam: Beam transmitted in the second medium when an ultrasonic beam is incident at an acute angle on the interface between two media having different sound speeds.[7,22]

refraction: Change in direction of an acoustic wave as the ultrasonic beam passes from one medium into another having different acoustic speeds. A change in both direction and mode occurs at acute angles of incidence. At small angles of incidence, the original mode and a converted mode may exist simultaneously in the second medium.[7]

refractive index: Ratio of the speed of the incident wave to that of a refracted wave. It is known as the refractive index of the second medium with respect to the first.[7]

reject: Minimize or eliminate low amplitude signals (such as electrical or material noise) so that other signals may be further amplified. This control can reduce vertical linearity.[7] Also called *suppression*.[22]

rejection level: Level above or below which a signal is an indication of a rejectable discontinuity.[7,22]

relevant indication: In nondestructive testing, an indication from a discontinuity requiring evaluation.[7]

repetition rate: Number of pulses generated or transmitted per unit of time (usually seconds).[7]

resolving power: Measure of the ability of an ultrasonic system to separate two signals close together in time or distance.[7,21]

resonance: Condition in which the frequency of a forcing vibration (ultrasonic wave) is the same as the natural vibration frequency of the propagation body (test object), possibly resulting in large amplitude vibrations.[7,21]

resonance technique: Method using the resonance principle for determining speed, thickness or presence of laminar discontinuities.[7]

resonant frequency: Frequency at which a body vibrates freely after being set in motion by some outside force.[7,21]

RF display: See *radio frequency display.*

ringing signals: (1) Closely spaced multiple signals caused by multiple reflections in a thin material. (2) Signals caused by continued vibration of a transducer.[7,22]

ringing technique: Test technique for bonded structures in which unbonds are indicated by increased amplitude of ringing signals.[7,22]

ringing time: Time that the mechanical vibrations of a transducer continue after the electrical pulse has stopped.[7,22]

roof angle: In a dual-element delay line transducer, the tilt angle by which the transducer elements of the delay line are oriented to direct the beams of the two elements to intersect at a specified zone in the medium.[7]

S

SAM: scanning acoustic microscope.

saturation: Condition in which high amplitude signals on a display screen do not increase with increased gain and appear flattened.[7]

scanning: Movement of the transducer over the surface of the test object in a controlled manner so as to achieve complete coverage. May be either a contact or immersion technique.[7]

scattering: Uncontrolled reflection of ultrasonic waves by small discontinuities or surface irregularities.[7]

schlieren system: Optical system used for visual display of an ultrasonic beam passing through a transparent medium.[7,22]

search unit: See *transducer.*

self-coupling transducer: Contact transducer that allows testing with a liquid couplant.

send/receive transducer: Transducer consisting of two piezoelectric elements mounted side by side separated by an acoustic barrier. One element transmits; one receives.[7,21]

sensitivity: Ability of signal to change with small changes of measured quantity.

sensor: Device that detects a material property or mechanical behavior (such as radiation or displacement) and converts it to an electrical signal. *Probe; transducer.*

shadow: Region in a test object that cannot be reached by ultrasonic energy traveling in a given direction. Shadows are caused by geometry or the presence of intervening large discontinuities.[7]

shear wave: See *transverse wave.*

shoe: Device used to adapt a straight beam transducer for use in a specific type of testing, including angle beam or surface wave tests and tests on curved surfaces.[7,22] See also *wedge.*

SH wave: *Transverse horizontal wave.*

SI (International System of Units): Measurement system using decimals in which the following seven units are considered basic: meter, mole, kilogram, second, ampere, kelvin and candela.[10,17]

signal: Physical quantity, such as electrical voltage, that contains information.[10,20]

signal-to-noise ratio: Ratio of signal amplitude (responses that contain information) to baseline noise amplitude (responses that contain no information). See also *noise.*[10,20]

skip distance: In angle beam tests of plate or pipe, the distance from the sound entry point to the exit point on the same surface after reflection from the back surface.[7] Also called V *path.*[22]

Snell's law: Physical law that defines the relationship between the angle of incidence and the angle of refraction.

SNR: See *signal-to-noise ratio.*

SNT-TC-1A: See *Recommended Practice No. SNT-TC-1A.*

specific acoustic impedance: Acoustic impedance in a particular test object or a defined volume of a specified material. See also *acoustic impedance; characteristic acoustic impedance.*

specification: Set of instructions or standards invoked by a specific customer to govern the results or performance of a specific set of tasks or products.[10]

spectrum: Amplitude distribution of frequencies in a signal.[7]

spectrum response: Amplification (gain) of a receiver over a range of frequencies.[7]

spherical wave: Wave in which points of the same phase lie on surfaces of concentric spheres.[7,23]

spurious echo: General term denoting any indication that cannot be associated with a discontinuity or boundary at the location displayed.[7] Also called *parasitic echo.*

squint angle: Angle by which the ultrasonic beam axis deviates from the probe axis.[7]

squirter: See *water column.*

standard: (1) Reference object used as a basis for comparison or calibration. (2) Concept established by authority, custom or agreement to serve as a model or rule in the measurement of quantity or the establishment of a practice or procedure.[7,22]

standing wave: Wave in which the energy flux is zero at all points. Such waves result from the interaction of similar waves traveling in opposite directions as when reflected waves meet advancing waves. A particular case is that of waves in a body whose thickness is an integral multiple of half-wavelengths, as in resonance testing.[7,21,22]

stiffness: Slope of curve of stress to strain, described by Young's modulus of elasticity. Compare *hardness.*

straight beam: Ultrasonic wave traveling normal to the test surface.[7,22]

suppression: See *reject.*

surface wave: See *rayleigh wave.*

SV wave: *Shear vertical wave.*

sweep: Uniform and repeated movement of a spot across the display screen to form the horizontal baseline.[7] Also called *time base.*

sweep delay: (1) Delay in time of starting the sweep after the initial pulse. (2) Control for adjusting the time.[7,22] Also called *time delay.*

sweep length: Length of time or distance represented by the horizontal baseline on an A-scan.[7,22]

T

test surface: Surface of the test object at which the ultrasonic energy enters or is detected.[7]

threshold: Voltage level setting of an instrument that causes it to register only signals greater or less than a specified magnitude.[10,20] This threshold may be adjustable, fixed or floating.[16]

through-transmission technique: Test technique in which ultrasonic energy is transmitted through the test object and received by a second transducer on the opposite side. Changes in received signal amplitude are taken as indications of variations in material continuity.[7]

time base: See *sweep.*

time delay: See *sweep delay.*

time differential: See *delta* t.

time of flight: Time for an acoustic wave to travel between two points. For example, the time required for a pulse to travel from the transmitter to the receiver via diffraction at a discontinuity edge or along the surface of the test object.[7]

tone burst: Wave train consisting of several cycles of the same frequency.[7]

transducer: (1) Device that converts mechanical energy to electrical output or vice versa. (2) Piezoelectric device that converts attributes of the stress-strain field of an acoustic wave into an electrical signal of voltage versus time. *Sensor; probe*.[16]

transducer, differential: Piezoelectric twin-element or dual-pole transducer, the output poles of which are isolated from the case and are at a floating potential.[16]

transducer element: In an ultrasonic *transducer*, the piezoelectric crystal to be coupled to the test surface. Also called the *crystal*.

transducer, flat response: Transducer whose frequency response has no resonance or characteristic response within its specified frequency band.[16]

transducer relative sensitivity: Response of the transducer to a given source.[16]

transducer, resonant: Transducer that uses the mechanical amplification due to a resonant frequency (or several close resonant frequencies) to give high sensitivity in a narrow band, typically ±10 percent of the principal resonant frequency at the –3 dB points.[16]

transducer, single-ended: Piezoelectric single-element transducer, the output pole of which is isolated from the case, the other pole being at the same potential as the case.[16]

transducer, wide band: Transducer whose response to surface displacements is flat over a wide frequency range.

transfer function: Description of changes to the waves arising as they propagate through the medium or, for a transducer, the relationship between the transducer output signal and the physical parameters of the acoustic wave at the transducer.[16]

transmission angle: Incident angle of a transmitted ultrasonic beam. It is zero degrees when the beam is perpendicular (normal) to the test surface.[7,21]

transmission characteristics: Test object characteristics that influence the passage of ultrasonic energy, including scattering, attenuation or surface conditions.[7]

transmission technique: See *through-transmission technique*.

transmitter: (1) Transducer that emits ultrasonic energy. (2) Electrical circuits that generate the signals emitted by the transducer.[7]

transverse horizontal (polarized) wave: Transverse wave in which the particle vibration is parallel to the incidence surface.[7]

transverse vertical (polarized) wave: Transverse wave in which the plane of vibration is normal to the incidence surface.[7]

transverse wave: Type of wave in which the particle motion is perpendicular to the direction of propagation.[7,22] Also called *shear wave*.

transverse wave transducer: Transducer that generates transverse waves in a test object.

two-transducer technique: See *pitch catch technique*.

U

ultrasonic absorption: Damping or dissipation of ultrasonic waves as they pass through a medium.[7,21] See also *attenuation coefficient*.

ultrasonic spectroscopy: Analysis of the frequency content of an acoustic wave. Generally performed mathematically using a fast fourier transform.[7]

ultrasonic spectrum: Usually the frequency range from 20 kHz to 50 MHz but may extend much higher in special applications.[7]

ultrasonic: Of or relating to acoustic vibration frequencies greater than about 20 kHz.[7,22]

ultrasonic testing: Method of nondestructive testing, using acoustic waves at inaudibly high frequencies at the interrogating energy.

UT: Abbreviation for the ultrasonic method of nondestructive testing.[7,22]

V

vertical limit: Maximum useful readable level of vertical indication on an A-scan.[7]

vertical linearity: See *linearity, amplitude*.

video presentation: Display presentation in which radiofrequency signals have been rectified and usually filtered.[7,22]

V path: See *skip distance*.

W

water column: Tube filled with water and attached to the front of a transducer to couple an ultrasonic beam to a test object. A delay line between the initial pulse and the front surface signal. Also serves as a coupling device.[7] See also *delay line.*

water jet: Unsupported stream of water carrying ultrasonic signals between the transducer and the test object surface.[7] Also called a *squirter* or *water column.*

water path: In immersion testing or with a water column, the distance from the transducer face to the test object's front surface.[7,22]

wave interference: Production of a series of maxima and minima of sound pressure as a consequence of the superposition of waves having different phases.[7,22]

wave train: Series of waves or groups of waves passing along the same course at regular intervals.[7]

wavefront: In a wave disturbance, the locus of points having the same phase.[7,22]

waveguide: Device to transmit elastic energy from a test object to a remote transducer — for example, a wire joined at one end to a test object and at the other end to a transducer.

wavelength: Distance needed in the propagation direction for a wave to go through a complete cycle.[7,21]

wear face: Protective material on the face of a transducer to prevent wear of the piezoelectric element.[7,22]

wedge: Device used to direct ultrasonic energy into a test object at an acute angle.[7,22] See also *shoe.*

wheel transducer: Device that couples ultrasonic energy to a test object through the rolling contact area of a wheel containing a liquid and one or more transducers.[7,22]

wrap around: Display of misleading ultrasonic reflections from a previously transmitted pulse because of excessive pulse repetition frequency.[7,24] See also *ghost.*

Part 2. Symbols

c = speed of sound in air (meter per second)
D = diameter (meter)
dB = decibel
E = Young's modulus of elasticity
f = frequency (hertz)
R, r = reflection coefficient
T = transmission coefficient
t = time (second)
V = volt
v = velocity (meter per second)
Z = impedance (pascal second per meter)
α = attenuation
ε = strain
λ = wavelength (meter)
θ = angle (radian)
ρ = density (kilogram per cubic meter)
σ = Poisson's ratio; stress (pascal)

References

1. *Nondestructive Testing Handbook,* second edition: Vol. 1, *Leak Testing.* Columbus, OH: American Society for Nondestructive Testing (1982).
2. *Nondestructive Testing Handbook,* second edition: Vol. 2, *Liquid Penetrant Tests.* Columbus, OH: American Society for Nondestructive Testing (1982).
3. *Nondestructive Testing Handbook,* second edition: Vol. 3, *Radiography and Radiation Testing.* Columbus, OH: American Society for Nondestructive Testing (1985).
4. *Nondestructive Testing Handbook,* second edition: Vol. 4, *Electromagnetic Testing.* Columbus, OH: American Society for Nondestructive Testing (1986).
5. *Nondestructive Testing Handbook,* second edition: Vol. 5, *Acoustic Emission Testing.* Columbus, OH: American Society for Nondestructive Testing (1987).
6. *Nondestructive Testing Handbook,* second edition: Vol. 6, *Magnetic Particle Testing.* Columbus, OH: American Society for Nondestructive Testing (1989).
7. *Nondestructive Testing Handbook,* second edition: Vol. 7, *Ultrasonic Testing.* Columbus, OH: American Society for Nondestructive Testing (1991).
8. *Nondestructive Testing Handbook,* second edition: Vol. 8, *Visual and Optical Testing.* Columbus, OH: American Society for Nondestructive Testing (1993).
9. *Nondestructive Testing Handbook,* second edition: Vol. 9, *Special Nondestructive Testing Methods.* Columbus, OH: American Society for Nondestructive Testing (1995).
10. *Nondestructive Testing Handbook,* second edition: Vol. 10, *Nondestructive Testing Overview.* Columbus, OH: American Society for Nondestructive Testing (1996).
11. *Nondestructive Testing Handbook,* third edition: Vol. 1, *Leak Testing.* Columbus, OH: American Society for Nondestructive Testing (1998).
12. *Nondestructive Testing Handbook,* third edition: Vol. 2, *Liquid Penetrant Testing.* Columbus, OH: American Society for Nondestructive Testing (2000).
13. *Nondestructive Testing Handbook,* third edition: Vol. 3, *Infrared and Thermal Testing.* Columbus, OH: American Society for Nondestructive Testing (2001).
14. *Nondestructive Testing Handbook,* third edition: Vol. 4, *Radiographic Testing.* Columbus, OH: American Society for Nondestructive Testing (2002).
15. *Nondestructive Testing Handbook,* third edition: Vol. 5, *Electromagnetic Testing.* Columbus, OH: American Society for Nondestructive Testing (2004).
16. *Nondestructive Testing Handbook,* third edition: Vol. 6, *Acoustic Emission Testing.* Columbus, OH: American Society for Nondestructive Testing (2005).
17. *IEEE Standard Dictionary of Electrical and Electronic Terms.* New York, NY: Wiley-Interscience, for the Institute of Electrical and Electronics Engineers (1984).
18. API RP 5A5, *Recommended Practice for Field Inspection of New Casing, Tubing, and Plain End Drill Pipe,* sixth edition. Washington, DC: American Petroleum Institute (1999).
19. *Annual Book of ASTM Standards:* Section 3, *Metals Test Methods and Analytical Procedures.* Vol. 03.03, *Nondestructive Testing.* West Conshohocken, PA: ASTM International (2001).
20. ASTM E 268-81, *Definitions Approved for Use by Agencies of the Department of Defense as Part of Federal Test Method Standard No. 151b and for Listing in the DoD Index of Specifications and Standards.* West Conshohocken, PA: ASTM International (1981).
21. Weismantel, E.E. et al. "Glossary of Terms Frequently Used in Nondestructive Testing." *Materials Evaluation.* Vol. 33, No. 4. Columbus, OH: American Society for Nondestructive Testing (April 1975): p 42A-44A.
22. TO33B-1-1 (NAVAIR 01-1A-16) TM43-0103, *Nondestructive Testing Methods.* Washington, DC: United States Department of Defense, United States Air Force (June 1984): p 1.25.

23. "Ultrasonic Flaw Detection." *The Glossary of Terms Used in Nondestructive Testing.* British Standard 3683, Part 4. London, England: British Standards Institute (1985). Superseded by EN 1330-4, *Nondestructive Terminology*: Part 4, "Terms Used in Ultrasonic Testing." Brussels, Belgium: European Committee for Standardization (2000).

24. MIL-STD-371, *Glossary of Terms and Definitions for Ultrasonic Testing Procedures.* Washington, DC: United States Department of Defense, United States Army (October 1987).

Index

carbon-to-carbon structures
material test issues in aerospace applications, 495
ultrasonic assessment of impact damage to space shuttle thermal
protection, 522-523
ultrasonic material inspection in aerospace applications, 504
carriage, ultrasonic immersion system, 413-414
castings
bibliography, 424
material production inspection in aerospace applications, 504
material test issues in aerospace applications, 495
ultrasonic testing in marine industry, 542
ultrasonic tests with closely positioned transducers, 236
cast iron
ultrasonic mechanical property characterization, 331
cellulose gums
couplants for ultrasonic contact testing, 223
central certification, 22
cepstrum processing
ultrasonic spectroscopy application, 162
ceramics
acoustic microscopy, 548
air coupled transducers, 131
piezoelectric materials, 60
ultrasonic material characterization, 322
ultrasonic testing of advanced structural, 358-368
ultrasonic testing of green state, 358-359
ultrasonic testing of sintered, 359-362
certification, 16-22
CGS (centimeter-gram-second) units, 30
characteristic length, and fracture toughness, 333
chemical and petroleum applications, 427
internal rotary ultrasonic testing, 429-430
ultrasonic inservice testing of offshore structures, 444-453
ultrasonic testing in chemical and petroleum industry, 428-431
ultrasonic testing in processing plants, 427, 432-438
ultrasonic testing of petroleum pipes, 441-443
ultrasonic testing of storage tanks, 439-440
chemical industry, 428
chemical spot testing, 12
chewing gum
couplant for ultrasonic contact testing, 223
Christoffel's equations, 42
civil structures
ultrasonic testing of wood and structural steel, 476, 477
cladding
ultrasonic testing in processing plants, 432-433
ultrasonic testing with dual-element transducers, 235
ultrasonic testing with electromagnetic acoustic transducers, 120-121
clustering
ultrasonic signal processing applications, 168-170
coatings
material test issues in aerospace applications, 495
ultrasonic testing assessment, 378-379
cobalt
ultrasonic testing of ingots, 401
cobalt alloys
ultrasonic testing of ingots, 401
coefficient of autocorrelation and correlation, ultrasonic signal processing, 151
coiflet wavelet, 163
cold reheat line, 458
cold shuts
ultrasonic testing of marine industry castings, 542
Columbia Accident Investigation Board, 522-523
composite laminates
discontinuities in, 184-285
focused beam ultrasonic tests, 299
pulse echo immersion ultrasonic testing, 273
ultrasonic immersion testing, 285
ultrasonic testing, 380-390
composite materials. See also carbon, ceramic, graphite
acoustic microscopy, 547-548
acoustoultrasonic testing of interlaminar shear strength, 339-340
angle beam ultrasonic immersion testing, 293-295
increasing use in aircraft, 500
material production inspection in aerospace applications, 499-503
pulse echo contact ultrasonic testing, 207-208, 212, 215-216
as replacement for steel and iron, and need for nondestructive testing, 3
ultrasonic immersion scanning, 284-288
ultrasonic immersion testing, 284-288
ultrasonic inservice inspection of aircraft, 514
ultrasonic inservice testing of aircraft, 507

ultrasonic mechanical property characterization, 336-337
ultrasonic spectroscopy of Space Station flywheel rotors, 521-522
ultrasonic testing of space systems for fatigue and thermal
damage, 516-519
composite tubing
ultrasonic immersion testing, 285-288
compressional waves, 482
concealed cut, See ply gap
concrete
moisture and curing conditions, 483-485
ultrasonic testing of highway bridge, 476, 477
ultrasonic testing of structural, 481-487
ultrasonic wave speed in, 481, 483
condensers
in power plants, 459
ultrasonic testing of fossil power plant turbine, 472
confined space, 22
consultants
for managing ultrasonic testing programs, 14
contact ultrasonic testing systems, 179, 262, 299
continuous girder bridge
ultrasonic testing, 476
continuous time fourier transform, 145-146
continuous wave bond testers, 193
continuous wavelet transform, 162
continuous wave phase comparison techniques, 193
contoured surfaces
contoured ultrasonic transducer shoes to fit, 221
laser ultrasound advantages, 107
sonic position encoding device, 210
ultrasonic immersion testing interpretation, 277-278
convolution
ultrasonic signal processing application, 149, 153-154
copper
acoustic parameters, 43
reflected field amplitude for copper layered steel half space, 49, 50
ultrasonic characterization of grain size of heat treated, 328
copper nickel alloys
ultrasonic inservice inspection of condensers in power plants, 459
corner welds
ultrasonic testing in marine industry, 542
correlation coefficient, 151
corrosion. See also corrosion; stress corrosion cracking; thickness testing
angle beam ultrasonic immersion testing of composites, 295
C-scan mapping in chemical industry, 431
detection using nondestructive testing, 2
material test issues in aerospace applications, 495
and nuclear power plant life, 465
ultrasonic field testing of bridges, 478
ultrasonic inservice inspection in power plants, 458
ultrasonic inservice inspection of aircraft, 512-513
ultrasonic inservice testing of offshore structures, 445-446, 451-452
ultrasonic testing in chemical and petroleum applications, 436
ultrasonic testing of fossil plant boilers, 466, 467
ultrasonic testing of fossil plant steam lines and headers, 469
ultrasonic testing of steel structures, 477
ultrasonic thickness testing in marine industry, 543
couplant path length, 262
couplants, for ultrasonic transducers
contact systems, 221-224
immersion systems, 262
coupling
operating techniques to ensure good coupling in ultrasonic testing, 223-
224
piezoelectric materials, 64-65, 71
in ultrasonic spectroscopy, 159
cracks. See also stress corrosion cracking
acoustic microscopy, 544
aerospace applications, ultrasonic testing in, 494
angle beam contact testing, 217
angle beam immersion testing, 290, 291
A-scan sensitivity, 179-180
detection using nondestructive testing, 2
fossil plant boilers, ultrasonic testing of, 467-468
highway bridges, ultrasonic testing of, 477
lamb wave applications, 100
liquid penetrant indication, 8
marine industry castings, ultrasonic testing of, 542
material test issues in aerospace applications, 495
phased array ultrasonic testing applications, 248
straight beam contact pulse echo tests, 206

heat resistant glass
    acoustic parameters, 43
heat treating scale
    ultrasonic indications from, 283
hertz (Hz), 32, 36
high frequency acoustics, 24
high frequency air coupled transducers, 131-132
high frequency piston generator, 24
high-speed self-aligning electromagnetic acoustic transducer probes, 127-128
high temperature
    ultrasonic testing standoffs, 222
    ultrasonic testing with electromagnetic acoustic transducers, 121-122
high temperature bolts
    ultrasonic testing of fossil power plant turbine, 471-472
highway bridges
    acoustic emission monitoring of floor beam, 10
    ultrasonic field testing, 478-480
    ultrasonic testing, 476-477
holes
    ultrasonic inservice inspection of aircraft, 514
holography, 12
honey
    couplant for ultrasonic contact testing, 223
honeycomb structures
    material test issues in aerospace applications, 495
    ultrasonic inservice inspection of aircraft, 514
    ultrasonic material inspection in aerospace applications, 503-504
    ultrasonic testing of adhesive bonds, 372
Hooke's law, 41
hot tears
    ultrasonic testing of marine industry castings, 542
hydrogen entrapment
    ultrasonic tests of steel and wrought alloys, 400
hydrostatic pressure testing, 2

I

ice
    acoustic parameters, 43
image analysis, 164
immersion macroscanning, 315
immersion tanks, 267
immersion ultrasonic testing systems, 262, 299. *See also* pulse echo immersion
        ultrasonic test systems
    advantages of, 263, 501
    angle beam techniques, 289-295
    composite materials, 284-288
    coupling devices, 267-269
    early development of, 29
    focused beam techniques, 296-299
    loss of back surface reflection, 275-276
    metals, 401-403
    through-transmission tests, 265
impact damage
    aerospace material test issues, 495
    characteristic parameters in filament wound tubes, 288
    pulse echo immersion ultrasonic testing, 273
    space shuttle thermal protection, 522-523
    ultrasonic immersion testing of composites, 287
impedance matching layers, air coupled transducers, 132
impedance matching networks
    and transducer characterization, 69
    ultrasonic testing application, 83
impulse function, 152
inclusions
    acoustic microscopy, 544
    A-scan sensitivity, 179-180
    material test issues in aerospace applications, 495
    ultrasonic immersion testing interpretation of indications from rotor
        wheels, 281-282
    ultrasonic material inspection in aerospace applications, 501, 504
    ultrasonic testing advantages and limitations, 496
    ultrasonic testing of rolled aluminum plates, 406
    ultrasonic tests of steel and wrought alloys, 400
incomplete penetration
    ultrasonic field testing of bridges, 478
index distance, 414
indirect pitch catch ultrasonic testing technique, 230-231
indirect transmission technique, 482, 483

inductance
    in equivalent circuit of piezoelectric element, 66
    ultrasonic transducers, 69-71
industrial applications, *See* particular industries
industrial production ultrasonic testing systems, 184
infrared testing, 11-12
infrastructure applications
    ultrasonic testing, 475-487
    ultrasonic testing of structural concrete, 481-487
    ultrasonic testing of wood and structural steel, 476-480
ingots
    discontinuities in, 400-401
    ultrasonic testing procedures, 401
    ultrasonic tests of steel and wrought alloys, 400
in-house programs
    for managing ultrasonic testing programs, 14
initial pulse, 272
inservice testing, 9
    inservice ultrasonic testing of offshore structures, 444-453
    ultrasonic inservice inspection in power plants, 458-460
    ultrasonic testing in marine industry, 542-543
    ultrasonic testing of aircraft, 507-515
instrumentation, for ultrasonic testing, 177. *See also* A-scan ultrasonic
        equipment; B-scan ultrasonic equipment; C-scan ultrasonic equipment
    acoustic microscopes, 192
    for aluminum testing, 414-415
    amplitude and transit time systems, 178-180
    amplitude systems, 178
    basic send/receive instrumentation, 182-190
    calibration, 194-198
    continuous wave technique, 192-193
    equipment classification, 178
    general purpose, 188
    instrument control effects, 183
    modular, 184, 189-190
    multiple-transducer techniques, 418-419
    operation in large testing systems, 193
    portable, 184, 185-188
    reference reflectors, 194-195
    scanning approaches, 178-181
    special purpose, 184-185, 191-193
    straight beam tests, 202-203
    and transducer characterization, 68-69
    types, 184
interface echo, 445
interface triggering
    in general purpose ultrasonic test equipment, 188, 189
    in portable ultrasonic test equipment, 185
interlaced scanning, 244
interlaminar shear strength
    acoustoultrasonic testing, 339-340
interleaving, 149
International Institute of Welding (IIW) reference block, 196, 197-198
    angle beam contact testing application, 217, 218
International Organization for Standardization (ISO) , 19, 22
    ISO 2400, 19
    ISO 4386-1, 19
    ISO 5577, 19
    ISO 5948, 19
    ISO 7963, 19
    ISO 9303, 19
    ISO 9305, 19
    ISO 9712, 22
    ISO 9764, 19
    ISO 9765, 19
    ISO 10124, 19
    ISO 10332, 19
    ISO 10375, 19
    ISO 10423, 19
    ISO 10543, 19
    ISO 11496, 19
    ISO 12094, 19
    ISO 12710, 19
    ISO 12715, 19
    ISO 13663, 19
    ISO 17640, 19
    ISO 18175, 19
    ISO 22825, 19
International Space Station
    ultrasonic spectroscopy of flywheel rotors, 521-522
    ultrasonic testing applications, 516

magnesium
    acoustic parameters, 43
    ultrasonic wavelength, 497
magnesium alloys
    as replacement for steel and iron, and need for nondestructive testing, 3
magnetic particle testing, 8
    fossil power plant turbines, 470
    petroleum pipes, 441
magnetization
    effect on ultrasonic elastic property measurement, 322
magnetoelasticity, 323
magnetostrictive effect, 25
main bang signal, 272
manipulator, ultrasonic immersion system, 413-414
manual scanning, 204
Manufacturers Standardization Society of the Vale and Fittings Industry
    MSS SP-94, 17
    standards for ultrasonic testing, 17
marine industry applications, 541-543
    ultrasonic detection of submarines, 25, 26, 28
martensitic stainless steel
    acoustic parameters, 43
matching layers, air coupled transducers, 130
    impedance materials layers, 132
    materials for, 132
material identification, 2, 12
material property characterization, 305
    acoustoultrasonic testing for mechanical properties, 338-342
    laser ultrasonic applications, 113-114
    microstructure and diffuse discontinuities, 324-330
    ultrasonic testing applications, 306-318
    ultrasonic testing for elastic properties, 319-323
    ultrasonic testing for mechanical properties, 331-337
materials characterization, 2, 307
    ultrasonic testing application, 308-318
maximum entropy spectrum analysis
    ultrasonic spectroscopy application, 162
maximum likelihood spectrum analysis
    ultrasonic spectroscopy application, 162
mechanical impedance, 61
    air, 129
mechanical losses
    piezoelectric materials, 66
mechanical position encoding, 209
mechanical properties
    acoustoultrasonic characterization, 338-342
    sintered ceramics, 359
    ultrasonic characterization, 306, 331-337
mechanical scanning, 209-210
medical applications
    B-scan ultrasonic testing applicable to, 264
    ultrasonic moving transducer tests, 252
membranes
    ultrasonic contact coupling applications, 222
metal composite laminates
    angle beam ultrasonic immersion testing, 295
metals applications, 399
    ultrasonic multiple-transducer techniques, 418-422
    ultrasonic testing of primary aluminum, 406-417
    ultrasonic testing of steel and wrought alloys, 400-405
metals fabrication
    ultrasonic testing at high temperature using electromagnetic acoustic transducers, 122
methods, 2
methyl methacrylate
    wedges for angle beam transducers, 75, 76, 77
microelectronic packaging applications
    acoustic microscopes, 192
microstructure, 2, 306
    effect of mechanical and thermal processes, 212
    and ultrasonic attenuation, 326-327
    ultrasonic characterization, 324-330
    and ultrasonic speed, 325-326
    whisker reinforced ceramics, 362
military specifications, 16
    MIL-A-8344, 530-531
    MIL-HDBK-1823, 531, 534
    MIL-HDBK-5 B, 531
    MIL-STD-1530, 530-531
    MIL-W-22759/34, 520

minimum distance classifier
    ultrasonic signal processing applications, 171
modular industrial ultrasonic testing instruments, 184
modular ultrasonic testing instruments, 189-190
moiré imaging, 12
moisture ingress
    material test issues in aerospace applications, 495
molybdenum
    acoustic parameters, 43
molybdenum alloy
    acoustic parameters of wrought, 43
monolithic linear phased transducer arrays, 242
morphology, 306, 324
mosaic phased array ultrasonic testing, 238
mother wavelet, 162, 163
multibeam satellite pulse observation technique, 235
multiclass problems
    ultrasonic signal processing applications, 171-172
multidiscriminant analysis
    ultrasonic signal processing applications, 171-172
multiparametric scanning, 317
multiple discriminant analysis
    ultrasonic signal processing applications, 172
multiple-transducer ultrasonic testing techniques
    metals testing, 418-419
    pulse echo contact ultrasonic test systems, 229-237
multiplexers
    ultrasonic testing application, 82, 229
multipliers, for SI units, 30-31
multizone ultrasonic technique, 419, 420

N

narrow band instrumentation, 183
National Aeronautics and Space Administration (NASA)
    damage tolerance approach, 530, 531
    ultrasonic testing of space systems, 516
National Electrical Safety Code, 22
National Electric Code, 22
natural waveguides, 101
naval brass
    acoustic parameters of, 43
network analyzers
    ultrasonic spectroscopy application, 159-160
neural networks
    ultrasonic signal processing applications, 172-173
newton per square meter, 31
nickel
    acoustic parameters, 43
    angle beam immersion ultrasonic testing of tubes, 292
    ultrasonic characterization of grain size of heat treated, 328
    ultrasonic wavelength, 497
nickel alloys
    ultrasonic testing of ingots, 401
nickel alloy UNS N07520
    acoustoultrasonic creep damage assessment of space system turbine, 524-525
nickel chromium alloy
    acoustic parameters of wrought, 43
no entry areas, 22
nondestructive material characterization, 2
nondestructive testing
    applications, 4
    defined, 2
    methods classification, 4-7
    methods overview, 7-12
    objectives, 5
    purposes, 2-4
    reliability, 530-534
    test object, 5-7
    value of, 7
nonmetallic inclusions
    ultrasonic tests of steel and wrought alloys, 400
nonperiodic waves, 38
normalization
    ultrasonic signal processing, 154
nozzles
    ultrasonic testing in nuclear power plants, 461, 464

porosity
angle beam ultrasonic immersion testing of composites, 295
A-scan sensitivity, 180
detection using nondestructive testing, 2
effect on ultrasonic microstructure characterization, 325
and elastic constants, 320-321
material test issues in aerospace applications, 495
pulse echo contact imaging of butt welds, 227
ultrasonic characterization, 329
ultrasonic material inspection in aerospace applications, 501
ultrasonic testing advantages and limitations, 496
ultrasonic testing of composite laminates, 380
ultrasonic testing of marine industry castings, 542
ultrasonic testing of rolled aluminum plates, 406, 415-416
porous solids, 319
portable ultrasonic testing instruments, 184, 185-188
portable ultrasonic wave speed testing units, 482
portland cement
ultrasonic testing of structural, 481
power boilers
ultrasonic inservice inspection in power plants, 458
power cepstrum
ultrasonic spectroscopy application, 162
precipitation
ultrasonic characterization, 329
prefixes, for SI units, 31
pressure coupling, for ultrasonic contact testing, 223
pressure units, 31-32
pressure vessels
phased array ultrasonic testing applications, 248-249
ultrasonic scanning of welds, 93
ultrasonic testing in processing plants, 432, 436-438
ultrasonic testing of nuclear reactor, 461-462
pressure wave, 36, 52
pressurized water nuclear reactors
ultrasonic testing, 461
ultrasonic testing of piping systems, 462-463
probability density function analysis
ultrasonic signal processing applications, 166-168
probability of detection, 530-532
probe, 15
processing plants
ultrasonic testing, 432-438
proof testing, 2
ultrasonic testing of joints, 505
ultrasonic testing of structures, 309
propylene glycol
couplant for ultrasonic contact testing, 223
proveup inspections
ultrasonic testing of petroleum pipes, 441
pulse, 182
pulse amplitude, 187
pulse echo contact ultrasonic test systems, 201, 299
angle beam contact testing, 217-220
butt weld imaging, 225-228
coupling media for, 221-224
moving transducers, 250-252
multiple-transducer techniques, 229-237
phased arrays, 238-249
straight beam pulse echo tests, 202-216
test frequency selection, 212-214
pulse echo immersion ultrasonic test systems, 299
amplitude of extraneous reflections, 272
back surface reflection amplitude, 271-272
frequency domain analysis, 273
summary of techniques, 299
test parameters, 271-273
time of flight, 272-273
pulse echo time-of-flight (TOF) scanning, 272-273, 501
chemical industry applications, 431
pulse echo ultrasonic test systems, 99, 262
adhesive bond testing, 371-373
calibration, 194-198
early development of, 29
for materials characterization, 309-312
scanning approaches, 178-188
send/receive instrumentation, 182-190
special purpose equipment, 191-193
pulse generator, 69
pulse repetition frequency, 187

pulsers
operation, 180-184
options, 180
and transducer characterization, 69
pumps
ultrasonic inservice inspection of condensers in power plants, 459
ultrasonic testing in processing plants, 432

Q

qualification, 16-22
quantization, 148
quartz
acoustic parameters, 43
early ultrasonic transducer tests, 26
piezoelectric material, 60
quasifocus point, paintbrush transducers, 412
quasilongitudinal wave modes, 40
quasi transverse wave modes, 40

R

radar, 2
radian, 32
radio astronomy, 2
radiofrequency amplifiers
ultrasonic testing application, 87
radiographic testing, 9-10
inservice testing of aircraft, 507
railroad axles
ultrasonic testing, 538-540
railroad industry applications, 535
ultrasonic testing of axles, 538-540
ultrasonic testing of rail track, 535-538
ultrasonic testing of wheels, 540
ultrasonic testing with moving electromagnetic acoustic transducers, 125-127
railroad wheels
testing with moving electromagnetic acoustic transducers, 126-127
ultrasonic material characterization, 323
rail track
testing with moving electromagnetic acoustic transducers, 125-126
ultrasonic material characterization, 323
ultrasonic testing, 535-538
ultrasonic thickness testers, early devices, 29
random signals, 144-145
range
adjustment in calibration, 194
range estimating
angle beam contact testing, 218
Rayleigh (Lord Rayleigh, John William Strutt), 24
rayleigh angle, 46
rayleigh disk, 24
rayleigh (surface) waves, 24, 39-40, 101, 220
first uses in testing, 29
leaky, 46-47, 49, 299
propagation in isotropic materials, 43-45
rear surface. See back surface
receiver saturation avoidance, 188
recertification, 21
recrystallization
ultrasonic characterization, 329
rectangular gate function, 149
reference blocks, ultrasonic. See reference standards
reference line, 403
reference signal, 153
reference standards, ultrasonic. See also calibration blocks
aerospace, 499
bonding, 515
calibration blocks for ultrasonic testing systems, 195-198
ingot ultrasonic testing, 401
for interpretation of immersion ultrasonic test indications, 274-275
petroleum pipes, 442
reflectors for calibrating ultrasonic testing systems, 194-195
refineries, 428
reflection
of ultrasonic waves at plane boundary in stress free media, 52-56
reflection, of ultrasonic waves, See ultrasonic wave reflection
reflection amplitude, ultrasonic waves, 497
reflection coefficients, ultrasonic waves, 53, 496
common materials, 497

sweep
    adjustment in calibration, 194
    instrument controls, 183, 186
    options, 180
sweep generator
    ultrasonic pulse echo test systems, 182
symlet wavelet, 163
symmetric lamb waves, 100
synchronizers, 180
synthetic aperture focusing, ultrasonic testing
    bibliography, 258
    described, 250-252
    technique, 112-113, 229, 250-252, 485-486
system amplifier
    ultrasonic spectroscopy application, 159

T

tailored welds
    phased array ultrasonic testing, 249
tandem transducer ultrasonic testing, 232-233
tanks
    ultrasonic water level determination in marine industry, 543
tap testing, 12
    adhesive bond testing, 369-370
    bonded joints, 505
techniques, 2
telephone, 25
temperature
    and elastic constants, 321
tensile strength
    ultrasonic measurement, 331-333
test blocks, ultrasonic. *See* reference standards
test object, 2
    nondestructive testing methods classified by, 5-7
tetragonal zirconia polycrystalline (TZP)
    ultrasonic testing, 364
texture
    effect on ultrasonic elastic property measurement, 319, 321, 322-323
    and stress, 322-323
texturing, 324
Theory of Sound (Rayleigh), 25
thermal coatings
    material test issues in aerospace applications, 495
thermal damage
    material test issues in aerospace applications, 495
    ultrasonic testing of fossil plant boilers, 466
    ultrasonic testing of space system composite materials, 516-519
thermal testing, 11-12
thickness gages, ultrasonic, *See* thickness measurement; ultrasonic thickness gages
thickness measurement. *See also* corrosion; erosion; ultrasonic thickness gages
    with electromagnetic acoustic transducers, 117-118
    instrumentation, 184-185
    laser ultrasonic, 111-112
    ultrasonic applications in marine industry, 542, 543
    ultrasonic detection of wall thinning in chemical and petroleum applications, 435-436
    ultrasonic inservice testing of offshore structures, 445
    ultrasonic testing advantages and limitations, 496
    ultrasonic testing of steel structures, 477
through arch truss bridge
    ultrasonic testing, 476
through-transmission ultrasonic testing technique, 99, 179, 229, 262, 299
    adhesive bonds, 371-373
    described, 230
    early experiments with, 26
    send/receive instrumentation, 188
    transducer alignment, 265-266
    for ultrasonic materials characterization, 312-313
    ultrasonic testing of reinforced concrete, 481
timber
    ultrasonic testing of highway bridge, 476
time corrected gain, 502
time correction gain, 414
time delay interferometric detection, 110
time-of-flight diffraction ultrasonic tests, 231-232
timer
    ultrasonic pulse echo test systems, 182
timing section, of pulse echo system, 186

titanium
    acoustic parameters, 43
    ultrasonic inservice inspection of condensers in power plants, 459
    ultrasonic interface transmission and reflection coefficients, 497
    ultrasonic material production inspection of billets in aerospace applications, 504
    ultrasonic mechanical property characterization, 331
    ultrasonic scanning of aerospace castings, 92
    ultrasonic testing of adhesive bonds on, 376
    ultrasonic wavelength, 497
titanium alloys
    ultrasonic characterization of grain size, 328
    ultrasonic toughness measurement, 334-335
titanium diboride
    ultrasonic testing of rolled aluminum inclusion, 406, 407
tomography. *See* ultrasonic tomography
tone burst pulsers, 78, 81
torque measurement technique, 434
torsional vibration, 320
toughness
    ultrasonic measurement, 333-336
tourmaline
    piezoelectric material, 60
track, railroad, *See* rail track
trains, *See* railroad industry applications
train wheels, *See* railroad wheels
tramp elements, 400
transducer array, 418
transducer characterization station, 68-69
transducer far field, 211
transducer near field, 210-211
transducers, 15. *See also* air coupled transducers; electromagnetic acoustic transducers
    alignment in through-transmission technique, 265-266
    configurations for multiple-transducer systems, 229
    effects of angle beam wedge, 74-77
    excitation, 78-87
    focal distance, 98-99
    focused, 95-96, 296-299
    generation and reception of ultrasound, 78-89
    history of development, 25-29
    instrumentation and transducer characterization, 68-69
    multiple-transducer ultrasonic techniques for metals, 418-422
    pencil shape focus, 99
    performance, 69-77
    sandwich, 26, 27
    shoes for contact testing, 221-222
    straight beam contact pulse echo tests, 202-203
    tests with closely positioned, 235-237
    for ultrasonic testing of aluminum alloys, 411-413
    ultrasonic thickness gages, 191-192
    underwater for ultrasonic testing of offshore structures, 449
transformer oil
    acoustic parameters, 43
transformers
    ultrasonic testing application, 83
transient signals, 145-146
transmission amplitude, ultrasonic waves, 497
transmission coefficient, ultrasonic waves, 496
transmit/receive switches
    timing and synchronization, 186-187
    ultrasonic testing application, 82
transportation applications
    lamb wave applications, 100
transverse horizontal waves
    reflection at plane boundary in stress free media, 53-54
    ultrasonic wave propagation, 49-51
transverse scanning technique, 414
transverse vertical waves
    reflection at plane boundary in stress free media, 54
transverse waves, 36, 39, 43
travel time mode conversion, 236
Treatise on Electricity (Maxwell), 25
tubes and tubing
    angle beam contact testing, 218
    angle beam immersion testing, 289-290
    angle beam immersion ultrasonic testing, 292
    internal rotary ultrasonic testing of chemical industry, 429-430
    laser ultrasonic thickness gaging in austenitic seamless tubes, 111
    phased array testing of seamless with electromagnetic acoustic transducers, 124-125

Figure Sources

Chapter 6. Ultrasonic Pulse Echo Contact Techniques

Figures 8-9 — Boeing Aerospace Company, Seattle, WA [formerly Douglas Aircraft Company, Long Beach, CA].

Figures 25b and 25c — General Electric Company, Schenectady, NY.

Chapter 12. Electric Power Applications of Ultrasonic Testing

Figures 1 and 3 — IHISw/Southwest Research Institute, ISwT, San Antonio, TX.

Figures 2 and 6 — IHISw, San Antonio, TX.

Figures 5, 7, 11 — Olympus NDT, Waltham, MA.

Chapter 14. Aerospace Applications of Ultrasonic Testing

Figures 30 to 45 — National Aeronautics and Space Administration, Cleveland, OH. Works of the United States government, not subject to copyright.